Developing Clinical Judgment

for Practical/Vocational Nursing Practice
and NGN Readiness

Developing Clinical Judgment

for Practical/Vocational Nursing Practice and NGN Readiness

DONNA D. IGNATAVICIUS
MS, RN, CNE, CNEcl, ANEF, FAADN

Speaker and Curriculum Consultant for Academic Nursing Programs
Founder, Boot Camp for Nurse Educators
President, DI Associates, Inc.
Littleton, Colorado

TAMI K. LITTLE
DNP, RN, CNE

Consultant for Academic Nursing Programs
LittleNurse, LLC
Las Vegas, Nevada;
Formerly, Corporate Director of Nursing
Vista College
Richardson, Texas

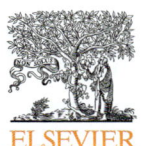

ELSEVIER

SECOND EDITION

Elsevier
3251 Riverport Lane
St. Louis, Missouri 63043

Notice

Practitioners and researchers must always rely on their own experience and knowledge in evaluating and using any information, methods, compounds or experiments described herein. Because of rapid advances in the medical sciences, in particular, independent verification of diagnoses and drug dosages should be made. To the fullest extent of the law, no responsibility is assumed by Elsevier, authors, editors or contributors for any injury and/or damage to persons or property as a matter of products liability, negligence or otherwise, or from any use or operation of any methods, products, instructions, or ideas contained in the material herein.

Previous edition copyrighted 2022.

Executive Content Strategist: Lee Henderson
Director, Content Development: Ellen Wurm-Cutter
Senior Content Development Specialist: Laura Goodrich
Publishing Services Manager: Catherine Jackson
Senior Project Manager: Jodi Willard
Design Direction: Amy Buxton

Typeset by GW Tech

Printed in India

Last digit is the print number: 9 8 7 6 5 4 3 2 1

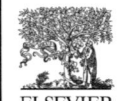 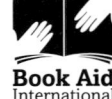

Working together
to grow libraries in
developing countries

www.elsevier.com • www.bookaid.org

Preface

Purpose of This Workbook

In 2023, the National Council of State Boards of Nursing (NCSBN) implemented the Next-Generation NCLEX® Examination (NGN) for nursing licensure based on its new model of clinical judgment. This one-of-a-kind workbook is designed to help students enrolled in prelicensure programs for licensed practical nursing/licensed vocational nursing (LPN/LVN) practice to:

- Develop clinical judgment skills for LPN/LVN practice to ensure patient safety and readiness for entry into practice.
- Prepare for success on the NGN through practical thinking exercises in which students apply clinical reasoning (cognitive) skills to make appropriate clinical judgments.

This book is intended for students to use throughout their nursing program. Thinking exercises are available for all major areas of clinical specialty practice, with a heavy emphasis on the care of older adults. Each exercise provides common client situations with multiple NGN-style test items that LPNs/LVNs will likely encounter. For many thinking exercises, the clinical situation evolves into continuing care, requiring the student to address changing client conditions.

Organization of This Workbook

This student-friendly workbook is organized by nursing concepts but is easy to use in any type of prelicensure LPN/LVN nursing program; it is divided into four distinct parts for a total of 23 chapters. Each health condition throughout the book consists of multiple thinking exercises for student practice, including at least two Unfolding Case Studies followed by one or more Stand-Alone items:

Part 1 (Chapters 1 and 2). Chapter 1 provides an introduction to clinical judgment as a primary skill needed by practicing nurses. Chapter 2 offers tips for answering the practical thinking exercises in the workbook.

Part 2 (Chapters 3 to 10). This section focuses on thinking exercises that address nursing care for young and middle-age clients experiencing commonly occurring medical-surgical and mental health problems.

Part 3 (Chapters 11 to 19). This section includes thinking exercises that focus on coordinating care for older adults who have commonly occurring health conditions.

Part 4 (Chapters 20 to 23). The last section focuses on thinking exercises that address commonly occurring health conditions experienced by obstetric-newborn and pediatric clients.

Answer Key. The last section of this workbook presents the answers, rationales, and clinical judgment cognitive skills for each thinking exercise. In addition, students are provided with reference pages, where they can read more about each health problem.

References. At the end of the book is the list of textbook citations that are used for reference for the thinking exercises.

In summary, the second edition of *Developing Clinical Judgment for Practical/Vocational Nursing Practice and NGN Readiness* is an excellent learning resource focused exclusively on developing the clinical judgment skills needed for LPN/LVN student success in practice readiness and on the NGN.

Donna D. "Iggy" Ignatavicius

Tami K. Little

*To my husband, Charles, who has lovingly supported me in my writing and consultation for four decades; to all the nursing educators who are passionate about facilitating learning; and to all of the nursing students who are passionate about thinking-in-action like a nurse! — **DDI***

*Many thanks to the faculty, students, and administrators who have challenged me to seek new opportunities and make positive contributions to nursing education, and to my loving husband, Michael, who patiently endures my compulsive work ethic and constantly provides essential support, encouragement, and advice. — **TKL***

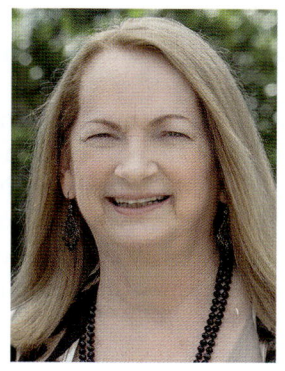

Donna D. Ignatavicius received her diploma in nursing from the Peninsula General School of Nursing in Salisbury, Maryland. After working as a charge nurse in medical-surgical nursing, she became an instructor in staff development at the University of Maryland Medical Center. She then received her BSN from the University of Maryland School of Nursing. For 5 years she taught in several schools of nursing, including an LPN program, while working toward her MS in Nursing, which she received in 1981. Donna then taught in the BSN program at the University of Maryland, after which she continued to pursue her interest in gerontology and accepted the position of Director of Nursing at a major skilled-nursing facility. Since that time, she has served as a nurse educator in several associate degree and baccalaureate nursing programs. Through her consulting activities, faculty development workshops, and international nursing education conferences (such as Boot Camp for Nurse Educators®), Donna is nationally recognized as an expert in nursing education. She is currently the President of DI Associates, Inc. (http://www.diassociates.com/), a company dedicated to improving health care through education and consultation for faculty. Well known as a prolific author of multiple nursing books, the 11th edition of her *Medical-Surgical Nursing: Concepts for Clinical Judgment and Collaborative Care* won a 2024 AJN first-place award in medical-surgical nursing. Her *Developing Clinical Judgment for Professional Nursing Practice and NGN Readiness* won a 2024 AJN second-place award in nursing education. In recognition of her contributions to the field, Donna was inducted as a charter Fellow of the prestigious Academy of Nursing Education (ANEF) in 2007, received her initial Certified Nurse Educator (CNE) credential in 2016 (recertified in 2021), and earned her Certified Academic Clinical Nurse Educator (CNEcl) credential in 2020. In 2022, Donna was inducted as a Fellow into the Academy of Associate Degree Nursing (FAADN).

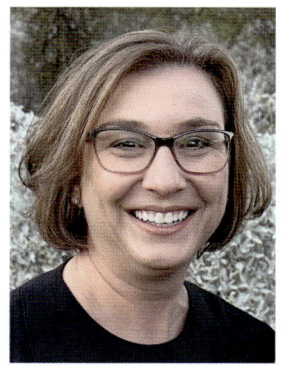

Tami K. Little started her career as a critical care nurse after achieving a BSN from the University of Arizona. She worked at several major medical institutions throughout the country for many years before returning to school for an MSN with an emphasis on nursing education. She began working as an adjunct clinical instructor for a local community college and methodically advanced to full-time faculty, program coordinator, dean of nursing, and corporate/national director of nursing within several academic institutions. Tami has facilitated student learning and managed academic programs at various levels including practical/vocational nursing as well as associate, baccalaureate, and master's degree programs. Tami achieved a Doctor of Nursing Practice (DNP) degree with a focus on systems leadership from Rush University, retains Registered Nurse licensure in several states, and maintains ongoing certification as a Certified Nurse Educator (CNE). Tami is also a nursing education consultant (LittleNurse, LLC) focused on the implementation and advancement of nursing education programs throughout the country.

Acknowledgments

Publishing a textbook would not be possible without the combined efforts of many people. With that in mind, we would like to extend our deepest gratitude to the many people who were such an integral part of this journey.

The staff of Elsevier has, as always, provided meaningful guidance and support throughout every step of the planning, writing, revision, and production of this new title. Executive Content Strategist Lee Henderson worked closely with us from the early stages of this title to help shape the second edition of this project. Content Development Specialist Dominque McPherson then worked with us from vision to publication. Senior Project Manager Jodi Willard was, as always, an absolute joy with whom to work. Her unwavering attention to detail, flexibility, and conscientiousness helped to make this title consistently readable while making the production process incredibly smooth.

Our acknowledgments would not be complete without recognizing the dedicated team of Education Solutions Consultants and other key members of the Sales and Marketing staff who helped put this book into your hands.

Contents

PART 1

Introduction to Clinical Judgment

CHAPTER 1

Clinical Judgment: Building on the Clinical Problem-Solving Process

Learning Outcomes

1. Explain why the National Council of State Boards of Nursing (NCSBN) added a focus on clinical judgment as part of the Next-Generation NCLEX® (NGN).
2. Identify the six NCSBN cognitive (thinking) skills needed to make safe clinical judgments.

Key Terms

Clinical judgment The observed outcome of critical thinking and decision making. It is an iterative process that uses nursing knowledge to observe and assess presenting situations, identify a prioritized client concern, and generate the best possible evidence-based solutions in order to deliver safe client care.

Clinical problem-solving process (nursing process) A scientific approach to client care that includes data collection, planning, implementation, and evaluation.

Clinical reasoning The cognitive (thinking) process of identifying a client's actual or potential problems or needs, collecting and analyzing client assessment data, hypothesizing and performing nursing actions, and evaluating and reflecting on the actions to determine if they were effective.

At this point in your nursing program, you have likely learned about the clinical problem-solving process that is used by practical/vocational nurses to provide safe, client-centered care in a variety of health care settings. Depending on the state or province where your program is located, you may refer to this process as the *nursing process*. This chapter will help you build on what you know about the clinical problem-solving process (nursing process) and explain why the nursing profession currently supports clinical judgment as the best standard for making clinical decisions. This workbook focuses on helping you learn how to use thinking skills to make sound clinical judgments in a variety of clinical situations to keep clients safe.

Brief Review of the Clinical Problem-Solving Process

The clinical problem-solving process (nursing process) is a systematic method for problem solving that nurses use to make safe, client-centered care decisions. It has been used since the 1960s as the gold standard to guide nursing practice and has been measured on the nursing licensure examinations (NCLEX®) for many years. State and provincial regulatory bodies, such as state boards of nursing, have since differentiated the role of the registered nurse (RN) and licensed practical nurse/licensed vocational nurse (LPN/LVN) related to the nursing process (NCSBN, 2023).

Table 1.1 Comparison of the RN and LPN/LVN Role Using the Nursing Process

Step of the Nursing Process	RN Role	LPN/LVN Role
Assessment	Performs a comprehensive client assessment	Collects and organizes client data (NCSBN, 2023)
Analysis	Interprets assessment data to identify client problems	Primarily an RN function, but may assist in the identification of health needs for clients across the life span
Planning	Develops a plan of care to meet desired or expected client outcomes	Contributes to the plan of care to meet desired or expected client outcomes
Implementation	Uses knowledge, skills, and abilities to meet the needs of clients requiring promotion, maintenance, and/or restoration of health	Performs competencies and skills needed to care for clients with commonly occurring health problems that have predictable outcomes (NCSBN, 2023)
Evaluation	Assesses the client's response to interventions to determine if desired or expected outcomes are met and if changes are needed in the plan of care	In coordination with the RN, measures the progress toward the desired or expected client outcomes

LPN/LVN, Licensed practical nurse/licensed vocational nurse; *RN,* registered nurse.

As you might expect, using a problem-solving approach for the nursing process requires thinking and reasoning. In the 1990s, the concept of critical thinking was introduced in nursing practice and nursing education. Since that time, experts have agreed that nurses use many types of thinking, including creative and analytical thinking, to make the best evidence-based decisions for their clients.

Clinical reasoning is also an important concept needed for the nursing process. In their landmark study, Benner et al. (2010) stated that clinical reasoning is the process of thinking about a client situation *in a specific context* while considering client and family concerns. A more recent definition by Joplin-Gonzales & Rounds (2022) states that **clinical reasoning** is the cognitive (thinking) process of identifying a client's actual or potential problems or needs, collecting and analyzing client assessment data, hypothesizing and performing nursing actions, and evaluating and reflecting on the actions to determine if they were effective.

The National Council of State Boards of Nursing (NCSBN) combined these concepts and defined the **clinical problem-solving process (nursing process)** for the LPN/LVN as "a scientific approach to client care that includes data collection [assessment], planning, implementation and evaluation" (NCSBN, 2023, p. 4). This definition is currently an Integrated Process for the NCLEX-PN® and does not include the analysis. However, in actual nursing practice, the LPN/LVN may use all of the steps of the process (Table 1.1).

Expanding From the Nursing Process to Clinical Judgment

In 2006, Tanner presented findings from classic meta-analysis research that examined how practicing nurses actually think and make clinical decisions. The researcher found that nurses use *clinical judgment* skills more than the nursing process and become more competent in these skills with experience and confidence. Tanner also found that making sound clinical judgments requires thinking skills such as clinical reasoning and critical thinking. These skills include:

- *Noticing* a client situation or changes in the situation triggers the nurse to collect more data for an accurate and thorough assessment. Noticing is affected by what the nurse brings to the situation, such as knowledge, ethical perspective, and expectations.
- *Interpreting* client findings requires the nurse to analyze the data to determine the client's problem(s).

- *Responding* requires the nurse to take actions or monitor the client based on current evidence to prevent, detect early, or resolve client problem(s).
- *Reflecting* on the situation allows the nurse to determine the client's status and think about what the nurse learned that can be used in another clinical situation.

In some ways, Tanner's components are distinctly different from the nursing process steps. For example, *Noticing* is the trigger that informs the nurse to perform the assessment. The *Interpreting* component involves identifying the client's problems and encourages the nurse to communicate effectively with appropriate health care team members. *Responding* may require implementing one or more specific actions or frequently monitoring a client's clinical situation. *Reflecting* not only includes evaluating the results of client care, but it also allows the nurse to examine the actions implemented to address the clinical situation.

The National League for Nursing (NLN) included *nursing judgment* as one of its four new nursing graduate competencies for all types of nursing programs. The NLN states that nursing judgment encompasses three processes: critical thinking, clinical judgment, and integration of best evidence into practice. Nurses use these processes when they make sound decisions about client care. More specifically, the use of nursing judgment involves these specific skills (www.nln.org):

- Processing information
- Thinking critically
- Evaluating the evidence
- Applying relevant knowledge
- Using problem-solving skills
- Reflecting on the situation

The National Council of State Boards of Nursing (NCSBN) Clinical Judgment Cognitive Skills

The NCSBN is responsible for the design and content of the registered and practical nursing licensure examinations known as the NCLEX-RN® and NCLEX-PN®, respectively. Over the past few years, the NCSBN conducted a study to determine if the current nursing licensure examinations for entry into practice are adequate to ensure that new nurses are competent in clinical judgment skills to protect the public. Older NCLEX® test item types have not measured all of the cognitive (thinking) skills needed to make sound clinical judgment but rather have focused on the more basic nursing process (Dickison et al., 2019). These test items measure only whether new graduates are *minimally safe* to practice, such as the examples in Box 1.1. The NCSBN study showed that although knowledge is essential, it is not enough to ensure safe clinical judgment. Put another way, having knowledge does not mean that a nurse has good clinical judgment skills. However, making good clinical judgments requires adequate nursing knowledge (Dickison et al., 2019).

As a result of the study, the NCSBN made major changes in the nursing licensure examinations, called the Next-Generation NCLEX® (NGN), that include *measuring* new graduates' competence in clinical judgment. In one of their first steps toward meeting that outcome and based on an extensive literature review, the NCSBN defined **clinical judgment** as the observed outcome of critical thinking and decision making. It is "an iterative [repeating] process that uses nursing knowledge to observe and assess presenting situations, identify a prioritized client concern, and generate the best possible evidence-based solutions in order to deliver safe client care" (NCSBN, 2023, p. 4).

The 2023 NCLEX-PN® Test Plan includes clinical judgment as an additional Integrated Process with the six thinking skills needed to make sound judgments. Using case scenarios that present more complex client information, the thinking skills that you will need to use to make sound clinical judgments include:

- **Recognize Cues (What matters most and now?)**
  Cues are elements of client data that provide important information for the nurse as a basis for making clinical decisions. In a clinical situation, determine which data are *relevant* (directly related to client outcomes or the priority of care) versus *irrelevant* (unrelated to client outcomes or the

---

Box 1.1 Examples of Current NCLEX-PN® Test Item Formats

Multiple-Choice Test Item

A client is admitted to the memory care unit with a diagnosis of Alzheimer disease. Which action by the nurse is the most important when caring for the client?

A. Be sure that the client receives environmental stimulation.
B. Reorient the client every time the nurse enters the room.
C. Protect the client and keep the client safe.
D. Use validation therapy when communicating with the client.

To answer this test item, the student or graduate only needs to know that ensuring safety is essential when caring for a client with dementia. Choice C is the best response. Having this knowledge does not guarantee clinical judgment ability.

Select All That Apply Item

A nurse is caring for a client who has heart failure. Which signs and symptoms would the nurse expect when collecting and organizing data? **Select all that apply.**

A. Shortness of breath
B. Lower extremity edema
C. Bruising on the chest and abdomen
D. Increased respiratory rate
E. Bounding radial pulse

To answer this test item, the student or graduate only needs to know the common signs and symptoms of a client who has heart failure. Choices A, B, D, and E are the correct responses. Bruising (Choice C) is not common in clients who have heart disease but is often found in clients who have clotting problems. Having this knowledge does not guarantee clinical judgment ability.

---

priority of care). Decide which data are the *most* important and require immediate follow-up by the nurse.

- **Analyze Cues (What could it mean?)**
  Consider the cues in the context of the client history and situation. Think about how the identified relevant cues relate to the client's condition or history. Identify cues that support a particular pattern in the situation, and determine why certain cues are more concerning to the nurse than others. Determine what could be going on in the situation and what client condition(s) is (are) suspected.

- **Prioritize Hypotheses (Where do I start?)**
  Consider all possibilities about what is occurring in the client situation. Consider their urgency and risk for the client. Determine which explanations are *most likely* and *most serious* and why to identify the priority for care.

- **Generate Solutions (What can I do?)**
  Identify expected client outcomes. Using the priority or priorities identified, plan specific actions that could achieve the desirable outcomes. Consider which actual or potential actions should be *avoided* or are *contraindicated* because they could be harmful for the client in the given situation.

- **Take Actions (What will I do?)**
  Decide which nursing action(s) will address the highest priorities of care, and determine in which priority the action(s) will be implemented. Actions can include, but are not limited to, collecting additional data, documentation, requesting primary health care provider orders, performing nursing skills, health teaching, additional client monitoring, and coordinating with health care team members.

- **Evaluate Outcomes (Did it help?)**
  Evaluate the actual client outcomes in the situation, and compare them to the desired or expected outcomes. Determine which client findings indicate an improvement or a decline in the client's condition. Decide if the selected nursing actions were effective or ineffective.

Table 1.2 Comparison of the Nursing Process, Tanner's Model of Clinical Judgment, and NCSBN Clinical Judgment Cognitive Skills

Nursing Process (AAPIE) (NCLEX-PN® Test Plan)	Tanner's Model of Clinical Judgment	Clinical Judgment Cognitive Skills (NCLEX-PN® Test Plan)
Assessment	Noticing	Recognize Cues
Analysis	Interpreting	Analyze Cues
Analysis	Interpreting	Prioritize Hypotheses
Planning	Responding	Generate Solutions
Implementation	Responding	Take Actions
Evaluation	Reflecting	Evaluate Outcomes

Table 1.2 shows a comparison of the nursing process, Tanner's model of clinical judgment, and the NCSBN clinical judgment cognitive skills. Chapter 2 in this workbook presents examples of the thinking exercises used in this book and how to approach them to determine the correct responses using clinical judgment thinking skills. These thinking exercises are very similar to proposed test item formats that you will have on the NCLEX®.

References

Asterisk (*) indicates a classic or definitive work on this subject.

*Benner, P., Sutphen, M., Leonard, V., & Day, L. (2010). Educating nurses: A call for radical transformation. San Francisco: Jossey-Bass.

Dickison, P., Haerling, K. A., & Lasater, K. (2019). Integrating the National Council of State Boards of Nursing Clinical Judgment Model into nursing educational frameworks. *Journal of Nursing Education*, 58(2), 72–78.

Joplin-Gonzales, P. & Rounds, L. (2022). The essential elements of clinical reasoning. *Nurse Educator*, 47(6), E145–E149.

National Council of State Boards of Nursing (NCSBN). (2023). NCLEX-PN® Examination: Test plan for the National Council Licensure Examination for Practical Nurses. Chicago: Author.

*Tanner, C. A. (2006). Thinking like a nurse: A research-based model of clinical judgment. *Journal of Nursing Education*, 45, 204–211.

Introduction to the New Next-Generation NCLEX® (NGN) Item Types

Learning Outcomes

1. Differentiate the new NGN test item formats used as thinking exercises in this workbook.
2. Identify tips for success when using the six clinical judgment (CJ) thinking skills to answer various types of thinking exercises in this workbook.

All nurses need to make sound clinical judgments to keep clients safe. As introduced in Chapter 1, the National Council of State Boards of Nursing (NCSBN) developed an evidence-based CJ model. This new model was the basis for a major NCSBN study on how to measure the CJ ability of new nursing graduates on the national licensure exams (NCLEX®) to ensure public safety. As a result of the study, a variety of new test item types were added to the NCLEX-RN® and NCLEX-PN® in April 2023. These new licensure exams are referred to as the Next-Generation NCLEX® (NGN).

This chapter will help you learn how to apply CJ and "think-in-action like a nurse" using a variety of practice thinking exercises that are very similar to the new NGN test items. Tips for applying the CJ cognitive (thinking) skills to correctly answer these thinking exercises are also provided.

CJ thinking skills are mental processes that are required for appropriate and sound clinical judgment. As introduced in Chapter 1, these skills include:

- Recognize Cues: *What matters most and now?*
- Analyze Cues: *What could it mean?*
- Prioritize Hypotheses: *Where do I start?*
- Generate Solutions: *What can I do?*
- Take Actions: *What will I do?*
- Evaluate Outcomes: *Did it help?*

The clinical case exercises in this workbook will help you apply the six thinking (cognitive) skills of the NCSBN's Clinical Judgment Measurement Model (NCJMM) using a variety of new NGN test item formats. Like the NGN items on the NCLEX®, this workbook's thinking exercises are presented in Unfolding Case Studies and as Stand-Alone items across the life span and across all specialties.

The answers and rationales for the correct responses to the thinking exercises are provided in the last section of this workbook. Please note that the reference pages provided for each exercise do not necessarily contain the answers but rather provide the knowledge that is needed as a basis for answering them. The CJ thinking skill needed to answer each exercise is also identified.

Unfolding Case Study Thinking Exercises

Unfolding Case Studies present a client situation that changes over time—over minutes, hours, or days. Like the new NGN items, each Unfolding Case Study thinking exercise in this workbook includes six questions to measure each of the six CJ thinking skills. To represent a more authentic clinical situation, client information is organized and presented under one or more tabs of a medical record. Any of these tabs may be used and include:

- Orders
- Nurses' Notes
- Progress Notes
- Laboratory Results

- Diagnostic Results
- Vital Signs
- History and Physical
- Nursing Flow Sheet

Box 2.1 lists the new item types organized by category used in NGN Unfolding Case Studies and this workbook.

The following examples present at least one test item example for each NGN item category. The answer, rationale, CJ thinking skill, and reference are provided immediately after each example.

Highlight Items

Highlight items require you to use a marker (print version) or mouse (computer version) to select the answer to the question within a client's medical record. This type of item is used to determine your ability to Recognize Cues or Evaluate Outcomes. The example in Box 2.2 is a Highlight In-Text test item that could begin an Unfolding Case Study. The other type of highlight test item, Highlight In-Table items, typically ask you to identify relevant lab or vital sign data presented in a table or flow sheet within a client situation.

Box 2.1   Test Item Types Used in NGN Unfolding Case Studies

- Highlight items
  - Highlight In-Text
  - Highlight In-Table
- Drag-and-Drop items
  - Drag-and-Drop Cloze
  - Drag-and-Drop Rationale
- Matrix items
  - Matrix Multiple Response
  - Matrix Multiple Choice
- Drop-Down items
  - Drop-Down Cloze
  - Drop-Down Rationale
  - Drop-Down Table
- Extended Multiple Response items
  - Extended Multiple Grouping
  - Extended Select All That Apply
  - Extended Select N

Box 2.2   Highlight Thinking Exercise Example

The nurse has collected data for an 83-year-old client admitted to the acute orthopedic unit. Highlight the client findings below that require **immediate** follow-up.

History and Physical	Nurses' Notes	Orders	Laboratory Results

0805: Client had a right open reduction and internal fixation (ORIF) of the hip yesterday following a fall at home. Alert but does not respond verbally to questions. Restless and picking at covers. Lung sounds clear with no adventitious breath sounds; S_1 and S_2 present. Hypoactive bowel sounds present $\times$ 4. Right hip dressing dry and intact. Yells when right leg touched. Capillary refill >3 sec bilaterally. No palpable right pedal pulse; 1+ left pedal pulse. Right foot cooler and ash gray compared with left foot. VS: T 98.6°F (37°C); HR 92 beats/min; RR 20 breaths/min; BP 166/90 mm Hg; SpO$_2$ 95% at 2 L/min O$_2$ via NC. FSBG 288 mg/dL (16 mmol/L). Client has history of diabetes mellitus, hypertension, and osteoporosis.

Continued

Box 2.2 Highlight Thinking Exercise Example—cont'd

Answer

History and Physical	Nurses' Notes	Orders	Laboratory Results

0805: Client had a right open reduction and internal fixation (ORIF) of the hip yesterday following a fall at home. Alert but does not respond verbally to questions. Restless and picking at covers. Lung sounds clear with no adventitious breath sounds; S_1 and S_2 present. Hypoactive bowel sounds present $\times$ 4. Right hip dressing dry and intact. Yells when right leg touched. Capillary refill >3 sec bilaterally. No palpable right pedal pulse; 1+ left pedal pulse. Right foot cooler and ash gray compared with left foot. VS: T 98.6°F (37°C); HR 92 beats/min; RR 20 breaths/min; BP 166/90 mm Hg; SpO_2 95% at 2 L/min O_2 via NC. FSBG 288 mg/dL (16 mmol/L). Client has history of diabetes mellitus, hypertension, and osteoporosis.

Rationale

This thinking exercise is asking you to *Recognize Cues* by identifying the relevant client findings that need immediate follow-up by the nurse and health care team at this time. The client findings indicate that the right leg may have peripheral circulation problems as indicated by an absent pulse, slowed capillary refill (should be <3 sec), ash gray color (which suggests pallor in clients with dark skin tones), and coolness. These findings are of immediate concern because the client may develop worsening neurovascular compromise. The elevated blood pressure, yelling when the leg is touched, and restlessness could be caused by acute pain, which needs to be managed immediately to promote comfort and prevent the development of long-term persistent pain. Acute pain requires attention by the nurse at this time. The finger stick blood glucose (FSBG) value is of immediate concern because it is well above normal range and needs to be controlled to prevent a diabetic emergency and/or poor healing. The oxygen saturation is within normal limits and needs to be routinely monitored rather than followed up as an immediate concern for the nurse at this time. The other vital sign findings are within normal limits.

CJ Thinking Skill: Recognize Cues

Reference: Linton & Matteson, 2023, pp. 923–928

Drag-and-Drop Items

Drag-and-Drop items require you to select the correct answer(s) from a list of word choices and move them via the computer mouse to fill in one to three blanks to complete one or two sentences. In this workbook, you'll need to select the correct answer and fill in the blank(s). Drag-and-Drop items can assess your ability to use most of the CJ thinking skills. Using the same Nurses' Note entry for the older adult who had a right hip ORIF, the example in Box 2.3 is a Drag-and-Drop Rationale item to assess your ability to Analyze Cues. Note that any type of NGN Rationale item typically includes the terms "as evidenced by," "due to," or "because."

Box 2.3 Drag-and-Drop Thinking Exercise Example

The nurse is caring for an 83-year-old client admitted to the acute orthopedic unit.

History and Physical	Nurses' Notes	Orders	Laboratory Results

0805: Client had a right open reduction and internal fixation (ORIF) of the hip yesterday following a fall at home. Alert but does not respond verbally to questions. Restless and picking at covers. Lung sounds clear with no adventitious breath sounds; S_1 and S_2 present. Hypoactive bowel sounds present $\times$ 4. Right hip dressing dry and intact. Yells when right leg touched. Capillary refill >3 sec bilaterally. No palpable right pedal pulse; 1+ left pedal pulse. Right foot cooler and ash gray compared with left foot. VS: T 98.6°F (37°C); HR 92 beats/min; RR 20 breaths/min; BP 166/90 mm Hg; SpO_2 95% at 2 L/min O_2 via NC. FSBG 288 mg/dL (16 mmol/L). Client has history of diabetes mellitus, hypertension, and osteoporosis.

The nurse has reviewed the collected client data with the registered nurse (RN). Complete the following sentence by selecting from the list of word choices below.

Box 2.3 Drag-and-Drop Thinking Exercise Example—cont'd

The client likely has **[Word Choice]** in the right leg as evidenced by **[Word Choice]** and **[Word Choice]**.

WORD CHOICES
Chronic (persistent) pain
Impaired circulation
Absent pedal pulse
Elevated blood pressure
Cool, ash gray skin
Restlessness

Answer:

The client likely has **impaired circulation** in the right leg as evidenced by **absent pedal pulse** and **cool, ash gray skin**.

Rationale

This thinking exercise is asking you to *Analyze Cues* by collaborating with the RN to interpret the client's relevant findings to determine what they mean. Clients who have fractures or reduction of fractures are at risk for inadequate peripheral circulation in the affected extremity. Evidence of impaired circulation includes coolness, pallor (or ash gray color in dark brown or black skin), weak or absent distal pulses, and sluggish capillary refill. The client is experiencing acute pain rather than chronic (persistent) pain due to surgery the day before. Restlessness and vital sign changes are typical in clients who have acute pain.

CJ Thinking Skill: Analyze Cues

Reference: Linton & Matteson, 2023, pp. 923–928

Tip for CJ Success

Be sure to consider all skin tones for a variety of clients across the life span. For example, hyperpigmentation is common when dark skin is inflamed; erythema or redness is seen in clients who have lighter skin. The skin appears ash gray in clients with dark skin tones due to lack of blood flow; pallor is seen in clients who have lighter skin.

Matrix Items

Matrix test items may be used to assess several CJ thinking skills. For example, to measure *Generate Solutions,* you may be given a list of nursing actions and asked to determine if each action would be Indicated or Not Indicated for the client situation presented. In this case, you would select one choice or the other—Indicated or Not Indicated (Matrix Multiple Choice item). In other client situations, you may be asked to select more than one choice (Matrix Multiple Response item). The Matrix thinking exercise in Box 2.4 assesses your ability to *Evaluate Outcomes* to identify if the nurse's actions were Effective or Not Effective.

Box 2.4 Matrix Thinking Exercise Example

The nurse is caring for a 74-year-old client in the rehabilitation unit.

History and Physical	Nurses' Notes	Orders	Laboratory Results

1130: Admitted for rehab following left total knee arthroplasty. Alert and oriented × 2 (person and place). Reminded to use call light when needing to get out of bed. Family states client became delirious after surgery for about 24 hours and could not recall her name. Client states understanding of safety instructions. Lung sounds clear with no adventitious breath sounds; S_1 and S_2 present. Bowel sounds present × 4. Left knee incision dry and intact with swelling and extensive bruising. Grimaces when left leg touched; states pain is 5/10. Capillary refill <3 sec bilaterally. Able to move all extremities, but very cautious with left leg. VS: T 98.6°F (37°C); HR 85 beats/min; RR 18 breaths/min; BP 126/80 mm Hg; SpO_2 95% on RA. Pain medication given at 1215.

1430: Alert and oriented × 2 (person and place). Reports pain at 3/10 prior to PT. PT and OT consults for evaluation complete. PT reported client frequently stood up from wheelchair without prompting and assistance; fell × 1 without apparent injury (see PT note).

Continued

Box 2.4 Matrix Thinking Exercise Example—cont'd

The nurse has reviewed client findings with the RN. For each current client finding, indicate whether the client is improving or worsening.

CLIENT FINDINGS	IMPROVING	WORSENING
Alert and oriented × 2		
States understanding of safety instructions		
Fell in PT due to standing without prompting or assistance		
Reports pain at 3/10 prior to PT		

Answer

CLIENT FINDINGS	IMPROVING	WORSENING
Alert and oriented × 2	✗	
States understanding of safety instructions	✗	
Fell in PT due to standing without prompting or assistance		✗
Reports pain at 3/10 prior to PT	✗	

Rationale

This thinking exercise is asking you to *Evaluate Outcomes* by determining if current assessment findings indicate if the client's delirium and pain have improved or worsened. Delirium is acute confusion that can occur in older adults after surgery due to pain, anesthesia, drug therapy, and the trauma of the procedure. This mental health condition is reversible for most clients when these causes are resolved. In addition to confusion, the client often has behavioral or emotional manifestations, such as yelling, agitation, and aggression. Being oriented × 2 is an improvement from what the client experienced in the hospital according to family. The client also indicated understanding of safety instructions. Both of these findings indicate that the client is improving. The client's report of pain is also improving as it decreased from 5/10 to 3/10. The fall during the physical therapy evaluation, though, shows that the client apparently forgot the safety instructions. There is no indication that the client fell while in the hospital, so this event demonstrates that the client's condition is worsening and the client now has a high risk of falling.

CJ Thinking Skill: Evaluate Outcomes
Reference: Morrison-Valfre, 2023, pp. 194–194

Drop-Down Items

Drop-Down test items are similar to Drag-and-Drop items because both require you to complete one or two sentences or a table. When answering these items on a computer-based test, you would click on each blank with the mouse to view a list of options to fill in the blank. In this printed workbook, each blank is numbered when needed to ensure that you select from the appropriate list of options. Drag-and-Drop items can assess your ability to apply most of the CJ thinking skills. The example in Box 2.5 is a Drag-and-Drop Cloze item in sentence format.

Box 2.5 Drop-Down Thinking Exercise Example

The nurse is caring for a 53-year-old client in the urgent care center.

History and Physical	Progress Notes	Diagnostic Results	Laboratory Results

0830: Came to center with report of increasing productive cough, chest discomfort, anorexia, extreme fatigue, fever, and chills for the past few days. Frequently coughs excessively, which sometimes causes choking and vomiting. Has missed the past 2 days of work. No significant medical history except for smoking 2 to 3 packs of cigarettes for the past 35 years. Has never had any vaccines for common respiratory infections. VS: T 102.8°F (39.3°C); HR 96 beats/min; RR 23 breaths/min; BP 102/56 mm Hg; SpO_2 94% on RA. Denies dyspnea or labored breathing.

The nurse has reviewed the collected client data with the RN. Complete the following sentence by selecting from the lists of options below.

The *priority* for the client's care at this time is to **[Select]**.

OPTIONS
Improve fatigue
Improve nutrition
Manage dehydration
Prevent airway obstruction
Improve oxygenation

Answer

The *priority* for the client's care at this time is to **prevent airway obstruction**.

Rationale

This thinking exercise is asking you to *Prioritize Hypotheses* to determine what you would do first when caring for this client. The client has a productive cough with excessive sputum that has caused choking and vomiting. Therefore airway obstruction is a potential complication. Using the ABCs to prioritize care, *A* is for airway, *B* is for breathing, and *C* is for circulation. Therefore preventing airway obstruction is more important than improving oxygenation and is the priority for client care. The client is not experiencing dyspnea; the SpO_2 is slightly below the normal minimum range of 95%, but the client is not symptomatic. The client's fatigue, nutrition, and possible dehydration need to be addressed, but not before the ABCs.

CJ Thinking Skill: Prioritize Hypotheses
Reference: Linton & Matteson, 2023, pp. 509–513

Extended Multiple Response Items

Extended Multiple Response test items may be used to measure any of the CJ thinking skills. For this type of item, you need to select the correct responses from a list of choices to answer the question. You might recognize this type of question as the Select All That Apply (SATA) item with 5 or 6 choices because it has been part of the NCLEX® for many years. The SATA and Select N items on the NGN now have 5 to 10 choices. A newer type of Extended Multiple Response item presents a table with groups of choices from which to select as the correct answer (Extended Multiple Grouping). The example in Box 2.6 assesses the CJ thinking skill of *Generate Solutions*.

Box 2.6 Extended Multiple Response Thinking Exercise Example

The nurse is caring for a 47-year-old client in the acute surgical unit.

History and Physical	Nurses' Notes	Diagnostic Results	Laboratory Results

1645: Returned from partial thyroidectomy late this morning. Resting in semi-Fowler position with O_2 at 3 L/min via NC. IV of NS infusing at 100 mL/h. No nausea or vomiting, but has not yet voided. Reports throat pain as 7/10. Neck surgical dressing dry and intact. Has hoarseness at times, and swallowing frequently. Breath sounds clear in all lung fields; no respiratory distress. VS: T 98°F (36.7°C); HR 82 beats/min; RR 18 breaths/min; BP 106/58 mm Hg; SpO_2 99% on O_2.

1800: Postop lab results posted.

History and Physical	Nurses' Notes	Diagnostic Results	Laboratory Results
Serum Laboratory Test and Reference Range		**Today (1300)**	
Blood urea nitrogen (BUN) (10–20 mg/dL [3.6–7.1 mmol/L])		12 mg/dL (4.29 mmol/L)	
Creatinine (Cr) (M: 0.6–1.2 mg/dL [53–106 mmol/L]; F: 0.5–1.1 mg/dL [44–97 µmol/L])		0.8 mg/dL (70.74 µmol/L)	
Sodium (Na) (136–145 mEq/L [136–145 mmol/L])		142 mEq/L (142 mmol/L)	
Potassium (K) (3.5–5.0 mEq/L [3.5–5.0 mmol/L])		4.3 mEq/L (4.3 mmol/L)	
Calcium (Ca) (9.0–10.5 mg/dL [2.25–2.62 mmol/L])		9.9 mg/dL (2.47 mmol/L)	

The nurse is contributing to the plan of care. Which of the following potential actions would be appropriate for the nurse to take? **Select all that apply.**

O Report the client's frequent swallowing to the RN immediately.
O Administer the prescribed analgesic as soon as possible.
O Monitor the client for muscle twitching and tingling.
O Request an order for oral potassium.
O Check behind the client's neck for bleeding.
O Place the client in a flat position to increase blood pressure.
O Teach the client that hoarseness is usually temporary.

Answer

✗ Report the client's frequent swallowing to the RN immediately.
✗ Administer the prescribed analgesic as soon as possible.
✗ Monitor the client for muscle twitching and tingling.
O Request an order for oral potassium.
✗ Check behind the client's neck for bleeding.
O Place the client in a flat position to increase blood pressure.
✗ Teach the client that hoarseness is usually temporary.

Rationale

This thinking exercise is assessing your ability to *Generate Solutions* appropriate for the client after surgery. The most important nursing action would be to report the client's frequent swallowing to the RN to assess for blood trickling into the throat (internal bleeding). External bleeding would also be assessed by checking behind the client's neck for moisture. The nurse would give the prescribed analgesic because the client reports a pain level of 7/10, indicating uncontrolled surgical pain. The desired pain level for most clients is 2/10 to 3/10. The nurse would assess for signs of potentially decreasing serum calcium, including tetany (muscle twitching) and tingling, especially around the mouth, in case there was parathyroid injury during surgery. However, according to the laboratory profile, the first postoperative serum calcium level was within normal limits. Temporary hoarseness is not unusual for clients having thyroid removal because the laryngeal nerve can become irritated. Oral potassium is not indicated because there is no evidence that the client has hypokalemia. The client is not hypotensive and needs to be in a sitting position to facilitate breathing.

CJ Thinking Skill: Generate Solutions
Reference: Linton & Matteson, 2023, pp. 986–988

Stand-Alone Thinking Exercises

In addition to Unfolding Case Study thinking exercises, each chapter of this workbook includes at least two Stand-Alone thinking exercises to simulate those items on the NGN and help you develop CJ skills. A Stand-Alone thinking exercise presents a client situation in a medical record format at one point in time as either a Bow-Tie or Trend item.

Bow-Tie Items

A Bow-Tie item presents a client situation followed by a bowtie-looking figure with three parts, and it typically measures your ability to apply all six CJ thinking skills. For each part of the thinking exercise, you will select the correct response from a list of options, as shown in Box 2.7.

Box 2.7 Bow-Tie Thinking Exercise Example

The nurse is caring for an 81-year-old client in the urgent care center.

History and Physical	**Nurses' Notes**	Orders	Laboratory Results

1605: Client brought to urgent care by family for evaluation of new-onset acute back pain that is preventing the client from using a walker to ambulate as usual and be ADL independent. Client alert and oriented × 4. When asked questions, client looks at family while answering. Makes little eye contact with nurse. States has been living with family for about 6 months since the client's partner died. No adventitious breath sounds. Abdomen soft, and bowel sounds present × 4. Several old bruises of varying shape, size, and age on back and chest. Client reports bruising is from falls that occurred during the past few weeks. States being very clumsy due to "getting old." Kyphosis and protruding spinal processes tender when palpated gently. Rates back pain as 8/10. Moves all extremities slowly. Capillary refill >3 sec; no dependent edema.

The nurse reviews the collected data with the RN. Complete the diagram by identifying from the choices below to specify what potential condition the client is likely experiencing, **2** nursing actions that are appropriate to take, and **2** parameters the nurse should monitor to assess the client's progress.

Actions to Take	Potential Complication	Parameters to Monitor
Prepare to teach client and family about prescribed drug therapy	Major depressive disorder	Indication of suicidal ideation
Conduct a more focused interview with the client in private without family	Delirium	ADL function
Express own feelings of anger about possible abuse to client	Elder abuse	Mood and affect
Question family about their ability to be adequate caregivers	Alzheimer disease	Decision-making ability
Inform the client that if abuse occurred, a referral to Adult Protective Services is required by law		Ability to ambulate

Continued

Box 2.7 Bow-Tie Thinking Exercise Example—cont'd

Answer

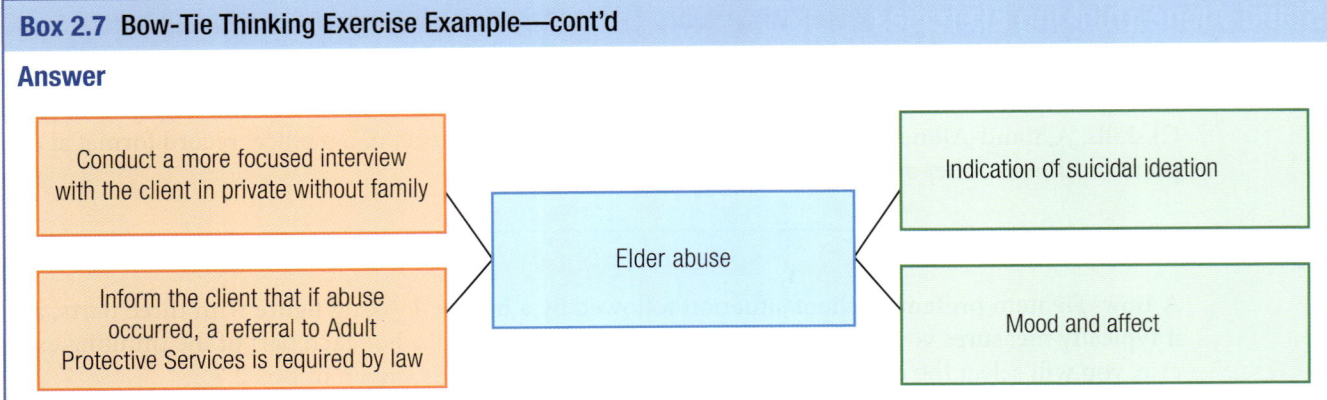

Rationale

The client is alert and oriented × 4, indicating that the client does not demonstrate acute (delirium) or chronic confusion (dementia such as Alzheimer disease). When asked questions, the client looked at family while answering and made little eye contact with the nurse. Several old bruises of varying shape, size, and age were observed on the client's back and chest, suggesting that the client was physically (and possibly emotionally) abused. When abuse is suspected, the nurse interviews the client in private and away from the family. Because the client is visiting a community center like urgent care, the nurse also informs the client that abuse is reportable to Adult Protective Services or a similar organization as required by law. The nurse should not express personal feelings about the client situation or accuse the family of being inadequate as caregivers. At this time, there is no evidence that the client has major depressive disorder, but the client's mood and affect need to be monitored. A client who is abused can become depressed and possibly have suicidal ideation. The client's ADL function and mobility will likely return to baseline when the acute back pain is adequately managed. The client is cognitively intact and should be able to make appropriate decisions.
CJ Thinking Skills: Recognize Cues, Analyze Cues, Prioritize Hypotheses, Generate Solutions, Take Actions, Evaluate Outcomes
Reference: Morrison-Valfre, 2023, p. 307

Trend Items

The Trend item shown in Box 2.8 is unique in that the client assessment data presented in the medical record are trended over time—minutes, hours, or days. The actual question related to the client situation may be any of the 12 item types that are used in Unfolding Case Studies and measure one or more CJ thinking skills.

Box 2.8 Trend Thinking Exercise Example

The nurse is caring for a 40-year-old client who had a cesarean section at 33 weeks' gestation. The nurse has reviewed the collected data with the RN.

Nurses' Notes	Vital Signs	Orders	Laboratory Results
Parameter	9/21 (Day of Delivery)	9/22 (Yesterday)	9/23 (Today)
Temperature	98.6°F (37°C)	98.6°F (37°C)	98.6°F (37°C)
Heart rate	90 beats/min	88 beats/min	94 beats/min
Respirations	18 breaths/min	20 breaths/min	20 breaths/min
Blood pressure	188/104 mm Hg	156/106 mm Hg	148/102 mm Hg
SpO_2	100% (on O_2)	97% (on RA)	98% (on RA)
Pain	7/10	4/10	3/10

Box 2.8 Trend Thinking Exercise Example—cont'd

The nurse reviews the collected data with the RN. Complete the following sentence by selecting from the list of word choices below.

The **priority** for nursing care is to manage the client's **[Word Choice]**.

WORD CHOICES
Fever
Tachycardia
Hypertension
Pain

Answer

The **priority** for nursing care is to manage the client's **hypertension**.

Rationale

The client likely has gestational hypertension, which is defined as development of a blood pressure greater than 140/90 mm Hg in a previously normotensive client after 20 weeks' gestation. This client continues to have an elevated blood pressure, which can lead to preeclampsia in the immediate postpartum period, although the blood pressure is slowly decreasing each day at this point. The nurse would monitor the client for severe headache, seizures, and protein in the urine. Therefore this client condition is the priority for nursing and collaborative care. The client does not have a fever or tachycardia, although the body temperature and heart rate have increased slightly. The client's pain seems to be managed because the client reports a 3/10.
CJ Thinking Skill: Recognize Cues, Analyze Cues, Prioritize Hypotheses
Reference: Leifer & Little, 2023, pp. 99–100

Applying the Clinical Judgment Thinking Skills

Clinical judgment can be learned through thinking exercises to apply nursing knowledge to clinical practice using a variety of client situations. Consider the client findings in Box 2.2.

Based on the assessment findings in this example, first determine which findings are relevant or important to the nurse in the client situation at this time. To Recognize Cues as a cognitive skill of clinical judgment in this thinking exercise, you need knowledge of:

- Normal physiologic and psychosocial changes associated with aging
- Adult normal or usual range for vital signs
- Signs and symptoms of adequate peripheral circulation
- Normal ranges for lab values

Tip for CJ Success

To help identify the clinical cues that are of greatest concern to the nurse, determine which findings are unusual or abnormal for the client situation.

To apply that knowledge, you likely selected the following *relevant* cues from the case study example that require immediate follow-up. The italicized phrases explain why these cues are the most important and require immediate attention.

- Blood pressure = 166/90 mm Hg *(increased above normal range)*
- Restless and picking at covers *(may suggest pain, hypoxia, or delirium)*
- Yells when right leg is touched *(surgical care painful when touched)*
- No palpable right pedal pulse; left pedal pulse present *(peripheral pulses should be present and equal in both legs)*
- Right foot cooler and ash gray compared with left foot *(temperature and color should be similar in both legs and feet)*
- FSBG = 288 mg/dL (16 mmol/L) *(increased above normal range)*

The next CJ thinking skill is to *Analyze Cues*. Analyzing or interpreting the meaning of the client findings in this case requires you to have knowledge of:

- Normal postoperative expectations
- Common postoperative complications of hip ORIF
- Normal range for FSBG and vital signs

Based on your interpretation, you then need to *Prioritize Hypotheses*. For this thinking skill, consider all possibilities about what is happening in the case, and then determine the *most likely* explanations and priority needs. The clinical cues in the case study reveal that the client is *most likely* experiencing an orthopedic surgical complication, which is possible decreased blood circulation in the right (surgical) leg as evidenced by the right foot being cooler and ash gray compared with the left foot; there is also no pedal pulse that the nurse can feel in the right foot. The client's elevated blood pressure and restlessness could be due to acute pain, hypoxia, or a history of hypertension. In addition, the FSBG value is above the normal range because surgery and trauma are stressors, especially for a client who has diabetes. The priorities for this client's care would be to:

#1 Improve circulation in the surgical (right) leg.

#2 Reduce the client's acute pain.

#3 Manage the client's elevated blood glucose.

The fourth thinking skill is to *Generate Solutions* that will meet desired or expected client outcomes. Collaborate with the RN to outline the desired outcomes in this situation, which are that the client will have:

- Sufficient peripheral circulation in both lower extremities.
- Adequate pain control (2–3/10).
- Vital signs within usual parameters.
- An FSBG within normal limits.

Consider which actual or potential nursing actions will meet these outcomes. Consider which ones should be *avoided* or are *contraindicated*. Remember that some actions could be harmful for the client in the given situation. This thinking skill requires you to have knowledge of how to care for the client and with which members of the health care team you will need to coordinate that care.

Tip for CJ Success

To effectively *Generate Solutions*, first collaborate with the RN to determine what expected outcomes are essential for the client. Then assist in planning solutions or actions that will meet these outcomes to contribute the plan of care.

When considering possible actions, recall that poor lower extremity circulation is an arterial problem. This means that elevating the client's left leg will *decrease* peripheral circulation and can potentially cause harm. Possible nursing actions based on best practice (and not in priority order) might include:

- Notify the surgeon regarding peripheral circulation changes.
- Check the right pedal pulse with a Doppler ultrasound device.
- Administer an analgesic as prescribed to manage pain.
- Administer regular insulin as prescribed to lower blood glucose.
- Avoid elevating the left leg.

The fifth CJ thinking skill is to *Take Actions*. Collaborate with the RN to determine the order of priority of the actions you want to take from the list of possible actions (solutions). Priorities are determined by factors such as urgency, difficulty, or complexity of the client's situation. As identified earlier, to meet the client's identified needs, the priority approach to care would be to:

1. Improve peripheral circulation in the surgical (right) leg.
2. Reduce the client's acute pain.
3. Manage the client's elevated blood glucose.

Based on these priorities, the nurse's actions would include:

1. Check the right pedal pulse with a Doppler ultrasound device.
2. Avoid elevating the right leg.
3. Notify the surgeon regarding peripheral circulation.
4. Administer an analgesic as prescribed to manage pain.
5. Administer regular insulin as prescribed to lower blood glucose.

> ### Tip for CJ Success
> When deciding on actions to take and in what order of priority, think about which client problems are potentially life- or limb-threatening and the urgency of each problem. Notifying the primary health care provider is not usually the most important action because there are always other actions that you can take first as an LPN/LVN.

The last thinking skill is to *Evaluate Outcomes* by collecting and reviewing data on the client's current condition after nursing actions have been implemented. Remember that the desired outcomes were that the client will:

- Have adequate peripheral circulation in both lower extremities.
- Have adequate pain control (2–3/10).
- Have vital signs within usual range for the client.
- Have an FSBG within normal range.

If the client met these outcomes, the nursing actions would be *effective*. If the outcomes were not met, then the actions would be *not effective*.

Clinical Judgment for Young and Middle-Aged Adults Experiencing Commonly Occurring Health Conditions

PART 2

CHAPTER 3

Client Conditions Affecting Perfusion

Unfolding Case Study 3.1

Thinking Exercise 3.1.1

The nurse is caring for a 47-year-old client at an outpatient endoscopy center. Highlight the client findings that require **immediate** follow-up.

History and Physical	Nurses' Notes	Orders	Laboratory Results

1150: Client arrives for routine colostomy and cancer screening. Health history includes hypertension, dyslipidemia, and iron deficiency anemia. Client reports nonadherence to antihypertensive drugs due to fear that they will cause sexual dysfunction. Alert and oriented × 4, but appears restless; reports, "my vision seems foggy around the edges." Heart tones regular. Respirations are equal with lung fields clear throughout upon auscultation. Abdomen soft, round, and nontender. Bowel sounds present in all quadrants. Client confirms completing procedural preparations, stating "I haven't had anything to eat or drink besides the laxative preparation, which I finished early this morning. Currently, I feel nauseous, and I may vomit." VS: T 98.4°F (36.9°C), HR 104 beats/min, BP 194/138 mm Hg, RR 14 breaths/min, SpO$_2$ 95% on RA. Client reports headache at the back of the head, rated 6/10.

Thinking Exercise 3.1.2

The nurse is caring for a 47-year-old client at an outpatient endoscopy center.

History and Physical	Nurses' Notes	Orders	Laboratory Results

1150: Client arrives for routine colostomy and cancer screening. Health history includes hypertension, dyslipidemia, and iron deficiency anemia. Client reports nonadherence to antihypertensive drugs due to fear that they will cause sexual dysfunction. Alert and oriented × 4, but appears restless; reports, "my vision seems foggy around the edges." Heart tones regular. Respirations are equal with lung fields clear throughout upon auscultation. Abdomen soft, round, and nontender. Bowel sounds present in all quadrants. Client confirms completing procedural preparations, stating "I haven't had anything to eat or drink besides the laxative preparation, which I finished early this morning. Currently, I feel nauseous, and I may vomit." VS: T 98.4°F (36.9°C), HR 104 beats/min, BP 194/138 mm Hg, RR 14 breaths/min, SpO$_2$ 95% on RA. Client reports headache at the back of the head, rated 6/10.

For each client finding listed below, determine if the finding is consistent with the health conditions of anemia, hypertensive crisis, or hypoglycemia. Some findings may be consistent with more than one condition.

CLIENT FINDINGS	ANEMIA	HYPERTENSIVE CRISIS	HYPOGLYCEMIA
Blurred vision			
Restless			
Headache			
Nausea			
Tachycardia			

Thinking Exercise 3.1.3

The nurse is caring for a 47-year-old client at an outpatient endoscopy center.

History and Physical	Nurses' Notes	Orders	Laboratory Results

1150: Client arrives for routine colostomy and cancer screening. Health history includes hypertension, dyslipidemia, and iron deficiency anemia. Client reports nonadherence to antihypertensive drugs due to fear that they will cause sexual dysfunction. Alert and oriented × 4, but appears restless; reports, "my vision seems foggy around the edges." Heart tones regular. Respirations are equal with lung fields clear throughout upon auscultation. Abdomen soft, round, and nontender. Bowel sounds present in all quadrants. Client confirms completing procedural preparations, stating "I haven't had anything to eat or drink besides the laxative preparation, which I finished early this morning. Currently, I feel nauseous, and I may vomit." VS: T 98.4°F (36.9°C), HR 104 beats/min, BP 194/138 mm Hg, RR 14 breaths/min, SpO$_2$ 95% on RA. Client reports headache at the back of the head, rated 6/10.

1205: Client remains alert and oriented × 4 and confirms not taking prescribed antihypertensive drugs for 5 to 6 days. Skin is dry with usual pigmentation, and extremities are warm with palpable pulses at 2+ throughout. VS: HR 105 beats/min, BP 194/139 mm Hg, RR 16 breaths/min, SpO$_2$ 95% on RA. FSBG 92 mg/dL (5.1 mmol/L). Denies chest discomfort and shortness of breath.

The nurse reviews collected data (Nurses' Note at 1205) with the registered nurse. Complete the following sentences by selecting from the lists of options below.

The client is **most likely** experiencing **1 [Select]**. Without immediate treatment, the client is at **high** risk for **2 [Select]**, **3 [Select]**, and **4 [Select]**.

OPTIONS FOR 1	OPTIONS FOR 2	OPTIONS FOR 3	OPTIONS FOR 4
Anemia	Cardiac failure	Hypovolemia	Ketoacidosis
Hypertension crisis	Pulmonary edema	Acute kidney injury	Respiratory failure
Hypoglycemia	Seizures	Sepsis	Stroke

Thinking Exercise 3.1.4

The nurse is caring for a 47-year-old client at an outpatient endoscopy center.

History and Physical	Nurses' Notes	Orders	Laboratory Results

1150: Client arrives for routine colostomy and cancer screening. Health history includes hypertension, dyslipidemia, and iron deficiency anemia. Client reports nonadherence to antihypertensive drugs due to fear that they will cause sexual dysfunction. Alert and oriented × 4, but appears restless; reports, "my vision seems foggy around the edges." Heart tones regular. Respirations are equal with lung fields clear throughout upon auscultation. Abdomen soft, round, and nontender. Bowel sounds present in all quadrants. Client confirms completing procedural preparations, stating "I haven't had anything to eat or drink besides the laxative preparation, which I finished early this morning. Currently, I feel nauseous, and I may vomit." VS: T 98.4°F (36.9°C), HR 104 beats/min, BP 194/138 mm Hg, RR 14 breaths/min, SpO$_2$ 95% on RA. Client reports headache at the back of the head, rated 6/10.

1205: Client remains alert and oriented × 4 and confirms not taking prescribed antihypertensive drugs for 5 to 6 days. Skin is dry with usual pigmentation, and extremities are warm with palpable pulses at 2+ throughout. VS: HR 105 beats/min, BP 194/139 mm Hg, RR 16 breaths/min, SpO$_2$ 95% on RA. FSBG 92 mg/dL (5.1 mmol/L). Denies chest discomfort and shortness of breath.

The nurse collaborates with the registered nurse and contributes to the client's plan of care. Select whether the following potential nursing actions are indicated or not indicated for the client at this time.

POTENTIAL NURSING ACTIONS	INDICATED	NOT INDICATED
Frequently assess for changes in level of consciousness		
Establish peripheral venous access		
Keep the head of the bed at less than 30 degrees		
Insert an indwelling urinary catheter		
Place oral airway and suction equipment at the bedside		

Thinking Exercise 3.1.5

The nurse is caring for a 47-year-old client at an outpatient endoscopy center.

History and Physical	Nurses' Notes	Orders	Laboratory Results

1150: Client arrives for routine colostomy and cancer screening. Health history includes hypertension, dyslipidemia, and iron deficiency anemia. Client reports nonadherence to antihypertensive drugs due to fear that they will cause sexual dysfunction. Alert and oriented × 4, but appears restless; reports, "my vision seems foggy around the edges." Heart tones regular. Respirations are equal with lung fields clear throughout upon auscultation. Abdomen soft, round, and nontender. Bowel sounds present in all quadrants. Client confirms completing procedural preparations, stating "I haven't had anything to eat or drink besides the laxative preparation, which I finished early this morning. Currently, I feel nauseous, and I may vomit." VS: T 98.4°F (36.9°C), HR 104 beats/min, BP 194/138 mm Hg, RR 14 breaths/min, SpO_2 95% on RA. Client reports headache at the back of the head, rated 6/10.

1205: Client remains alert and oriented × 4 and confirms not taking prescribed antihypertensive drugs for 5 to 6 days. Skin is dry with usual pigmentation, and extremities are warm with palpable pulses at 2+ throughout. VS: HR 105 beats/min, BP 194/139 mm Hg, RR 16 breaths/min, SpO_2 95% on RA. FSBG 92 mg/dL (5.1 mmol/L). Denies chest discomfort and shortness of breath.

1215: Provider at bedside. Orders received.

History and Physical	Nurses' Notes	Orders	Laboratory Results

1215:
- Reschedule colonoscopy procedure after cleared by cardiologist
- Supplemental O_2 to keep SpO_2 >94%
- Vital signs every 15 minutes
- Continuous pulse oximetry monitoring
- 12-lead ECG
- Labetalol 20 mg IV × 1 dose for hypertension, repeat dose after 15 minutes if SBP >120 mm Hg
- Furosemide 20 mg PO × 1 dose for hypertension

The nurse assists with implementation of the client's plan of care. Select the **3** nursing actions that the nurse would plan to implement **immediately**.

○ Administer the prescribed furosemide dose
○ Assist the medical technician to obtain an ECG
○ Collaborate with the RN to administer IV labetalol
○ Consult with the cardiologist
○ Delegate 15-minute vital signs to assistive personnel
○ Implement continuous pulse oximetry
○ Initiate O_2 therapy at 2 L/min via NC
○ Obtain vital signs before and after each dose of labetalol

Thinking Exercise 3.1.6

The nurse is caring for a 47-year-old client at an outpatient endoscopy center.

History and Physical	Nurses' Notes	Orders	Laboratory Results

1150: Client arrives for routine colostomy and cancer screening. Health history includes hypertension, dyslipidemia, and iron deficiency anemia. Client reports nonadherence to antihypertensive drugs due to fear that they will cause sexual dysfunction. Alert and oriented × 4, but appears restless; reports, "my vision seems foggy around the edges." Heart tones regular. Respirations are equal with lung fields clear throughout upon auscultation. Abdomen soft, round, and nontender. Bowel sounds present in all quadrants. Client confirms completing procedural preparations, stating "I haven't had anything to eat or drink besides the laxative preparation, which I finished early this morning. Currently, I feel nauseous, and I may vomit." VS: T 98.4°F (36.9°C), HR 104 beats/min, BP 194/138 mm Hg, RR 14 breaths/min, SpO_2 95% on RA. Client reports headache at the back of the head, rated 6/10.

1205: Client remains alert and oriented × 4 and confirms not taking prescribed antihypertensive drugs for 5 to 6 days. Skin is dry with usual pigmentation, and extremities are warm with palpable pulses at 2+ throughout. VS: HR 105 beats/min, BP 194/139 mm Hg, RR 16 breaths/min, SpO_2 95% on RA. FSBG 92 mg/dL (5.1 mmol/L). Denies chest discomfort and shortness of breath.

1215: Provider at bedside. Orders received.

1400: Labetalol administered × 2 doses at 1220 and 1240. Furosemide administered at 1245. Client resting with eyes closed. Easily aroused and oriented × 4. Heart tones regular. Client denies chest pain or shortness of breath, but observed breathing effort has increased with use of accessory muscles. Coarse crackles auscultated in bilateral lower lung fields. Abdomen soft, round, and nontender. Bowel sounds present in all quadrants. Client reports feelings of nausea have subsided. Client voided 140 mL of dark amber urine. VS: HR 82 beats/min, BP 156/116 mm Hg, RR 19 breaths/min, SpO_2 98% on 2 L/min O_2 via NC. Client reports pain, rated 4/10, stating "My headache is starting to decrease."

The nurse reviews the client findings with the registered nurse. Which of the following findings indicate **worsening** of the client's condition? **Select all that apply.**

- ○ Accessory muscle use when breathing
- ○ Coarse crackles auscultated in bilateral lungs
- ○ HR 82 beats/min
- ○ Headache rated 4/10
- ○ Resting with eyes closed
- ○ RR 19 breaths/min
- ○ SpO_2 98% on 2 L/min O_2 via NC
- ○ Voided 140 mL of dark amber urine

Unfolding Case Study 3.2

Thinking Exercise 3.2.1

The nurse is caring for a 56-year-old client on a medical-surgical unit.

History and Physical	Nurses' Notes	Orders	Progress Notes

0730: Alert and oriented × 4 and follows all commands. Reports, "I got a couple hours of sleep before the laboratory technician arrived to take my blood early this morning." Heart tones regular. Respirations are symmetrical and unlabored. Chest anteroposterior to transverse diameter ratio approximately 1:1. Lung fields clear throughout upon auscultation. Abdomen soft, round, and nontender. Bowel sounds present in all quadrants. VS: T 98.8°F (37.1°C), HR 62 beats/min, BP 124/68 mm Hg, RR 12 breaths/min, SpO_2 96% on RA. Client denies pain.

0910: Client uses call light to request assistance and is found sitting up in bed with emesis basin on lap. Approximately 250 mL of yellowish-green emesis with remnants of breakfast present in basin. Client reports feeling "tightness" in the chest and then suddenly needing to vomit. Pale and diaphoretic. Respirations labored with use of accessory muscles. Dyspnea present and unrelieved by sitting in the high Fowler position or leaning forward against the bedside table. Client states, "I feel like I am being smothered. I can't seem to get comfortable or get enough air." VS: HR 92 beats/min, BP 146/88 mm Hg, RR 22 breaths/min, SpO_2 89% on RA. Pain rated 8/10 in chest and left shoulder.

Select the **4** client findings that require **immediate** follow-up.
- ○ Blood pressure
- ○ Chest diameter ratio
- ○ Dyspnea
- ○ Emesis
- ○ Pain
- ○ Pale and diaphoretic
- ○ SpO$_2$ level

Thinking Exercise 3.2.2

The nurse is caring for a 56-year-old client on a medical-surgical unit.

History and Physical	Nurses' Notes	Orders	Progress Notes

Medical History:
- Hypertension
- Gastroesophageal reflux disease
- BMI 31: Height 67 inches (170 cm), Weight 198 lb (90 kg)

Allergies: NKDA

Medications:
- Amlodipine
- Famotidine
- Lisinopril

Social History: Client is married with two children and manages a retail store. Reports diet primarily consists of fast-food meals, daily alcohol use of 4 to 6 beers, and a 20-pack-year history of tobacco use via cigarette smoking.

History and Physical	Nurses' Notes	Orders	Progress Notes

0730: Alert and oriented × 4 and follows all commands. Reports, "I got a couple hours of sleep before the laboratory technician arrived to take my blood early this morning." Heart tones regular. Respirations are symmetrical and unlabored. Chest anteroposterior to transverse diameter ratio approximately 1:1. Lung fields clear throughout upon auscultation. Abdomen soft, round, and nontender. Bowel sounds present in all quadrants. VS: T 98.8°F (37.1°C), HR 62 beats/min, BP 124/68 mm Hg, RR 12 breaths/min, SpO$_2$ 96% on RA. Client denies pain.

0910: Client uses call light to request assistance and is found sitting up in bed with emesis basin on lap. Approximately 250 mL of yellowish-green emesis with remnants of breakfast present in basin. Client reports feeling "tightness" in the chest and then suddenly needing to vomit. Pale and diaphoretic. Respirations labored with use of accessory muscles. Dyspnea present and unrelieved by sitting in the high Fowler position or leaning forward against the bedside table. Client states, "I feel like I am being smothered. I can't seem to get comfortable or get enough air." VS: HR 92 beats/min, BP 146/88 mm Hg, RR 22 breaths/min, SpO$_2$ 89% on RA. Pain rated 8/10 in chest and left shoulder.

The nurse reviews client findings and health history data with the registered nurse. Which of the following conditions is the client potentially experiencing? **Select all that apply.**
- ○ Acute coronary syndrome
- ○ Alcohol withdrawal
- ○ Emphysema
- ○ Gastroesophageal reflux disease
- ○ Hyperosmolar hyperglycemia nonketotic syndrome
- ○ Pulmonary embolism

Thinking Exercise 3.2.3

The nurse is caring for a 56-year-old client on a medical-surgical unit.

History and Physical	Nurses' Notes	Orders	Progress Notes

Medical History:
- Hypertension
- Gastroesophageal reflux disease
- BMI 31: Height 67 inches (170 cm), Weight 198 lb (90 kg)

Allergies: NKDA

Medications:
- Amlodipine
- Famotidine
- Lisinopril

Social History: Client is married with two children and manages a retail store. Reports diet primarily consists of fast-food meals, daily alcohol use of 4 to 6 beers, and a 20-pack-year history of tobacco use via cigarette smoking.

History and Physical	Nurses' Notes	Orders	Progress Notes

0730: Alert and oriented × 4 and follows all commands. Reports, "I got a couple hours of sleep before the laboratory technician arrived to take my blood early this morning." Heart tones regular. Respirations are symmetrical and unlabored. Chest anteroposterior to transverse diameter ratio approximately 1:1. Lung fields clear throughout upon auscultation. Abdomen soft, round, and nontender. Bowel sounds present in all quadrants. VS: T 98.8°F (37.1°C), HR 62 beats/min, BP 124/68 mm Hg, RR 12 breaths/min, SpO_2 96% on RA. Client denies pain.

0910: Client uses call light to request assistance and is found sitting up in bed with emesis basin on lap. Approximately 250 mL of yellowish-green emesis with remnants of breakfast present in basin. Client reports feeling "tightness" in the chest and then suddenly needing to vomit. Pale and diaphoretic. Respirations labored with use of accessory muscles. Dyspnea present and unrelieved by sitting in the high Fowler position or leaning forward against the bedside table. Client states, "I feel like I am being smothered. I can't seem to get comfortable or get enough air." VS: HR 92 beats/min, BP 146/88 mm Hg, RR 22 breaths/min, SpO_2 89% on RA. Pain rated 8/10 in chest and left shoulder.

0915: Rapid response team at bedside. Administered nitroglycerin sublingual × 1 and antacid suspension orally. O_2 administered at 4 L/min via NC.

0920: Pain continues, rated 8/10 in chest and left shoulder. No wheezing or adventitious sounds auscultated in lung fields. Dyspnea unrelieved by sitting in the high Fowler position or leaning forward against the bedside table. 12-lead ECG demonstrates sinus tachycardia with ST-segment depression and T-wave inversion. VS: HR 95 beats/min, BP 151/88 mm Hg, RR 18 breaths/min, SpO_2 97% on 4 L/min O_2 via NC.

The nurse reviews the Nurses' Notes from 0915 and 0920 with the registered nurse. Complete the following sentence by selecting from the list of word choices below.

The nurse recognizes that the client is *most likely* experiencing [**Word Choice**] as evidenced by [**Word Choice**] and [**Word Choice**].

WORD CHOICES
Acute coronary syndrome
BMI 31
Chest pain not relieved with nitroglycerin
ECG rhythm changes
Emphysema exacerbation
Gastroesophageal reflux disease
Shortness of breath with exertion

Thinking Exercise 3.2.4

The nurse is caring for a 56-year-old client on a medical-surgical unit.

History and Physical	Nurses' Notes	Orders	Progress Notes

Medical History:
- Hypertension
- Gastroesophageal reflux disease
- BMI 31: Height 67 inches (170 cm), Weight 198 lb (90 kg)

Allergies: NKDA

Medications:
- Amlodipine
- Famotidine
- Lisinopril

Social History: Client is married with two children and manages a retail store. Reports diet primarily consists of fast-food meals, daily alcohol use of 4 to 6 beers, and a 20-pack-year history of tobacco use via cigarette smoking.

History and Physical	Nurses' Notes	Orders	Progress Notes

0730: Alert and oriented × 4 and follows all commands. Reports, "I got a couple hours of sleep before the laboratory technician arrived to take my blood early this morning." Heart tones regular. Respirations are symmetrical and unlabored. Chest anteroposterior to transverse diameter ratio approximately 1:1. Lung fields clear throughout upon auscultation. Abdomen soft, round, and nontender. Bowel sounds present in all quadrants. VS: T 98.8°F (37.1°C), HR 62 beats/min, BP 124/68 mm Hg, RR 12 breaths/min, SpO_2 96% on RA. Client denies pain.

0910: Client uses call light to request assistance and is found sitting up in bed with emesis basin on lap. Approximately 250 mL of yellowish-green emesis with remnants of breakfast present in basin. Client reports feeling "tightness" in the chest and then suddenly needing to vomit. Pale and diaphoretic. Respirations labored with use of accessory muscles. Dyspnea present and unrelieved by sitting in the high Fowler position or leaning forward against the bedside table. Client states, "I feel like I am being smothered. I can't seem to get comfortable or get enough air." VS: HR 92 beats/min, BP 146/88 mm Hg, RR 22 breaths/min, SpO_2 89% on RA. Pain rated 8/10 in chest and left shoulder.

0915: Rapid response team at bedside. Administered nitroglycerin sublingual × 1 and antacid suspension orally. O_2 administered at 4 L/min via NC.

0920: Pain continues, rated 8/10 in chest and left shoulder. No wheezing or adventitious sounds auscultated in lung fields. Dyspnea unrelieved by sitting in the high Fowler position or leaning forward against the bedside table. 12-lead ECG demonstrates sinus tachycardia with ST-segment depression and T-wave inversion. VS: HR 95 beats/min, BP 151/88 mm Hg, RR 18 breaths/min, SpO_2 97% on 4 L/min O_2 via NC.

The nurse collaborates with the registered nurse and contributes to the client's plan of care. Select whether the following potential nursing actions are indicated or not indicated for the client at this time.

POTENTIAL NURSING ACTIONS	INDICATED	NOT INDICATED
Administer second dose of nitroglycerin sublingual		
Ask spouse to remain in the waiting room		
Establish peripheral venous access		
Initiate continuous cardiac monitoring		
Request order for IV pain medication		

Thinking Exercise 3.2.5

The nurse is caring for a 56-year-old client on a medical-surgical unit.

History and Physical	Nurses' Notes	Orders	Progress Notes

0730: Alert and oriented × 4 and follows all commands. Reports, "I got a couple hours of sleep before the laboratory technician arrived to take my blood early this morning." Heart tones regular. Respirations are symmetrical and unlabored. Chest anteroposterior to transverse diameter ratio approximately 1:1. Lung fields clear throughout upon auscultation. Abdomen soft, round, and nontender. Bowel sounds present in all quadrants. VS: T 98.8°F (37.1°C), HR 62 beats/min, BP 124/68 mm Hg, RR 12 breaths/min, SpO_2 96% on RA. Client denies pain.

0910: Client uses call light to request assistance and is found sitting up in bed with emesis basin on lap. Approximately 250 mL of yellowish-green emesis with remnants of breakfast present in basin. Client reports feeling "tightness" in the chest and then suddenly needing to vomit. Pale and diaphoretic. Respirations labored with use of accessory muscles. Dyspnea present and unrelieved by sitting in the high Fowler position or leaning forward against the bedside table. Client states, "I feel like I am being smothered. I can't seem to get comfortable or get enough air." VS: HR 92 beats/min, BP 146/88 mm Hg, RR 22 breaths/min, SpO_2 89% on RA. Pain rated 8/10 in chest and left shoulder.

0915: Rapid response team at bedside. Administered nitroglycerin sublingual × 1 and antacid suspension orally. O_2 administered at 4 L/min via NC.

0920: Pain continues, rated 8/10 in chest and left shoulder. No wheezing or adventitious sounds auscultated in lung fields. Dyspnea unrelieved by sitting in the high Fowler position or leaning forward against the bedside table. 12-lead ECG demonstrates sinus tachycardia with ST-segment depression and T-wave inversion. VS: HR 95 beats/min, BP 151/88 mm Hg, RR 18 breaths/min, SpO_2 97% on 4 L/min O_2 via NC.

History and Physical	Nurses' Notes	Orders	Progress Notes

0930:
- Aspirin 325 mg orally every day to prevent clot formation
- Case management consultation for cardiac rehabilitation services
- Continuous ECG monitoring
- Laboratory tests: CBC, BMP, Cardiac troponin T, Cardiac troponin I
- Morphine 2 mg IV every 20 minutes PRN, chest pain
- Nitroglycerin sublingual PRN chest pain, may repeat every 5 minutes × 3 doses
- Signed consent for percutaneous coronary intervention (PCI)
- Supplemental O_2 to keep SpO_2 >94%

The nurse assists with implementation of the client's plan of care. Complete the following sentence by selecting from the lists of options below.

The nurse would *prioritize* **1 [Select]** and **2 [Select]** so the client may be urgently transported to the **3 [Select]**.

OPTIONS FOR 1	OPTIONS FOR 2	OPTIONS FOR 3
Administration of aspirin	Case management	Cardiac catheterization lab
ECG monitoring	Elimination of chest pain	Intensive care unit
Laboratory tests	Informed consent	Cardiac rehabilitation center

Thinking Exercise 3.2.6—Pharmacology

The nurse is caring for a 56-year-old client on a medical-surgical unit.

History and Physical	Nurses' Notes	Orders	Progress Notes

Day 1

0730: Client is alert and oriented × 4 and follows all commands. Reports, "I got a couple hours of sleep before the laboratory technician arrived to take my blood early this morning." Heart tones regular. Respirations are symmetrical and unlabored. Chest anteroposterior to transverse diameter ratio approximately 1:1. Lung fields clear throughout upon auscultation. Abdomen soft, round, and nontender. Bowel sounds present in all quadrants. VS: T 98.8°F (37.1°C), HR 62 beats/min, BP 124/68 mm Hg, RR 12 breaths/min, SpO_2 96% on RA. Client denies pain.

0910: Client uses call light to request assistance and is found sitting up in bed with emesis basin on lap. Approximately 250 mL of yellowish-green emesis with remnants of breakfast present in basin. Client reports feeling "tightness" in the chest and then suddenly needing to vomit. Pale and diaphoretic. Respirations labored with use of accessory muscles. Dyspnea present and unrelieved by sitting in the high Fowler position or leaning forward against the bedside table. Client states, "I feel like I am being smothered. I can't seem to get comfortable or get enough air." VS: HR 92 beats/min, BP 146/88 mm Hg, RR 22 breaths/min, SpO_2 89% on RA. Pain rated 8/10 in chest and left shoulder.

0915: Rapid response team at bedside. Administered nitroglycerin sublingual × 1 and antacid suspension orally. O_2 administered at 4 L/min via NC.

0920: Pain continues, rated 8/10 in chest and left shoulder. No wheezing or adventitious sounds auscultated in lung fields. Dyspnea unrelieved by sitting in the high Fowler position or leaning forward against the bedside table. 12-lead ECG demonstrates sinus tachycardia with ST-segment depression and T-wave inversion. VS: HR 95 beats/min, BP 151/88 mm Hg, RR 18 breaths/min, SpO_2 97% on 4 L/min O_2 via NC.

0950: Report given to cardiac catheterization nurse, and personal items packed for anticipated transfer to intensive care unit after PCI.

Day 5
1335: Client prepared for discharge home after successful PCI procedure and reopening of occluded coronary artery. Follow-up appointments scheduled with cardiologist. Cardiac rehabilitation and discharge teaching provided.

The nurse reviews collected data with the registered nurse and reinforces teaching with the client. Select whether the following client statements indicate understanding or no understanding of discharge teaching provided.

CLIENT STATEMENTS	UNDERSTANDING	NO UNDERSTANDING
"Chest pain may occur with activity, so I will always carry nitroglycerin tablets and contact EMS if pain is not relieved after 3 doses."		
"I don't like fish, but I plan to eat more walnuts and food items that contain soybeans."		
"I will begin exercising every day by walking around my city block 3 times."		
"My heart wouldn't need to work so hard if I lost some weight and stopped smoking."		
"Spices, garlic, and onions can add flavor to my food without adding more sodium."		
"Wearing a telemetry monitor when I exercise will help me become more active in a safe manner."		

Stand-Alone Thinking Exercise 3.1

A nurse is caring for a 36-year-old client at a community clinic.

History and Physical	Nurses' Notes	Orders	Laboratory Results

1655: Client is alert and oriented × 4. Appearance is disheveled, hair and clothing is wet, and coat is inappropriately thin for the current weather. Client states, "I wasn't expecting the weather to change. Yesterday it was sunny and warm, and today it is cold and raining." Respirations are equal and unlabored. Lung fields clear to auscultation. Heart tones regular. Skin cool to touch. Scleral and conjunctival jaundice present in bilateral eyes. Right lower extremity with 2+ pitting edema, hyperpigmentation, and multiple open ulcerations. Right pedal and dorsalis pedis pulses weak but palpable through edema. Client reports a chronic dull ache in the right calf that feels better when the leg is raised. Medical alert bracelet on client's left wrist indicates a history of type 2 diabetes mellitus and sickle cell anemia. VS: T 102.1°F (38.9°C), HR 104 beats/min, BP 124/54 mm Hg, RR 16 breaths/min, SpO$_2$ 96% on RA. Client reports pain in bilateral upper extremities at 9/10 and discomfort in chest and abdomen at 5/10. Client denies tobacco or alcohol use.

1715: Client assisted to change into dry clothing provided by the clinic. Point-of-care blood tests completed.

History and Physical	Nurses' Notes	Orders	Laboratory Results
Serum Laboratory Tests and Reference Ranges		**1715**	
Red blood cell (RBC) count (4.7–6.1 × 10^6/mm^3 [4.7–6.1 × 10^{12}/L])		4.6 × 10^6/mm^3 (4.6 × 10^{12}/L)	
White blood cell (WBC) count (5000–10,000/mm^3 [5–10 × 10^9/L])		20,000/mm^3 (20 × 10^9/L)	
Glucose (74–106 mg/dL [4.1–5.9 mmol/L])		189 mg/dL (10.5 mmol/L)	
Blood urea nitrogen (BUN) (10–20 mg/dL [3.6–7.1 mmol/L])		58 mg/dL (20.7 mmol/L)	
Creatinine (0.7–1.3 mg/dL [61.89–114.95 μmol/L])		1.1 mg/dL (97.26 μmol/L)	

The nurse reviews the collected data and collaborates with the registered nurse. Complete the diagram by identifying from the choices below to specify what potential condition the client is likely experiencing, **2** nursing actions that are appropriate to take, and **2** parameters the nurse should monitor to assess the client's progress.

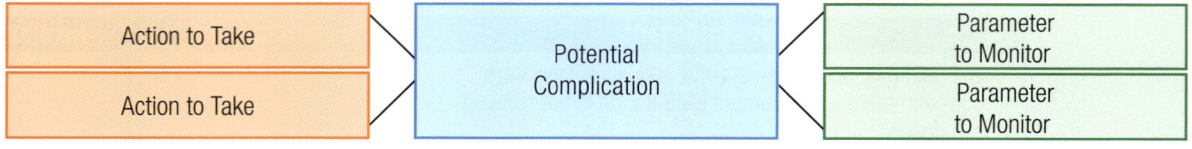

Action to Take			
Action to Take	Potential Complication	Parameter to Monitor	Parameter to Monitor

Actions to Take	Potential Conditions	Parameters to Monitor
Administer hydroxyurea	Arterial embolism	Blood glucose
Apply supplemental O$_2$ via NC	Cirrhosis	Intake and output
Initiate IV fluids	Diabetic ketoacidosis (DKA)	Pulse strength and rhythm
Obtain wound cultures from right leg ulcers	Sickle cell crisis	Red blood cell count
Administer pain medication		Vital signs

Stand-Alone Thinking Exercise 3.2

The nurse is caring for a 55-year-old client at an acute cardiac rehabilitation center following coronary bypass surgery. To plan the most appropriate care, the nurse reviews relevant client findings recorded on the Nursing Flow Sheet and collaborates with the registered nurse.

History and Physical	Nurses' Notes	Nursing Flow Sheet	Laboratory Results
Vital Signs	**0600**	**1130**	**1600**
T	98.6°F (37°C)	98.8°F (37.1°C)	99.1°F (37.2°C)
HR	89 beats/min	86 beats/min	43 beats/min
RR	13 breaths/min	14 breaths/min	18 breaths/min
BP	138/46 mm Hg	140/50 mm Hg	82/42 mm Hg
SpO_2	98% on 2 L/min O_2 via NC	98% on 2 L/min O_2 via NC	92% on 2 L/min O_2 via NC
Pain	3/10 surgical incision	0/10	8/10 substernal chest, reports dyspnea and light-headedness

Complete the following sentences by selecting from the lists of options below.

Based on assessment findings and medical history, the client is *most likely* experiencing **1 [Select]**. The nurse would **2 [Select]** in anticipation of **3 [Select]** and prepare for **4 [Select]** if the client's condition does not improve.

OPTIONS FOR 1	OPTIONS FOR 2	OPTIONS FOR 3	OPTIONS FOR 4
Cardiac arrest	Evaluate for an iodine allergy	Atropine administration	Defibrillation
Pulmonary embolism	Insert a peripheral venous device	Cardiopulmonary resuscitation	Thrombolytic therapy
Symptomatic bradycardia	Lower the head of the bed	Computed tomography pulmonary angiogram	Transcutaneous pacing

Stand-Alone Thinking Exercise 3.3

A nurse is caring for a 48-year-old client on a medical-surgical unit who has a history of hyperthyroidism.

History and Physical	Nurses' Notes	Orders	Laboratory Results

0915: Client ambulates to toilet independently and uses call bell to notify nursing staff of light-headedness and dyspnea upon safety returning to the bed. Client is alert and oriented × 4. Appears restless and fidgeting in bed. Facial features symmetrical with bilateral swelling around eyes. Respirations equal but labored. Lung fields clear upon auscultation. Heart tones irregular. Skin warm and diaphoretic. Pulses bounding and irregular. No peripheral edema noted. Abdomen soft and flat with bowel sounds present throughout. Client ate whole-grain cereal and fresh berries for breakfast. VS: T 100.1°F (37.8°C), HR 120 beats/min, BP 92/36 mm Hg, RR 18 breaths/min, SpO_2 96% on RA. Client denies pain but states, "it feels like my heart is racing."

0920: 12-Lead ECG completed at bedside; Results—Irregular rhythm with atrial rate of 410 beats/min and ventricular rate of 122 beats/min.

The nurse reviews the collected data and collaborates with the registered nurse. Complete the diagram by identifying from the choices below to specify what potential condition the client is likely experiencing, **2** nursing actions that are appropriate to take, and **2** parameters the nurse should monitor to assess the client's progress.

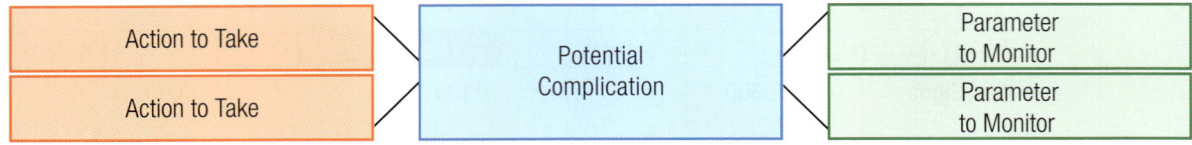

Actions to Take	Potential Conditions	Parameters to Monitor
Administer drugs to correct the cardiac rhythm and control the pulse rate	Anaphylactic reaction	Angioedema
Apply a cool, damp cloth to the client's face and eyes	Atrial fibrillation	Level of orientation
Assist the RN to administer IV epinephrine to prevent airway constriction	Cardiomyopathy	Thyroid hormone levels
Obtain an informed consent for percutaneous coronary intervention.	Thyroid storm	Urine output
Teach the client about anticoagulation therapy		White blood cell count

Client Conditions Affecting Gas Exchange

Unfolding Case Study 4.1

Thinking Exercise 4.1.1

A nurse is caring for a 55-year-old client in the emergency department. Highlight the client findings that require **immediate** follow-up.

History and Physical	Nurses' Notes	Orders	Laboratory Results

1115: Alert and oriented × 4, but unable to speak full sentences due to shortness of breath. Client's spouse is at bedside and states, "Feelings of breathlessness with moderate activity started several days ago. It has progressively worsened to difficulty breathing at rest and an inability to sleep at night." Heart tones regular and pulses palpable throughout. Client denies chest pain. Bilateral lower extremity 2+ pitting edema present. Barrel chest; wheezing and bilateral rhonchi auscultated in lung fields. Productive cough present with a large amount of yellow-green sputum. Abdomen soft and obese with normal bowel sounds. VS: T 97.3°F (36.2°C), HR 84 beats/min, RR 24 breaths/min, BP 109/56 mm Hg, SpO$_2$ 90% on 2 L/min O$_2$ via NC.

Thinking Exercise 4.1.2

A nurse is caring for a 55-year-old client in the emergency department.

History and Physical	Nurses' Notes	Orders	Laboratory Results

Medical History:
- Chronic obstructive pulmonary disease (COPD)
- Hypertension
- Hyperlipidemia
- Morbid obesity

Allergies: NKDA
Medications:
- Hydralazine
- Hydrochlorothiazide
- Albuterol MDI
- Ipratropium MDI
- Aspirin
- Rosuvastatin

Social History: 30 years of smoking tobacco, which was stopped 5 years ago due to increasing shortness of breath. Denies alcohol or illicit drug use.

History and Physical	Nurses' Notes	Orders	Laboratory Results

1115: Alert and oriented × 4, but unable to speak full sentences due to shortness of breath. Client's spouse is at bedside and states, "Feelings of breathlessness with moderate activity started several days ago. It has progressively worsened to difficulty breathing at rest and an inability to sleep at night." Heart tones regular and pulses palpable throughout. Client denies chest pain. Bilateral lower extremity 2+ pitting edema present. Barrel chest; wheezing and bilateral rhonchi auscultated in lung fields. Productive cough present with a large amount of yellow-green sputum. Abdomen soft and obese with normal bowel sounds. VS: T 97.3°F (36.2°C), HR 84 beats/min, RR 24 breaths/min, BP 109/56 mm Hg, SpO$_2$ 90% on 2 L/min O$_2$ via NC.

The nurse reviews the client findings and health history with the registered nurse. Which of the following conditions is the client potentially experiencing? **Select all that apply.**

○ Acute COPD exacerbation
○ Acute severe asthma
○ Heart failure
○ Gastroesophageal reflux disease
○ Liver cirrhosis
○ Pneumonia

Thinking Exercise 4.1.3

A nurse is caring for a 55-year-old client in the emergency department.

History and Physical	Nurses' Notes	Orders	Laboratory Results

Medical History:
- Chronic obstructive pulmonary disease (COPD)
- Hypertension
- Hyperlipidemia
- Morbid obesity

Allergies: NKDA

Medications:
- Hydralazine
- Hydrochlorothiazide
- Albuterol MDI
- Ipratropium MDI
- Aspirin
- Rosuvastatin

Social History: 30 years of smoking tobacco, which was stopped 5 years ago due to increasing shortness of breath. Denies alcohol or illicit drug use.

History and Physical	Nurses' Notes	Orders	Laboratory Results

1115: Alert and oriented × 4, but unable to speak full sentences due to shortness of breath. Client's spouse is at bedside and states, "Feelings of breathlessness with moderate activity started several days ago. It has progressively worsened to difficulty breathing at rest and an inability to sleep at night." Heart tones regular and pulses palpable throughout. Client denies chest pain. Bilateral lower extremity 2+ pitting edema present. Barrel chest; wheezing and bilateral rhonchi auscultated in lung fields. Productive cough present with a large amount of yellow-green sputum. Abdomen soft and obese with normal bowel sounds. VS: T 97.3°F (36.2°C), HR 84 beats/min, RR 24 breaths/min, BP 109/56 mm Hg, SpO_2 90% on 2 L/min O_2 via NC.

The nurse reviews the collected client data and collaborates with the registered nurse. Complete the following sentence by selecting from the lists of options below.

The nurse recognizes that the client is most likely experiencing **1 [Select]**. The nurse would prioritize **2 [Select]** and **3 [Select]** to improve gas exchange.

OPTIONS FOR 1	OPTIONS FOR 2	OPTIONS FOR 3
Acute COPD exacerbation	Antibiotic therapy	Airway clearance
Congestive heart failure	Breathing techniques	Cardiac rehabilitation
Pneumonia	Fluid restrictions	Supplemental oxygenation

Thinking Exercise 4.1.4

A nurse is caring for a 55-year-old client in the emergency department.

History and Physical	Nurses' Notes	Orders	Laboratory Results

Medical History:
- Chronic obstructive pulmonary disease (COPD)
- Hypertension
- Hyperlipidemia
- Morbid obesity

Allergies: NKDA

Medications:
- Hydralazine
- Hydrochlorothiazide
- Albuterol MDI
- Ipratropium MDI
- Aspirin
- Rosuvastatin

Social History: 30 years of smoking tobacco, which was stopped 5 years ago due to increasing shortness of breath. Denies alcohol or illicit drug use.

History and Physical	Nurses' Notes	Orders	Laboratory Results

1115: Alert and oriented × 4, but unable to speak full sentences due to shortness of breath. Client's spouse is at bedside and states, "Feelings of breathlessness with moderate activity started several days ago. It has progressively worsened to difficulty breathing at rest and an inability to sleep at night." Heart tones regular and pulses palpable throughout. Client denies chest pain. Bilateral lower extremity 2+ pitting edema present. Barrel chest; wheezing and bilateral rhonchi auscultated in lung fields. Productive cough present with a large amount of yellow-green sputum. Abdomen soft and obese with normal bowel sounds. VS: T 97.3°F (36.2°C), HR 84 beats/min, RR 24 breaths/min, BP 109/56 mm Hg, SpO$_2$ 90% on 2 L/min O$_2$ via NC.

The nurse collaborates with the registered nurse and contributes to the client's plan of care. Select whether the following potential nursing actions are indicated or not indicated for the client at this time.

POTENTIAL NURSING INTERVENTIONS	INDICATED	NOT INDICATED
Place the client in an upright position with the head of the bed elevated		
Use supplemental oxygen to keep oxygen saturation levels at 88% to 92%		
Perform nasotracheal suction to clear the client's airway		
Assist the care team to obtain an arterial blood sample to assess ABGs		
Encourage the client to remain out of bed for 3 hours twice a day		

Thinking Exercise 4.1.5—Pharmacology

A nurse is caring for a 55-year-old client in the emergency department.

History and Physical	Nurses' Notes	Orders	Laboratory Results

Medical History:
- Chronic obstructive pulmonary disease (COPD)
- Hypertension
- Hyperlipidemia
- Morbid obesity

Allergies: NKDA

Medications:
- Hydralazine
- Hydrochlorothiazide
- Albuterol MDI
- Ipratropium MDI
- Aspirin
- Rosuvastatin

Social History: 30 years of smoking tobacco, which was stopped 5 years ago due to increasing shortness of breath. Denies alcohol or illicit drug use.

History and Physical	Nurses' Notes	Orders	Laboratory Results

1115: Alert and oriented × 4, but unable to speak full sentences due to shortness of breath. Client's spouse is at bedside and states, "Feelings of breathlessness with moderate activity started several days ago. It has progressively worsened to difficulty breathing at rest and an inability to sleep at night." Heart tones regular and pulses palpable throughout. Client denies chest pain. Bilateral lower extremity 2+ pitting edema present. Barrel chest; wheezing and bilateral rhonchi auscultated in lung fields. Productive cough present with a large amount of yellow-green sputum. Abdomen soft and obese with normal bowel sounds. VS: T 97.3°F (36.2°C), HR 84 beats/min, RR 24 breaths/min, BP 109/56 mm Hg, SpO_2 90% on 2 L/min O_2 via NC.

1140: Provider at bedside. Orders received.

History and Physical	Nurses' Notes	Orders	Laboratory Results

1140:
- Admit to medical-surgical unit
- Supplemental O_2 to keep SpO_2 at 88% to 92%
- Vital signs routine
- Arterial blood gas (ABG)
- Portable chest x-ray
- Albuterol 2.5 mg/ipratropium bromide 0.5 mg by nebulizer every 6 hours
- Budesonide 2 inhalations 2 times per day
- Guaifenesin 200 mg orally every 4 hours

The nurse reviews the orders and collaborates with the registered nurse in the implementation of the plan of care. For each prescribed medication, select nursing actions for the administration of each medication.

PRESCRIBED MEDICATIONS	NURSING ACTIONS
Albuterol 2.5 mg/ipratropium bromide 0.5 mg by nebulizer every 6 hours	O Assess the client's HR and rhythm prior to and during nebulizer treatments. O Report an increase in HR of 20 beats/min or more to the provider. O Encourage the client to suck on ice chips or hard candy.
Budesonide 2 inhalations 2 times per day	O Assess the client for signs and symptoms of pneumonia. O Assist the client to gargle and rinse the mouth with a nonalcoholic mouthwash after each dose. O Position the client with the head of the bed elevated at 30 degrees during administration of inhalants.
Guaifenesin 200 mg orally every 4 hours	O Administer 1 hour before or 2 hours after meals. O Promote fluid intake of 8 to 12 8-ounce glasses of water daily. O Use a humidifier when providing supplemental oxygen.

Thinking Exercise 4.1.6

A nurse is caring for a 55-year-old client on a medical-surgical unit.

History and Physical	Nurses' Notes	Orders	Laboratory Results

Medical History:
- Chronic obstructive pulmonary disease (COPD)
- Hypertension
- Hyperlipidemia
- Morbid obesity

Allergies: NKDA

Medications:
- Hydralazine
- Hydrochlorothiazide
- Albuterol MDI
- Ipratropium MDI
- Aspirin
- Rosuvastatin

Social History: 30 years of smoking tobacco, which was stopped 5 years ago due to increasing shortness of breath. Denies alcohol or illicit drug use.

History and Physical	Nurses' Notes	Orders	Laboratory Results

Emergency Department

1115: Alert and oriented × 4, but unable to speak full sentences due to shortness of breath. Client's spouse is at bedside and states, "Feelings of breathlessness with moderate activity started several days ago. It has progressively worsened to difficulty breathing at rest and an inability to sleep at night." Heart tones regular and pulses palpable throughout. Client denies chest pain. Bilateral lower extremity 2+ pitting edema present. Barrel chest; wheezing and bilateral rhonchi auscultated in lung fields. Productive cough present with a large amount of yellow-green sputum. Abdomen soft and obese with normal bowel sounds. VS: T 97.3°F (36.2°C), HR 84 beats/min, RR 24 breaths/min, BP 109/56 mm Hg, SpO_2 90% on 2 L/min O_2 via NC.

1140: Provider at bedside. Orders received.

1215: Radiology and laboratory tests completed. Albuterol/ipratropium nebulizer administered. VS: HR 88 beats/min, RR 20 breaths/min, BP 112/54 mm Hg, SpO_2 91% on 2 L/min O_2 via NC. Client prepared for transfer to medical-surgical unit.

Medical-Surgical Unit

1800: Client alert and oriented × 4. Appears comfortable in bed and answers questions in full sentences. Client states, "My breathing is better. I was able to walk to and from the bathroom without distress." Respirations equal and slightly labored. Expiratory wheezes auscultated in lung fields. VS: HR 75 beats/min, RR 16 breaths/min, BP 115/54 mm Hg, SpO_2 92% on 2 L/min O_2 via NC. Client denies pain. Health teaching provided in preparation for discharge home in the next day or two.

History and Physical	Nurses' Notes	Orders	Laboratory Results

1140:
- Admit to medical-surgical unit
- Supplemental O_2 to keep SpO_2 at 88% to 92%
- Vital signs routine
- Arterial blood gas (ABG)
- Portable chest x-ray
- Albuterol 2.5 mg/ipratropium bromide 0.5 mg by nebulizer every 6 hours
- Budesonide 2 inhalations 2 times per day
- Guaifenesin 200 mg orally every 4 hours

The nurse reviews collected data with the registered nurse and reinforces teaching with the client. Select whether the following client statements indicate understanding or no understanding of the discharge teaching provided.

CLIENT STATEMENTS	UNDERSTANDING	NO UNDERSTANDING
"I will perform controlled coughing exercises in the morning and at night before bed to help clear my lungs."		
"When I feel breathless, sitting forward in my chair and leaning against a table may help me catch my breath."		
"Taking my ipratropium inhaler routinely will help prevent symptoms of dyspnea."		
"When my breathing rate increases, I should hold a paper bag over my mouth and nose and try to take normal breaths."		
"Losing some weight may decrease my symptoms and help me tolerate more activity."		

Unfolding Case Study 4.2

Thinking Exercise 4.2.1

A nurse is caring for a 42-year-old client at an infusion center.

History and Physical	Nurses' Notes	Orders	Laboratory Results

0820: Third cycle of adjunctive chemotherapy for breast cancer initiated 20 minutes ago. Client is seated in a recliner with legs elevated and reports feelings of fatigue and generalized discomfort, rated 4/10. Client states pain level is acceptable and confirms pain goal of less than 6. Heart tones regular and radial pulses palpable 2+. Bilateral lower extremity edema present, right > left. Right calf reddened, warm, and tender when touched and with movement. Pedal pulses 1+ and capillary refill <3 seconds in both lower extremities. Auscultated lung fields clear throughout. Client denies chest pain, cough, or shortness of breath. Abdomen soft and round. Client reports having no appetite but attempts to eat small meals several times a day. VS: T 99.8°F (37.6°C), HR 72 beats/min, RR 14 breaths/min, BP 98/50 mm Hg, SpO_2 98% on RA. IV site clean and without signs of extravasation. Infusion continued.

0900: Client apprehensive and diaphoretic. Reports dyspnea and sharp, stabbing chest pain, rated 10/10. Wheezing and crackles noted on auscultation of the lungs. VS: T 101.1°F (38.4°C), HR 118 beats/min, RR 28 breaths/min, BP 128/66 mm Hg, SpO_2 88% on RA.

The nurse reviews collected data with the registered nurse. Which of the following client findings require **immediate** follow-up? **Select all that apply.**

- ○ Anorexia
- ○ Chest pain
- ○ Fatigue
- ○ Dyspnea
- ○ Body temperature
- ○ Pedal pulses
- ○ SpO_2

Thinking Exercise 4.2.2

A nurse is caring for a 42-year-old client at an infusion center.

History and Physical	Nurses' Notes	Orders	Laboratory Results

0820: Third cycle of adjunctive chemotherapy for breast cancer initiated 20 minutes ago. Client is seated in a recliner with legs elevated and reports feelings of fatigue and generalized discomfort, rated 4/10. Client states pain level is acceptable and confirms pain goal of less than 6. Heart tones regular and radial pulses palpable 2+. Bilateral lower extremity edema present, right > left. Right calf reddened, warm, and tender when touched and with movement. Pedal pulses 1+ and capillary refill <3 seconds in both lower extremities. Auscultated lung fields clear throughout. Client denies chest pain, cough, or shortness of breath. Abdomen soft and round. Client reports having no appetite but attempts to eat small meals several times a day. VS: T 99.8°F (37.6°C), HR 72 beats/min, RR 14 breaths/min, BP 98/50 mm Hg, SpO$_2$ 98% on RA. IV site clean and without signs of extravasation. Infusion continued.

0900: Client apprehensive and diaphoretic. Reports dyspnea and sharp, stabbing chest pain, rated 10/10. Wheezing and crackles noted on auscultation of the lungs. VS: T 101.1°F (38.4°C), HR 118 beats/min, RR 28 breaths/min, BP 128/66 mm Hg, SpO$_2$ 88% on RA.

The nurse reviews the collected data and collaborates with the registered nurse. Complete the following sentence by selecting from the lists of options below.

The nurse recognizes that the client is most likely experiencing **1 [Select]** as evidenced by **2 [Select]** and **3 [Select]**.

OPTIONS FOR 1	OPTIONS FOR 2	OPTIONS FOR 3
Pneumonia	Apprehension	Anorexia
Metastatic lung cancer	Lower extremity edema	Diaphoresis
Pulmonary embolism	Sudden onset of dyspnea	Stabbing chest pain

Thinking Exercise 4.2.3

A nurse is caring for a 42-year-old client at an infusion center.

History and Physical	Nurses' Notes	Orders	Laboratory Results

0820: Third cycle of adjunctive chemotherapy for breast cancer initiated 20 minutes ago. Client is seated in a recliner with legs elevated and reports feelings of fatigue and generalized discomfort, rated 4/10. Client states pain level is acceptable and confirms pain goal of less than 6. Heart tones regular and radial pulses palpable 2+. Bilateral lower extremity edema present, right > left. Right calf reddened, warm, and tender when touched and with movement. Pedal pulses 1+ and capillary refill <3 seconds in both lower extremities. Auscultated lung fields clear throughout. Client denies chest pain, cough, or shortness of breath. Abdomen soft and round. Client reports having no appetite but attempts to eat small meals several times a day. VS: T 99.8°F (37.6°C), HR 72 beats/min, RR 14 breaths/min, BP 98/50 mm Hg, SpO$_2$ 98% on RA. IV site clean and without signs of extravasation. Infusion continued.

0900: Client apprehensive and diaphoretic. Reports dyspnea and sharp, stabbing chest pain, rated 10/10. Wheezing and crackles noted on auscultation of the lungs. VS: T 101.1°F (38.4°C), HR 118 beats/min, RR 28 breaths/min, BP 128/66 mm Hg, SpO$_2$ 88% on RA.

The nurse reviews the collected client data and collaborates with the registered nurse. Complete the following sentence by selecting from the list of word choices below.

The nurse determines the *priority* for care at this time is to manage the client's **[Word Choice]**.

WORD CHOICES
Anxiety
Hypoxemia
Pain
Tachycardia

Thinking Exercise 4.2.4

A nurse is caring for a 42-year-old client at an infusion center.

History and Physical	Nurses' Notes	Orders	Laboratory Results

0820: Third cycle of adjunctive chemotherapy for breast cancer initiated 20 minutes ago. Client is seated in a recliner with legs elevated and reports feelings of fatigue and generalized discomfort, rated 4/10. Client states pain level is acceptable and confirms pain goal of less than 6. Heart tones regular and radial pulses palpable 2+. Bilateral lower extremity edema present, right > left. Right calf reddened, warm, and tender when touched and with movement. Pedal pulses 1+ and capillary refill <3 seconds in both lower extremities. Auscultated lung fields clear throughout. Client denies chest pain, cough, or shortness of breath. Abdomen soft and round. Client reports having no appetite but attempts to eat small meals several times a day. VS: T 99.8°F (37.6°C), HR 72 beats/min, RR 14 breaths/min, BP 98/50 mm Hg, SpO$_2$ 98% on RA. IV site clean and without signs of extravasation. Infusion continued.

0900: Client apprehensive and diaphoretic. Reports dyspnea and sharp, stabbing chest pain, rated 10/10. Wheezing and crackles noted on auscultation of the lungs. VS: T 101.1°F (38.4°C), HR 118 beats/min, RR 28 breaths/min, BP 128/66 mm Hg, SpO$_2$ 88% on RA.

0910: Chemotherapy infusion stopped. Supplemental oxygen initiated at 4 L/min via NC.

The nurse collaborates with the registered nurse and contributes to the client's plan of care. Select whether the following potential nursing actions are indicated or not indicated for the client at this time.

POTENTIAL NURSING ACTIONS	INDICATED	NOT INDICATED
Transfer the client to a bed, and position with the head of the bed elevated 30 degrees.		
Apply a continuous pulse oximetry device to assess oxygenation.		
Perform chest percussion to assist the client with expectoration.		
Monitor respiratory status including rate, effort, and lung sounds.		
Contact the provider and arrange an ambulance for transport to the hospital.		

Thinking Exercise 4.2.5

A nurse is caring for a 42-year-old client on an oncology unit.

History and Physical	Nurses' Notes	Orders	Laboratory Results

Ambulatory Infusion Center

0820: Third cycle of adjunctive chemotherapy for breast cancer initiated 20 minutes ago. Client is seated in a recliner with legs elevated and reports feelings of fatigue and generalized discomfort, rated 4/10. Client states pain level is acceptable and confirms pain goal of less than 6. Heart tones regular and radial pulses palpable 2+. Bilateral lower extremity edema present, right > left. Right calf reddened, warm, and tender when touched and with movement. Pedal pulses 1+ and capillary refill <3 seconds in both lower extremities. Auscultated lung fields clear throughout. Client denies chest pain, cough, or shortness of breath. Abdomen soft and round. Client reports having no appetite but attempts to eat small meals several times a day. VS: T 99.8°F (37.6°C), HR 72 beats/min, RR 14 breaths/min, BP 98/50 mm Hg, SpO_2 98% on RA. IV site clean and without signs of extravasation. Infusion continued.

0900: Client apprehensive and diaphoretic. Reports dyspnea and sharp, stabbing chest pain, rated 10/10. Wheezing and crackles noted on auscultation of the lungs. VS: T 101.1°F (38.4°C), HR 118 beats/min, RR 28 breaths/min, BP 128/66 mm Hg, SpO_2 88% on RA.

0910: Chemotherapy infusion stopped. Supplemental oxygen initiated at 4 L/min via NC.

0940: Client care transferred to ambulance personnel for transport to local hospital with orders for direct admission to an oncology unit. VS: T 99.9°F (37.7°C), HR 102 beats/min, RR 20 breaths/min, BP 118/58 mm Hg, SpO_2 94% on 4 L/min O_2 via NC.

Inpatient Oncology Unit

1030: Admitted to oncology unit. Client alert and oriented × 4. Denies chest pain but appears anxious; becomes breathless when speaking. Heart tones regular, skin warm and diaphoretic. Pulses palpable throughout. Tachypnea and labored respirations noted. SpO_2 95% on 4 L/min O_2 via NC. Crackles noted on auscultation. Orders received.

History and Physical	Nurses' Notes	Orders	Laboratory Results

1215:
- Continuous telemetry and pulse oximetry monitoring
- Routine vital signs
- Supplemental O_2 to keep SpO_2 > 94%
- Portable chest x-ray
- Laboratory tests: CBC, PT, aPTT, D-dimer, ABG
- 0.9% normal saline IV at 100 mL/h
- Heparin infusion per protocol
- Heart-healthy diet

The nurse reviews physician orders and collaborates with the registered nurse in the implementation of the client's plan of care. Select the **3** nursing actions that nurse would plan to implement **immediately**.

○ Apply a 5-lead telemetry monitor
○ Initiate a heparin infusion
○ Contact dietary for a lunch tray
○ Increase the supplemental oxygen rate
○ Assess vital signs
○ Obtain a wheelchair for a radiology test
○ Collaborate with the laboratory for serum blood tests

Thinking Exercise 4.2.6

A nurse is caring for a 42-year-old client on an oncology unit.

History and Physical	Nurses' Notes	Orders	Laboratory Results

Ambulatory Infusion Center

0820: Third cycle of adjunctive chemotherapy for breast cancer initiated 20 minutes ago. Client is seated in a recliner with legs elevated and reports feelings of fatigue and generalized discomfort, rated 4/10. Client states pain level is acceptable and confirms pain goal of less than 6. Heart tones regular and radial pulses palpable 2+. Bilateral lower extremity edema present, right > left. Right calf reddened, warm, and tender when touched and with movement. Pedal pulses 1+ and capillary refill <3 seconds in both lower extremities. Auscultated lung fields clear throughout. Client denies chest pain, cough, or shortness of breath. Abdomen soft and round. Client reports having no appetite but attempts to eat small meals several times a day. VS: T 99.8°F (37.6°C), HR 72 beats/min, RR 14 breaths/min, BP 98/50 mm Hg, SpO$_2$ 98% on RA. IV site clean and without signs of extravasation. Infusion continued.

0900: Client apprehensive and diaphoretic. Reports dyspnea and sharp, stabbing chest pain, rated 10/10. Wheezing and crackles noted on auscultation of the lungs. VS: T 101.1°F (38.4°C), HR 118 beats/min, RR 28 breaths/min, BP 128/66 mm Hg, SpO$_2$ 88% on RA.

0910: Chemotherapy infusion stopped. Supplemental oxygen initiated at 4 L/min via NC.

0940: Client care transferred to ambulance personnel for transport to local hospital with orders for direct admission to an oncology unit. VS: T 99.9°F (37.7°C), HR 102 beats/min, RR 20 breaths/min, BP 118/58 mm Hg, SpO$_2$ 94% on 4 L/min O$_2$ via NC.

Inpatient Oncology Unit

1030: Admitted to oncology unit. Client alert and oriented × 4. Denies chest pain but appears anxious; becomes breathless when speaking. Heart tones regular, skin warm and diaphoretic. Pulses palpable throughout. Tachypnea and labored respirations noted. SpO$_2$ 95% on 4 L/min O$_2$ via NC. Crackles noted on auscultation. Orders received.

1800: Client alert and oriented × 4. Resting comfortably in bed when not disturbed. Follows commands and moves all extremities. Normal sinus rhythm; skin warm and dry. Bilateral lower extremity edema present, right > left. Radial and pedal pulses 2+. Respirations equal and unlabored. Crackles noted on auscultation of lung fields. Client denies chest pain and shortness of breath. Abdomen soft and round. Bowel sounds hypoactive in all quadrants. Peripheral venous device sites in right forearm and left AC are clean, dry, and without signs of extravasation. Heparin infusing per protocol. VS: T 99.8°F (37.6°C), HR 88 beats/min, RR 18 breaths/min, BP 109/50 mm Hg, SpO$_2$ 98% on 4 L/min O$_2$ via NC. Client reports generalized discomfort, rated 4/10.

The nurse reviews the oncology unit Nurses' Notes and assists in evaluating the client's status. For each data collection finding, select whether the finding indicates that the client's status has improved or has not improved.

DATA COLLECTION FINDING	IMPROVED	NOT IMPROVED
Heart rate		
Lung sounds		
Oxygen saturation		
Pain		
Respiratory rate		

Stand-Alone Thinking Exercise 4.1

A nurse is caring for a 31-year-old client at an urgent care facility.

History and Physical	Nurses' Notes	Orders	Laboratory Results

2250: Friend brought client to center due to persistent and worsening dyspnea. Medical history includes allergic contact dermatitis, asthma, and iron deficiency anemia. Alert and oriented × 4 and speaks in short phrases due to breathlessness. Client states, "We were at a concert. It was very smoky. I started having difficulty beathing. We left the concert. It is getting worse, not better." Respirations labored with use of accessory muscles. Expiratory wheezes auscultated in lung fields. Client denies cough, nasal drainage, or recent infection. Heart tones regular. Skin warm and diaphoretic. Pulses 2+ and equal throughout. Bilateral jugular veins distended. Abdomen soft, round, and nontender. Bowel sounds present in all quadrants. VS: T 98.7°F (37°C), HR 93 beats/min, RR 25 breaths/min, BP 130/62 mm Hg, SpO_2 94% on RA. Client denies pain but reports chest tightness.

The nurse reviews the collected data and collaborates with the registered nurse. Complete the diagram by selecting from the choices below to specify what potential condition the client is likely experiencing, **2** nursing actions that are appropriate to take, and **2** parameters the nurse would monitor to assess the client's progress.

Action to Take		Parameter to Monitor
Action to Take	Potential Complication	Parameter to Monitor

Actions to Take	Potential Conditions	Parameters to Monitor
Obtain a sputum culture	Acute severe asthma	Depth and quality of respirations
Apply supplemental O_2 via NC	Anxiety-induced hyperventilation	Intake and output
Administer an albuterol nebulizer treatment	Acute bronchitis	Sputum consistency and color
Teach the client breathing techniques	Allergic rhinitis	White blood cell count
Obtain peripheral venous access		Vital signs

Stand-Alone Thinking Exercise 4.2

A nurse is caring for a 48-year-old client at a medical-surgical unit.

History and Physical	Nurses' Notes	Orders	Nursing Flow Sheet

1345: Client arrives from PACU after an open cholecystectomy and exploratory laparotomy. Medical history includes chronic obstructive pulmonary disease and 20 years of cigarette smoking. Drowsy but able to arouse and oriented × 4. Speech clear and appropriate. Follows all commands. Heart tones regular and pulses 2+ throughout. Skin warm and dry. Respirations equal and unlabored. Lung fields clear throughout. Client denies chest pain and dyspnea. Abdomen soft and round. Hypoactive bowel sounds present in all quadrants. Abdominal incision covered with clean dressing. Jackson Pratt (JP) drain to bulb suction with serous sanguineous drainage. Indwelling urinary catheter secured to right inner thigh and draining dark yellow urine to gravity. Right antecubital peripheral venous device present; site clean and dry with no signs of extravasation. 0.9% normal saline infusing at 100 mL/h. Client reports pain at surgical site rated 4/10.

1530: Client sleeping. Easily aroused and oriented × 4. Client reports surgical site rated 8/10. Morphine 2 mg IV administered per PRN orders.

1840: Client drowsy but able to arouse. Client refuses dinner stating, "The pain has decreased, and I just want to sleep." Client's spouse at bedside and updated on plan of care.

2200: Client alert and oriented × 4. Spouse at bedside. Respirations equal and unlabored. Lung fields clear throughout. Abdominal incision intact with clean dressing. JP drain to bulb suction with serous sanguineous drainage. Indwelling urinary catheter draining yellow urine to gravity. Client reports pain at surgical site rated 6/10 but refuses pain medication stating "it makes me feel weird."

0600: Client sleeping. Easily aroused and oriented × 4. Client refuses to get out of bed and states, "It is too early; I promise to get up in a couple hours when my spouse comes to visit."

0810: Alert and oriented × 4. Spouse at bedside assisting client to eat breakfast. Heart tones regular and pulses palpable throughout. Fine crackles noted in bilateral lower lobes upon auscultation. Weak cough present. Client denies chest pain or dyspnea. Abdomen soft and tender when touched. Surgical incision well approximated with clean, dry dressing. JP drain to bulb suction with scant drainage. Indwelling urinary catheter draining yellow urine to gravity. Client denies pain at surgical site but grimaces with any movement and refuses to get out of bed. Client and spouse are educated on the importance of pain management.

1000: Client reports difficulty breathing. Tachypnea and shallow respirations present. Crackles noted in bilateral upper lung lobes, and diminished breath sounds noted in bilateral lower lobes.

History and Physical	Nurses' Notes	Orders	Nursing Flow Sheet	
	1400	**2200**	**0600**	**1000**
Vital Signs				
Temp	98.5°F (36.9°C)	98.9°F (37.1°C)	99.9°F (37.8°C)	100.2°F (37.8°C)
HR	69 beats/min	88 beats/min	92 beats/min	102 beats/min
BP	108/56 mm Hg	132/80 mm Hg	138/79 mm Hg	144/82 mm Hg
RR	12 breaths/min	15 breaths/min	18 breaths/min	24 breaths/min
SpO$_2$	99% on 2 L/min O$_2$ via NC	99% on 2 L/min O$_2$ via NC	95% on 2 L/min O$_2$ via NC	94% on 2 L/min O$_2$ via NC
Intake				
IV	1500 mL (from OR)	800 mL	800 mL	200 mL
Oral	—	120 mL	360 mL	—
Output				
Urinary	430 mL	595 mL	820 mL	120 mL
JP Drain	50 mL	30 mL	10 mL	—

The nurse collaborates with the registered nurse and contributes to the client's plan of care. Select whether the following potential nursing actions are indicated or not indicated for the client at this time.

POTENTIAL NURSING ACTIONS	INDICATED	NOT INDICATED
Assist the client to change position at least every 2 hours.		
Teach the client to hold a pillow firmly over the abdominal incision prior to performing coughing and deep breathing exercises.		
Encourage the client to perform coughing and deep breathing exercises every hour.		
Instruct the client to take a deep breath and then blow out the air through the incentive spirometer mouthpiece.		
Promote early ambulation by assisting the client to walk in the hallway several times daily.		
Collaborate with the client to properly manage pain with pharmacologic and nonpharmacologic therapies.		

CHAPTER 5

Client Conditions Affecting Mobility

Unfolding Case Study 5.1

Thinking Exercise 5.1.1

The nurse is caring for a 55-year-old client who had a right above-the-knee amputation (AKA).

History and Physical	Nurses' Notes	Orders	Laboratory Results

0745: Had right AKA yesterday afternoon due to complications of type 1 diabetes mellitus. Alert and oriented × 4. States "I'm so upset I can't drive for a long time." Right leg and foot pain described as sharp with a "pins and needles" feeling; reports pain rated 8/10. PCA shows inadequate dosing by the client. Breath sounds clear throughout lung fields; no dyspnea. Abdomen soft, round, and nontender. Skin dry with usual pigmentation. Saline lock in place. Bowel sounds present in all quadrants. Pulses 2+ except for left pedal pulse at 1+. Capillary refill >3 sec. Bulky dressing on right residual limb dry and intact. Small amount of blood-tinged drainage in Jackson-Pratt (JP) drain. VS: T 98.8°F (37.1°C), HR 94 beats/min and regular, RR 22 breaths/min, BP 118/64 mm Hg, SpO$_2$ 97% on RA. FSBG 108 mg/dL (5.99 mmol/L) at 0700. (Normal range 70-110 mg/dL [3.89–6.11 mmol/L].)

1130: Used PCA more often this morning; reports pain at 5/10. Moderate amount of new bright-red blood on surgical dressing. VS: T 98.8°F (37.1°C), HR 104 beats/min and regular, RR 26 breaths/min, BP 110/58 mm Hg, SpO$_2$ 96% on RA. FSBG 100 mg/dL (5.55 mmol/L). (Normal range 70–110 mg/dL [3.89–6.11 mmol/L].)

The nurse collects data from the client. Select the **3** client findings that require **immediate** follow-up.
- ○ Pain
- ○ Temperature
- ○ Heart rate
- ○ Respiratory rate
- ○ Blood pressure
- ○ SpO$_2$
- ○ Blood glucose
- ○ Blood on surgical dressing
- ○ Client's concern about driving

Thinking Exercise 5.1.2

The nurse is caring for a 55-year-old client who had a right above-the-knee amputation (AKA).

History and Physical	Nurses' Notes	Orders	Laboratory Results

0745: Had right AKA yesterday afternoon due to complications of type 1 diabetes mellitus. Alert and oriented × 4. States "I'm so upset I can't drive for a long time." Right leg and foot pain described as sharp with a "pins and needles" feeling; reports pain rated 8/10. PCA shows inadequate dosing by the client. Breath sounds clear throughout lung fields; no dyspnea. Abdomen soft, round, and nontender. Skin dry with usual pigmentation. Saline lock in place. Bowel sounds present in all quadrants. Pulses 2+ except for left pedal pulse at 1+. Capillary refill >3 sec. Bulky dressing on right residual limb dry and intact. Small amount of blood-tinged drainage in Jackson-Pratt (JP) drain. VS: T 98.8°F (37.1°C), HR 94 beats/min and regular, RR 22 breaths/min, BP 118/64 mm Hg, SpO$_2$ 97% on RA. FSBG 108 mg/dL (5.99 mmol/L) at 0700. (Normal range 70–110 mg/dL [3.89–6.11 mmol/L].)

1130: Used PCA more often this morning; reports pain at 5/10. Moderate amount of new bright-red blood on surgical dressing. VS: T 98.8°F (37.1°C), HR 104 beats/min and regular, RR 26 breaths/min, BP 110/58 mm Hg, SpO$_2$ 96% on RA via pulse oximetry. FSBG 100 mg/dL (5.55 mmol/L). (Normal range 70–110 mg/dL [3.89–6.11 mmol/L].)

The nurse reviews the collected data and collaborates with the registered nurse. Complete the following sentence by selecting from the list of word choices below.

The nurse should recognize that the client is likely experiencing [**Word Choice**] and [**Word Choice**].

WORD CHOICES
Infection
Hemorrhage
Hypoxia
Phantom limb pain
Acute compartment syndrome

Thinking Exercise 5.1.3

The nurse is caring for a 55-year-old client who had a right above-the-knee amputation (AKA).

History and Physical	Nurses' Notes	Orders	Laboratory Results

0745: Had right AKA yesterday afternoon due to complications of type 1 diabetes mellitus. Alert and oriented × 4. States "I'm so upset I can't drive for a long time." Right leg and foot pain described as sharp with a "pins and needles" feeling; reports pain rated 8/10. PCA shows inadequate dosing by the client. Breath sounds clear throughout lung fields. Abdomen soft, round, and nontender. Skin dry with usual pigmentation. Saline lock in place; no dyspnea. Bowel sounds present in all quadrants. Pulses 2+ except for left pedal pulse at 1+. Capillary refill >3 sec. Bulky dressing on right residual limb dry and intact. Small amount of blood-tinged drainage in Jackson-Pratt (JP) drain. VS: T 98.8°F (37.1°C), HR 94 beats/min and regular, RR 22 breaths/min, BP 118/64 mm Hg, SpO_2 97% on RA. FSBG 108 mg/dL (5.99 mmol/L) at 0700. (Normal range 70–110 mg/dL [3.89–6.11 mmol/L].)

1130: Used PCA more often this morning; reports pain at 5/10. Moderate amount of new bright-red blood on surgical dressing. VS: T 98.8°F (37.1°C), HR 104 beats/min and regular, RR 26 breaths/min, BP 110/58 mm Hg, SpO_2 96% on RA via pulse oximetry. FSBG 100 mg/dL (5.55 mmol/L). (Normal range 70–110 mg/dL [3.89–6.11 mmol/L].)

The nurse reviews the collected client data and collaborates with the registered nurse. Complete the following sentence by selecting from the lists of options below.

The nurse determines the *priority* for care at this time is to manage the client's **1 [Select]** as evidenced by **2 [Select]** and **3 [Select]**.

OPTIONS FOR 1	OPTIONS FOR 2	OPTIONS FOR 3
Pain	Self-report of pain	Blood on dressing
Infection	Elevated heart rate	Elevated blood glucose
Hemorrhage	Elevated temperature	Decreased SpO_2

Thinking Exercise 5.1.4

The nurse is caring for a 55-year-old client who had a right above-the-knee amputation (AKA).

History and Physical	Nurses' Notes	Orders	Laboratory Results

0745: Had right AKA yesterday afternoon due to complications of type 1 diabetes mellitus. Alert and oriented × 4. States "I'm so upset I can't drive for a long time." Right leg and foot pain described as sharp with a "pins and needles" feeling; reports pain rated 8/10. PCA shows inadequate dosing by the client. Breath sounds clear throughout lung fields; no dyspnea. Abdomen soft, round, and nontender. Skin dry with usual pigmentation. Saline lock in place. Bowel sounds present in all quadrants. Pulses 2+ except for left pedal pulse at 1+. Capillary refill >3 sec. Bulky dressing on right residual limb dry and intact. Small amount of blood-tinged drainage in Jackson-Pratt (JP) drain. VS: T 98.8°F (37.1°C), HR 94 beats/min and regular, RR 22 breaths/min, BP 118/64 mm Hg, SpO_2 97% on RA. FSBG 108 mg/dL (5.99 mmol/L) at 0700. (Normal range 70–110 mg/dL [3.89–6.11 mmol/L].)

1130: Used PCA more often this morning; reports pain at 5/10. Moderate amount of new bright-red blood on surgical dressing. VS: T 98.8°F (37.1°C), HR 104 beats/min and regular, RR 26 breaths/min, BP 110/58 mm Hg, SpO_2 96% on RA via pulse oximetry. FSBG 100 mg/dL (5.55 mmol/L). (Normal range 70–110 mg/dL [3.89–6.11 mmol/L].)

The nurse collaborates with the registered nurse and contributes to the client's plan of care. Select whether the following potential nursing actions are indicated or not indicated for the client at this time.

POTENTIAL NURSING ACTIONS	INDICATED	NOT INDICATED
Apply a pressure dressing over the surgical dressing		
Keep the right residual limb flat on the bed		
Monitor vital signs every 8 hours		
Maintain bedrest for the rest of the day		

Thinking Exercise 5.1.5

The nurse is caring for a 55-year-old client who had a right above-the-knee amputation (AKA).

History and Physical	Nurses' Notes	Orders	Laboratory Results

0745: Had right AKA yesterday afternoon due to complications of type 1 diabetes mellitus. Alert and oriented × 4. States "I'm so upset I can't drive for a long time." Right leg and foot pain described as sharp with a "pins and needles" feeling; reports pain rated 8/10. PCA shows inadequate dosing by the client. Breath sounds clear throughout lung fields; no dyspnea. Abdomen soft, round, and nontender. Skin dry with usual pigmentation. Saline lock in place. Bowel sounds present in all quadrants. Pulses 2+ except for left pedal pulse at 1+. Capillary refill >3 sec. Bulky dressing on right residual limb dry and intact. Small amount of blood-tinged drainage in Jackson-Pratt (JP) drain. VS: T 98.8°F (37.1°C), HR 94 beats/min and regular, RR 22 breaths/min, BP 118/64 mm Hg, SpO_2 97% on RA. FSBG 108 mg/dL (5.99 mmol/L) at 0700. (Normal range 70–110 mg/dL [3.89–6.11 mmol/L].)

1130: Used PCA more often this morning; reports pain at 5/10. Moderate amount of new bright-red blood on surgical dressing. VS: T 98.8°F (37.1°C), HR 104 beats/min and regular, RR 26 breaths/min, BP 110/58 mm Hg, SpO_2 96% on RA via pulse oximetry. FSBG 100 mg/dL (5.55 mmol/L). (Normal range 70–110 mg/dL [3.89–6.11 mmol/L].)

1145: Surgeon notified about changes in vital signs and new bright-red blood on dressing. Plans to examine client in the next hour.

The nurse assists with implementation of the client's plan of care. Which of the following actions would the nurse take at this time? **Select all that apply.**

○ Elevate the right residual limb on 1 to 2 pillows.
○ Check under the residual limb for bleeding.
○ Apply a heat compress to the right residual limb.
○ Apply a pressure dressing over the surgical dressing.
○ Mark and label the area where blood is located on the dressing.
○ Monitor vital signs every 1 to 2 hours.
○ Start peripheral IV fluids.
○ Maintain bedrest today.

Thinking Exercise 5.1.6

The nurse is caring for a 55-year-old client who had a right above-the-knee amputation (AKA).

History and Physical	Nurses' Notes	Orders	Laboratory Results

0745: Had right AKA yesterday afternoon due to complications of type 1 diabetes mellitus. Alert and oriented × 4. States "I'm so upset I can't drive for a long time." Right leg and foot pain described as sharp with a "pins and needles" feeling; reports rated 8/10. PCA shows inadequate dosing by the client. Breath sounds clear throughout lung fields; no dyspnea. Abdomen soft, round, and nontender. Skin dry with usual pigmentation. Saline lock in place. Bowel sounds present in all quadrants. Pulses 2+ except for left pedal pulse at 1+. Capillary refill >3 sec. Bulky dressing on right residual limb dry and intact. Small amount of blood-tinged drainage in Jackson-Pratt (JP) drain. VS: T 98.8°F (37.1°C), HR 94 beats/min and regular, RR 22 breaths/min, BP 118/64 mm Hg, SpO_2 97% on RA. FSBG 108 mg/dL (5.99 mmol/L) at 0700. (Normal range 70–110 mg/dL [3.89–6.11 mmol/L].)

1130: Used PCA more often this morning; reports pain at 5/10. Moderate amount of new bright-red blood on surgical dressing. VS: T 98.8°F (37.1°C), HR 104 beats/min and regular, RR 26 breaths/min, BP 110/58 mm Hg, SpO_2 96% on RA via pulse oximetry. FSBG 100 mg/dL (5.55 mmol/L). (Normal range 70–110 mg/dL [3.89–6.11 mmol/L].)

1145: Surgeon notified about changes in vital signs and new bright-red blood on dressing. Plans to examine client in the next hour.

1155: Right residual limb elevated on 2 pillows and wrapped in pressure dressing over surgical dressing. No blood or dampness under surgical limb. Peripheral IV fluids started via saline lock. Client to stay in bed today. PCA discontinued.

1340: VS: T 98.6°F (37°C), HR 86 beats/min and regular, RR 18 breaths/min, BP 122/76 mm Hg, SpO_2 97% on RA. States right foot pain is becoming very painful at 10/10, even after taking prescribed oral analgesic. No new bleeding noted on surgical dressing.

The nurse reviews the most recent nurses' notes and is assisting to evaluate the client's condition based on collected data. For each data collection finding, select whether the finding indicates that the client's condition has improved or worsened.

DATA COLLECTION FINDING	IMPROVED	WORSENED
Heart rate		
Pain intensity		
Respiratory rate		
Blood pressure		
Bleeding from surgical site		

Unfolding Case Study 5.2

Thinking Exercise 5.2.1

The nurse is caring for a 47-year-old client in the acute postsurgical unit.

History and Physical	Nurses' Notes	Orders	Laboratory Results

1955: Client brought to emergency department early this morning after being struck by a truck on a downtown street resulting in fractures of the pelvis and left fibula. Multiple bruises on entire left leg with tire mark imprint on left lower leg. History of type 2 diabetes mellitus and peptic ulcer disease. Drowsy but oriented × 4; reports pain rated 4/10 after pain med administered. Breath sounds clear throughout lung fields; no dyspnea. Skin dry with usual pigmentation. Peripheral IV of 5%D/0.45%NS infusing at 100 mL/h. Bowel sounds present in all quadrants. Distal pulses 2+ bilaterally. Capillary refill <3 sec. Moves and feels toes on both feet. Left leg splint in place and leg elevated on pillow. Urinary catheter draining clear yellow urine. VS: T 98°F (36.7°C), HR 78 beats/min and regular, RR 16 breaths/min, BP 112/60 mm Hg, SpO2 98% on RA.

0810: Reports increasing pain not being relieved as well as earlier after pain med administered. States left lower leg and foot are throbbing and tingling. Left foot more pale and cooler than right foot. Left pedal pulse 1+; right pedal pulse 2+. VS: T 98°F (36.7°C), HR 89 beats/min and regular, RR 20 breaths/min, BP 126/74 mm Hg, SpO2 97% on RA. Surgeon notified and additional pain med given per new orders. Pillow under affected leg removed. Distal dressing cut and splint loosened per surgeon's request. Will continue to monitor.

1322: Reports left leg and foot pain at 9/10. Pain med given less than 1 hour ago. Left foot pale and cool; somewhat mottled. Left pedal pulse absent. Capillary refill left foot >3 sec. Difficulty moving and feeling toes. VS: T 98.6°F (37°C), HR 96 beats/min and regular, RR 20 breaths/min, BP 130/82 mm Hg, SpO2 97% on RA.

The nurse collects data from the client. Select the **3** client findings that require **immediate** follow-up.

- Pain level
- Absent pedal pulse
- Heart rate
- Respiratory rate
- Blood pressure
- Capillary refill
- Cool, pale left foot

Thinking Exercise 5.2.2

The nurse is caring for a 47-year-old client in the acute postsurgical unit.

History and Physical	Nurses' Notes	Orders	Laboratory Results

1955: Client brought to emergency department early this morning after being struck by a truck on a downtown street resulting in fractures of the pelvis and left fibula. Multiple bruises on entire left leg with tire mark imprint on left lower leg. History of type 2 diabetes mellitus and peptic ulcer disease. Drowsy but oriented × 4; reports pain rated 4/10 after pain med administered. Breath sounds clear throughout lung fields; no dyspnea. Skin dry with usual pigmentation. Peripheral IV of 5%D/0.45%NS infusing at 100 mL/h. Bowel sounds present in all quadrants. Distal pulses 2+ bilaterally. Capillary refill <3 sec. Moves and feels toes on both feet. Left leg splint in place and leg elevated on pillow. Urinary catheter draining clear yellow urine. VS: T 98°F (36.7°C), HR 78 beats/min and regular, RR 16 breaths/min, BP 112/60 mm Hg, SpO2 98% on RA.

0810: Reports increasing pain not being relieved as well as earlier after pain med administered. States left lower leg and foot are throbbing and tingling. Left foot more pale and cooler than right foot. Left pedal pulse 1+; right pedal pulse 2+. VS: T 98°F (36.7°C), HR 89 beats/min and regular, RR 20 breaths/min, BP 126/74 mm Hg, SpO2 97% on RA. Surgeon notified and additional pain med given per new orders. Pillow under affected leg removed. Distal dressing cut and splint loosened per surgeon's request. Will continue to monitor.

1322: Reports left leg and foot pain at 9/10. Pain med given less than 1 hour ago. Left foot pale and cool; somewhat mottled. Left pedal pulse absent. Capillary refill left foot >3 sec. Difficulty moving and feeling toes. VS: T 98.6°F (37°C), HR 96 beats/min and regular, RR 20 breaths/min, BP 130/82 mm Hg, SpO2 97% on RA.

The nurse reviews the collected data and collaborates with the registered nurse. Complete the following sentence by selecting from the list of word choices below.

The nurse should recognize that the client is likely experiencing **[Word Choice]**.

WORD CHOICES
Substance withdrawal
Deep vein thrombosis
Compartment syndrome
Peripheral vascular disease

Thinking Exercise 5.2.3

The nurse is caring for a 47-year-old client in the acute postsurgical unit.

History and Physical	Nurses' Notes	Orders	Laboratory Results

1955: Client brought to emergency department early this morning after being struck by a truck on a downtown street resulting in fractures of the pelvis and left fibula. Multiple bruises on entire left leg with tire mark imprint on left lower leg. History of type 2 diabetes mellitus and peptic ulcer disease. Drowsy but oriented × 4; reports pain rated 4/10 after pain med administered. Breath sounds clear throughout lung fields; no dyspnea. Skin dry with usual pigmentation. Peripheral IV of 5%D/0.45%NS infusing at 100 mL/h. Bowel sounds present in all quadrants. Distal pulses 2+ bilaterally. Capillary refill <3 sec. Moves and feels toes on both feet. Left leg splint in place and leg elevated on pillow. Urinary catheter draining clear yellow urine. VS: T 98°F (36.7°C), HR 78 beats/min and regular, RR 16 breaths/min, BP 112/60 mm Hg, SpO$_2$ 98% on RA.

0810: Reports increasing pain not being relieved as well as earlier after pain med administered. States left lower leg and foot are throbbing and tingling. Left foot more pale and cooler than right foot. Left pedal pulse 1+; right pedal pulse 2+. VS: T 98°F (36.7°C), HR 89 beats/min and regular, RR 20 breaths/min, BP 126/74 mm Hg, SpO$_2$ 97% on RA. Surgeon notified and additional pain med given per new orders. Pillow under affected leg removed. Distal dressing cut and splint loosened per surgeon's request. Will continue to monitor.

1322: Reports left leg and foot pain at 9/10. Pain med given less than 1 hour ago. Left foot pale and cool; somewhat mottled. Left pedal pulse absent. Capillary refill left foot >3 sec. Difficulty moving and feeling toes. VS: T 98.6°F (37°C), HR 96 beats/min and regular, RR 22 breaths/min, BP 130/82 mm Hg, SpO$_2$ 97% on RA.

The nurse reviews the collected client data and collaborates with the registered nurse. Complete the following sentence by selecting from the lists of options below.

The nurse determines the *priority* for care at this time is to manage the client's **1 [Select]** as evidenced by **2 [Select]** and **3 [Select]**.

OPTIONS FOR 1	OPTIONS FOR 2	OPTIONS FOR 3
Left leg/foot pain	Pale, cool left foot	Tachycardia
Left leg pressure	Elevated blood pressure	Increased respirations
Left leg thrombosis	Report of 9/10 pain	Absent left pedal pulse

Thinking Exercise 5.2.4

The nurse is caring for a 47-year-old client in the acute postsurgical unit.

History and Physical	Nurses' Notes	Orders	Laboratory Results

1955: Client brought to emergency department early this morning after being struck by a truck on a downtown street resulting in fractures of the pelvis and left fibula. Multiple bruises on entire left leg with tire mark imprint on left lower leg. History of type 2 diabetes mellitus and peptic ulcer disease. Drowsy but oriented × 4; reports pain rated 4/10 after pain med administered. Breath sounds clear throughout lung fields; no dyspnea. Skin dry with usual pigmentation. Peripheral IV of 5%D/0.45%NS infusing at 100 mL/h. Bowel sounds present in all quadrants. Distal pulses 2+ bilaterally. Capillary refill <3 sec. Moves and feels toes on both feet. Left leg splint in place and leg elevated on pillow. Urinary catheter draining clear yellow urine. VS: T 98°F (36.7°C), HR 78 beats/min and regular, RR 16 breaths/min, BP 112/60 mm Hg, SpO$_2$ 98% on RA.

0810: Reports increasing pain not being relieved as well as earlier after pain med administered. States left lower leg and foot are throbbing and tingling. Left foot more pale and cooler than right foot. Left pedal pulse 1+; right pedal pulse 2+. VS: T 98°F (36.7°C), HR 89 beats/min and regular, RR 20 breaths/min, BP 126/74 mm Hg, SpO$_2$ 97% on RA. Surgeon notified and additional pain med given per new orders. Pillow under affected leg removed. Distal dressing cut and splint loosened per surgeon's request. Will continue to monitor.

1322: Reports left leg and foot pain at 9/10. Pain med given less than 1 hour ago. Left foot pale and cool; somewhat mottled. Left pedal pulse absent. Capillary refill left foot >3 sec. Difficulty moving and feeling toes. VS: T 98.6°F (37°C), HR 96 beats/min and regular, RR 22 breaths/min, BP 130/82 mm Hg, SpO$_2$ 97% on RA.

The nurse collaborates with the registered nurse and contributes to the client's plan of care. Which of the following potential actions would be appropriate for the nurse to take at this time? **Select all that apply**.

O Elevate the affected leg on 2 pillows.
O Increase the rate of peripheral IV fluids.
O Start oxygen therapy via nasal cannula.
O Notify the surgeon about the most recent client findings.
O Apply heat to the affected lower leg to promote circulation.
O Request an order for additional analgesia to manage the client's pain.
O Prepare the client for a potential fasciotomy to relieve leg pressure.

Thinking Exercise 5.2.5

The nurse is caring for a 47-year-old client in the acute postsurgical unit.

History and Physical	Nurses' Notes	Orders	Laboratory Results

1955: Client brought to emergency department early this morning after being struck by a truck on a downtown street resulting in fractures of the pelvis and left fibula. Multiple bruises on entire left leg with tire mark imprint on left lower leg. History of type 2 diabetes mellitus and peptic ulcer disease. Drowsy but oriented × 4; reports pain rated 4/10 after pain med administered. Breath sounds clear throughout lung fields; no dyspnea. Skin dry with usual pigmentation. Peripheral IV of 5%D/0.45%NS infusing at 100 mL/h. Bowel sounds present in all quadrants. Distal pulses 2+ bilaterally. Capillary refill <3 sec. Moves and feels toes on both feet. Left leg splint in place and leg elevated on pillow. Urinary catheter draining clear yellow urine. VS: T 98°F (36.7°C), HR 78 beats/min and regular, RR 16 breaths/min, BP 112/60 mm Hg, SpO$_2$ 98% on RA.

0810: Reports increasing pain not being relieved as well as earlier after pain med administered. States left lower leg and foot are throbbing and tingling. Left foot more pale and cooler than right foot. Left pedal pulse 1+; right pedal pulse 2+. VS: T 98°F (36.7°C), HR 89 beats/min and regular, RR 20 breaths/min, BP 126/74 mm Hg, SpO$_2$ 97% on RA. Surgeon notified and additional pain med given per new orders. Pillow under affected leg removed. Distal dressing cut and splint loosened per surgeon's request. Will continue to monitor.

1322: Reports left leg and foot pain at 9/10. Pain med given less than 1 hour ago. Left foot pale and cool; somewhat mottled. Left pedal pulse absent. Capillary refill left foot >3 sec. Difficulty moving and feeling toes. VS: T 98.6°F (37°C), HR 96 beats/min and regular, RR 22 breaths/min, BP 130/82 mm Hg, SpO$_2$ 97% on RA.

1330: Surgeon notified and will examine client within next hour. Client received additional pain med per order.

1410: Surgeon in to examine client. Explained need for emergent fasciotomy to relieve leg pressure and restore circulation to injured leg.

1850: Returned from OR with bulky surgical dressing, two Jackson-Pratts draining small amount bloody drainage, and fiberglass splint with elastic wrap extending entire left leg. Alert and oriented × 4; dozing at times. Breath sounds clear throughout lung fields; no dyspnea. Skin dry with usual pigmentation. Left pedal pulse 1+; foot warmer and less pale when compared with presurgical status. Can move left toes slightly but sensation not yet returned. Urinary catheter draining clear, light-yellow urine. VS: T 98.6°F (37°C), HR 76 beats/min and regular, RR 16 breaths/min, BP 110/62 mm Hg, SpO$_2$ 100% on 3 L/min O$_2$ via NC. Peripheral IV intact and infusing per order.

The nurse assists with implementation of the client's plan of care. For each body system, select the nursing actions that are appropriate as part of the client's postoperative care.

BODY SYSTEM	NURSING ACTION
Cardiovascular	○ Take and record vital signs every 2–4 hours per protocol ○ Perform a circulation check on the left foot every 2–4 hours per surgeon protocol ○ Empty and record JP drainage every 8–12 hours per agency protocol
Respiratory	○ Monitor SpO$_2$ and titrate supplemental oxygen per surgeon protocol ○ Encourage deep breathing every hour while awake ○ Encourage use of an incentive spirometer every 8 hours
Neurologic	○ Assess pain level with other vital signs ○ Document the location and quality of pain for each assessment ○ Monitor for substance withdrawal behaviors

Thinking Exercise 5.2.6

The nurse is caring for a 47-year-old client in the acute postsurgical unit.

History and Physical	Nurses' Notes	Orders	Laboratory Results

1955: Client brought to emergency department early this morning after being struck by a truck on a downtown street resulting in fractures of the pelvis and left fibula. Multiple bruises on entire left leg with tire mark imprint on left lower leg. History of type 2 diabetes mellitus and peptic ulcer disease. Drowsy but oriented × 4; reports pain rated 4/10 after pain med administered. Breath sounds clear throughout lung fields; no dyspnea. Skin dry with usual pigmentation. Peripheral IV of 5%D/0.45%NS infusing at 100 mL/h. Bowel sounds present in all quadrants. Distal pulses 2+ bilaterally. Capillary refill <3 sec. Moves and feels toes on both feet. Left leg splint in place and leg elevated on pillow. Urinary catheter draining clear yellow urine. VS: T 98°F (36.7°C), HR 78 beats/min and regular, RR 16 breaths/min, BP 112/60 mm Hg, SpO$_2$ 98% on RA.

0810: Reports increasing pain not being relieved as well as earlier after pain med administered. States left lower leg and foot are throbbing and tingling. Left foot more pale and cooler than right foot. Left pedal pulse 1+; right pedal pulse 2+. VS: T 98°F (36.7°C), HR 89 beats/min and regular, RR 20 breaths/min, BP 126/74 mm Hg, SpO$_2$ 97% on RA. Surgeon notified and additional pain med given per new orders. Pillow under affected leg removed. Distal dressing cut and splint loosened per surgeon's request. Will continue to monitor.

1322: Reports left leg and foot pain at 9/10. Pain med given less than 1 hour ago. Left foot pale and cool; somewhat mottled. Left pedal pulse absent. Capillary refill left foot >3 sec. Difficulty moving and feeling toes. VS: T 98.6°F (37°C), HR 96 beats/min and regular, RR 22 breaths/min, BP 130/82 mm Hg, SpO$_2$ 97% on RA.

1330: Surgeon notified and will examine client within next hour. Client received additional pain med per order.

1410: Surgeon in to examine client. Explained need for emergent fasciotomy to relieve leg pressure and restore circulation to injured leg.

1850: Returned from OR with bulky surgical dressing, two Jackson-Pratts draining small amount bloody drainage, and fiberglass splint with elastic wrap extending entire left leg. Alert and oriented × 4; dozing at times. Reports pain at 3/10. Breath sounds clear throughout lung fields; no dyspnea. Skin dry with usual pigmentation. Left pedal pulse 1+; foot warmer and less pale when compared with presurgical status. Can move left foot and toes slightly, but sensation not yet returned. Urinary catheter draining clear, light-yellow urine. VS: T 98.6°F (37°C), HR 76 beats/min and regular, RR 16 breaths/min, BP 110/62 mm Hg, SpO$_2$ 100% on 3 L/min O$_2$ via NC. Peripheral IV intact and infusing per order.

2 Days Later
1230: Client has reported increasing burning heel pain for the past 24 hours that has not responded to multimodal pain protocol. Surgeon removed splint to examine foot and dressing. 3 cm × 2 cm necrotic area on left heel. Draining thick tan exudate with foul odor. Unable to determine wound depth.

The nurse is assisting to evaluate the client's condition based on the most recent collected data. For each data collection finding, select whether the finding indicates that the client's condition has improved or worsened after the fasciotomy.

DATA COLLECTION FINDING	IMPROVED	WORSENED
Reports pain at 3/10		
Left pedal pulse 1+		
Foot and toe movement		
Vital signs		
Skin integrity of injured foot		

Unfolding Case Study 5.3

Thinking Exercise 5.3.1

The nurse is caring for a 21-year-old client in the acute rehabilitation unit. Highlight the client findings that require **immediate** follow-up.

History and Physical	Nurses' Notes	Orders	Laboratory Results

1550: Client admitted yesterday for acute rehabilitation program following cervical (C7–C8) spinal cord injury resulting from diving into a shallow pool. Evaluated yesterday by PT and OT. Alert and oriented × 4; reports pain rated 2/10 after pain med administered. Anterior neck surgical incision intact and healing. Halo fixator in place; no redness or drainage around screws. Breath sounds clear throughout lung fields; no dyspnea. Skin dry with usual pigmentation. Bowel sounds present in all quadrants. Abdomen soft, round, and nondistended. Urinary catheter draining medium-yellow urine with sediment. High-top shoes and antiembolism stockings in place. VS: T 98.6°F (37°C), HR 82 beats/min and regular, RR 18 breaths/min, BP 118/56 mm Hg, SpO$_2$ 95% on RA. Scheduled for first PT session to begin mobility training at 1600.

1815: Reports developing severe "pounding" frontal headache about 10 minutes ago. Face and neck flushed and diaphoretic. States vision is blurred and nose suddenly began feeling "stuffy." VS: T 99°F (37.2°C), HR 58 beats/min and regular, RR 22 breaths/min, BP 194/116 mm Hg, SpO$_2$ 94% on RA.

Thinking Exercise 5.3.2

The nurse is caring for a 21-year-old client in the acute rehabilitation unit.

History and Physical	Nurses' Notes	Orders	Laboratory Results

1550: Client admitted yesterday for acute rehabilitation program following cervical (C7–C8) spinal cord injury resulting from diving into a shallow pool. Evaluated yesterday by PT and OT. Alert and oriented × 4; reports pain rated 2/10 after pain med administered. Anterior neck surgical incision intact and healing. Halo fixator in place; no redness or drainage around screws. Breath sounds clear throughout lung fields; no dyspnea. Skin dry with usual pigmentation. Bowel sounds present in all quadrants. Abdomen soft, round, and nondistended. Urinary catheter draining medium-yellow urine with sediment. High-top shoes and antiembolism stockings in place. VS: T 98.6°F (37°C), HR 82 beats/min and regular, RR 18 breaths/min, BP 118/56 mm Hg, SpO$_2$ 95% on RA. Scheduled for first PT session to begin mobility training at 1600.

1815: Reports developing severe "pounding" frontal headache about 10 minutes ago. Face and neck flushed and diaphoretic. States vision is blurred and nose suddenly began feeling "stuffy." VS: T 99°F (37.2°C), HR 58 beats/min and regular, RR 22 breaths/min, BP 194/116 mm Hg, SpO$_2$ 94% on RA.

The nurse reviews the collected data and collaborates with the registered nurse. Complete the following sentence by selecting from the list of word choices below.

The nurse should recognize that the client is likely experiencing [**Word Choice**].

WORD CHOICES
Spasticity
Spinal shock
Neurogenic shock
Autonomic dysreflexia

Thinking Exercise 5.3.3

The nurse is caring for a 21-year-old client in the acute rehabilitation unit.

History and Physical	Nurses' Notes	Orders	Laboratory Results

1550: Client admitted yesterday for acute rehabilitation program following cervical (C7–C8) spinal cord injury resulting from diving into a shallow pool. Evaluated yesterday by PT and OT. Alert and oriented × 4; reports pain rated 2/10 after pain med administered. Anterior neck surgical incision intact and healing. Halo fixator in place; no redness or drainage around screws. Breath sounds clear throughout lung fields; no dyspnea. Skin dry with usual pigmentation. Bowel sounds present in all quadrants. Abdomen soft, round, and nondistended. Urinary catheter draining medium-yellow urine with sediment. High-top shoes and antiembolism stockings in place. VS: T 98.6°F (37°C), HR 82 beats/min and regular, RR 18 breaths/min, BP 118/56 mm Hg, SpO$_2$ 95% on RA. Scheduled for first PT session to begin mobility training at 1600.

1815: Reports developing severe "pounding" frontal headache about 10 minutes ago. Face and neck flushed and diaphoretic. States vision is blurred and nose suddenly began feeling "stuffy." VS: T 99°F (37.2°C), HR 58 beats/min and regular, RR 22 breaths/min, BP 194/116 mm Hg, SpO$_2$ 94% on RA.

The nurse reviews the collected client data and collaborates with the registered nurse. Complete the following sentence by selecting from the lists of options below.

The nurse determines the *priority* for care at this time is to manage the client's **1 [Select]** because the client could develop a(n) **2 [Select]**.

OPTIONS FOR 1	OPTIONS FOR 2
Headache pain	Stroke
Blood pressure	Aneurysm
Heart rate	Pulmonary embolus

Thinking Exercise 5.3.4

The nurse is caring for a 21-year-old client in the acute rehabilitation unit.

History and Physical	Nurses' Notes	Orders	Laboratory Results

1550: Client admitted yesterday for acute rehabilitation program following cervical (C7–C 8) spinal cord injury resulting from diving into a shallow pool. Evaluated yesterday by PT and OT. Alert and oriented × 4; reports pain rated 2/10 after pain med administered. Anterior neck surgical incision intact and healing. Halo fixator in place; no redness or drainage around screws. Breath sounds clear throughout lung fields; no dyspnea. Skin dry with usual pigmentation. Bowel sounds present in all quadrants. Abdomen soft, round, and nondistended. Urinary catheter draining medium-yellow urine with sediment. High-top shoes and antiembolism stockings in place. VS: T 98.6°F (37°C), HR 82 beats/min and regular, RR 18 breaths/min, BP 118/56 mm Hg, SpO$_2$ 95% on RA. Scheduled for first PT session to begin mobility training at 1600.

1815: Reports developing severe "pounding" frontal headache about 10 minutes ago. Face and neck flushed and diaphoretic. States vision is blurred and nose suddenly began feeling "stuffy." VS: T 99°F (37.2°C), HR 58 beats/min and regular, RR 22 breaths/min, BP 194/116 mm Hg, SpO$_2$ 94% on RA.

The nurse collaborates with the registered nurse and contributes to the client's plan of care. Which of the following potential actions would be appropriate for the nurse to take at this time? **Select all that apply**.

○ Lower the head of the client's bed to a flat position.
○ Check the indwelling urinary catheter tubing for kinks.
○ Administer an analgesic medication.
○ Ask the client about bowel habits, especially constipation.
○ Notify the health care provider immediately.

Thinking Exercise 5.3.5

The nurse is caring for a 21-year-old client in the acute rehabilitation unit.

History and Physical	Nurses' Notes	Orders	Laboratory Results

1550: Client admitted yesterday for acute rehabilitation program following cervical (C7–C8) spinal cord injury resulting from diving into a shallow pool. Evaluated yesterday by PT and OT. Alert and oriented $\times$ 4; reports pain rated 2/10 after pain med administered. Anterior neck surgical incision intact and healing. Halo fixator in place; no redness or drainage around screws. Breath sounds clear throughout lung fields; no dyspnea. Skin dry with usual pigmentation. Bowel sounds present in all quadrants. Abdomen soft, round, and nondistended. Urinary catheter draining medium-yellow urine with sediment. High-top shoes and antiembolism stockings in place. VS: T 98.6°F (37°C), HR 82 beats/min and regular, RR 18 breaths/min, BP 118/56 mm Hg, SpO$_2$ 95% on RA. Scheduled for first PT session to begin mobility training at 1600.

1815: Reports developing severe "pounding" frontal headache about 10 minutes ago. Face and neck flushed and diaphoretic. States vision is blurred and nose suddenly began feeling "stuffy." VS: T 99°F (37.2°C), HR 58 beats/min and regular, RR 22 breaths/min, BP 194/116 mm Hg, SpO$_2$ 94% on RA.

1820: Client placed in sitting position. States feeling very nauseated. No kinks or occlusions in urinary catheter. Reports having daily bowel movement with bowel training program. Health care provider notified of client's condition. Orders received.

History and Physical	Nurses' Notes	Orders	Laboratory Results

1820:
- Check BP every 5 minutes until systolic blood pressure (SBP) is less than 150 mm Hg.
- Bedside bladder scan; notify health care provider if residual urine is greater than 100 mL.
- POC urine test for bacteria; if positive, send sample to lab for C&S.
- Immediate-release nifedipine 10 mg; repeat in 30 minutes if SBP is not less than 150 mm Hg.
- Monitor client for seizure activity.
- Notify ICU of possible transfer if BP does not stabilize.

The nurse assists with implementation of the client's plan of care. Select the **1** order the nurse should implement **first.**

○ Check BP every 5 minutes.
○ Perform a bladder scan.
○ Test urine for the presence of bacteria.
○ Administer immediate-release nifedipine.
○ Monitor the client for seizure activity.
○ Notify the ICU of a possible transfer.

Thinking Exercise 5.3.6

The nurse is caring for a 21-year-old client in the acute rehabilitation unit.

History and Physical	Nurses' Notes	Orders	Laboratory Results

1550: Client admitted yesterday for acute rehabilitation program following cervical (C7–C8) spinal cord injury resulting from diving into a shallow pool. Evaluated yesterday by PT and OT. Alert and oriented × 4; reports pain rated 2/10 after pain med administered. Anterior neck surgical incision intact and healing. Halo fixator in place; no redness or drainage around screws. Breath sounds clear throughout lung fields; no dyspnea. Skin dry with usual pigmentation. Bowel sounds present in all quadrants. Abdomen soft, round, and nondistended. Urinary catheter draining medium-yellow urine with sediment. High-top shoes and antiembolism stockings in place. VS: T 98.6°F (37°C), HR 82 beats/min and regular, RR 18 breaths/min, BP 118/56 mm Hg, SpO$_2$ 95% on RA. Scheduled for first PT session to begin mobility training at 1600.

1815: Reports developing severe "pounding" frontal headache about 10 minutes ago. Face and neck flushed and diaphoretic. States vision is blurred and nose suddenly began feeling "stuffy." VS: T 99°F (37.2°C), HR 58 beats/min and regular, RR 22 breaths/min, BP 194/116 mm Hg, SpO$_2$ 94% on RA.

1820: Client placed in sitting position. States feeling very nauseated. No kinks or occlusions in urinary catheter. Reports having daily bowel movement with bowel training program. Health care provider notified of client's condition. Orders received.

1825: IR nifedipine given. BP 182/106 mm Hg.

1830: Urine negative for bacteria. BP 164/100 mm Hg. No neurologic changes.

1845: Bladder scan residual urine 60 mL; BP 174/106 mm Hg. No neurologic changes. ICU notified of possible transfer if BP does not stabilize. Client reports less blurred vision. Flushing and diaphoresis starting to decrease.

1855: HR 76 beats/min and regular. BP 148/90 mm Hg. No neurologic changes, blurred vision, or flushing of face and neck. Reports continued nausea.

History and Physical	Nurses' Notes	Orders	Laboratory Results

1820:
- Check BP every 5 minutes until systolic blood pressure (SBP) is less than 150 mm Hg.
- Bedside bladder scan; notify the health care provider if residual urine is greater than 100 mL.
- POC urine test for bacteria; if positive, send sample to lab for C&S.
- Immediate-release nifedipine 10 mg; repeat in 30 minutes if SBP is not less than 150 mm Hg.
- Monitor client for seizure activity.
- Notify ICU of possible transfer if BP does not stabilize.

The nurse is assisting to evaluate the client's condition based on the most recent collected data. For each data collection finding, select whether the finding indicates that the client's condition has improved or not improved.

DATA COLLECTION FINDING	IMPROVED	NOT IMPROVED
Vision		
Flushing		
Nausea		
Heart rate		
Blood pressure		

Stand-Alone Thinking Exercise 5.1

The nurse is caring for a 34-year-old client in a family practice office.

History and Physical	Nurses' Notes	Orders	Laboratory Results

0830: Client seeking health care today due to experiencing severe fatigue, anorexia, unintended weight loss, increasing muscle aches, morning stiffness (over 1 hour), and painful, swollen hand and ankle joints for over 3 months. Initially thought these findings were the result of working long hours at night in a local meat packing plant. Stands most of the work shift with only one short break. Cares for 2 school-age children as a single parent, but recently asked family to help out due to fatigue and pain. Client has missed work more often in the past 2 months due to fatigue and is afraid of losing job. Currently reports finger joint pain rated 6/10. Alert and oriented × 4. Breath sounds clear throughout lung fields; no dyspnea. Skin very dry; skin on hands cracking in several places. MCPs (knuckles) on both hands slightly swollen, warm, and red. Both ankles with 2+ nonpitting edema; no warmth or redness and are not as achy as hands. VS: T 98.6°F (37°C), HR 80 beats/min and regular, RR 18 breaths/min, BP 122/75 mm Hg, SpO$_2$ 98% on RA.

The nurse reviews the collected data and collaborates with the registered nurse. Complete the diagram by selecting from the choices below to specify what potential condition the client is likely experiencing, **2** nursing actions that are appropriate to take, and **2** parameters the nurse would monitor to assess the client's progress.

Action to Take		
Action to Take	Potential Complication	Parameter to Monitor
		Parameter to Monitor

Actions to Take	Potential Conditions	Parameters to Monitor
Reinforce teaching about drug therapy	Osteoporosis	Uric acid
Reinforce teaching about a low-purine diet	Rheumatoid arthritis	Presence of nodules
Reinforce teaching about the importance of rest balanced with exercise	Osteoarthritis	Joint pain
Reinforce teaching about bisphosphonates	Acute gout	Weight
Reinforce teaching about the client's need to change jobs as soon as possible		Fatigue

Stand-Alone Thinking Exercise 5.2

The nurse is caring for a 42-year-old client who has a follow-up visit with the neurologist.

History and Physical	Nurses' Notes	Orders	Laboratory Results

Medical History:
- Multiple sclerosis (diagnosed 10 years ago)
- Hypothyroidism (diagnosed 6 years ago)
- BMI 28.4, height 5 ft 6 in (66 in) (167.6 cm), weight 176 lb (79.8 kg)

Allergies: No known drug allergies

Medications:
- Glatiramer acetate 20 mg subcutaneously each day
- Oxybutynin 5 mg orally three times a day
- Levothyroxine 50 mcg orally each morning

Social History: Client is married with 2 adolescent children in high school. Reports that worsening multiple sclerosis has affected marriage and was considering separation. Has a housekeeper who cleans once a week; the children help out with household chores and cooking. Started drinking 1 to 2 glasses of wine most evenings to help relax before bed, but had several falls.

History and Physical	Nurses' Notes	Orders	Laboratory Results

1545: Follow-up 6-month visit for multiple sclerosis (MS). Alert and oriented × 4. States had to start using a cane a few weeks ago due to recently falling several times at home. No longer able to drive due to increased muscle spasticity and pain. Reports diplopia (double vision) worse than 6 months ago. Breath sounds clear throughout lung fields; no dyspnea. Bowel sounds present × 4. Abdomen soft, round, and nondistended. Can move all extremities, but left arm and leg weaker than right. Pulses 2+ bilaterally. Capillary refill <3 sec. VS: T 98°F (36.7°C), HR 80 beats/min and regular, RR 18 breaths/min, BP 120/74 mm Hg, SpO$_2$ 97% on RA.

The nurse reviews the collected data and collaborates with the registered nurse. Complete the diagram by selecting from the choices below to specify what potential condition the client is *most* at risk for, **2** nursing actions that are appropriate to take, and **2** parameters the client, family, and nurse would monitor to assess the client's progress.

Action to Take		Potential Complication		Parameter to Monitor
Action to Take				Parameter to Monitor

Actions to Take	Potential Conditions Most At Risk		Parameters to Monitor
Refer the client for evaluation by physical therapy	Contractures		Frequency of falls
Reinforce teaching about ways to prevent infection	Incontinence		Use of ambulatory aids
Reinforce teaching about performing range-of-motion exercises	ADL dependence		ADL ability
Remind the client to wear contact lenses to help decrease diplopia	Falls		Urinary function
Remind the client to avoid drinking alcohol			Frequency of infections

Client Conditions Affecting Glucose Regulation

Unfolding Case Study 6.1

Thinking Exercise 6.1.1

The nurse is caring for a 31-year-old client in the emergency department (ED).

History and Physical	Nurses' Notes	Orders	Laboratory Results

2020: Family brought client to ED due to new-onset nausea and vomiting, abdominal discomfort, headache, and fatigue. Client states craving water more than usual; has been voiding in frequent large amounts. Medical history includes type 1 diabetes mellitus (DM) for over 15 years, substance use disorder (has been "clean" for almost 2 years), and bipolar disorder. Alert and oriented × 4. Breath sounds clear throughout lung fields. Fruity smelling breath. Client states has not been carefully following the prescribed diabetic diet but knows when and what to eat. Abdomen soft, round, and nontender. Skin dry with usual pigmentation. Bowel sounds present in all quadrants. VS: T 100.8°F (38.2°C), HR 102 beats/min and irregular, RR 28 breaths/min, BP 88/46 mm Hg, SpO_2 96% on RA. FSBG 528 mg/dL (29.3 mmol/L). (Normal range 70–110 mg/dL [3.89–6.11 mmol/L].)

The nurse collects data from the client. Which of the following client findings require **immediate** follow-up? **Select all that apply.**

O Nausea and vomiting
O Blood glucose level
O Fatigue
O Body temperature
O SpO_2
O Respiratory rate

Thinking Exercise 6.1.2

The nurse is caring for a 31-year-old client in the emergency department.

History and Physical	Nurses' Notes	Orders	Laboratory Results

2020: Family brought client to ED due to new-onset nausea and vomiting, abdominal discomfort, headache, and fatigue. Client states craving water more than usual; has been voiding in frequent large amounts. Medical history includes type 1 diabetes mellitus (DM) for over 15 years, substance use disorder (has been "clean" for almost 2 years), and bipolar disorder. Alert and oriented × 4. Breath sounds clear throughout lung fields. Fruity smelling breath. Client states has not been carefully following the prescribed diabetic diet but knows when and what to eat. Abdomen soft, round, and nontender. Skin dry with usual pigmentation. Bowel sounds present in all quadrants. VS: T 100.8°F (38.2°C), HR 102 beats/min and irregular, RR 28 breaths/min, BP 88/46 mm Hg, SpO_2 96% on RA. FSBG 528 mg/dL (29.3 mmol/L). (Normal range 70–110 mg/dL [3.89–6.11 mmol/L].)

The nurse reviews the collected client data and collaborates with the registered nurse. Complete the following sentence by selecting from the list of word choices below.

The nurse recognizes that the client is likely experiencing early **[Word Choice]**.

WORD CHOICES
Infection
Alcohol poisoning
Diabetic ketoacidosis
Hyperosmolar hyperglycemic nonketotic syndrome

Thinking Exercise 6.1.3

The nurse is caring for a 31-year-old client in the emergency department.

History and Physical	Nurses' Notes	Orders	Laboratory Results

2020: Family brought client to ED due to new-onset nausea and vomiting, abdominal discomfort, headache, and fatigue. Client states craving water more than usual; has been voiding in frequent large amounts. Medical history includes type 1 diabetes mellitus (DM) for over 15 years, substance use disorder (has been "clean" for almost 2 years), and bipolar disorder. Alert and oriented × 4. Breath sounds clear throughout lung fields. Fruity smelling breath. Client states has not been carefully following the prescribed diabetic diet but knows when and what to eat. Abdomen soft, round, and nontender. Skin dry with usual pigmentation. Bowel sounds present in all quadrants. VS: T 100.8°F (38.2°C), HR 102 beats/min and irregular, RR 28 breaths/min, BP 88/46 mm Hg, SpO$_2$ 96% on RA. FSBG 528 mg/dL (29.3 mmol/L). (Normal range 70–110 mg/dL [3.89–6.11 mmol/L].)

The nurse reviews the collected client data and collaborates with the registered nurse. Complete the following sentence by selecting from the lists of options below.

The nurse determines the *priority* for care at this time is to manage the client's **1 [Select]** as evidenced by **2 [Select]** and **3 [Select]**.

OPTIONS FOR 1	OPTIONS FOR 2	OPTIONS FOR 3
Hyperglycemia	Tachycardia	Fruity breath
Dehydration	Tachypnea	Hypotension
Nausea and vomiting	Hypoxia	Diuresis

Thinking Exercise 6.1.4

The nurse is caring for a 31-year-old client in the emergency department.

History and Physical	Nurses' Notes	Orders	Laboratory Results

2020: Family brought client to ED due to new-onset nausea and vomiting, abdominal discomfort, headache, and fatigue. Client states craving water more than usual; has been voiding in frequent large amounts. Medical history includes type 1 diabetes mellitus (DM) for over 15 years, substance use disorder (has been "clean" for almost 2 years), and bipolar disorder. Alert and oriented × 4. Breath sounds clear throughout lung fields. Fruity smelling breath. Client states has not been carefully following the prescribed diabetic diet but knows when and what to eat. Abdomen soft, round, and nontender. Skin dry with usual pigmentation. Bowel sounds present in all quadrants. VS: T 100.8°F (38.2°C), HR 102 beats/min and irregular, RR 28 breaths/min, BP 88/46 mm Hg, SpO$_2$ 95% on RA. FSBG 528 mg/dL (29.3 mmol/L). (Normal range 70–110 mg/dL [3.89–6.11 mmol/L].)

2050: Stat labs drawn; urinalysis sent to lab. Peripheral venous access established.

The nurse collaborates with the registered nurse and contributes to the client's plan of care. Select whether the following potential nursing actions are indicated or not indicated for the client at this time.

POTENTIAL NURSING ACTIONS	INDICATED	NOT INDICATED
Monitor IV fluid infusion of 5% dextrose/normal saline.		
Monitor the client's heart rate and rhythm.		
Monitor serum electrolyte levels.		
Begin supplemental oxygen via nasal cannula.		
Monitor FSBG levels during IV regular insulin administration.		

Thinking Exercise 6.1.5

The nurse is caring for a 31-year-old client in the emergency department.

History and Physical	Nurses' Notes	Orders	Laboratory Results

Emergency Department:
2020: Family brought client to ED due to new-onset nausea and vomiting, abdominal discomfort, headache, and fatigue. Client states craving water more than usual; has been voiding in frequent large amounts. Medical history includes type 1 diabetes mellitus (DM) for over 15 years, substance use disorder (has been "clean" for almost 2 years), and bipolar disorder. Alert and oriented × 4. Breath sounds clear throughout lung fields. Fruity smelling breath. Client states has not been carefully following the prescribed diabetic diet but knows when and what to eat. Abdomen soft, round, and nontender. Skin dry with usual pigmentation. Bowel sounds present in all quadrants. VS: T 100.8°F (38.2°C), HR 102 beats/min and irregular, RR 28 breaths/min, BP 88/46 mm Hg, SpO2 95% on RA. FSBG 528 mg/dL (29.3 mmol/L). (Normal range 70–110 mg/dL [3.89–6.11 mmol/L].)

2050: Stat labs drawn; urinalysis sent to lab. Peripheral venous access established.

2145: IV regular insulin infusion started per protocol. Cardiac monitoring initiated. Labs entered and provider notified. VS: 100°F (37.8°C), HR 98 beats/min and irregular, RR 22 breaths/min, BP 106/58 mm Hg, SpO2 96% on RA. FSBG 326 mg/dL (18.09 mmol/L).

Acute Medical Unit:
2230: Transferred to acute medical unit for continued care.

History and Physical	Nurses' Notes	Orders	Laboratory Results
Serum Laboratory Tests and Reference Ranges		**2050**	
Potassium (3.5–5.0 mEq/L [3.5–5.0 mmol/L])		6.4 mEq/L (6.4 mmol/L)	
Sodium (136–145 mEq/L [136–145 mmol/L])		127 mEq/L (127 mmol/L)	
Glucose (74–106 mg/dL [4.1–5.9 mmol/L])		512 mg/dL (28.4 mmol/L)	
Blood urea nitrogen (BUN) (10–20 mg/dL [3.6–7.1 mmol/L])		58 mg/dL (20.7 mmol/L)	
Creatinine (0.7–1.3 mg/dL [61.89–114.95 µmol])		1.1 mg/dL (97.26 µmol/L)	

The nurse reviews the most recent nurses' notes and is assisting to evaluate the client's condition based on the collected data. Select the **5** actions that the nurse would potentially implement.
○ Continue to monitor and record blood glucose levels frequently per agency protocol.
○ Encourage water and other appropriate fluids as tolerated.
○ Record fluid intake and urine output per agency protocol.
○ Increase supplemental oxygen from 3 L/min to 4 L/min via NC.
○ Maintain continuous cardiac monitoring.
○ Insert an indwelling urinary catheter for hourly monitoring.
○ Collaborate with the registered nurse regarding potassium administration.

The nurse is caring for a 31-year-old client in the emergency department.

History and Physical	Nurses' Notes	Orders	Laboratory Results

Emergency Department:
2020: Family brought client to ED due to new-onset nausea and vomiting, abdominal discomfort, headache, and fatigue. Client states craving water more than usual; has been voiding in frequent large amounts. Medical history includes type 1 diabetes mellitus (DM) for over 15 years, substance use disorder (has been "clean" for almost 2 years), and bipolar disorder. Alert and oriented × 4. Breath sounds clear throughout lung fields. Fruity smelling breath. Client states has not been carefully following the prescribed diabetic diet but knows when and what to eat. Abdomen soft, round, and nontender. Skin dry with usual pigmentation. Bowel sounds present in all quadrants. VS: T 100.8°F (38.2°C), HR 102 beats/min and irregular, RR 28 breaths/min, BP 88/46 mm Hg, SpO$_2$ 95% on RA. FSBG 528 mg/dL (29.3 mmol/L). (Normal range 70–110 mg/dL [3.89–6.11 mmol/L].)

2050: Stat labs drawn; urinalysis sent to lab. Peripheral venous access established.

2145: IV regular insulin infusion started per protocol. Cardiac monitoring initiated. Labs entered and provider notified. VS: 100°F (37.8°C), HR 98 beats/min and irregular, RR 22 breaths/min, BP 106/58 mm Hg, SpO$_2$ 96% on RA. FSBG 326 mg/dL (18.09 mmol/L).

Acute Medical Unit:
2230: Transferred to acute medical unit for continued care.

0030: Alert and oriented × 4. IV regular insulin and fluids infusing per protocol. VS: 99°F (37.2°C), HR 89 beats/min and irregular, RR 20 breaths/min, BP 118/66 mm Hg, SpO$_2$ 97% on RA. FSBG 275 mg/dL (15.26 mmol/L).

The nurse reviews the most recent nurses' notes and is assisting to evaluate the client's condition based on the collected data. For each data collection finding, select whether the finding indicates that the client's status has improved or is unchanged.

DATA COLLECTION FINDING	IMPROVED	UNCHANGED
Blood glucose		
Cardiac rhythm		
Temperature		
Blood pressure		

Unfolding Case Study 6.2

The nurse is caring for a 23-year-old client at the urgent care center. Highlight the client findings that require **immediate** follow-up.

History and Physical	Nurses' Notes	Orders	Laboratory Results

1435: Friend brought client to center due to new-onset signs and symptoms including shakiness, irritability, lightheadedness, and diaphoresis. Medical history includes anorexia nervosa, anemia, and recent diagnosis of type 1 diabetes mellitus (DM). Alert and oriented × 3 (person, place, and event). Breath sounds clear throughout lung fields. Client states has not eaten today except for a protein bar at around 0730. Abdomen soft, round, and nontender. Skin cool and very moist. Bowel sounds present in all quadrants. Able to move all extremities; cap refill <3 sec. VS: T 98.6°F (37°C), HR 58 beats/min and irregular, RR 18 breaths/min, BP 92/56 mm Hg, SpO$_2$ 96% on RA. FSBG 50 mg/dL (2.77 mmol/L). (Normal range 70–110 mg/dL [3.89–6.11 mmol/L].) Reported height 5 ft 10 inches (178 cm), reported weight 110 lb (49.9 kg).

Thinking Exercise 6.2.2

The nurse is caring for a 23-year-old client at the urgent care center.

History and Physical	Nurses' Notes	Orders	Laboratory Results

1435: Friend brought client to center due to new-onset signs and symptoms including shakiness, irritability, light-headedness, and diaphoresis. Medical history includes anorexia nervosa, anemia, and recent diagnosis of type 1 diabetes mellitus (DM). Alert and oriented × 3 (person, place, and event). Breath sounds clear throughout lung fields. Client states has not eaten today except for a protein bar at around 0730. Abdomen soft, round, and nontender. Skin cool and very moist. Bowel sounds present in all quadrants. Able to move all extremities; cap refill <3 sec. VS: T 98.6°F (37°C), HR 58 beats/min and irregular, RR 18 breaths/min, BP 92/56 mm Hg, SpO$_2$ 96% on RA. FSBG 50 mg/dL (2.77 mmol/L). (Normal range 70–110 mg/dL [3.89–6.11 mmol/L].) Reported height 5 ft 10 inches (1.78 m), reported weight 110 lb (49.9 kg).

The nurse reviews the collected client data and collaborates with the registered nurse. Complete the following sentence by selecting from the lists of options below

The nurse recognizes that the client is experiencing **1 [Select]** as evidenced by the client's **2 [Select]** and **3 [Select]**.

OPTIONS FOR 1	OPTIONS FOR 2	OPTIONS FOR 3
Diabetic ketoacidosis	FSBG	Anemia
Acute hypoglycemia	Heart rate	Blood pressure
Acute ischemic stroke	Body weight	Diaphoresis

Thinking Exercise 6.2.3

The nurse is caring for a 23-year-old client at the urgent care center.

History and Physical	Nurses' Notes	Orders	Laboratory Results

1435: Friend brought client to center due to new-onset signs and symptoms including shakiness, irritability, light-headedness, and diaphoresis. Medical history includes anorexia nervosa, anemia, and recent diagnosis of type 1 diabetes mellitus (DM). Alert and oriented × 3 (person, place, and event). Breath sounds clear throughout lung fields. Client states has not eaten today except for a protein bar at around 0730. Abdomen soft, round, and nontender. Skin cool and very moist. Bowel sounds present in all quadrants. Able to move all extremities; cap refill <3 sec. VS: T 98.6°F (37°C), HR 58 beats/min and irregular, RR 18 breaths/min, BP 92/56 mm Hg, SpO$_2$ 96% on RA. FSBG 50 mg/dL (2.77 mmol/L). (Normal range 70–110 mg/dL [3.89–6.11 mmol/L].) Reported height 5 ft 10 inches (1.78 m), reported weight 110 lb (49.9 kg).

The nurse reviews the collected client data and collaborates with the registered nurse. Complete the following sentence by selecting from the list of word choices below.

The nurse determines the *priority* for care is to manage the client's [**Word Choice**].

WORD CHOICES
Anorexia nervosa
Dehydration
Hypoglycemia
Neurologic changes

Thinking Exercise 6.2.4

The nurse is caring for a 23-year-old client at the urgent care center.

History and Physical	Nurses' Notes	Orders	Laboratory Results

1435: Friend brought client to center due to new-onset signs and symptoms including shakiness, irritability, light-headedness, and diaphoresis. Medical history includes anorexia nervosa, anemia, and recent diagnosis of type 1 diabetes mellitus (DM). Alert and oriented × 3 (person, place, and event). Breath sounds clear throughout lung fields. Client states has not eaten today except for a protein bar at around 0730. Abdomen soft, round, and nontender. Skin cool and very moist. Bowel sounds present in all quadrants. Able to move all extremities; cap refill <3 sec. VS: T 98.6°F (37°C), HR 58 beats/min and irregular, RR 18 breaths/min, BP 92/56 mm Hg, SpO$_2$ 96% on RA. FSBG 50 mg/dL (2.77 mmol/L). (Normal range 70–110 mg/dL [3.89–6.11 mmol/L].) Reported height 5 ft 10 inches (1.78 m), reported weight 110 lb (49.9 kg).

1445: History and physical performed by provider. Client states "I took two doses of lispro today—one before breakfast and one before lunch. I was working and didn't have time to have any lunch yet."

The nurse collaborates with the registered nurse and contributes to the client's plan of care. Select whether the following potential nursing actions are indicated or not indicated for the client at this time.

POTENTIAL NURSING ACTIONS	INDICATED	NOT INDICATED
Administer subcutaneous glucagon per agency protocol.		
Give 15 g of fast-acting carbohydrates such as 4 oz (120 mL) of apple juice.		
Start 50 mL of 50% dextrose IV per agency protocol.		
Retest FSBG following the initial intervention to treat hypoglycemia.		

Thinking Exercise 6.2.5

The nurse is caring for a 23-year-old client at the urgent care center.

History and Physical	Nurses' Notes	Orders	Laboratory Results

1435: Friend brought client to center due to new-onset signs and symptoms including shakiness, irritability, light-headedness, and diaphoresis. Medical history includes anorexia nervosa, anemia and recent diagnosis of type 1 diabetes mellitus (DM). Alert and oriented × 3 (person, place, and event). Breath sounds clear throughout lung fields. Client states has not eaten today except for a protein bar at around 0730. Abdomen soft, round, and nontender. Skin cool and very moist. Bowel sounds present in all quadrants. Able to move all extremities; cap refill <3 sec. VS: T 98.6°F (37°C), HR 58 beats/min and irregular, RR 18 breaths/min, BP 92/56 mm Hg, SpO$_2$ 96% on RA. FSBG 50 mg/dL (2.77 mmol/L). (Normal range 70–110 mg/dL [3.89–6.11 mmol/L].) Reported height 5 ft 10 inches (1.78 m), reported weight 110 lb (49.9 kg).

1445: History and physical performed by provider. Client states "I took two doses of lispro today—one before breakfast and one before lunch. I was working and didn't have time to have any lunch yet."

The nurse assists with implementation of the client's plan of care. Select the **2** actions the nurse should implement at this time.

○ Establish peripheral intravenous access.
○ Administer subcutaneous glucagon per agency protocol.
○ Give 15 g of fast-acting carbohydrates such as 4 oz (120 mL) of apple juice.
○ Provide discharge teaching about diabetes to improve glucose control.
○ Retest FSBG following the initial intervention to treat hypoglycemia.

Thinking Exercise 6.2.6—Pharmacology

The nurse is caring for a 23-year-old client at the urgent care center.

History and Physical	Nurses' Notes	Orders	Laboratory Results

1435: Friend brought client to center due to new-onset signs and symptoms including shakiness, irritability, light-headedness, and diaphoresis. Medical history includes anorexia nervosa, anemia, and recent diagnosis of type 1 diabetes mellitus (DM). Alert and oriented × 3 (person, place, and event). Breath sounds clear throughout lung fields. Client states has not eaten today except for a protein bar at around 0730. Abdomen soft, round, and nontender. Skin cool and very moist. Bowel sounds present in all quadrants. Able to move all extremities; cap refill <3 sec. VS: T 98.6°F (37°C), HR 58 beats/min and irregular, RR 18 breaths/min, BP 92/56 mm Hg, SpO$_2$ 96% on RA. FSBG 50 mg/dL (2.77 mmol/L). (Normal range 70–110 mg/dL [3.89–6.11 mmol/L].) Reported height 5 ft 10 inches (1.78 m), reported weight 110 lb (49.9 kg).

1445: History and physical performed by provider. Client states "I took two doses of lispro today—one before breakfast and one before lunch. I was working and didn't have time to have any lunch yet."

1450: Drank 4 oz (120 mL) of apple juice.

1510: FSBG 72 mg/dL (3.99 mmol/L). After glucose tested, ate package of peanut butter crackers. Alert and oriented × 4. States feeling less shaky and light-headed. Skin continues to be cool and moist.

1530: Health teaching provided to prepare for discharge to home.

The nurse reviews the collected client data with the registered nurse and reinforces teaching with the client. Select whether the following client statements indicate understanding or no understanding of the discharge teaching provided.

CLIENT STATEMENTS	UNDERSTANDING	NO UNDERSTANDING
"I need to more carefully follow the prescribed diet to control this disorder."		
"I should follow up with my primary care provider to monitor my hemoglobin A1c."		
"I should carry some hard candies with me in case my sugar drops too low."		
"I plan to get an insulin pump, which will control my diabetes."		
"I should keep injectable glucagon on hand just in case."		

Unfolding Case Study 6.3

Thinking Exercise 6.3.1

The nurse is caring for a 59-year-old client in the family practice office.

History and Physical	Nurses' Notes	Orders	Laboratory Results

Medical History:
- Hypertension (diagnosed 3 years ago)
- Hypercholesteremia (diagnosed 3 years ago)
- Type 2 DM (diagnosed 5 years ago)
- Gastroesophageal reflux disease (for many years)
- Eczema (worsened in past few weeks and is reason for office visit)
- BMI 33.8, height 6 ft (183 cm), weight 249 lb (112.9 kg)

Allergies: Sulfa (urticaria)

Medications:
- Amlodipine
- Famotidine
- Losartan
- Lovastatin
- Metformin

Social History: Client is married with no children and works 2 days a week as a security guard. Retired from a manufacturing supervisor position. Reports diet primarily consists of meats and starches, although has been eating more salads lately. Able to verbalize prescribed diet needed to help control BP and glucose. Hobbies include watching television and cooking for wife, who works remotely full-time as a tutor.

History and Physical	Nurses' Notes	Orders	Laboratory Results

1435: Requested office visit for worsening eczema (primarily on legs) and increasing fatigue since having COVID-19 3 months ago. Alert and oriented × 4. Breath sounds clear throughout lung fields. Abdomen soft, round, and nontender. Bowel sounds present in all quadrants. Able to move all extremities; finger joints arthritic with bony nodules. Cap refill >3 sec. Pulses present at 2+, except for pedal pulses, which are not palpable. Varicose veins on both lower legs. Skin dry and warm. Peppery, itchy rash with crusty reddened patches on both lower legs. VS: T 98.6°F (37°C), HR 88 beats/min and regular, RR 18 breaths/min, BP 184/100 mm Hg, SpO$_2$ 96% on RA. FSBG 450 mg/dL (24.98 mmol/L). (Normal range 70–110 mg/dL [3.89–6.11 mmol/L].) BMI 33.8.

The nurse reviews the collected client data with the registered nurse. Which of the following client findings require **immediate** follow-up? **Select all that apply.**

○ Fatigue
○ Varicose veins
○ Eczema on legs
○ Blood pressure
○ Heart rate
○ Blood glucose
○ BMI

Thinking Exercise 6.3.2

The nurse is caring for a 59-year-old client in the family practice office.

History and Physical	Nurses' Notes	Orders	Laboratory Results

Medical History:
- Hypertension (diagnosed 3 years ago)
- Hypercholesteremia (diagnosed 3 years ago)
- Type 2 DM (diagnosed 5 years ago)
- Gastroesophageal reflux disease (for many years)
- Eczema (worsened in past few weeks and is reason for office visit)
- BMI 33.8, height 6 ft (183 cm), weight 249 lb (112.9 kg)

Allergies: Sulfa (urticaria)

Medications:
- Amlodipine
- Famotidine
- Losartan
- Lovastatin
- Metformin

Social History: Client is married with no children and works 2 days a week as a security guard. Retired from a manufacturing supervisor position. Reports diet primarily consists of meats and starches, although has been eating more salads lately. Able to verbalize prescribed diet needed to help control BP and glucose. Hobbies include watching television and cooking for wife, who works remotely full-time as a tutor.

History and Physical	Nurses' Notes	Orders	Laboratory Results

1435: Requested office visit for worsening eczema (primarily on legs) and increasing fatigue since having COVID-19 3 months ago. Alert and oriented × 4. Breath sounds clear throughout lung fields. Abdomen soft, round, and nontender. Bowel sounds present in all quadrants. Able to move all extremities; finger joints arthritic with bony nodules. Cap refill >3 sec. Pulses present at 2+, except for pedal pulses, which are not palpable. Varicose veins on both lower legs. Skin dry and warm. Peppery, itchy rash with crusty reddened patches on both lower legs. VS: T 98.6°F (37°C), HR 88 beats/min and regular, RR 18 breaths/min, BP 184/100 mm Hg, SpO$_2$ 96% on RA. FSBG 450 mg/dL (24.98 mmol/L). (Normal range 70–110 mg/dL [3.89–6.11 mmol/L].) BMI 33.8.

1450: Physical examination by provider; review of lab results drawn 2 days ago. Most labs within normal range. Hemoglobin A1c 10.8% (normal range 4%–5.9%).

The nurse reviews the collected client data and collaborates with the registered nurse. Complete the following sentence by selecting from the list of word choices below.

The nurse recognizes that the client is most at risk for developing **[Word Choice]** and **[Word Choice]**.

WORD CHOICES
Sepsis
Obesity
Stroke
Diabetic ketoacidosis
Hyperosmolar hyperglycemic nonketotic syndrome

Thinking Exercise 6.3.3

The nurse is caring for a 59-year-old client in the family practice office.

History and Physical	Nurses' Notes	Orders	Laboratory Results

Medical History:
- Hypertension (diagnosed 3 years ago)
- Hypercholesteremia (diagnosed 3 years ago)
- Type 2 DM (diagnosed 5 years ago)
- Gastroesophageal reflux disease (for many years)
- Eczema (worsened in past few weeks and is reason for office visit)
- BMI 33.8, height 6 ft (183 cm), weight 249 lb (112.9 kg)

Allergies: Sulfa (urticaria)

Medications:
- Amlodipine
- Famotidine
- Losartan
- Lovastatin
- Metformin

Social History: Client is married with no children and works 2 days a week as a security guard. Retired from a manufacturing supervisor position. Reports diet primarily consists of meats and starches, although has been eating more salads lately. Able to verbalize prescribed diet needed to help control BP and glucose. Hobbies include watching television and cooking for wife, who works remotely full-time as a tutor.

History and Physical	Nurses' Notes	Orders	Laboratory Results

1435: Requested office visit for worsening eczema (primarily on legs) and increasing fatigue since having COVID-19 3 months ago. Alert and oriented × 4. Breath sounds clear throughout lung fields. Abdomen soft, round, and nontender. Bowel sounds present in all quadrants. Able to move all extremities; finger joints arthritic with bony nodules. Cap refill >3 sec. Pulses present at 2+, except for pedal pulses, which are not palpable. Varicose veins on both lower legs. Skin dry and warm. Peppery, itchy rash with crusty reddened patches on both lower legs. VS: T 98.6°F (37°C), HR 88 beats/min and regular, RR 18 breaths/min, BP 184/100 mm Hg, SpO$_2$ 96% on RA. FSBG 450 mg/dL (24.98 mmol/L). (Normal range 70–110 mg/dL [3.89–6.11 mmol/L].) BMI 33.8.

1450: Physical examination by provider; review of lab results drawn 2 days ago. Most labs within normal range. Hemoglobin A1c 10.8% (normal range 4%–5.9%).

The nurse reviews the collected client data and collaborates with the registered nurse. Select the **2** priorities for the client's care at this time.
- ○ Treating the eczema
- ○ Providing health teaching about diet
- ○ Managing the hypertension
- ○ Treating the fatigue
- ○ Decreasing the blood glucose level

Thinking Exercise 6.3.4

The nurse is caring for a 59-year-old client in the family practice office.

History and Physical	Nurse's Notes	Orders	Laboratory Results

Medical History:
- Hypertension (diagnosed 3 years ago)
- Hypercholesteremia (diagnosed 3 years ago)
- Type 2 DM (diagnosed 5 years ago)
- Gastroesophageal reflux disease (for many years)
- Eczema (worsened in past few weeks and is reason for office visit)
- BMI 33.8, height 6 ft (183 cm), weight 249 lb (112.9 kg)

Allergies: Sulfa (urticaria)

Medications:
- Amlodipine
- Famotidine
- Losartan
- Lovastatin
- Metformin

Social History: Client is married with no children and works 2 days a week as a security guard. Retired from a manufacturing supervisor position. Reports diet primarily consists of meats and starches, although has been eating more salads lately. Able to verbalize prescribed diet that is needed to help control BP and glucose. Hobbies include watching television and cooking for wife, who works remotely full-time as a tutor.

History and Physical	Nurses' Notes	Orders	Laboratory Results

1435: Requested office visit for worsening eczema (primarily on legs) and increasing fatigue since having COVID-19 3 months ago. Alert and oriented × 4. Breath sounds clear throughout lung fields. Abdomen soft, round, and nontender. Bowel sounds present in all quadrants. Able to move all extremities; finger joints arthritic with bony nodules. Cap refill >3 sec. Pulses present at 2+, except for pedal pulses, which are not palpable. Varicose veins on both lower legs. Skin dry and warm. Peppery, itchy rash with crusty reddened patches on both lower legs. VS: T 98.6°F (37°C), HR 88 beats/min and regular, RR 18 breaths/min, BP 184/100 mm Hg, SpO$_2$ 96% on RA. FSBG 450 mg/dL (24.98 mmol/L). (Normal range 70–110 mg/dL [3.89–6.11 mmol/L].) BMI 33.8.

1450: Physical examination by provider; review of lab results drawn 2 days ago. Most labs within normal range. Hemoglobin A1c 10.8% (normal range 4%–5.9%).

The nurse collaborates with the registered nurse and contributes to the client's plan of care. For each body system, select the potential nursing actions that are appropriate as part of the client's plan of care.

BODY SYSTEM/PROCESS	POTENTIAL NURSING ACTIONS
Endocrine	○ Reinforce teaching about new diabetic medication to replace metformin. ○ Give the client a fast-acting insulin bolus in the office. ○ Teach the client about the need to wear an emergency ID card, bracelet, or necklace.
Cardiovascular	○ Schedule a cardiac catheterization procedure. ○ Explain the need to increase the daily antihypertensive drug dosage. ○ Schedule vascular studies of the lower extremities.
Nutrition	○ Refer the client to a registered dietitian nutritionist. ○ Explain the relationship of BMI to glucose control. ○ Reinforce teaching about the need for regular exercise.

Thinking Exercise 6.3.5—Pharmacology

The nurse is caring for a 59-year-old client in the family practice office.

History and Physical	Nurses' Notes	Orders	Laboratory Results

Medical History:
- Hypertension (diagnosed 3 years ago)
- Hypercholesteremia (diagnosed 3 years ago)
- Type 2 DM (diagnosed 5 years ago)
- Gastroesophageal reflux disease (for many years)
- Eczema (worsened in past few weeks and is reason for office visit)
- BMI 33.8, height 6 ft (183 cm), weight 249 lb (112.9 kg)

Allergies: Sulfa (urticaria)

Medications:
- Amlodipine
- Famotidine
- Losartan
- Lovastatin
- Metformin

Social History: Client is married with no children and works 2 days a week as a security guard. Retired from a manufacturing supervisor position. Reports diet primarily consists of meats and starches, although has been eating more salads lately. Able to verbalize prescribed diet needed to help control BP and glucose. Hobbies include watching television and cooking for wife, who works remotely full-time as a tutor.

History and Physical	Nurse's Notes	Orders	Laboratory Results

1435: Requested office visit for worsening eczema (primarily on legs) and increasing fatigue since having COVID-19 3 months ago. Alert and oriented × 4. Breath sounds clear throughout lung fields. Abdomen soft, round, and nontender. Bowel sounds present in all quadrants. Able to move all extremities; finger joints arthritic with bony nodules. Cap refill >3 sec. Pulses present at 2+, except for pedal pulses, which are not palpable. Varicose veins on both lower legs. Skin dry and warm. Peppery, itchy rash with crusty reddened patches on both lower legs. VS: T 98.6°F (37°C), HR 88 beats/min and regular, RR 18 breaths/min, BP 184/100 mm Hg, SpO_2 96% on RA. FSBG 450 mg/dL (24.98 mmol/L). (Normal range 70–110 mg/dL [3.89–6.11 mmol/L].) BMI 33.8.

1450: Physical examination by provider; review of lab results drawn 2 days ago. Most labs within normal range. Hemoglobin A1c 10.8% (normal range 4%–5.9%).

1530: Rx for increased dose of amlodipine from 5 to 10 mg. Discontinued metformin; to begin empagliflozin 10 mg orally each day. Reinforced teaching about new diabetic medication. Reminded to follow prescribed diabetic diet and exercise on a regular basis to lose weight and gain glucose control. Reviewed signs and symptoms of diabetic emergencies. Scheduled for vascular studies of lower extremities next Friday. Follow-up office visit scheduled for 1 month.

The nurse collaborates with the registered nurse and assists with implementation of the client's plan of care. Which of the following statements would the nurse include when reinforcing health teaching about empagliflozin? **Select all that apply.**

○ "This drug works to eliminate excess glucose through your urine."
○ "You may gain weight while taking this drug."
○ "Report any symptoms of urinary tract infection such as burning and frequency."
○ "You will need follow-up laboratory testing to check your electrolyte levels."
○ "This drug will help decrease your hemoglobin A1c level to 7% or lower.
○ "This drug will help reduce your risk of long-term complications of diabetes."

Thinking Exercise 6.3.6

The nurse is caring for a 59-year-old client in the family practice office.

History and Physical	Nurses' Notes	Orders	Laboratory Results

Medical History:
- Hypertension (diagnosed 3 years ago)
- Hypercholesteremia (diagnosed 3 years ago)
- Type 2 DM (diagnosed 5 years ago)
- Gastroesophageal reflux disease (for many years)
- Eczema (worsened in past few weeks and is reason for office visit)
- BMI 33.8, height 6 ft (183 cm), weight 249 lb (112.9 kg)

Allergies: Sulfa (urticaria)

Medications:
- Amlodipine
- Famotidine
- Losartan
- Lovastatin
- Metformin

Social History: Client is married with no children and works 2 days a week as a security guard. Retired from a manufacturing supervisor position. Reports diet primarily consists of meats and starches, although has been adding more salads lately. Able to verbalize prescribed diet needed to help control BP and glucose. Hobbies include watching television and cooking for wife, who works remotely full-time as a tutor.

History and Physical	Nurses' Notes	Orders	Laboratory Results

1435: Requested office visit for worsening eczema (primarily on legs) and increasing fatigue since having COVID-19 3 months ago. Alert and oriented × 4. Breath sounds clear throughout lung fields. Abdomen soft, round, and nontender. Bowel sounds present in all quadrants. Able to move all extremities; finger joints arthritic with bony nodules. Cap refill >3 sec. Pulses present at 2+, except for pedal pulses, which are not palpable. Varicose veins on both lower legs. Skin dry and warm. Peppery, itchy rash with crusty reddened patches on both lower legs. VS: T 98.6°F (37°C), HR 88 beats/min and regular, RR 18 breaths/min, BP 184/100 mm Hg, SpO$_2$ 96% on RA. FSBG 450 mg/dL (24.98 mmol/L). (Normal range 70–110 mg/dL [3.89–6.11 mmol/L].) BMI 33.8.

1450: Physical examination by provider; review of lab results drawn 2 days ago. Most labs within normal range. Hemoglobin A1c 10.8% (normal range 4%–5.9%).

1530: Rx for increased dose of amlodipine from 5 mg to 10 mg. Discontinued metformin; to begin empagliflozin 10 mg orally each day. Reinforced teaching about new diabetic medication. Reminded to follow prescribed diabetic diet and exercise on a regular basis to lose weight and gain glucose control. Reviewed signs and symptoms of diabetic emergencies. Scheduled for vascular studies of lower extremities next Friday. Follow-up office visit scheduled for 1 month.

1-Month Follow-up Visit:
1020: Follow-up visit for poor diabetic and blood pressure control diagnosed last month. Medication changes and health teaching provided at last visit. Laboratory results from yesterday show hemoglobin A1c decreased to 8.9%. VS: T 98.6°F (37°C), HR 86 beats/min and regular, RR 20 breaths/min, BP 142/86 mm Hg, SpO$_2$ 96% on RA. Non-fasting FSBG 128 mg/dL (7.10 mmol/L). (Normal range 70–110 mg/dL [3.89–6.11 mmol/L].) Weight decreased to 230 lb (104.3 kg). BMI 31.2. Reports following diet and exercising regularly since last visit. No UTI or other side effects resulting from medication changes.

The nurse reviews the most recent nurses' notes and is assisting to evaluate the client's condition based on the collected data. For each data collection finding, select whether the finding indicates that the client's status has improved or is unchanged.

DATA COLLECTION FINDING	IMPROVED	UNCHANGED
Hemoglobin A1c		
Blood pressure		
FSBG		
Heart rate		
Body weight		

Stand-Alone Thinking Exercise 6.1

The nurse is caring for a 44-year-old client in the emergency department (ED).

History and Physical	Nurses' Notes	Orders	Laboratory Results

1810: Homeless client living in tent encampment brought to ED via ambulance after being found unconscious by a community outreach worker, who called 911. Client had no apparent injury. FSBG 41 mg/dL (2.28 mmol/L); peripheral IV access obtained by first responders. Medical history not known; client smells strongly of alcohol, is thin and bony, and is dirty with a strong odor. Stuporous and responds with groans when pain stimulus induced. PERRLA. Breath sounds clear throughout lung fields. Abdomen soft and concave. Bowel sounds present in all quadrants. Point-of-care ultrasound examination shows no internal injury or bleeding. 2+ pulses with pedal pulses of 1+; cap refill <3 sec. VS: T 99.4°F (37.4°C), HR 100 beats/min and regular, RR 22 breaths/min, BP 164/92 mm Hg, SpO_2 95% on RA. FSBG 48 mg/dL (2.66 mmol/L). (Normal range 70–110 mg/dL [3.89–6.11 mmol/L].)

The nurse reviews the collected client data and collaborates with the registered nurse. Complete the diagram by selecting from the choices below to specify what potential condition the client is likely experiencing, **2** nursing actions that are appropriate to take, and **2** parameters the nurse would monitor to assess the client's progress.

Action to Take		Potential Complication		Parameter to Monitor
Action to Take				Parameter to Monitor

Actions to Take	Potential Conditions	Parameters to Monitor
Obtain orders for total parenteral nutrition	Protein-calorie malnutrition	Blood glucose
Start supplemental O_2 via NC	Acute ischemic stroke	Intake and output
Give 50 mL of 50% IV dextrose solution	Closed traumatic brain injury	Level of consciousness
Monitor FSBG frequently during treatment	Acute hypoglycemia	Heart rate
Administer subcutaneous glucagon per protocol		Blood pressure

Stand-Alone Thinking Exercise 6.2

The nurse is caring for a 58-year-old client who has had type 2 DM for over 20 years. The client is being seen today for follow-up at the outpatient clinic.

History and Physical	Nurses' Notes	Orders	Laboratory Results
Serum Laboratory Tests and Reference Ranges		**Results Today (1000)**	**Results 30 Days Ago**
Blood urea nitrogen (BUN) (10–20 mg/dL [3.6–7.1 mmol/L])		71 mg/dL (25.35 mmol/L)	33 mg/dL (11.78 mmol/L)
Creatinine (0.7–1.3 mg/dL [61.89–114.95 µmol/L])		1.3 mg/dL (114.95 µmol/L)	1.1 mg/dL (97.26 µmol/L)
Glucose (74–106 mg/dL [4.1–5.9 mmol/L])		512 mg/dL (28.42 mmol/L)	450 mg/dL (24.98 mmol/L)
Potassium (3.5–5.0 mEq/L [3.5–5.0 mmol/L])		4.7 mEq/L (4.7 mmol/L)	4.8 mEq/L (4.8 mmol/L)
Sodium (136 –145 mEq/L [136–145 mmol/L])		150 mEq/L (150 mmol/L)	142 mEq/L (142 mmol/L)
Chloride (98–106 mEq/L [98–106 mmol/L])		103 mEq/L (103 mmol/L)	102 mEq/L (102 mmol/L)
Bicarbonate (23–30 mEq/L [23–30 mmol/L])		21 mEq/L (21 mmol/L)	25 mEq/L (25 mmol/L)

The nurse reviews the collected client data and collaborates with the registered nurse. Complete the following sentence by selecting from the list of word choices below.

The nurse recognizes that the client is at high risk for **[Word Choice]**.

WORD CHOICES
Chronic kidney disease
Metabolic alkalosis
Diabetic ketoacidosis
Hyperosmolar hyperglycemic nonketotic syndrome

Unfolding Case Study 7.1

Thinking Exercise 7.1.1

The nurse is caring for a 20-year-old client in the emergency department (ED).

History and Physical	Nurses' Notes	Orders	Laboratory Results

0820: Client in the ED with parents. Alert and oriented × 4. Speech clear and appropriate. Reports experiencing abdominal discomfort and nausea beginning after dinner last night and vomiting, which started in the early morning. Parent confirms client vomited multiple times. Emesis contained food particles at first, and then large amounts of liquid were expelled. Skin warm and dry. Pulses palpable with irregular rhythm. Respirations equal, and lung fields clear throughout. Abdomen distended with visible peristalsis. Multiple scars present on abdomen from pedestrian-vehicular accident and small bowel resection 5 years ago. Bowel sounds hyperactive and high-pitched in upper quadrants. Tenderness and guarding present with light palpation. Last bowel movement yesterday morning with soft, normal-size stools. Client reports feeling bloated and passing flatulence. Denies use of alcohol or illicit drugs. No recent illnesses or other medical conditions. VS: T 100.7°F (38.1°C), HR 97 beats/min, RR 18 breaths/min, BP 95/46 mm Hg, SpO$_2$ 98% on RA. Generalized abdominal pain rated 5/10. Pain does not radiate and does not worsen with coughing, food, or beverage.

0825: Projectile vomiting. Dark green, bile-colored emesis, 500 mL collected in bag. Client attempted to get out of bed to change soiled clothing, became light-headed, and needed assistance to remain upright. Client positioned safely back in bed. Oral care and clean gown provided.

The nurse reviews collected client data with the registered nurse. Which of the following data collection findings require **immediate** follow-up? **Select all that apply**.

○ Blood pressure
○ Cardiac rhythm
○ Flatulence
○ Light-headedness
○ Pain
○ Respirations
○ Temperature
○ Vomiting

Thinking Exercise 7.1.2

The nurse is caring for a 20-year-old client in the emergency department.

History and Physical	Nurses' Notes	Orders	Laboratory Results

0820: Client in the ED with parents. Alert and oriented × 4. Speech clear and appropriate. Reports experiencing abdominal discomfort and nausea beginning after dinner last night and vomiting, which started in the early morning. Parent confirms client vomited multiple times. Emesis contained food particles at first, and then large amounts of liquid were expelled. Skin warm and dry. Pulses palpable with irregular rhythm. Respirations equal, and lung fields clear throughout. Abdomen distended with visible peristalsis. Multiple scars present on abdomen from pedestrian-vehicular accident and small bowel resection 5 years ago. Bowel sounds hyperactive and high-pitched in upper quadrants. Tenderness and guarding present with light palpation. Last bowel movement yesterday morning with soft, normal-size stools. Client reports feeling bloated and passing flatulence. Denies use of alcohol or illicit drugs. No recent illnesses or other medical conditions. VS: T 100.7°F (38.1°C), HR 97 beats/min, RR 18 breaths/min, BP 95/46 mm Hg, SpO$_2$ 98% on RA. Generalized abdominal pain rated 5/10. Pain does not radiate and does not worsen with coughing, food, or beverage.

0825: Projectile vomiting. Dark green, bile-colored emesis, 500 mL collected in bag. Client attempted to get out of bed to change soiled clothing, became light-headed, and needed assistance to remain upright. Client positioned safely back in bed. Oral care and clean gown provided.

The nurse reviews collected client data with the registered nurse. For each data collection finding listed below, determine if the finding is consistent with the health conditions of acute appendicitis, acute pancreatitis, or small bowel obstruction. Some findings may be consistent with more than one condition.

DATA COLLECTION FINDINGS	ACUTE APPENDICITIS	ACUTE PANCREATITIS	SMALL BOWEL OBSTRUCTION
Abdominal pain			
Hyperactive, high-pitched bowel sounds			
Nausea and vomiting			
Fever			
Flatulence			

Thinking Exercise 7.1.3

The nurse is caring for a 20-year-old client in the emergency department.

History and Physical	Nurses' Notes	Orders	Laboratory Results

0820: Client in the ED with parents. Alert and oriented × 4. Speech clear and appropriate. Reports experiencing abdominal discomfort and nausea beginning after dinner last night and vomiting, which started in the early morning. Parent confirms client vomited multiple times. Emesis contained food particles at first, and then large amounts of liquid were expelled. Skin warm and dry. Pulses palpable with irregular rhythm. Respirations equal, and lung fields clear throughout. Abdomen distended with visible peristalsis. Multiple scars present on abdomen from pedestrian-vehicular accident and small bowel resection 5 years ago. Bowel sounds hyperactive and high-pitched in upper quadrants. Tenderness and guarding present with light palpation. Last bowel movement yesterday morning with soft, normal-size stools. Client reports feeling bloated and passing flatulence. Denies use of alcohol or illicit drugs. No recent illnesses or other medical conditions. VS: T 100.7°F (38.1°C), HR 97 beats/min, RR 18 breaths/min, BP 95/46 mm Hg, SpO$_2$ 98% on RA. Generalized abdominal pain rated 5/10. Pain does not radiate and does not worsen with coughing, food, or beverage.

0825: Projectile vomiting. Dark green, bile-colored emesis, 500 mL collected in bag. Client attempted to get out of bed to change soiled clothing, became light-headed, and needed assistance to remain upright. Client positioned safely back in bed. Oral care and clean gown provided.

0830: Phlebotomy technician at bedside. Blood drawn for serum laboratory tests.

History and Physical	Nurses' Notes	Orders	Laboratory Results
Serum Laboratory Test and Reference Range		0855	
Complete Blood Count (CBC)			
Red blood cell (RBC) count (4.7–6.1 × 10^6/mm^3 [4.7–6.1 × 10^{12}/_])		5.8 × 10^6/mm^3 (5.8 × 10^{12}/L)	
White blood cell (WBC) count (5000–10,000/mm^3 [5–10 × 10^9/L])		6500/mm^3 (6.5 × 10^9/L)	
Platelet count (150,000–450,000/mm^3 [150–450 × 10^9/L])		250,000/mm^3 (250 × 10^9/L)	
Other Serum Tests			
C-reactive protein (<1.0 mg/dL [<10 mg/L])		0.8 mg/dL (8 mg/L)	

The nurse reviews the collected client data and collaborates with the registered nurse. Complete the following sentence by selecting from the list of word choices below.

The nurse recognizes that the client is ***most likely*** experiencing **[Word Choice]**. The client is at the highest risk for **[Word Choice]** and **[Word Choice]**.

WORD CHOICES
Acute appendicitis
Anemia
Ascites
Dehydration
Electrolyte imbalance
Pancreatitis
Small bowel obstruction

Thinking Exercise 7.1.4

The nurse is caring for a 20-year-old client in the emergency department.

History and Physical	Nurses' Notes	Orders	Laboratory Results

0820: Client in the ED with parents. Alert and oriented × 4. Speech clear and appropriate. Reports experiencing abdominal discomfort and nausea beginning after dinner last night and vomiting, which started in the early morning. Parent confirms client vomited multiple times. Emesis contained food particles at first, and then large amounts of liquid were expelled. Skin warm and dry. Pulses palpable with irregular rhythm. Respirations equal, and lung fields clear throughout. Abdomen distended with visible peristalsis. Multiple scars present on abdomen from pedestrian-vehicular accident and small bowel resection 5 years ago. Bowel sounds hyperactive and high-pitched in upper quadrants. Tenderness and guarding present with light palpation. Last bowel movement yesterday morning with soft, normal-size stools. Client reports feeling bloated and passing flatulence. Denies use of alcohol or illicit drugs. No recent illnesses or other medical conditions. VS: T 100.7°F (38.1°C), HR 97 beats/min, RR 18 breaths/min, BP 95/46 mm Hg, SpO$_2$ 98% on RA. Generalized abdominal pain rated 5/10. Pain does not radiate and does not worsen with coughing, food, or beverage.

0825: Projectile vomiting. Dark green, bile-colored emesis, 500 mL collected in bag. Client attempted to get out of bed to change soiled clothing, became light-headed, and needed assistance to remain upright. Client positioned safely back in bed. Oral care and clean gown provided.

0830: Phlebotomy technician at bedside. Blood drawn for serum laboratory tests.

History and Physical	Nurses' Notes	Orders	Laboratory Results

Serum Laboratory Test and Reference Range	0855
Complete Blood Count (CBC)	
Red blood cell (RBC) count (4.7–6.1 $\times$ 10^6/mm^3 [4.7–6.1 $\times$ 10^{12}/L])	5.8 $\times$ 10^6/mm^3 (5.8 $\times$ 10^{12}/L)
White blood cell (WBC) count (5000–10,000/mm^3 [5–10 $\times$ 10^9/L])	6500/mm^3 (6.5 $\times$ 10^9/L)
Platelet count (150,000–450,000/mm^3 [150–450 $\times$ 10^9/L])	250,000/mm^3 (250 $\times$ 10^9/L)
Other Serum Tests	
C-reactive protein (<1.0 mg/dL [<10 mg/L])	0.8 mg/dL (8 mg/L)

The nurse collaborates with the registered nurse and contributes to the client's plan of care. Select whether the following potential nursing actions are indicated or not indicated for the client at this time.

POTENTIAL NURSING ACTIONS	INDICATED	NOT INDICATED
Insert a nasogastric tube and connect to suction.		
Infuse isotonic fluids via peripheral venous access.		
Request a breakfast tray with bland foods.		
Monitor intake and output.		
Prepare for an abdominal computed tomography (CT) scan.		

Thinking Exercise 7.1.5

The nurse is caring for a 20-year-old client in the emergency department.

History and Physical	Nurses' Notes	Orders	Laboratory Results

Emergency Department

0820: Client in the ED with parents. Alert and oriented $\times$ 4. Speech clear and appropriate. Reports experiencing abdominal discomfort and nausea beginning after dinner last night and vomiting, which started in the early morning. Parent confirms client vomited multiple times. Emesis contained food particles at first, and then large amounts of liquid were expelled. Skin warm and dry. Pulses palpable with irregular rhythm. Respirations equal, and lung fields clear throughout. Abdomen distended with visible peristalsis. Multiple scars present on abdomen from pedestrian-vehicular accident and small bowel resection 5 years ago. Bowel sounds hyperactive and high-pitched in upper quadrants. Tenderness and guarding present with light palpation. Last bowel movement yesterday morning with soft, normal-size stools. Client reports feeling bloated and passing flatulence. Denies use of alcohol or illicit drugs. No recent illnesses or other medical conditions. VS: T 100.7°F (38.1°C), HR 97 beats/min, RR 18 breaths/min, BP 95/46 mm Hg, SpO$_2$ 98% on RA. Generalized abdominal pain rated 5/10. Pain does not radiate and does not worsen with coughing, food, or beverage.

0825: Projectile vomiting. Dark green, bile-colored emesis, 500 mL collected in bag. Client attempted to get out of bed to change soiled clothing, became light-headed, and needed assistance to remain upright. Client positioned safely back in bed. Oral care and clean gown provided.

0830: Phlebotomy technician at bedside. Blood drawn for serum laboratory tests.

0900: Physician at bedside. Orders received.

0910: Client alert and oriented $\times$ 4. Right forearm peripheral venous device inserted, and IV fluids started. Nasogastric tube inserted; placement confirmed with portable x-ray. NG tube clamped for client transport to radiology for abdominal CT scan. VS: T 100.8°F (38.2°C), HR 99 beats/min, RR 17 breaths/min, BP 93/44 mm Hg, SpO$_2$ 98% on RA.

Medical-Surgical Unit

0940: Client arrived at medical-surgical unit after radiology scan. Report received from ER nurse. NG tube connected to low continuous suction. Immediate drainage 800 mL dark green bile. VS: T 100.5°F (38°C), HR 96 beats/min, RR 15 breaths/min, BP 97/46 mm Hg, SpO$_2$ 96% on RA. Reports abdominal pain rated 7/10. Additional laboratory results from 0855 blood draw available.

History and Physical	Nurses' Notes	Orders	**Laboratory Results**
Serum Laboratory Test and Reference Range		0855	

Complete Blood Count (CBC)

Red blood cell (RBC) count (4.7–6.1 $\times$ 10^6/mm^3 [4.7–6.1 $\times$ 10^{12}/L])	5.8 $\times$ 10^6/mm^3 (5.8 $\times$ 10^{12}/L)
White blood cell (WBC) count (5000–10,000/mm^3 [5–10 $\times$ 10^9/L])	6500/mm^3 (6.5 $\times$ 10^9/L)
Platelet count (150,000–450,000/mm^3 [150–450 $\times$ 10^9/L])	250,000/mm^3 (250 $\times$ 10^9/L)

Other Serum Tests

C-reactive protein (<1.0 mg/dL [<10 mg/L])	0.8 mg/dL (8 mg/L)
Glucose (74–106 mg/dL [4.1–5.9 mmol/L])	88 mg/dL (4.9 mmol/L)
Blood urea nitrogen (BUN) (10–20 mg/dL [3.6–7.1 mmol/L])	62 mg/dL (22.1 mmol/L)
Creatinine (0.7–1.3 mg/dL [61.89–114.95 µmol/L])	0.9 mg/dL (79.6 µmol/L)
Sodium (136–145 mEq/L [136–145 mmol/L])	148 mEq/L (148 mmol/L)
Potassium (3.5–5 mEq/L [3.5–5 mmol/L])	3.2 mEq/L (3.2 mmol/L)

History and Physical	Nurses' Notes	**Orders**	Laboratory Results

0900:
- Admit to medical-surgical unit
- NPO
- Supplemental O_2 to keep SpO_2 > 94%
- Laboratory tests (previously collected): CBC, BMP, lipase, C-reactive protein
- Abdominal CT scan; evaluate for possible intestinal obstruction
- 0.9% normal saline at 150 mL/h
- Nasogastric tube to low continuous suction
- Continuous ECG
- Strict intake and output
- Monitor and replace electrolytes per protocol
- Morphine sulfate 2 mg IV every 4 hours as needed

The nurse reviews the collected client data and collaborates with the registered nurse. Complete the following sentence by selecting from the lists of options below.

The nurse would *prioritize* the administration of **1 [Select]** and monitoring for **2 [Select]**.

OPTIONS FOR 1	OPTIONS FOR 2
Morphine sulfate IV	Cardiac dysrhythmias
Oxygen at 2 L/min via NC	Hypoxemia
Potassium chloride IV	Pain relief

Thinking Exercise 7.1.6

The nurse is caring for a 20-year-old client in the emergency department.

History and Physical	Nurses' Notes	Orders	Laboratory Results

Emergency Department

0820: Client in the ED with parents. Alert and oriented × 4. Speech clear and appropriate. Reports experiencing abdominal discomfort and nausea beginning after dinner last night and vomiting, which started in the early morning. Parent confirms client vomited multiple times. Emesis contained food particles at first, and then large amounts of liquid were expelled. Skin warm and dry. Pulses palpable with irregular rhythm. Respirations equal, and lung fields clear throughout. Abdomen distended with visible peristalsis. Multiple scars present on abdomen from pedestrian-vehicular accident and small bowel resection 5 years ago. Bowel sounds hyperactive and high-pitched in upper quadrants. Tenderness and guarding present with light palpation. Last bowel movement yesterday morning with soft, normal-size stools. Client reports feeling bloated and passing flatulence. Denies use of alcohol or illicit drugs. No recent illnesses or other medical conditions. VS: T 100.7°F (38.1°C), HR 97 beats/min, RR 18 breaths/min, BP 95/46 mm Hg, SpO$_2$ 98% on RA. Generalized abdominal pain rated 5/10. Pain does not radiate and does not worsen with coughing, food, or beverage.

0825: Projectile vomiting. Dark green, bile-colored emesis, 500 mL collected in bag. Client attempted to get out of bed to change soiled clothing, became light-headed, and needed assistance to remain upright. Client positioned safely back in bed. Oral care and clean gown provided.

0830: Phlebotomy technician at bedside. Blood drawn for serum laboratory tests.

0900: Physician at bedside. Orders received.

0910: Client alert and oriented × 4. Right forearm peripheral venous device inserted, and IV fluids started. Nasogastric tube inserted; placement confirmed with portable x-ray. NG tube clamped for client transport to radiology for CT scan. VS: T 100.8°F (38.2°C), HR 99 beats/min, RR 17 breaths/min, BP 93/44 mm Hg, SpO$_2$ 98% on RA.

Medical-Surgical Unit

0940: Client arrived at medical-surgical unit after radiology scan. Report received from ER nurse. NG tube connected to low continuous suction. Immediate drainage, 800 mL dark green bile. VS: T 100.5°F (38°C), HR 96 beats/min, RR 15 breaths/min, BP 97/46 mm Hg, SpO$_2$ 96% on RA. Reports abdominal pain rated 7/10. Additional laboratory results from 0855 blood draw available.

1200: Client sleeping, arouses easily. NG tube draining light-green fluid to low continuous suction. Peripheral venous device intact; site clean and without infiltration. Infusing normal saline and potassium replacements as prescribed. ECG shows sinus rhythm with occasional PVCs. Client voided 350 mL clear, yellow urine via bedpan. VS: T 100.1°F (37.8°C), HR 83 beats/min, RR 12 breaths/min, BP 106/52 mm Hg, SpO$_2$ 98% on RA. After receiving pain medication, the client reports 2/10 abdominal pain.

1400: Client is alert and oriented × 4. Parents remain at bedside. Denies nausea. Heart tones regular, and ECG presents normal sinus rhythm. Skin warm and diaphoretic. Respirations equal. Abdomen rigid to touch. No bowel sounds noted. NG tube to continuous low suction. Client reports sudden onset of sharp abdominal pain rated 10/10. VS: T 101.2°F (38.4°C), HR 99 beats/min, RR 16 breaths/min, BP 132/59 mm Hg, SpO$_2$ 98% on RA.

The nurse reviews nurses' notes from 1200 and 1400 and collaborates with the registered nurse to evaluate the client's status. For each data collection finding, select whether the finding indicates that the client's status has improved or not improved.

DATA COLLECTION FINDINGS	IMPROVED	NOT IMPROVED
Abdominal pain		
Blood pressure		
Cardiac rhythm		
Fever		
Urine output		

Unfolding Case Study 7.2

Thinking Exercise 7.2.1

The nurse is caring for a 48-year-old client at a medical-surgical unit after an exploratory laparotomy.

History and Physical	Nurses' Notes	Laboratory Results	Nursing Flow Sheet

Surgical Day

1430: Client arrived from postanesthesia care unit. Health history includes type 2 diabetes mellitus, hypertension, and obesity. Alert and oriented × 4. Follows commands and moves extremities appropriately. Respirations equal and unlabored. Bilateral upper lobes clear, and lower lobes diminished on auscultation. Heart tones regular, pulses palpable throughout. Peripheral venous devices present in each arm; 0.9% NS infusing at 100 mL/h with no signs of infiltration present. Abdomen large and soft. Bowel sounds hypoactive in all quadrants. Midline abdominal incision covered with dry dressing, no drainage present. Indwelling urinary catheter draining clear-yellow urine to gravity. Reinforced deep breathing and coughing exercises. Client accurately demonstrates use of incentive spirometer and abdominal splinting. Patient-controlled anesthesia (PCA) device set as prescribed. Client denies pain.

Postoperative Day 1

0730: Client drowsy, easily aroused, and oriented × 4. Skin warm and dry. 1+ pitting edema present in bilateral lower extremities. Heart tones regular, bilateral radial pulses bounding, and pedal pulses palpable throughout. Respirations labored. Crackles noted throughout lung fields on auscultation. Client splints abdomen and performs deep breathing and coughing exercises. Expectorates pale, frothy secretions. Abdomen large, round, and soft. Bowel sounds hypoactive in all quadrants. Client reports passing small amounts of flatulence. No bowel movement. Midline abdominal incision well approximated, redness and swelling present around umbilicus, normal temperature, no drainage noted on dressing. Client reports incisional pain rated 3/10. Client demonstrates appropriate use of PCA. Indwelling urinary catheter draining dark-amber urine to gravity. Discussed daily plan including out of bed for breakfast. Client states being too tired to get out of bed and does not feel like eating breakfast.

History and Physical	Nurses' Notes	Laboratory Results	Nursing Flow Sheet

		Medical-Surgical Unit		
Vital Signs	Postanesthesia Care Unit	Surgical Day 1430	Surgical Day 2000	Postoperative Day 1 0730
T	98.1°F (36.7°C)	98.5°F (36.9°C)	98.7°F (37° C)	98.9°F (37.1°C)
HR	72 beats/min	80 beats/min	86 beats/min	92 beats/min
BP	88/45 mm Hg	110/49 mm Hg	118/50 mm Hg	143/72 mm Hg
RR	12 breaths/min	14 breaths/min	12 breaths/min	18 breaths/min
SpO$_2$	96%	98%	98%	94%
O$_2$	40% facemask	4 L/min via NC	2 L/min via NC	2 L/min via NC
Intake				
IV	2500 mL	–	550 mL	1150 mL
Oral	–	–	240 mL	360 mL
Output				
Urinary	–	300 mL	150 mL	200 mL
Approximate blood loss	1750 mL	–	–	–

Complete the following sentence by selecting from the list of word choices below.

The client's [**Word Choice**] and [**Word Choice**] are *most concerning* and must be followed up by the nurse immediately.

WORD CHOICES
Abdominal incision
Bounding radial pulses
Pain level
Pitting edema
Pulmonary congestion
Urine output

Thinking Exercise 7.2.2

The nurse is caring for a 48-year-old client at a medical-surgical unit after an exploratory laparotomy.

History and Physical	Nurses' Notes	Laboratory Results	Nursing Flow Sheet

Surgical Day

1430: Client arrived from postanesthesia care unit. Health history includes type 2 diabetes mellitus, hypertension, and obesity. Alert and oriented × 4. Follows commands and moves extremities appropriately. Respirations equal and un-labored. Bilateral upper lobes clear, and lower lobes diminished on auscultation. Heart tones regular, pulses palpable throughout. Peripheral venous devices present in each arm; 0.9% NS infusing at 100 mL/h with no signs of infiltration present. Abdomen large and soft. Bowel sounds hypoactive in all quadrants. Midline abdominal incision covered with dry dressing, no drainage present. Indwelling urinary catheter draining clear-yellow urine to gravity. Reinforced deep breathing and coughing exercises. Client accurately demonstrates use of incentive spirometer and abdominal splinting. Patient-controlled anesthesia (PCA) device set as prescribed. Client denies pain.

Postoperative Day 1

0730: Client drowsy, easily aroused, and oriented × 4. Skin warm and dry. 1+ pitting edema present in bilateral lower extremities. Heart tones regular, bilateral radial pulses bounding, and pedal pulses palpable throughout. Respirations labored. Crackles noted throughout lung fields on auscultation. Client splints abdomen and performs deep breathing and coughing exercises. Expectorates pale, frothy secretions. Abdomen large, round, and soft. Bowel sounds hypoactive in all quadrants. Client reports passing small amounts of flatulence. No bowel movement. Midline abdominal incision well approximated, redness and swelling present around umbilicus, normal temperature, no drainage noted on dressing. Client reports incisional pain rated 3/10. Client demonstrates appropriate use of PCA. Indwelling urinary catheter draining dark-amber urine to gravity. Discussed daily plan including out of bed for breakfast. Client states being too tired to get out of bed and does not feel like eating breakfast.

History and Physical	Nurses' Notes	Laboratory Results	Nursing Flow Sheet

		Medical-Surgical Unit		
	Postanesthesia Care Unit	Surgical Day 1430	Surgical Day 2000	Postoperative Day 1 0730
Vital Signs				
T	98.1°F (36.7°C)	98.5°F (36.9°C)	98.7°F (37°C)	98.9°F (37.1°C)
HR	72 beats/min	80 beats/min	86 beats/min	92 beats/min
BP	88/45 mm Hg	110/49 mm Hg	118/50 mm Hg	143/72 mm Hg
RR	12 breaths/min	14 breaths/min	12 breaths/min	18 breaths/min
SpO$_2$	96%	98%	98%	94%
O$_2$	40% facemask	4 L/min via NC	2 L/min via NC	2 L/min via NC
Intake				
IV	2500 mL	–	550 mL	1150 mL
Oral	–	–	240 mL	360 mL
Output				
Urinary	–	300 mL	150 mL	200 mL
Approximate blood loss	1750 mL	–	–	–

History and Physical	Nurses' Notes	**Laboratory Results**	Nursing Flow Sheet

Serum Laboratory Test and Reference Range	Preoperative	Postoperative Day 1
Red blood cell (RBC) count (4.7–6.1×10^6/mm³ [4.7–6.1×10^{12}/L])	5.3×10^6/mm³ (5.3×10^{12}/L)	4.9×10^6/mm³ (4.9×10^{12}/L)
White blood cell (WBC) count (5000–$10,000$/mm³ [5–10×10^9/L])	6000/mm³ (6×10^9/L)	9500/mm³ (9.5×10^9/L)
Platelet count ($150,000$–$450,000$/mm³ [150–450×10^9/L])	$300,000$/mm³ (300×10^9/L)	$350,000$/mm³ (350×10^9/L)
Glucose (74–106 mg/dL [4.1–5.9 mmol/L])	148 mg/dL (8.2 mmol/L)	226 mg/dL (12.6 mmol/L)
Blood urea nitrogen (BUN) (10–20 mg/dL [3.6–7.1 mmol/L])	24 mg/dL (8.5 mmol/L)	55 mg/dL (19.6 mmol/L)
Creatinine (0.7–1.3 mg/dL [61.89–114.95 µmol/L])	1.3 mg/dL (114.9 µmol/L)	1.8 mg/dL (159.2 µmol/L)
Sodium (136–145 mEq/L [136–145 mmol/L])	142 mEq/L (142 mmol/L)	138 mEq/L (138 mmol/L)
Potassium (3.5–5 mEq/L [3.5–5 mmol/L])	4.2 mEq/L (4.2 mmol/L)	4.8 mEq/L (4.8 mmol/L)
HbA1c (4%–5.9%)	8.2%	—

The nurse reviews the collected client data and collaborates with the registered nurse. Complete the following sentence by selecting from the lists of options below.

The nurse recognizes that the client is *most likely* experiencing **1 [Select]** as manifested by **2 [Select]** and **3 [Select]**.

OPTIONS FOR 1	OPTIONS FOR 2	OPTIONS FOR 3
Acute kidney injury (AKI)	Hyperglycemia	BUN and creatinine levels
Hyperglycemic hyperosmolar state (HHS)	Hypoactive bowel sounds	RBC and WBC counts
Paralytic ileus	Oliguria	Serum glucose level

Thinking Exercise 7.2.3

The nurse is caring for a 48-year-old client at a medical-surgical unit after an exploratory laparotomy.

History and Physical	**Nurses' Notes**	Laboratory Results	Nursing Flow Sheet

Surgical Day

1430: Client arrived from postanesthesia care unit. Health history includes type 2 diabetes mellitus, hypertension, and obesity. Alert and oriented × 4. Follows commands and moves extremities appropriately. Respirations equal and unlabored. Bilateral upper lobes clear, and lower lobes diminished on auscultation. Heart tones regular, pulses palpable throughout. Peripheral venous devices present in each arm; 0.9% NS infusing at 100 mL/h with no signs of infiltration present. Abdomen large and soft. Bowel sounds hypoactive in all quadrants. Midline abdominal incision covered with dry dressing, no drainage present. Indwelling urinary catheter draining clear-yellow urine to gravity. Reinforced deep breathing and coughing exercises. Client accurately demonstrates use of incentive spirometer and abdominal splinting. Patient-controlled anesthesia (PCA) device set as prescribed. Client denies pain.

Postoperative Day 1

0730: Client drowsy, easily aroused, and oriented × 4. Skin warm and dry. 1+ pitting edema present in bilateral lower extremities. Heart tones regular, bilateral radial pulses bounding, and pedal pulses palpable throughout. Respirations labored. Crackles noted throughout lung fields on auscultation. Client splints abdomen and performs deep breathing and coughing exercises. Expectorates pale, frothy secretions. Abdomen large, round, and soft. Bowel sounds hypoactive in all quadrants. Client reports passing small amounts of flatulence. No bowel movement. Midline abdominal incision well approximated, redness and swelling present around umbilicus, normal temperature, no drainage noted on dressing. Client reports incisional pain rated 3/10. Client demonstrates appropriate use of PCA. Indwelling urinary catheter draining dark-amber urine to gravity. Discussed daily plan including out of bed for breakfast. Client states being too tired to get out of bed and does not feel like eating breakfast.

History and Physical		Nurses' Notes	Laboratory Results	Nursing Flow Sheet
		Medical-Surgical Unit		
	Postanesthesia Care Unit	Surgical Day 1430	Surgical Day 2000	Postoperative Day 1 0730
Vital Signs				
T	98.1°F (36.7°C)	98.5°F (36.9°C)	98.7°F (37°C)	98.9°F (37.1°C)
HR	72 beats/min	80 beats/min	86 beats/min	92 beats/min
BP	88/45 mm Hg	110/49 mm Hg	118/50 mm Hg	143/72 mm Hg
RR	12 breaths/min	14 breaths/min	12 breaths/min	18 breaths/min
SpO$_2$	96%	98%	98%	94%
O$_2$	40% facemask	4 L/min via NC	2 L/min via NC	2 L/min via NC
Intake				
IV	2500 mL	–	550 mL	1150 mL
Oral	–	–	240 mL	360 mL
Output				
Urinary	–	300 mL	150 mL	200 mL
Approximate blood loss	1750 mL	–	–	–

History and Physical	Nurses' Notes	Laboratory Results	Nursing Flow Sheet
Serum Laboratory Test and Reference Range	Preoperative	Postoperative Day 1	
Red blood cell (RBC) count ($4.7–6.1 \times 10^6$/mm^3 [$4.7–6.1 \times 10^{12}$/L])	5.3×10^6/mm^3 (5.3×10^{12}/L)	4.9×10^6/mm^3 (4.9×10^{12}/L)	
White blood cell (WBC) count (5,000–10,000/mm^3 [$5–10 \times 10^9$/L])	6000/mm^3 (6×10^9/L)	9500/mm^3 (9.5×10^9/L)	
Platelet count (150,000–450,000/mm^3 [$150–450 \times 10^9$/L])	300,000/mm^3 (300×10^9/L)	350,000/mm^3 (350×10^9/L)	
Glucose (74–106 mg/dL [4.1–5.9 mmol/L])	148 mg/dL (8.2 mmol/L)	226 mg/dL (12.6 mmol/L)	
Blood urea nitrogen (BUN) (10–20 mg/dL [3.6–7.1 mmol/L])	24 mg/dL (8.5 mmol/L)	55 mg/dL (19.6 mmol/L)	
Creatinine (0.7–1.3 mg/dL [61.89–114.95 µmol/L])	1.3 mg/dL (114.9 µmol/L)	1.8 mg/dL (159.2 µmol/L)	
Sodium (136–145 mEq/L [136–145 mmol/L])	142 mEq/L (142 mmol/L)	138 mEq/L (138 mmol/L)	
Potassium (3.5–5 mEq/L [3.5–5 mmol/L])	4.2 mEq/L (4.2 mmol/L)	4.8 mEq/L (4.8 mmol/L)	
HbA1c (4%–5.9%)	8.2%	–	

The client is diagnosed with acute kidney injury. Select the **3** priority conditions for this client based on documented data.

O Anemia
O Bone fractures
O Fluid volume excess
O Hyperglycemia
O Inadequate nutrition
O Peripheral neuropathy
O Uremic halitosis

Thinking Exercise 7.2.4

The nurse is caring for a 48-year-old client at a medical-surgical unit after an exploratory laparotomy.

History and Physical	Nurses' Notes	Laboratory Results	Nursing Flow Sheet

Surgical Day

1430: Client arrived from postanesthesia care unit. Health history includes type 2 diabetes mellitus, hypertension, and obesity. Alert and oriented × 4. Follows commands and moves extremities appropriately. Respirations equal and un-labored. Bilateral upper lobes clear, and lower lobes diminished on auscultation. Heart tones regular, pulses palpable throughout. Peripheral venous devices present in each arm; 0.9% NS infusing at 100 mL/h with no signs of infiltration present. Abdomen large and soft. Bowel sounds hypoactive in all quadrants. Midline abdominal incision covered with dry dressing, no drainage present. Indwelling urinary catheter draining clear-yellow urine to gravity. Reinforced deep breathing and coughing exercises. Client accurately demonstrates use of incentive spirometer and abdominal splinting. Patient-controlled anesthesia (PCA) device set as prescribed. Client denies pain.

Postoperative Day 1

0730: Client drowsy, easily aroused, and oriented × 4. Skin warm and dry. 1+ pitting edema present in bilateral lower extremities. Heart tones regular, bilateral radial pulses bounding, and pedal pulses palpable throughout. Respirations labored. Crackles noted throughout lung fields on auscultation. Client splints abdomen and performs deep breathing and coughing exercises. Expectorates pale, frothy secretions. Abdomen large, round, and soft. Bowel sounds hypoactive in all quadrants. Client reports passing small amounts of flatulence. No bowel movement. Midline abdominal incision well approximated, redness and swelling present around umbilicus, normal temperature, no drainage noted on dressing. Client reports incisional pain rated 3/10. Client demonstrates appropriate use of PCA. Indwelling urinary catheter drains dark-amber urine to gravity. Discussed daily plan including out of bed for breakfast. Client states being too tired to get out of bed and does not feel like eating breakfast.

History and Physical	Nurses' Notes	Laboratory Results	Nursing Flow Sheet

		Medical-Surgical Unit		
Vital Signs	Postanesthesia Care Unit	Surgical Day 1430	Surgical Day 2000	Postoperative Day 1 0730
T	98.1°F (36.7°C)	98.5°F (36.9°C)	98.7°F (37°C)	98.9°F (37.1°C)
HR	72 beats/min	80 beats/min	86 beats/min	92 beats/min
BP	88/45 mm Hg	110/49 mm Hg	118/50 mm Hg	143/72 mm Hg
RR	12 breaths/min	14 breaths/min	12 breaths/min	18 breaths/min
SpO$_2$	96%	98%	98%	94%
O$_2$	40% facemask	4 L/min via NC	2 L/min via NC	2 L/min via NC
Intake				
IV	2500 mL	–	550 mL	1150 mL
Oral	–	–	240 mL	360 mL
Output				
Urinary	–	300 mL	150 mL	200 mL
Approximate blood loss	1750 mL	–	–	–

History and Physical	Nurses' Notes	Laboratory Results	Nursing Flow Sheet

Serum Laboratory Test and Reference Range	Preoperative	Postoperative Day 1
Red blood cell (RBC) count (4.7–6.1 × 10^6/mm^3 [4.7–6.1 × 10^{12}/L])	5.3 × 10^6/mm^3 (5.3 × 10^{12}/L)	4.9 × 10^6/mm^3 (4.9 × 10^{12}/L)
White blood cell (WBC) count (5000–10,000/mm^3 [5–10 × 10^9/L])	6000/mm^3 (6 × 10^9/L)	9500/mm^3 (9.5 × 10^9/L)
Platelet count (150,000–450,000/mm^3 [150–450 × 10^9/L])	300,000/mm^3 (300 × 10^9/L)	350,000/mm^3 (350 × 10^9/L)
Glucose (74–106 mg/dL [4.1–5.9 mmol/L])	148 mg/dL (8.2 mmol/L)	226 mg/dL (12.6 mmol/L)
Blood urea nitrogen (BUN) (10–20 mg/dL [3.6–7.1 mmol/L])	24 mg/dL (8.5 mmol/L)	55 mg/dL (19.6 mmol/L)
Creatinine (0.7–1.3 mg/dL [61.89–114.95 µmol/L])	1.3 mg/dL (114.9 µmol/L)	1.8 mg/dL (159.2 µmol/L)
Sodium (136–145 mEq/L [136–145 mmol/L])	142 mEq/L (142 mmol/L)	138 mEq/L (138 mmol/L)
Potassium (3.5–5 mEq/L [3.5–5 mmol/L])	4.2 mEq/L (4.2 mmol/L)	4.8 mEq/L (4.8 mmol/L)
HbA1c (4%–5.9%)	8.2%	–

The nurse collaborates with the registered nurse and contributes to the client's plan of care. For each priority condition, select the potential nursing actions that are appropriate as part of the client's plan of care.

PRIORITY CONDITIONS	POTENTIAL NURSING ACTIONS
Fluid volume excess	○ Administer a diuretic, such as spironolactone ○ Restrict fluid intake ○ Continuously assess and document fluid status
Hyperglycemia	○ Administer oral antihyperglycemic medications ○ Frequently monitor blood glucose levels ○ Monitor for urinary ketones
Inadequate nutrition	○ Assess food intake during every shift ○ Collaborate with a registered dietitian nutritionist (RDN) ○ Provide supplemental nutrition if needed

Thinking Exercise 7.2.5

The nurse is caring for a 48-year-old client at a medical-surgical unit after an exploratory laparotomy.

History and Physical	Nurses' Notes	Laboratory Results	Nursing Flow Sheet

Surgical Day

1430: Client arrived from postanesthesia care unit. Health history includes type 2 diabetes mellitus, hypertension, and obesity. Alert and oriented × 4. Follows commands and moves extremities appropriately. Respirations equal and un-labored. Bilateral upper lobes clear, and lower lobes diminished on auscultation. Heart tones regular, pulses palpable throughout. Peripheral venous devices present in each arm; 0.9% NS infusing at 100 mL/h with no signs of infiltration present. Abdomen large and soft. Bowel sounds hypoactive in all quadrants. Midline abdominal incision covered with dry dressing, no drainage present. Indwelling urinary catheter draining clear-yellow urine to gravity. Reinforced deep breathing and coughing exercises. Client accurately demonstrates use of incentive spirometer and abdominal splinting. Patient-controlled anesthesia (PCA) device set as prescribed. Client denies pain.

Postoperative Day 1

0730: Client drowsy, easily aroused, and oriented × 4. Skin warm and dry. 1+ pitting edema present in bilateral lower extremities. Heart tones regular, bilateral radial pulses bounding, and pedal pulses palpable throughout. Respirations labored. Crackles noted throughout lung fields on auscultation. Client splints abdomen and performs deep breathing and coughing exercises. Expectorates pale, frothy secretions. Abdomen large, round, and soft. Bowel sounds hypoactive in all quadrants. Client reports passing small amounts of flatulence. No bowel movement. Midline abdominal incision well approximated, redness and swelling present around umbilicus, normal temperature, no drainage noted on dressing. Client reports incisional pain rated 3/10. Client demonstrates appropriate use of PCA. Indwelling urinary catheter drains dark-amber urine to gravity. Discussed daily plan including out of bed for breakfast. Client states being too tired to get out of bed and does not feel like eating breakfast.

0820: Physician at bedside. Orders received. Intravenous fluids discontinued. Furosemide 20 mg IV administered. Registered dietitian nutritionist consult initiated. Client oriented × 4. Remains in bed for breakfast, eating less than 50% of meal. Fluids restricted to 1500 mL daily.

1130: Client requests a glass of iced water, stating "My mouth is so dry. I can't believe I am only allowed a liter and a half of fluid today. That won't be enough."

The nurse collaborates with the registered nurse and contributes to the client's plan of care. Which of the following actions would the nurse take for the client? **Select all that apply**.

O Assist the client to identify desired fluids to drink throughout the day.
O Collaborate with the client to develop a plan for fluid intake.
O Encourage the client to suck on ice chips as desired to prevent dry mouth.
O Explain the purpose of fluid restriction and the goals of the current treatment plan.
O Offer oral care with swish-and-spit mouthwash to moisten oral mucosa.
O Only allow fluids with meals to ensure that restrictions are not exceeded.
O Provide a glass of iced water with directions to sip it slowly throughout the day.
O Suggest eating foods higher in sodium to retain ingested fluids.

Thinking Exercise 7.2.6

The nurse is caring for a 48-year-old client at a medical-surgical unit after an exploratory laparotomy. Highlight data collection findings in the 1400 Nurses' Notes and Nursing Flow Sheet that demonstrate the client's status is improving.

History and Physical	Nurses' Notes	Laboratory Results	Nursing Flow Sheet

Surgical Day

1430: Client arrived from postanesthesia care unit. Health history includes type 2 diabetes mellitus, hypertension, and obesity. Alert and oriented × 4. Follows commands and moves extremities appropriately. Respirations equal and unlabored. Bilateral upper lobes clear, and lower lobes diminished on auscultation. Heart tones regular, pulses palpable throughout. Peripheral venous devices present in each arm; 0.9% NS infusing at 100 mL/h with no signs of infiltration present. Abdomen large and soft. Bowel sounds hypoactive in all quadrants. Midline abdominal incision covered with dry dressing, no drainage present. Indwelling urinary catheter draining clear-yellow urine to gravity. Reinforced deep breathing and coughing exercises. Client accurately demonstrates use of incentive spirometer and abdominal splinting. Patient-controlled anesthesia (PCA) device set as prescribed. Client denies pain.

Postoperative Day 1

0730: Client drowsy, easily aroused, and oriented × 4. Skin warm and dry. 1+ pitting edema present in bilateral lower extremities. Heart tones regular, bilateral radial pulses bounding, and pedal pulses palpable throughout. Respirations labored. Crackles noted throughout lung fields on auscultation. Client splints abdomen and performs deep breathing and coughing exercises. Expectorates pale, frothy secretions. Abdomen large, round, and soft. Hypoactive bowel sounds in all quadrants. Client reports passing small amounts of flatulence. No bowel movement. Midline abdominal incision well approximated, redness and swelling present around umbilicus, normal temperature, no drainage noted on dressing. Client reports incisional pain rated 3/10. Client demonstrates appropriate use of PCA. Indwelling urinary catheter drains dark-amber urine to gravity. Discussed daily plan including out of bed for breakfast. Client states being too tired to get out of bed and does not feel like eating breakfast.

0820: Physician at bedside. Orders received. Intravenous fluids discontinued. Furosemide 20 mg IV administered. Registered dietitian nutritionist consult initiated. Client oriented × 4. Remains in bed for breakfast, eating less than 50% of meal. Fluids restricted to 1500 mL daily.

1130: Client requests a glass of iced water, stating "My mouth is so dry. I can't believe I am only allowed a liter and a half of fluid today. That won't be enough."

1400: Client alert and oriented × 4. Skin warm and dry. Nonpitting edema present in bilateral lower extremities. Heart tones regular, and pulses palpable throughout. Respirations equal and unlabored. Crackles noted in bilateral lower lobes of lungs on auscultation. Abdomen large, round, and soft. Bowel sounds present in all quadrants. Client reports passing flatulence. No bowel movement. Midline abdominal incision well approximated, redness and swelling present around umbilicus, normal temperature, no drainage noted on dressing. Client splints abdomen, uses incentive spirometer, and performs deep breathing and coughing exercises. Dry cough: No sputum expectorated. Client reports incisional pain rated 2/10 with breathing exercises; demonstrates appropriate use of PCA. Indwelling urinary catheter draining clear-yellow urine to gravity.

	History and Physical	Nurses' Notes	Laboratory Results	Nursing Flow Sheet	
			Medical-Surgical Unit		
	Postanesthesia Care Unit	Surgical Day 1430	Surgical Day 2000	Postoperative Day 1 0730	Postoperative Day 1 1400
Vital Signs					
T	98.1°F (36.7°C)	98.5°F (36.9°C)	98.7°F (37°C)	98.9°F (37.1°C)	98.7°F (37°C)
HR	72 beats/min	80 beats/min	86 beats/min	92 beats/min	86 beats/min
BP	88/45 mm Hg	110/49 mm Hg	118/50 mm Hg	143/72 mm Hg	114/69 mm Hg
RR	12 breaths/min	14 breaths/min	12 breaths/min	18 breaths/min	14 breaths/min
SpO_2	96%	98%	98%	94%	98%
O_2	40% facemask	4 L/min via NC	2 L/min via NC	2 L/min via NC	2 L/min via NC
Intake					
IV	2500 mL	–	550 mL	1150 mL	100 mL
Oral	–	–	240 mL	360 mL	450 mL
Output					
Urinary	–	300 mL	150 mL	200 mL	720 mL
Approximate blood loss	1750 mL	–	–	–	–

Stand-Alone Thinking Exercise 7.1

The nurse is caring for a 46-year-old client after an abdominoperineal resection with sigmoid colostomy placement for rectal cancer.

History and Physical	Nurses' Notes	Orders	Laboratory Results

Postoperative Day 2

0740: Client is alert and oriented × 4. Heart tones regular, and pulses palpable throughout. Skin warm and dry. Nonpitting, dependent edema present in bilateral lower extremities. Right forearm, peripheral venous device intact, site clean and without infiltration. 0.9% NS infusing at 50 mL/h with morphine patient-controlled anesthesia (PCA). Settings on PCA pump verified, and client verbalizes appropriate understanding and utilization of PCA. Respirations equal and unlabored. Upper lung fields clear, and lower lung fields diminished upon auscultation. Client demonstrates correct use of incentive spirometer. Abdomen large, round, and soft. Bowel sounds present in all quadrants. Stoma present in lower left abdomen with clear ostomy pouch intact. The stoma stump is edematous and bright red with dark purple discoloration along the lower and right edges. Ostomy pouch filled with air. Light brown thick liquid stool is also present. Voids without difficulty in bathroom. Urine is clear, yellow, and odorless. VS: 99.9°F (37.7°C), HR 69 beats/min, RR 14 breaths/min, BP 132/54 mm Hg, SpO_2 97% on RA. Reports abdominal tenderness at stoma site, rated 4/10. Daily weight: 290 lb (131.8 kg). Preoperative weight: 293 lb (133.2 kg).

The nurse reviews the collected client data and collaborates with the registered nurse. Complete the diagram by selecting from the choices below to specify what potential condition the client is likely experiencing, **2** nursing actions that are appropriate to take, and **2** parameters the nurse would monitor to assess the client's progress.

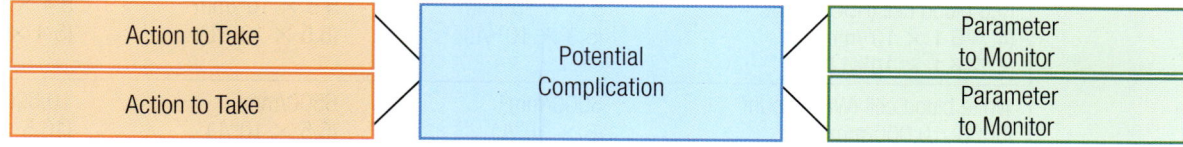

Actions to Take	Potential Conditions	Parameters to Monitor
Empty the client's ostomy pouch	Excessive flatulence	Color and integrity of the client's stoma
Encourage intake of foods high in fiber	Fluid imbalance	Lung fields for pulmonary congestion
Discontinue the morphine PCA	Stoma necrosis	Peristomal skin for presence of excoriation
Recommend increasing the IV fluid rate	Opioid-induced respiratory depression	Respiration rate and depth
Report client findings to the surgeon		Skin temperature, moisture, and turgor

Stand-Alone Thinking Exercise 7.2

The nurse is caring for a 28-year-old client in a gynecology outpatient clinic.

History and Physical	Nurses' Notes	Orders	Laboratory Results

1530: Client presents for routine checkup at 26 weeks' gestation. Alert and oriented × 4. Reports general fatigue, stating "I haven't been sleeping well due to needing to urinate multiple times each night." Heart tones regular, and pulses palpable throughout. Skin warm and diaphoretic. Respirations equal and unlabored. Lung fields clear throughout. Abdomen round. Bowel sounds present in all quadrants. Client reports feeling nauseated with abdominal discomfort over the past few days. Last bowel movement was this morning with usual stool. Client also reports experiencing a burning sensation when urinating. VS: 101.2°F (38.4°C), HR 102 beats/min, RR 16 breaths/min, BP 129/61 mm Hg, SpO$_2$ 99% on RA. Client reports back pain, rated 6/10 in the right flank and 3/10 in the left flank. Fetal heart tones regular, and HR 140 beats/min. Client reports fetus is active and moves frequently.

History and Physical	Nurses' Notes	Orders	Laboratory Results
Serum Laboratory Test and Reference Range	**20 Weeks' Gestation**	**24 Weeks' Gestation**	**26 Weeks' Gestation**
Serum Labs			
Red blood cell (RBC) count (4.7–$6.1 \times 10^6/mm^3$ [4.7–$6.1 \times 10^{12}/L$])	$5.3 \times 10^6/mm^3$ ($5.3 \times 10^{12}/L$)	$5.5 \times 10^6/mm^3$ ($5.5 \times 10^{12}/L$)	$5.4 \times 10^6/mm^3$ ($5.4 \times 10^{12}/L$)
White blood cell (WBC) count (5000–$10,000/mm^3$ [5–$10 \times 10^9/L$])	$6000/mm^3$ ($6 \times 10^9/L$)	$6500/mm^3$ ($6.5 \times 10^9/L$)	$10,500/mm^3$ ($10.5 \times 10^9/L$)
Platelet count ($150,000$–$450,000/mm^3$ [150–$450 \times 10^9/L$])	$250,000/mm^3$ ($25 \times 10^9/L$)	$260,000/mm^3$ ($260 \times 10^9/L$)	$255,000/mm^3$ ($255 \times 10^9/L$)
Glucose (74–106 mg/dL [4.1–5.9 mmol/L])	85 mg/dL (4.8 mmol/L)	88 mg/dL (4.9 mmol/L)	92 mg/dL (5.1 mmol/L)
Blood urea nitrogen (BUN) (10–20 mg/dL [3.6–7.1 mmol/L])	15 mg/dL (5.36 mmol/L)	17 mg/dL (6.1 mmol/L)	32 mg/dL (11.4 mmol/L)
Creatinine (0.7–1.3 mg/dL [61.89–114.95 µmol/L])	0.9 mg/dL (79.6 µmol/L)	1.1 mg/dL (97.2 µmol/L)	1.4 mg/dL (123.8 µmol/L)
Sodium (136–145 mEq/L [136–145 mmol/L])	139 mEq/L (139 mmol/L)	140 mEq/L (140 mmol/L)	145 mEq/L (145 mmol/L)
Potassium (3.5–5 mEq/L [3.5–5 mmol/L])	4.2 mEq/L (4.2 mmol/L)	4.6 mEq/L (4.6 mmol/L)	4.5 mEq/L (4.5 mmol/L)
Urinary Labs			
Color/Appearance (amber yellow/clear)	Pale yellow, clear	Amber yellow, clear	Amber, cloudy
pH (4.6–8)	5.8	6	7.9
Specific gravity (1.005–1.03)	1.01	1.012	1.02
Glucose (negative)	Negative	120 mg/dL	128 mg/dL
Ketones (negative)	Negative	Negative	Negative
Nitrates (negative)	Negative	Negative	Positive
Leukocyte esterase (negative)	Negative	Negative	Positive

The nurse collaborates with the registered nurse and contributes to the client's plan of care. Select whether the following potential orders would be indicated or not indicated for the client at this time.

POTENTIAL ORDERS	INDICATED	NOT INDICATED
Acetaminophen for pain and fever management		
Blood culture and sensitivity		
Broad-spectrum antibiotic		
Fetal ultrasound		
Fluid restriction		
Serum HbA1c level		
Urine culture and sensitivity		

Client Conditions Affecting Reproduction

Unfolding Case Study 8.1

Thinking Exercise 8.1.1

The nurse is caring for a 46-year-old client at an ambulatory care clinic.

History and Physical	Nurses' Notes	Orders	Laboratory Results

1030: Female client with a G1P0 obstetric history presents with lower abdominal and back pain. Reports chronic dysmenorrhea that has recently worsened to extreme pain accompanied by episodes of nausea and fatigue. Client becomes tearful stating, "The pain doesn't seem to go away between my periods. I experience pain every time I urinate, and sex is so uncomfortable that I haven't been intimate in over 6 months." Denies unusual vaginal discharge and urinary frequency or urgency. Client confirms a monogamous partner and not using hormonal birth control since 28 years of age. Reports feeling safe at home and does not have any thoughts of self-harm. Denies smoking. Drinks 2 to 3 alcoholic beverages daily. VS: T 98.9°F (37.1°C), HR 89 beats/min, RR 14 breaths/min, BP 122/45 mm Hg, SpO$_2$ 98% on RA. Urine sample obtained for laboratory tests. Urine is dark yellow, clear, and without odor.

Complete the following sentence by selecting from the list of word choices below.

The nurse recognizes that the client's [**Word Choice**] and [**Word Choice**] require follow-up by the nurse and health care team.

WORD CHOICES
Alcohol use
Dysuria
Fatigue
Urine color
Pelvic pain

Thinking Exercise 8.1.2

The nurse is caring for a 46-year-old client at an ambulatory care clinic.

History and Physical	Nurses' Notes	Orders	Laboratory Results

1030: Female client with a G1P0 obstetric history presents with lower abdominal and back pain. Reports chronic dysmenorrhea that has recently worsened to extreme pain accompanied by episodes of nausea and fatigue. Client becomes tearful stating, "The pain doesn't seem to go away between my periods. I experience pain every time I urinate, and sex is so uncomfortable that I haven't been intimate in over 6 months." Denies unusual vaginal discharge and urinary frequency or urgency. Client confirms a monogamous partner and not using hormonal birth control since 28 years of age. Reports feeling safe at home and does not have any thoughts of self-harm. Denies smoking. Drinks 2 to 3 alcoholic beverages daily. VS: T 98.9°F (37.1°C), HR 89 beats/min, RR 14 breaths/min, BP 122/45 mm Hg, SpO$_2$ 98% on RA. Urine sample obtained for laboratory tests. Urine is dark yellow, clear, and without odor.

The nurse reviews the collected data with the registered nurse. For each data collection finding listed below, determine if the finding is consistent with the health conditions of endometriosis, interstitial cystitis, or pelvic inflammatory disease. Some findings may be consistent with more than one condition.

CLIENT FINDINGS	ENDOMETRIOSIS	INTERSTITIAL CYSTITIS	PELVIC INFLAMMATORY DISEASE
Pelvic pain not related to menstruation			
Dysmenorrhea			
Painful sexual intercourse (dyspareunia)			
Dysuria			

Thinking Exercise 8.1.3

The nurse is caring for a 46-year-old client at an ambulatory care clinic.

History and Physical	Nurses' Notes	Orders	Laboratory Results

1030: Female client with a G1P0 obstetric history presents with lower abdominal and back pain. Reports chronic dysmenorrhea that has recently worsened to extreme pain accompanied by episodes of nausea and fatigue. Client becomes tearful stating, "The pain doesn't seem to go away between my periods. I experience pain every time I urinate, and sex is so uncomfortable that I haven't been intimate in over 6 months." Denies unusual vaginal discharge and urinary frequency or urgency. Client confirms a monogamous partner and not using hormonal birth control since 28 years of age. Reports feeling safe at home and does not have any thoughts of self-harm. Denies smoking. Drinks 2 to 3 alcoholic beverages daily. VS: T 98.9°F (37.1°C), HR 89 beats/min, RR 14 breaths/min, BP 122/45 mm Hg, SpO$_2$ 98% on RA. Urine sample obtained for laboratory tests. Urine is dark yellow, clear, and without odor.

1150: Urinalysis results include hematuria but no signs of infection. Bedside ultrasonography completed; small pelvic masses visualized. Laparoscopy with tissue biopsy planned.

The nurse reviews the collected client data with the registered nurse. Complete the following sentence by selecting from the lists of options below.

The client is **most likely** experiencing **1 [Select]**. The nurse determines that the **priority** for care at this time is **2 [Select]**.

OPTIONS FOR 1	OPTIONS FOR 2
Endometriosis	Antibiotic therapy
Interstitial cystitis	Couples counseling
Pelvic inflammatory disease	Pain management

Thinking Exercise 8.1.4

The nurse is caring for a 46-year-old client at an ambulatory care clinic.

History and Physical	Nurses' Notes	Orders	Laboratory Results

Initial Clinic Visit

1030: Female client with a G1P0 obstetric history presents with lower abdominal and back pain. Reports chronic dysmenorrhea that has recently worsened to extreme pain accompanied by episodes of nausea and fatigue. Client becomes tearful stating, "The pain doesn't seem to go away between my periods. I experience pain every time I urinate, and sex is so uncomfortable that I haven't been intimate in over 6 months." Denies unusual vaginal discharge and urinary frequency or urgency. Client confirms a monogamous partner and not using hormonal birth control since 28 years of age. Reports feeling safe at home and does not have any thoughts of self-harm. Denies smoking. Drinks 2 to 3 alcoholic beverages daily. VS: T 98.9°F (37.1°C), HR 89 beats/min, RR 14 breaths/min, BP 122/45 mm Hg, SpO$_2$ 98% on RA. Urine sample obtained for laboratory tests. Urine is dark yellow, clear, and without odor.

1150: Urinalysis results include hematuria but no signs of infection. Bedside ultrasonography completed; small pelvic masses visualized. Laparoscopy with tissue biopsy planned.

Follow-up Clinic Visit—4 Weeks Later

0920: Client alert and oriented × 4. Appears anxious, holding partner's hand. Diagnostic results presented by provider, including laparoscopy and biopsy analysis that demonstrate multiple endometrial adhesions and implants present throughout abdomen. Client reports that pelvic pain continues to worsen and is limiting participation in daily activities. Treatment options discussed. Client and partner agree to a total abdominal hysterectomy with bilateral salpingo-oophorectomy and removal of abdominal adhesions. Presurgical care provided.

The nurse collaborates with the registered nurse and contributes to the client's plan of care. Select whether the following potential nursing actions are indicated or not indicated for the client at this time.

POTENTIAL NURSING ACTIONS	INDICATED	NOT INDICATED
Encourage expression of anxiety and concerns related to sexuality and reproduction.		
Discuss postoperative care including incentive spirometry, early ambulation, and pain management.		
Assess the client's understanding of the procedure, and answer questions as appropriate.		
Suggest the use of creams and lubricants to manage loss of libido or vaginal changes.		
Reinforce preoperative teaching focused on laboratory tests and preparations the night before surgery.		

Thinking Exercise 8.1.5

The nurse is caring for a 46-year-old client on a medical-surgical unit.

History and Physical	Nurses' Notes	Orders	Laboratory Results

Initial Clinic Visit

1030: Female client with a G1P0 obstetric history presents with lower abdominal and back pain. Reports chronic dysmenorrhea that has recently worsened to extreme pain accompanied by episodes of nausea and fatigue. Client becomes tearful stating, "The pain doesn't seem to go away between my periods. I experience pain every time I urinate, and sex is so uncomfortable that I haven't been intimate in over 6 months." Denies unusual vaginal discharge and urinary frequency or urgency. Client confirms a monogamous partner and not using hormonal birth control since 28 years of age. Reports feeling safe at home and does not have any thoughts of self-harm. Denies smoking. Drinks 2 to 3 alcoholic beverages daily. VS: T 98.9°F (37.1°C), HR 89 beats/min, RR 14 breaths/min, BP 122/45 mm Hg, SpO$_2$ 98% on RA. Urine sample obtained for laboratory tests. Urine is dark yellow, clear, and without odor.

1150: Urine analysis results include hematuria but no signs of infection. Bedside ultrasonography completed; small pelvic masses visualized. Laparoscopy with tissue biopsy ordered.

Follow-up Clinic Visit—4 Weeks Later

0920: Client alert and oriented × 4. Appears anxious, holding partner's hand. Diagnostic results presented by provider, including laparoscopy and biopsy analysis that demonstrate multiple endometrial adhesions and implants present throughout abdomen. Client reports that pelvic pain continues to worsen and is limiting participation in daily activities. Treatment options discussed. Client and partner agree to a total abdominal hysterectomy with bilateral salpingo-oophorectomy and removal of abdominal adhesions. Presurgical care provided.

Medical-Surgical Unit After Surgery

1800: Client arrives on unit after total abdominal hysterectomy with bilateral salpingo-oophorectomy and removal of abdominal adhesions. Alert and oriented × 4. Follows simple commands, and repositions self in bed. Heart tones normal. Skin warm and dry with pulses palpable throughout. Right AC peripheral vascular device with 0.9% NS at 100 mL/h. Respirations equal and unlabored. Lung fields clear upon auscultation. Bowel sounds hypoactive. Client tolerates sips of water without aspiration or nausea. Perineal pad in place with scant red drainage. Abdominal incision covered with dry dressing. VS: T 97.8°F (36.5°C), HR 82 beats/min, RR 16 breaths/min, BP 116/40 mm Hg, SpO$_2$ 98% on 4 L/min O$_2$ via NC. Reports incisional pain rated 4/10.

The nurse collaborates with the registered nurse and contributes to the client's plan of care. For each potential postoperative complication, select the potential nursing actions that are appropriate as part of the client's plan of care.

POTENTIAL POSTOPERATIVE COMPLICATIONS	POTENTIAL NURSING ACTIONS
Postoperative bleeding	○ Assess the client's abdominal dressing and perineal pad every hour. ○ Monitor vital signs every 12 hours and then once a shift until discharge. ○ Report vaginal bleeding that saturates more than one perineal pad per hour to the surgeon.
Urinary retention	○ Assist the client to the bathroom, and provide privacy and assistive measures to promote spontaneous voiding. ○ Record urinary output and the color, clarity, and odor of urine. ○ Teach the client to perform perineal hygiene after voiding and at least every 8 hours.
Pain	○ Administer analgesics as ordered. ○ Assess pain location, character, and severity. ○ Assist the client to brace the abdomen when performing breathing exercises.

Thinking Exercise 8.1.6

The nurse is caring for a 46-year-old client on a medical-surgical unit.

History and Physical	Nurses' Notes	Orders	Laboratory Results

Initial Clinic Visit

1030: Female client with a G1P0 obstetric history presents with lower abdominal and back pain. Reports chronic dysmenorrhea that has recently worsened to extreme pain accompanied by episodes of nausea and fatigue. Client becomes tearful stating, "The pain doesn't seem to go away between my periods. I experience pain every time I urinate, and sex is so uncomfortable that I haven't been intimate in over 6 months." Denies unusual vaginal discharge and urinary frequency or urgency. Client confirms a monogamous partner and not using hormonal birth control since 28 years of age. Reports feeling safe at home and does not have any thoughts of self-harm. Denies smoking. Drinks 2 to 3 alcoholic beverages daily. VS: T 98.9°F (37.1°C), HR 89 beats/min, RR 14 breaths/min, BP 122/45 mm Hg, SpO$_2$ 98% on RA. Urine sample obtained for laboratory tests. Urine is dark yellow, clear, and without odor.

1150: Urinalysis results include hematuria but no signs of infection. Bedside ultrasonography completed; small pelvic masses visualized. Laparoscopy with tissue biopsy planned.

Follow-up Clinic Visit—4 Weeks Later

0920: Client alert and oriented × 4. Appears anxious, holding partner's hand. Diagnostic results presented by provider, including laparoscopy and biopsy analysis that demonstrate multiple endometrial adhesions and implants present throughout abdomen. Client reports that pelvic pain continues to worsen and is limiting participation in daily activities. Treatment options discussed. Client and partner agree to a total abdominal hysterectomy with bilateral salpingo-oophorectomy and removal of abdominal adhesions. Presurgical care provided.

Medical-Surgical Unit After Surgery

1800: Client arrives on unit after total abdominal hysterectomy with bilateral salpingo-oophorectomy and removal of abdominal adhesions. Alert and oriented × 4. Follows simple commands, and repositions self in bed. Heart tones normal. Skin warm and dry with pulses palpable throughout. Right AC peripheral vascular device with 0.9% NS at 100 mL/h. Respirations equal and unlabored. Lung fields clear upon auscultation. Bowel sounds hypoactive. Client tolerates sips of water without aspiration or nausea. Perineal pad in place with scant red drainage. Abdominal incision covered with dry dressing. VS: T 97.8°F (36.5°C), HR 82 beats/min, RR 16 breaths/min, BP 116/40 mm Hg, SpO$_2$ 98% on 4 L/min O$_2$ via NC. Reports incisional pain rated 4/10.

Postoperative Day 2

0910: Client is alert and oriented × 4. Scheduled for discharge this morning.

The nurse reviews the collected client data with the registered nurse and reinforces discharge teaching with the client. Which client statements indicate **understanding** of the discharge teaching provided? **Select all that apply.**

○ "I will report any increased redness or drainage from my incision to the surgeon."

○ "Resting in bed for at least 1 week will minimize surgical complications and promote wound healing."

○ "I will avoid lifting anything more than 10 lb (4.5 kg) for the next 6 weeks."

○ "My menstrual periods may be irregular for the first few months after surgery."

○ "I will monitor my temperature and contact the surgeon if I have a fever at or above 100°F (37.8°C)."

○ "I may experience hot flashes, night sweats, and vaginal dryness due to the surgical procedure."

○ "If I experience any acute leg pain, swelling, or redness, I should contact the surgeon."

Unfolding Case Study 8.2

Thinking Exercise 8.2.1

The nurse is caring for a 47-year-old client in the emergency department (ED). Highlight the client findings that require **immediate** follow-up.

History and Physical	Nurses' Notes	Orders	Laboratory Results

1220: Male client presents with dysuria and hematuria. Client reports difficulty starting urination, unable to maintain a constant stream, and burning during urination. States, "I thought I should come to the emergency room when I noticed blood in my urine." Alert and oriented × 4. Reports recent fatigue and some expected weight loss. Heart tones regular, skin warm and dry, pulses palpable throughout. Bilateral lower extremity 1+ pitting edema present. Respirations equal and unlabored. Lung fields clear upon auscultation. Abdomen soft and flat with active bowel sounds in all quadrants. Last bowel movement this morning; soft, light-brown stool. Client reports recent rectal pressure and painful defecation. Denies penile discharge or blisters/sores on genitals or anus. VS: T 98.8°F (37.1°C), HR 72 beats/min, RR 14 breaths/min, BP 136/49 mm Hg, SpO$_2$ 98% on RA. Denies pain. The client is a tax accountant, lives alone, and is divorced with no children.

Thinking Exercise 8.2.2

The nurse is caring for a 47-year-old client in the emergency department.

History and Physical	Nurses' Notes	Orders	Laboratory Results

1220: Male client presents with dysuria and hematuria. Client reports difficulty starting urination, unable to maintain a constant stream, and burning during urination. States, "I thought I should come to the emergency room when I noticed blood in my urine." Alert and oriented × 4. Reports recent fatigue and some expected weight loss. Heart tones regular, skin warm and dry, pulses palpable throughout. Bilateral lower extremity 1+ pitting edema present. Respirations equal and unlabored. Lung fields clear upon auscultation. Abdomen soft and flat with active bowel sounds in all quadrants. Last bowel movement this morning; soft, light-brown stool. Client reports recent rectal pressure and painful defecation. Denies penile discharge or blisters/sores on genitals or anus. VS: T 98.8°F (37.1°C), HR 72 beats/min, RR 14 breaths/min, BP 136/49 mm Hg, SpO$_2$ 98% on RA. Denies pain. The client is a tax accountant, lives alone, and is divorced with no children.

The nurse reviews the collected data and collaborates with the registered nurse. Which of the following conditions is the client potentially experiencing? **Select all that apply.**

○ Benign prostatic hyperplasia

○ Constipation

○ Cystitis

○ Hemorrhoids

○ Prostate cancer

○ Sexually transmitted infection

○ Renal calculi

Thinking Exercise 8.2.3

The nurse is caring for a 47-year-old client in the emergency department.

History and Physical	Nurses' Notes	Orders	Laboratory Results

1220: Male client presents with dysuria and hematuria. Client reports difficulty starting urination, unable to maintain a constant stream, and burning during urination. States, "I thought I should come to the emergency room when I noticed blood in my urine." Alert and oriented × 4. Reports recent fatigue and some expected weight loss. Heart tones regular, skin warm and dry, pulses palpable throughout. Bilateral lower extremity 1+ pitting edema present. Respirations equal and unlabored. Lung fields clear upon auscultation. Abdomen soft and flat with active bowel sounds in all quadrants. Last bowel movement this morning; soft, light-brown stool. Client reports recent rectal pressure and painful defecation. Denies penile discharge or blisters/sores on genitals or anus. VS: T 98.8°F (37.1°C), HR 72 beats/min, RR 14 breaths/min, BP 136/49 mm Hg, SpO$_2$ 98% on RA. Denies pain. The client is a tax accountant, lives alone, and is divorced with no children.

1300: Provider at bedside and reviews diagnostic tests with the client. Blood test shows an elevated prostate-specific antigen (PSA) level, postvoid residual (PVR) volume bladder ultrasound shows 125 mL of urine retained, and physical exam confirms enlarged prostate gland and 1.8-mm prostate nodule. Outpatient transrectal prostate ultrasound with needle aspiration and biopsy scheduled. Fleet enema ordered for 2 hours prior to exam.

The nurse reviews the collected client data and collaborates with the registered nurse. Complete the following sentence by selecting from the lists of options below.

The nurse determines the *priority* for care at this time is to establish a **1 [Select]** for **2 [Select]**.

OPTIONS FOR 1	OPTIONS FOR 2
Clear pathway	Ambulation to the bathroom
Sterile field	Expressing concerns and asking questions
Therapeutic environment	Intermittent urinary catheterization

Thinking Exercise 8.2.4

The nurse is caring for a 47-year-old client in a medical-surgical unit.

History and Physical	Nurses' Notes	Orders	Laboratory Results

Initial ED Visit

1220: Male client presents with dysuria and hematuria. Client reports difficulty starting urination, unable to maintain a constant stream, and burning during urination. States, "I thought I should come to the emergency room when I noticed blood in my urine." Alert and oriented × 4. Reports recent fatigue and some expected weight loss. Heart tones regular, skin warm and dry, pulses palpable throughout. Bilateral lower extremity 1+ pitting edema present. Respirations equal and unlabored. Lung fields clear upon auscultation. Abdomen soft and flat with active bowel sounds in all quadrants. Last bowel movement this morning; soft, light-brown stool. Client reports recent rectal pressure and painful defecation. Denies penile discharge or blisters/sores on genitals or anus. VS: T 98.8°F (37.1°C), HR 72 beats/min, RR 14 breaths/min, BP 136/49 mm Hg, SpO$_2$ 98% on RA. Denies pain. The client is a tax accountant, lives alone, and is divorced with no children.

1300: Provider at bedside and reviews diagnostic tests with the client. Blood test shows an elevated prostate-specific antigen (PSA) level, postvoid bladder ultrasound shows 125 mL of urine retained, and physical exam confirms enlarged prostate gland and 1.8-mm prostate nodule. Outpatient transrectal prostate ultrasound with needle aspiration and biopsy scheduled. Fleet enema ordered for 2 hours prior to exam.

Clinic Visit After Transrectal Ultrasound and Biopsy

1000: Client alert and oriented × 4. Provider at bedside discussing diagnosis of advanced adenocarcinoma of the prostate and treatment options. Prostatectomy scheduled and preoperative teaching completed.

Postoperative Medical-Surgical Unit

1430: Client admitted to surgical unit after a robotic-assisted laparoscopic prostatectomy. Drowsy but arousable. Oriented × 4 and follows simple commands. Heart tones regular. Skin cool and dry and without edema. Pulses palpable throughout. Respirations equal and unlabored. Lung fields clear throughout. Abdomen soft and flat with hypoactive bowel sounds. Three small incisions are present on the abdomen and covered by 4 × 4 dressings. No incisional drainage noted. Indwelling urinary catheter secured to inner thigh and draining clear, pink-colored urine to gravity. VS: T 97.5°F (36.3°C), HR 88 beats/min, RR 12 breaths/min, BP 126/44 mm Hg, SpO$_2$ 98% on 4 L/min O$_2$ via NC. Client reports abdominal pain rated 6/10.

The nurse collaborates with the registered nurse and contributes to the client's plan of care. Which of the following orders would the nurse anticipate? **Select all that apply.**

○ Case manager consult for discharge home in the morning
○ Discontinue urinary catheter once ambulating
○ Docusate sodium 50 mg orally each day PRN
○ Monitor intake and output every shift
○ Oxybutynin 5 mg orally every 8 hours PRN
○ Patient-controlled anesthesia (PCA)
○ Sequential compression devices when in bed

Thinking Exercise 8.2.5

The nurse is caring for a 47-year-old client in a medical-surgical unit.

History and Physical	Nurses' Notes	Orders	Laboratory Results

Initial ED Visit

1220: Male client presents with dysuria and hematuria. Client reports difficulty starting urination, unable to maintain a constant stream, and burning during urination. States, "I thought I should come to the emergency room when I noticed blood in my urine." Alert and oriented × 4. Reports recent fatigue and some expected weight loss. Heart tones regular, skin warm and dry, pulses palpable throughout. Bilateral lower extremity 1+ pitting edema present. Respirations equal and unlabored. Lung fields clear upon auscultation. Abdomen soft and flat with active bowel sounds in all quadrants. Last bowel movement this morning; soft, light-brown stool. Client reports recent rectal pressure and painful defecation. Denies penile discharge or blisters/sores on genitals or anus. VS: T 98.8°F (37.1°C), HR 72 beats/min, RR 14 breaths/min, BP 136/49 mm Hg, SpO_2 98% on RA. Denies pain. The client is a tax accountant, lives alone, and is divorced with no children.

1300: Provider at bedside and reviews diagnostic tests with the client. Blood test shows an elevated prostate-specific antigen (PSA) level, postvoid bladder ultrasound shows 125 mL of urine retained, and physical exam confirms enlarged prostate gland and 1.8-mm prostate nodule. Outpatient transrectal prostate ultrasound with needle aspiration and biopsy scheduled. Fleet enema ordered for 2 hours prior to exam.

Clinic Visit After Transrectal Ultrasound and Biopsy

1000: Client alert and oriented × 4. Provider at bedside discussing diagnosis of advanced adenocarcinoma of the prostate and treatment options. Prostatectomy scheduled and preoperative teaching completed.

Postoperative Medical-Surgical Unit

1430: Client admitted to surgical unit after a robotic-assisted laparoscopic prostatectomy. Drowsy but arousable. Oriented × 4 and follows simple commands. Heart tones regular. Skin cool and dry and without edema. Pulses palpable throughout. Respirations equal and unlabored. Lung fields clear throughout. Abdomen soft and flat with hypoactive bowel sounds. Three small incisions are present on the abdomen and covered by 4 × 4 dressings. No incisional drainage noted. Indwelling urinary catheter secured to inner thigh and draining clear, pink-colored urine to gravity. VS: T 97.5°F (36.3°C), HR 88 beats/min, RR 12 breaths/min, BP 126/44 mm Hg, SpO_2 98% on 4 L/min O_2 via NC. Client reports abdominal pain rated 6/10.

1930: Client out of bed to chair with minimal assistance. Demonstrates appropriate use of PCA. Discharge planning discussed.

The nurse collaborates with the registered nurse and contributes to the client's plan of care. Select whether the following potential nursing actions are indicated or not indicated for the client at this time.

POTENTIAL NURSING ACTION	INDICATED	NOT INDICATED
Teach the client how to empty the indwelling urinary catheter collection bag.		
Demonstrate how to inspect the incisional sites for signs of infection.		
Obtain a blood sample for a postsurgical PSA blood test.		
Remove the wound closure tape, and cleanse each laparoscopic wound with sterile saline.		
Teach the client proper urinary meatus cleansing.		

Thinking Exercise 8.2.6

The nurse is caring for a 47-year-old client during a follow-up clinic visit.

History and Physical	Nurses' Notes	Orders	Laboratory Results

Initial ED Visit

1220: Male client presents with dysuria and hematuria. Client reports difficulty starting urination, unable to maintain a constant stream, and burning during urination. States, "I thought I should come to the emergency room when I noticed blood in my urine." Alert and oriented × 4. Reports recent fatigue and some expected weight loss. Heart tones regular, skin warm and dry, pulses palpable throughout. Bilateral lower extremity 1+ pitting edema present. Respirations equal and unlabored. Lung fields clear upon auscultation. Abdomen soft and flat with active bowel sounds in all quadrants. Last bowel movement this morning; soft, light-brown stool. Client reports recent rectal pressure and painful defecation. Denies penile discharge or blisters/sores on genitals or anus. VS: T 98.8°F (37.1°C), HR 72 beats/min, RR 14 breaths/min, BP 136/49 mm Hg, SpO$_2$ 98% on RA. Denies pain. The client is a tax accountant, lives alone, and is divorced with no children.

1300: Provider at bedside and reviews diagnostic tests with the client. Blood test shows an elevated prostate-specific antigen (PSA) level, postvoid bladder ultrasound presents 125 mL of urine retained, and physical exam confirms enlarged prostate gland and 1.8-mm prostate nodule. Outpatient transrectal prostate ultrasound with needle aspiration and biopsy scheduled. Fleet enema ordered for 2 hours prior to exam.

Clinic Visit After Transrectal Ultrasound and Biopsy

1000: Client alert and oriented × 4. Provider at bedside discussing diagnosis of advanced adenocarcinoma of the prostate and treatment options. Prostatectomy scheduled and preoperative teaching completed.

Postoperative Medical-Surgical Unit

1430: Client admitted to surgical unit after a robotic-assisted laparoscopic prostatectomy. Drowsy but arousable. Oriented × 4 and follows simple commands. Heart tones regular. Skin cool and dry and without edema. Pulses palpable throughout. Respirations equal and unlabored. Lung fields clear throughout. Abdomen soft and flat with hypoactive bowel sounds. Three small incisions are present on the abdomen and covered by 4 × 4 dressings. No incisional drainage noted. Indwelling urinary catheter secured to inner thigh and draining clear, pink-colored urine to gravity. VS: T 97.5°F (36.3°C), HR 88 beats/min, RR 12 breaths/min, BP 126/44 mm Hg, SpO$_2$ 98% on 4 L/min O$_2$ via NC. Client reports abdominal pain rated 6/10.

1930: Client out of bed to chair with minimal assistance. Demonstrates appropriate use of PCA. Discharge planning discussed.

Clinic Visit 6 Weeks After Surgery

0900: Client is alert and oriented × 4. Client reports is back to full-time work, continues to walk daily, and recently started going back to the gym and socializing with friends. Client expresses concern about inability to achieve an erection the previous week. Heart tones regular, skin warm and dry, pulses palpable throughout, no edema present. Respirations equal and unlabored. Lung fields clear upon auscultation. Abdomen soft and flat with active bowel sounds in all quadrants. Laparoscopic incisional sites are well approximated with no redness, swelling, or drainage. Last bowel movement this morning; soft, light-brown stool. Client reports taking a stool softener daily to prevent painful defecation, which was previously experienced. Denies dysuria, urinary hesitancy, and hematuria. Reports the need to urinate comes on quickly and sometimes unable to get to the toilet in time. VS: T 98.6°F (37°C), HR 70 beats/min and regular, RR 12 breaths/min, BP 132/47 mm Hg, SpO$_2$ 98% on RA. Denies pain.

The nurse reviews the most recent nurses' notes and is assisting to evaluate the client's condition based on the collected data. Complete the following sentence by selecting from the list of word choices below.

The nurse recognizes that the client is likely experiencing **[Word Choice]** and **[Word Choice]**, which indicates that the client is not progressing as expected.

WORD CHOICES
Activity intolerance
Constipation
Erectile dysfunction
Painful defecation
Urinary incontinence
Wound infection

Unfolding Case Study 8.3

Thinking Exercise 8.3.1

The nurse is caring for a 24-year-old client in the emergency department. Highlight the client findings that require **immediate** follow-up.

History and Physical	Nurses' Notes	Orders	Laboratory Results

0620: Client presents with dysuria and testicular pain. Reports symptoms started yesterday afternoon and noticed a creamy, green-colored discharge from his penis this morning. Alert and oriented × 4. Heart tones regular, skin warm and dry, pulses palpable throughout. Respirations equal and unlabored. Lung fields clear upon auscultation. Abdomen soft and flat with active bowel sounds in all quadrants. Last bowel movement yesterday morning. Client reports urinary frequency and urgency throughout the night. Testicles are swollen and tender to touch. No swelling, discoloration, or wounds present on penis or meatus. VS: T 99.9°F (37.7°C), HR 68 beats/min, RR 14 breaths/min, BP 127/42 mm Hg, SpO$_2$ 97% on RA. The client is single, works as a waiter, and is sexually active with more than one partner.

Thinking Exercise 8.3.2

The nurse is caring for a 24-year-old client in the emergency department.

History and Physical	Nurses' Notes	Orders	Laboratory Results

0620: Client presents with dysuria and testicular pain. Reports symptoms started yesterday afternoon and noticed a creamy, green-colored discharge from his penis this morning. Alert and oriented × 4. Heart tones regular, skin warm and dry, pulses palpable throughout. Respirations equal and unlabored. Lung fields clear upon auscultation. Abdomen soft and flat with active bowel sounds in all quadrants. Last bowel movement yesterday morning. Client reports urinary frequency and urgency throughout the night. Testicles are swollen and tender to touch. No swelling, discoloration, or wounds present on penis or meatus. VS: T 99.9°F (37.7°C), HR 68 beats/min, RR 16 breaths/min, BP 127/42 mm Hg, SpO$_2$ 97% on RA. The client is single, works as a waiter, and is sexually active with more than one partner.

The nurse reviews the collected client data with the registered nurse. Complete the following sentence by selecting from the list of word choices below.

The nurse recognizes that the client is likely experiencing **[Word Choice]**.

WORD CHOICES
Inguinal hernia
Prostatitis
Sexually transmitted infection
Urinary tract infection

Thinking Exercise 8.3.3

The nurse is caring for a 24-year-old client in the emergency department.

History and Physical	Nurses' Notes	Orders	Laboratory Results

0620: Client presents with dysuria and testicular pain. Reports symptoms started yesterday afternoon and noticed a creamy, green-colored discharge from his penis this morning. Alert and oriented × 4. Heart tones regular, skin warm and dry, pulses palpable throughout. Respirations equal and unlabored. Lung fields clear upon auscultation. Abdomen soft and flat with active bowel sounds in all quadrants. Last bowel movement yesterday morning. Client reports urinary frequency and urgency throughout the night. Testicles are swollen and tender to touch. No swelling, discoloration, or wounds present on penis or meatus. VS: T 99.9°F (37.7°C), HR 68 beats/min, RR 16 breaths/min, BP 127/42 mm Hg, SpO$_2$ 97% on RA. The client is single, works as a waiter, and is sexually active with more than one partner.

The nurse reviews the collected client data and collaborates with the registered nurse. Complete the following sentence by selecting from the lists of options below.

The nurse determines the *priority* for care at this time is to obtain **1 [Select]** prior to **2 [Select]**.

OPTIONS FOR 1	OPTIONS FOR 2
Client consent	Administering anti-infective agents
Names of recent sexual partners	Reporting the sexually transmitted infection to the local health department
Specimen for culture	Teaching safe sex practices

Thinking Exercise 8.3.4

The nurse is caring for a 24-year-old client in the emergency department.

History and Physical	Nurses' Notes	Orders	Laboratory Results

0620: Client presents with dysuria and testicular pain. Reports symptoms started yesterday afternoon and noticed a creamy, green-colored discharge from his penis this morning. Alert and oriented × 4. Heart tones regular, skin warm and dry, pulses palpable throughout. Respirations equal and unlabored. Lung fields clear upon auscultation. Abdomen soft and flat with active bowel sounds in all quadrants. Last bowel movement yesterday morning. Client reports urinary frequency and urgency throughout the night. Testicles are swollen and tender to touch. No swelling, discoloration, or wounds present on penis or meatus. VS: T 99.9°F (37.7°C), HR 68 beats/min, RR 16 breaths/min, BP 127/42 mm Hg, SpO$_2$ 97% on RA. The client is single, works as a waiter, and is sexually active with more than one partner.

0750: Client alert and oriented × 4. Ambulates to the bathroom independently. Food tray provided for breakfast. Physician at bedside to discuss diagnosis and treatments. Laboratory results confirm sexually transmitted infections: chlamydia and gonorrhea. Client states, "I need to get out of here. I can't be late for work."

The nurse collaborates with the registered nurse and contributes to the client's plan of care. Select whether the following potential nursing actions are indicated or not indicated for the client at this time.

POTENTIAL NURSING ACTIONS	INDICATED	NOT INDICATED
Assess the client's psychological response to being diagnosed with the sexually transmitted infections.		
Explain the risk for multiple sexually transmitted infections and other medical complications.		
Prepare the client for prostate and rectal examinations.		
Suggest wearing supportive underwear and applying an ice pack to the groin area to reduce testicular pain.		
Transfer the client to an inpatient acute care unit.		

Thinking Exercise 8.3.5

The nurse is caring for a 24-year-old client in the emergency department.

History and Physical	Nurses' Notes	Orders	Laboratory Results

0620: Client presents with dysuria and testicular pain. Reports symptoms started yesterday afternoon and noticed a creamy, green-colored discharge from his penis this morning. Alert and oriented × 4. Heart tones regular, skin warm and dry, pulses palpable throughout. Respirations equal and unlabored. Lung fields clear upon auscultation. Abdomen soft and flat with active bowel sounds in all quadrants. Last bowel movement yesterday morning. Client reports urinary frequency and urgency throughout the night. Testicles are swollen and tender to touch. No swelling, discoloration, or wounds present on penis or meatus. VS: T 99.9°F (37.7°C), HR 68 beats/min, RR 16 breaths/min, BP 127/42 mm Hg, SpO$_2$ 97% on RA. The client is single, works as a waiter, and is sexually active with more than one partner.

0750: Client alert and oriented × 4. Ambulates to the bathroom independently. Food tray provided for breakfast. Physician at bedside to discuss diagnosis and treatments. Laboratory results confirm sexually transmitted infections: chlamydia and gonorrhea. Client states, "I need to get out of here. I can't be late for work."

0800: Orders received.

History and Physical	Nurses' Notes	Orders	Laboratory Results

0800:
- Discharge home
- Follow up with primary health care provider
- Doxycycline 200 mg orally every day for 7 days
- Ceftriaxone 1000 mg IM

The nurse assists with implementation of the plan of care. Select the **2** actions that would be appropriate for the nurse to implement at this time.

○ Assess for allergies before administering antimicrobials.
○ Teach the client proper techniques for administering IM medication.
○ Advise the client to be retested for sexually transmitted infections in 3 to 4 months.
○ Schedule a follow-up appointment with the client's primary health care provider.
○ Teach the client to take the antibiotics until symptoms are eliminated.

Thinking Exercise 8.3.6

The nurse is caring for a 24-year-old client in the emergency department.

History and Physical	Nurses' Notes	Orders	Laboratory Results

0620: Client presents with dysuria and testicular pain. Reports symptoms started yesterday afternoon and a creamy-green colored discharge from his penis was noticed this morning. Alert and oriented × 4. Heart tones regular, skin warm and dry, pulses palpable throughout. Respirations equal and unlabored. Lung fields clear upon auscultation. Abdomen soft and flat with active bowel sounds in all quadrants. Last bowel movement yesterday morning. Client reports urinary frequency and urgency throughout the night. Testicles are swollen and tender to touch. No swelling, discoloration, or wounds present on penis or meatus. VS: T 99.9°F (37.7°C), HR 68 beats/min, RR 16 breaths/min, BP 127/42 mm Hg, SpO$_2$ 97% on RA. The client is single, works as a waiter, and is sexually active with more than one partner.

0750: Client alert and oriented × 4. Ambulates to the bathroom independently. Food tray provided for breakfast. Physician at bedside to discuss diagnosis and treatments. Laboratory results confirm sexually transmitted infections: chlamydia and gonorrhea. Client states, "I need to get out of here. I can't be late for work."

0800: Orders received.

The nurse reviews the collected client data with the registered nurse and reinforces discharge teaching with the client. Select whether the following client statements indicate understanding or no understanding of the discharge teaching provided.

CLIENT STATEMENTS	UNDERSTANDING	NO UNDERSTANDING
"I will use a latex condom when engaging in sexual activities that involve genital contact."		
"I should engage in oral sex because my sexually transmitted infections cannot be spread by oral-genital contact."		
"Decreasing the number of sexual partners will decrease my risk for future sexually transmitted infections."		
"Treatment will eliminate symptoms, but I will always have these sexually transmitted infections."		

Stand-Alone Thinking Exercise 8.1

The nurse is caring for a 38-year-old client at an ambulatory care clinic.

History and Physical	Nurses' Notes	Orders	Laboratory Results

1220: Client presents for a routine primary care visit. Health history includes stage III breast cancer with bilateral modified radical mastectomy 18 months ago. Alert and oriented × 4. Follows all commands, and moves all extremities with equal strength. Reports left arm discomfort, stating "My left arm has been stiff and achy over the past several weeks. It sounds strange, but it almost feels heavier than the right one." Heart tones regular with pulses palpable and equal throughout. Left upper extremity appears slightly large. No edema present. Skin warm and dry throughout. Bruising and scabbed wounds present around left knee. Client reports tripping when playing with daughters at the park. Respirations equal and unlabored. Lung fields clear upon auscultation. Client denies dyspnea and/or chest pain with activity. Abdomen soft and flat with active bowel sounds in all quadrants. Denies nausea and gastrointestinal issues. VS: T 99.5°F (37.5°C), HR 88 beats/min, RR 16 breaths/min, BP 122/45 mm Hg via right thigh, SpO$_2$ 100% on RA. Reports left shoulder and arm pain rated 4/10.

The nurse reviews the collected data and collaborates with the registered nurse. Complete the diagram by selecting from the choices below to specify what potential condition the client is likely experiencing, **2** nursing actions that are appropriate to take, and **2** parameters the nurse would monitor to assess the client's progress.

Action to Take		Potential Complication		Parameter to Monitor
Action to Take				Parameter to Monitor

Actions to Take	Potential Conditions	Parameters to Monitor
Administer sublingual nitroglycerin.	Angina	Circumference of each arm
Assess the client's electrocardiogram (ECG).	Carpal tunnel syndrome	Symptoms of altered body image
Elevate the client's arm above the level of the heart.	Lymphedema	Heart rate and rhythm
Obtain an order for a compression sleeve.	Wrist sprain	Pulse pressure
Place an ice pack on the client's wrist.		Signs of infection

CHAPTER 9

Client Conditions Affecting Mood and Affect

Unfolding Case Study 9.1

Thinking Exercise 9.1.1

The nurse is caring for a 58-year-old client at the psychiatric clinic. Highlight the client findings that require **immediate** follow-up.

History and Physical	Nurses' Notes	Orders	Laboratory Results

1145: Client brought to clinic by friend after concern that client was becoming isolated at home. Friend states that client recently "lost his wife, who was his best friend," and now is being evicted from a small apartment due to financial issues. Wife's health care bills were "overwhelming." Client's two adult children live out of state and seldom visit. Client states, "There's no need to worry about me; nothing really matters." Reports recent anorexia, insomnia, and irritable moods, especially in the mornings. Reports losing 30 lb (13.6 kg) in the past month. Other medical history includes substance use disorder (alcohol), hypertension, type 2 diabetes mellitus, H/O myocardial infarction, and early COPD. Alert and oriented × 4. VS: T 98.6°F (37°C), HR 78 beats/min and regular, RR 20 breaths/min, BP 126/82 mm Hg.

Thinking Exercise 9.1.2

The nurse is caring for a 58-year-old client at the psychiatric clinic.

History and Physical	Nurses' Notes	Orders	Laboratory Results

1145: Client brought to clinic by friend after concern that client was becoming isolated at home. Friend states that client recently "lost his wife, who was his best friend," and now is being evicted from a small apartment due to financial issues. Wife's health care bills were "overwhelming." Client's two adult children live out of state and seldom visit. Client states, "There's no need to worry about me; nothing really matters." Reports recent anorexia, insomnia, and irritable moods, especially in the mornings. Reports losing 30 lb (13.6 kg) in the past month. Other medical history includes substance use disorder (alcohol), hypertension, type 2 diabetes mellitus, H/O myocardial infarction, and early COPD. Alert and oriented × 4. VS: T 98.6°F (37°C), HR 78 beats/min and regular, RR 20 breaths/min, BP 126/82 mm Hg.

The nurse reviews the collected client data and collaborates with the registered nurse. Complete the following sentence by selecting from the list of word choices below.

The nurse recognizes that the client is likely experiencing [**Word Choice**].

WORD CHOICES
Schizophrenia spectrum disorder
Generalized anxiety disorder
Major depressive disorder
Bipolar disorder

Thinking Exercise 9.1.3

The nurse is caring for a 58-year-old client at the psychiatric clinic.

History and Physical	Nurses' Notes	Orders	Laboratory Results

1145: Client brought to clinic by friend after concern that client was becoming isolated at home. Friend states that client recently "lost his wife, who was his best friend," and now is being evicted from a small apartment due to financial issues. Wife's health care bills were "overwhelming." Client's two adult children live out of state and seldom visit. Client states, "There's no need to worry about me; nothing really matters." Reports recent anorexia, insomnia, and irritable moods, especially in the mornings. Reports losing 30 lb (13.6 kg) in the past month. Other medical history includes substance use disorder (alcohol), hypertension, type 2 diabetes mellitus, H/O myocardial infarction, and early COPD. Alert and oriented × 4. VS: T 98.6°F (37°C), HR 78 beats/min and regular, RR 20 breaths/min, BP 126/82 mm Hg.

The nurse reviews the collected client data and collaborates with the registered nurse. Complete the following sentence by selecting from the lists of options below.

The nurse determines the *priority* for care at this time is to ensure the client's **1 [Select]** because the client **2 [Select]** and **3 [Select]**.

OPTIONS FOR 1	OPTIONS FOR 2	OPTIONS FOR 3
Safety	Has been evicted	Is becoming isolated
Nutritional status	Feels worthless	Has lost weight
Financial security	Has anorexia	Has high-cost medical bills

Thinking Exercise 9.1.4

The nurse is caring for a 58-year-old client at the psychiatric clinic.

History and Physical	Nurses' Notes	Orders	Laboratory Results

1145: Client brought to ED by friend after concern that client was becoming isolated at home. Friend states that client recently "lost his wife, who was his best friend," and now is being evicted from a small apartment due to financial issues. Wife's health care bills were "overwhelming." Client's two adult children live out of state and seldom visit. Client states, "There's no need to worry about me; nothing really matters." Reports recent anorexia, insomnia, and irritable moods, especially in the mornings. Reports losing 30 lb (13.6 kg) in the past month. Other medical history includes substance use disorder (alcohol), hypertension, type 2 diabetes mellitus, H/O myocardial infarction, and early COPD. Alert and oriented × 4. VS: T 98.6°F (37°C), HR 78 beats/min and regular, RR 20 breaths/min, BP 126/82 mm Hg.

1210: Patient Health Questionnaire (PHQ-9) score = 14, indicating moderate depression. States that he has considered suicide several times since losing his wife and planned to use his hunting rifle.

The nurse collaborates with the registered nurse and contributes to the client's plan of care. Select whether the following potential nursing actions are indicated or not indicated for the client at this time.

POTENTIAL NURSING ACTIONS	INDICATED	NOT INDICATED
Transfer the client to an inpatient acute psychiatric facility.		
Reinforce health teaching about antidepressant drug therapy.		
Consult with a social worker to ensure a safe home environment.		
Assist the client in developing a safety plan.		
Assess the client's support systems.		

Thinking Exercise 9.1.5

The nurse is caring for a 58-year-old client at the psychiatric clinic.

History and Physical	Nurses' Notes	Orders	Laboratory Results

1145: Client brought to ED by friend after concern that client was becoming isolated at home. Friend states that client recently "lost his wife, who was his best friend," and now is being evicted from a small apartment due to financial issues. Wife's health care bills were "overwhelming." Client's two adult children live out of state and seldom visit. Client states, "There's no need to worry about me; nothing really matters." Reports recent anorexia, insomnia, and irritable moods, especially in the mornings. Reports losing 30 lb (13.6 kg) in the past month. Other medical history includes substance use disorder (alcohol), hypertension, type 2 diabetes mellitus, H/O myocardial infarction, and early COPD. Alert and oriented × 4. VS: T 98.6°F (37°C), HR 78 beats/min and regular, RR 20 breaths/min, BP 126/82 mm Hg.

1210: Patient Health Questionnaire (PHQ-9) score = 14, indicating moderate depression. States that he has considered suicide several times since losing his wife and planned to use his hunting rifle.

1220: Met with social worker to develop a safety plan. Lives on disability benefits from an accident as a railroad worker. Wife was primary household earner. Plans to live with a friend until financial situation improves. Given prescription for antidepressant drug.

The nurse assists with implementation of the client's plan of care. Which of the following questions are appropriate for the nurse to ask regarding the client's safety? **Select all that apply.**

O "Do you feel like hurting yourself at this time?"
O "Do you feel like hurting someone else at this time?"
O "Do you have a plan for paying your wife's medical bills?"
O "Do you have a plan for where to live after your eviction?"
O "Do you have a plan to hurt yourself now or in the future?"

Thinking Exercise 9.1.6

The nurse is caring for a 58-year-old client during a follow-up visit at the psychiatric clinic.

History and Physical	Nurses' Notes	Orders	Laboratory Results

Initial Psychiatric Clinic Visit

1145: Client brought to ED by friend after concern that client was becoming isolated at home. Friend states that client recently "lost his wife, who was his best friend," and now is being evicted from a small apartment due to financial issues. Wife's health care bills were "overwhelming." Client's two adult children live out of state and seldom visit. Client states, "There's no need to worry about me; nothing really matters." Reports recent anorexia, insomnia, and irritable moods, especially in the mornings. Reports losing 30 lb (13.6 kg) in the past month. Other medical history includes substance use disorder (alcohol), hypertension, type 2 diabetes mellitus, H/O myocardial infarction, and early COPD. Alert and oriented × 4. VS: T 98.6°F (37°C), HR 78 beats/min and regular, RR 20 breaths/min, BP 126/82 mm Hg.

1210: Patient Health Questionnaire (PHQ-9) score = 14, indicating moderate depression. States that he has considered suicide several times since losing his wife and planned to use his hunting rifle.

1220: Met with social worker to develop a safety plan. Receives disability benefits from an accident as a railroad worker. Wife was primary household earner. Plans to live with a friend until financial situation improves. Given prescription for antidepressant drug.

Four-Week Follow-up Psychiatric Clinic Visit

0905: Client has been taking antidepressant drug as prescribed for 4 weeks. Has been living with a friend and looking for a part-time job. No suicidal ideation or attempts. Worked out a plan with the hospital for paying wife's medical bills. Daughter visiting for 2 weeks. Client states (while smiling), "I found out yesterday I'm going to be a grandfather! I might be moving closer to my daughter to enjoy this new role." Has gained 4.4 lb (2 kg) since last visit, but reports continued problems with sleeping.

The nurse reviews the latest nurses' notes to evaluate the client's current status with findings from 4 weeks ago. For each data collection finding, select whether the finding indicates that the client's status has improved or not improved.

DATA COLLECTION FINDING	IMPROVED	NOT IMPROVED
Client safety		
Nutrition status		
Feelings of worthlessness		
Sleep		

Unfolding Case Study 9.2

Thinking Exercise 9.2.1

The nurse is caring for a 37-year-old client in the emergency department (ED).

History and Physical	Nurses' Notes	Orders	Laboratory Results

1800: Client brought to ED via ambulance after 911 call that client was walking in busy street wearing only underwear and carrying a large knife threatening to kill anyone who approached. Police called and client de-escalated until hospital arrival. Client's skin dirty and odorous. Staff member who recognized client from previous admissions verified that client has a long history of schizophrenia and frequently stops taking prescribed medication for illness. Also has history of intermittent substance use, including cocaine and methamphetamine. Recently completed inpatient drug rehabilitation program. Currently unhoused and unemployed. Client angrily talking to self. States, "Didn't you hear what he said? I have to get out of here to stop all those people. God picked me to decide who goes to heaven."

The nurse reviews the collected client data with the registered nurse. Select the **2** client findings that require **immediate** follow-up.
O Skin dirty and odorous
O Wearing only underwear
O History of schizophrenia
O Threatening to kill people
O History of substance use disorder
O Having auditory hallucinations

Thinking Exercise 9.2.2

The nurse is caring for a 37-year-old client in the emergency department.

History and Physical	Nurses' Notes	Orders	Laboratory Results

1800: Client brought to ED via ambulance after 911 call that client was walking in busy street wearing only underwear and carrying a large knife threatening to kill anyone who approached. Police called and client de-escalated until hospital arrival. Client's skin dirty and odorous. Staff member who recognized client from previous admissions verified that client has a long history of schizophrenia and frequently stops taking prescribed medication for illness. Also has history of intermittent substance use, including cocaine and methamphetamine. Recently completed inpatient drug rehabilitation program. Currently unhoused and unemployed. Client angrily talking to self. States, "Didn't you hear what he said? I have to get out of here to stop all those people. God picked me to decide who goes to heaven."

The nurse reviews the collected client data with the registered nurse. Complete the following sentence by selecting from the list of word choices below.

The nurse recognizes that the client is likely experiencing [**Word Choice**].

WORD CHOICES
Anxiety
Depression
Psychosis
Dementia

Thinking Exercise 9.2.3

The nurse is caring for a 37-year-old client in the emergency department.

History and Physical	Nurses' Notes	Orders	Laboratory Results

1800: Client brought to ED via ambulance after 911 call that client was walking in busy street wearing only underwear and carrying a large knife threatening to kill anyone who approached. Police called and client de-escalated until hospital arrival. Client's skin dirty and odorous. Staff member who recognized client from previous admissions verified that client has a long history of schizophrenia and frequently stops taking prescribed medication for illness. Also has history of intermittent substance use, including cocaine and methamphetamine. Recently completed inpatient drug rehabilitation program. Currently unhoused and unemployed. Client angrily talking to self. States, "Didn't you hear what he said? I have to get out of here to stop all those people. God picked me to decide who goes to heaven."

The nurse reviews the collected client data and collaborates with the registered nurse. Complete the following sentence by selecting from the lists of options below.

The nurse determines the *priority* for care at this time is to ensure **1 [Select]** because the client is **2 [Select]**.

OPTIONS FOR 1	OPTIONS FOR 2
Safety for self and others	Dirty and odorous
Infection prevention	Currently unhoused
Housing for the client	Threatening to kill people

Thinking Exercise 9.2.4

The nurse is caring for a 37-year-old client in the emergency department.

History and Physical	Nurses' Notes	Orders	Laboratory Results

1800: Client brought to ED via ambulance after 911 call that client was walking in busy street wearing only underwear and carrying a large knife threatening to kill anyone who approached. Police called and client de-escalated until hospital arrival. Client's skin dirty and odorous. Staff member who recognized client from previous admissions verified that client has a long history of schizophrenia and frequently stops taking prescribed medication for illness. Also has history of intermittent substance use, including cocaine and methamphetamine. Recently completed inpatient drug rehabilitation program. Currently unhoused and unemployed. Client angrily talking to self. States, "Didn't you hear what he said? I have to get out of here to stop all those people. God picked me to decide who goes to heaven."

1815: Client becoming increasingly agitated. Standing and threatening staff without weapon or other device that could cause injury.

The nurse collaborates with the registered nurse and contributes to the client's plan of care. Select whether the following potential nursing actions are indicated or not indicated for the client at this time.

POTENTIAL NURSING ACTIONS	INDICATED	NOT INDICATED
Contact the hospital administrator.		
Initiate a response code for agitation/potential violence.		
Speak in a low voice when communicating with the client.		
Restrain the client to prevent harm to self or others.		
Ask if the voices are telling the client to harm others.		

Thinking Exercise 9.2.5

The nurse is caring for a 37-year-old client in the emergency department.

History and Physical	Nurses' Notes	Orders	Laboratory Results

1800: Client brought to ED via ambulance after 911 call that client was walking in busy street wearing only underwear and carrying a large knife threatening to kill anyone who approached. Police called and client de-escalated until hospital arrival. Client's skin dirty and odorous. Staff member who recognized client from previous admissions verified that client has a long history of schizophrenia and frequently stops taking prescribed medication for illness. Also has history of intermittent substance use, including cocaine and methamphetamine. Recently completed inpatient drug rehabilitation program. Currently unhoused and unemployed. Client angrily talking to self. States, "Didn't you hear what he said? I have to get out of here to stop all those people. God picked me to decide who goes to heaven."

1815: Client becoming increasingly agitated. Standing and threatening staff without weapon or other device that could cause injury.

1820: Code Gray initiated for response by security and clinical psychiatric staff.

The nurse assists with implementation of the response team's verbal de-escalation plan. Which of the following actions are appropriate to ensure the safety of the client and staff? **Select all that apply.**

O Provide time for the client to verbalize the outburst.
O Actively listen to what the client is saying before responding.
O Remove any equipment or items that could be a source of injury.
O Ask any unnecessary staff to leave the immediate area.
O Try to redirect the client's attention away from the internal voices.
O Maintain a distance of 2 to 3 feet from the client.

Thinking Exercise 9.2.6

The nurse is caring for a 37-year-old client in the acute psychiatric unit who was admitted through the emergency department.

History and Physical	Nurses' Notes	Orders	Laboratory Results

Emergency Department
1800: Client brought to ED via ambulance after 911 call that client was walking in busy street wearing only underwear and carrying a large knife threatening to kill anyone who approached. Police called and client de-escalated until hospital arrival. Client's skin dirty and odorous. Staff member who recognized client from previous admissions verified that client has a long history of schizophrenia and frequently stops taking prescribed medication for illness. Also has history of intermittent substance use, including cocaine and methamphetamine. Recently completed inpatient drug rehabilitation program. Currently unhoused and unemployed. Client angrily talking to self. States, "Didn't you hear what he said? I have to get out of here to stop all those people. God picked me to decide who goes to heaven."

1815: Client becoming increasingly agitated. Standing and threatening staff without weapon or other device that could cause injury.

1820: Code Gray initiated for response by security and clinical psychiatric staff.

1935: Admitted to acute psychiatric unit for evaluation, drug therapy, and psychiatric therapy.

One Week After Admission to Acute Psychiatric Unit
0815: Client showered and dressed for breakfast. Preparing for group session at 0900.

0900: Participated in group therapy. States continuing to hear voices, but tries to ignore them and tells them to stop. No threats to self or others while in unit. Takes medications without resistance.

1010: Met with social worker, who arranged for client to stay in halfway house for at least 3 months as needed until more permanent housing obtained. Client states formerly receiving monthly disability check but not sure where they are being sent now. Social worker to follow up. Possible discharge this week.

The nurse reviews the most recent nurses' notes to compare the client's current findings with the behaviors documented in the ED last week. For each data collection finding, select whether the finding indicates that the client's status has improved or not improved.

DATA COLLECTION FINDING	IMPROVED	NOT IMPROVED
Attention to internal voices		
Dress and hygiene		
Communication with others		
Aggressive behaviors		

Unfolding Case Study 9.3

Thinking Exercise 9.3.1

The nurse is caring for a 22-year-old client at the psychiatric clinic.

History and Physical	Nurses' Notes	Orders	Laboratory Results

1130: Client brought to clinic by family with report of not eating or sleeping for the past 8 days at home. Has stayed isolated from the rest of the family, and refuses to participate in meals or other activities. Has been more irritable, restless, and louder than usual; uses excessive profanity when approached by family. At times, seems euphoric and impulsive, but changes rapidly to anger. Conversation and thinking seem disorganized, distracted, and difficult to follow. Client recently went with friends to a local shopping center and spent over $3000 using a credit card for clothes that were not needed. Client plans to meet and sing with Taylor Swift. History of generalized anxiety disorder, but no other medical or psychiatric history. Family history of major depressive disorder. Client alert and oriented × 2 (person and place only).

The nurse reviews the collected client data with the registered nurse. Which of the following client findings are the **most** concerning to the nurse? **Select all that apply.**

O Family history of major depressive disorder
O Alert and oriented × 2
O Isolated from family
O Has not eaten or slept for 8 days
O Irritable and using excessive profanity
O Mood changes from euphoria to anger
O Conversation difficult to follow
O History of generalized anxiety disorder

Thinking Exercise 9.3.2

The nurse is caring for a 22-year-old client at the psychiatric clinic.

History and Physical	Nurses' Notes	Orders	Laboratory Results

1130: Client brought to clinic by family with report of not eating or sleeping for the past 8 days at home. Has stayed isolated from the rest of the family, and refuses to participate in meals or other activities. Has been more irritable, restless, and louder than usual; uses excessive profanity when approached by family. At times, seems euphoric and impulsive, but changes rapidly to anger. Conversation and thinking seem disorganized, distracted, and difficult to follow. Client recently went with friends to a local shopping center and spent over $3000 using a credit card for clothes that were not needed. Client plans to meet and sing with Taylor Swift. History of generalized anxiety disorder, but no other medical or psychiatric history. Family history of major depressive disorder. Client alert and oriented × 2 (person and place only).

The nurse reviews the collected client data with the registered nurse. Complete the following sentence by selecting from the list of word choices below.

The nurse recognizes that the client is likely experiencing **[Word Choice]**.

WORD CHOICES
Acute mania
Severe anxiety
Major depressive disorder

Thinking Exercise 9.3.3

The nurse is caring for a 22-year-old client at the psychiatric clinic.

History and Physical	Nurses' Notes	Orders	Laboratory Results

1130: Client brought to clinic by family with report of not eating or sleeping for the past 8 days at home. Has stayed isolated from the rest of the family, and refuses to participate in meals or other activities. Has been more irritable, restless, and louder than usual; uses excessive profanity when approached by family. At times, seems euphoric and impulsive, but changes rapidly to anger. Conversation and thinking seem disorganized, distracted, and difficult to follow. Client recently went with friends to a local shopping center and spent over $3000 using a credit card for clothes that were not needed. Client plans to meet and sing with Taylor Swift. History of generalized anxiety disorder, but no other medical or psychiatric history. Family history of major depressive disorder. Client alert and oriented × 2 (person and place only).

The nurse reviews the collected client data and collaborates with the registered nurse. Complete the following sentence by selecting from the lists of options below.

The nurse determines the **priority** for care at this time is to prevent **1 [Select]** because the client **2 [Select]**.

OPTIONS FOR 1	OPTIONS FOR 2
Dehydration	Is disoriented
Malnutrition	Has not had food for 8 days
Injury	Is irritable, impulsive, and angry

Thinking Exercise 9.3.4

The nurse is caring for a 22-year-old client at the psychiatric clinic.

History and Physical	Nurses' Notes	Orders	Laboratory Results

Psychiatric Clinic

1130: Client brought to clinic by family with report of not eating or sleeping for the past 8 days at home. Has stayed isolated from the rest of the family, and refuses to participate in meals or other activities. Has been more irritable, restless, and louder than usual; uses excessive profanity when approached by family. At times, seems euphoric and impulsive, but changes rapidly to anger. Conversation and thinking seem disorganized, distracted, and difficult to follow. Client recently went with friends to a local shopping center and spent over $3000 using a credit card for clothes that were not needed. History of generalized anxiety disorder, but no other medical or psychiatric history. Family history of major depressive disorder. Client alert and oriented × 2 (person and place only).

1220: Discussed with family and client the need for short-term hospitalization at this time for client protection. Arrangements for transfer to local acute behavioral health unit completed.

Acute Behavioral Health Unit

1345: Client admitted for acute manic episode lasting more than 1 week. No history of bipolar disorder or acute mania. Client alert and oriented × 4. Admission assessment completed. Client and family educated about potential plan of care.

The nurse collaborates with the registered nurse and contributes to the client's plan of care. Select whether the following potential nursing actions are indicated or not indicated for the client at this time.

POTENTIAL NURSING ACTIONS	INDICATED	NOT INDICATED
Assess whether the client is a danger to self or others.		
Assess the family's understanding of the client's situation.		
Use a firm and calm approach to the client.		
Provide thorough explanations to the client.		
Monitor food intake and sleep pattern.		

Thinking Exercise 9.3.5

The nurse is caring for a 22-year-old client at the psychiatric clinic.

History and Physical	Nurses' Notes	Orders	Laboratory Results

Psychiatric Clinic

1130: Client brought to clinic by family with report of not eating or sleeping for the past 8 days at home. Has stayed isolated from the rest of the family, and refuses to participate in meals or other activities. Has been more irritable, restless, and louder than usual; uses excessive profanity when approached by family. At times, seems euphoric and impulsive, but changes rapidly to anger. Conversation and thinking seem disorganized, distracted, and difficult to follow. Client recently went with friends to a local shopping center and spent over $3000 using a credit card for clothes that were not needed. History of generalized anxiety disorder, but no other medical or psychiatric history. Family history of major depressive disorder. Client alert and oriented × 2 (person and place only).

1220: Discussed with family and client the need for short-term hospitalization at this time for client protection. Arrangements for transfer to local acute behavioral health unit completed.

Acute Behavioral Health Unit

1345: Client admitted for acute manic episode lasting more than 1 week. No history of bipolar disorder or acute mania. Client alert and oriented × 4. Admission assessment completed. Client and family educated about potential plan of care.

The nurse assists with implementation of the client's plan of care. Select the **4** actions that would be appropriate for the nurse to implement at this time.

○ Provide frequent rest periods.
○ Provide high-calorie fluids and finger foods.
○ Encourage the client to participate in structured group activities.
○ Decrease environmental stimuli when possible.
○ Provide one-on-one client observation on admission to ensure safety.

Thinking Exercise 9.3.6—Pharmacology

The nurse is caring for a 22-year-old client at the psychiatric clinic.

History and Physical	Nurses' Notes	Orders	Laboratory Results

Psychiatric Clinic

1130: Client brought to clinic by family with report of not eating or not sleeping for the past 8 days at home. Has stayed isolated from the rest of the family, and refuses to participate in meals or other activities. Has been more irritable, restless, and louder than usual; uses excessive profanity when approached by family. At times, seems euphoric and impulsive, but changes rapidly to anger. Conversation and thinking seem disorganized, distracted, and difficult to follow. Client recently went with friends to a local shopping center and spent over $3000 using a credit card for clothes that were not needed. History of generalized anxiety disorder, but no other medical or psychiatric history. Family history of major depressive disorder. Client alert and oriented × 2 (person and place only).

1220: Discussed with family and client the need for short-term hospitalization at this time for client protection. Arrangements for transfer to local acute behavioral health unit completed.

Acute Behavioral Health Unit

1345: Client admitted for acute manic episode lasting more than 1 week. No history of bipolar disorder or acute mania. Client alert and oriented × 4. Admission assessment completed. Client and family educated about potential plan of care.

1420: Lithium therapy initiated per orders. Client responding to firm, calm approach by staff. Agreed to engage in individual structured activity. Drinking high-calorie smoothie beverage.

The nurse reviews the collected client data with the registered nurse and reinforces teaching about lithium therapy with the client and family. Select whether the following client statements indicate understanding or no understanding of the health teaching provided.

CLIENT STATEMENTS	UNDERSTANDING	NO UNDERSTANDING
"My blood lithium levels will be monitored while I am taking this drug."		
"I will restrict my intake of fluids while taking this drug."		
"I know that I might gain weight while taking this drug."		
"I should take this drug with meals to help decrease stomach irritation."		

Stand-Alone Thinking Exercise 9.1

The nurse is caring for a 38-year-old client in the emergency department (ED).

History and Physical	Nurses' Notes	Orders	Laboratory Results

1150: Client brought to ED by neighbor and friend, although client did not want to seek health care. Client presents holding left arm that is bruised, swollen, and not aligned below the elbow. Reports pain rated 8/10. Crying and asking if children are okay. Neighbor states that client's children are being cared for by neighbor's family and are safe. Seems withdrawn and frightened. Has visited the ED seven times in the past year with a variety of conditions, including insomnia, unexplained bruises, lacerations, and injuries such as a fractured hand and dislocated shoulder. No other significant medical history. Client alert and oriented × 4. Breath sounds clear throughout lung fields; no dyspnea. Old bruising noted on back and right wrist. Bowel sounds present × 4. Abdomen soft and nondistended. VS: T 98.6°F (37°C), HR 70 beats/min and regular, RR 16 breaths/min, BP 112/64 mm Hg, SpO$_2$ 96% on RA.

1225: Partner arrived at ED demanding to take client home. Seems angry and trying to intimidate staff.

The nurse reviews the collected client data and collaborates with the registered nurse. Complete the diagram by selecting from the choices below to specify what potential condition the client is likely experiencing, **2** nursing actions that are appropriate to take, and **2** parameters the nurse would monitor to assess the client's progress.

Action to Take		Potential Complication		Parameter to Monitor
Action to Take				Parameter to Monitor

Actions to Take	Potential Conditions	Parameters to Monitor
Conduct a client interview in private	Substance use disorder	Neurologic assessment
Draw blood for drug testing	Intimate partner violence	Vital signs
Notify hospital security personnel	Major depressive disorder	Client safety
Recommend counseling services	Suicidal ideation	Development of a suicide plan
Contact child protective services (CPS)		Vital signs

Stand-Alone Thinking Exercise 9.2

The nurse is caring for a 46-year-old client in the psychiatric emergency services department.

History and Physical	Nurses' Notes	Orders	Laboratory Results

2340: Client brought to PES department by neighbors. Client yelling loudly using numerous profanities; states drank two 6-packs of beer and used marijuana this evening. Expresses anger that neighbors brought the client here. Neighbors report that client was waving a rifle outside their houses and threatening to kill anyone seen on the street. Client states was looking for the person who was "messing around with my people." Medical history includes morbid obesity, hypertension, type 2 diabetes mellitus, and hypercholesteremia. Mental health history includes attention deficit/hyperactivity disorder, major depressive disorder, and delusional disorder. Has had several episodes of threatening neighbors in the past for a variety of different reasons, but never carried a weapon when threatening. Client alert and oriented × 2 (person and place). Refuses admission assessment, and threatening staff to stay away. Physician notified.

The nurse reviews the collected client data and collaborates with the registered nurse. Complete the diagram by identifying from the choices below to specify what potential condition the client is likely experiencing, **2** nursing actions that are appropriate to take, and **2** parameters the nurse would monitor to assess the client's progress.

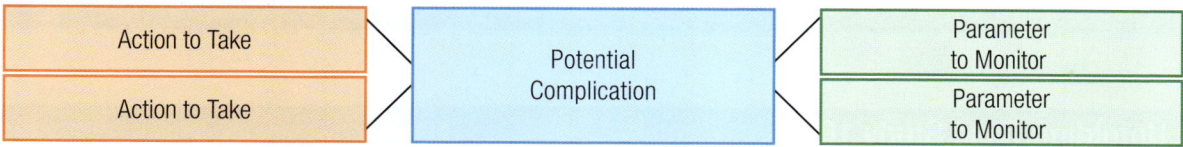

Actions to Take	Potential Conditions	Parameters to Monitor
Ask the client what the plan is	Antisocial personality disorder	Staff safety
Restrain the client	Generalized anxiety disorder	Vital signs
Offer antipsychotic medication to help calm the client	Major depressive disorder	Client safety
Recommend counseling services	Aggression and violence	Development of a suicide plan
Contact the hospital social worker		Blood alcohol level

Stand-Alone Thinking Exercise 9.3

The nurse reviews posted laboratory results in the emergency department for a 22-year-old client with a history of anorexia nervosa, major depressive disorder, and self-mutilation behaviors.

History and Physical	Nurses' Notes	Orders	Laboratory Results
Serum Laboratory Tests and Reference Ranges		1325	
Potassium (3.5–5.0 mEq/L [3.5–5.0 mmol/L])		2.7 mEq/L (2.7 mmol/L)	
Sodium (136–145 mEq/L [136–145 mmol/L])		132 mEq/L (132 mmol/L)	
Glucose (74–106 mg/dL [4.1–5.9 mmol/L])		59 mg/dL (3.3 mmol/L)	
Blood urea nitrogen (BUN) (10–20 mg/dL [3.6–7.1 mmol/L])		28 mg/dL (10 mmol/L)	
Creatinine (0.7–1.3 mg/dL [61.89–114.95 μmol/L])		1.5 mg/dL (132.63 μmol/L)	

The nurse reviews the collected client data and collaborates with the registered nurse. Complete the following sentence by selecting from the list of word choices below.

The nurse determines that the client is most at risk for **[Word Choice]** at this time.

WORD CHOICES
Acute kidney injury
Acute confusion
Cardiac dysrhythmias
Diabetic ketoacidosis

Client Conditions Resulting From Ineffective Coping

Unfolding Case Study 10.1

Thinking Exercise 10.1.1

The nurse is caring for a 40-year-old client at the mental health clinic.

History and Physical	Nurses' Notes	Orders	Progress Notes

1145: Client seeking health care due to worsening anxiety resulting from recent unexpected loss of job. Client is sole provider for family of 5, including 3 children younger than 6 years of age. Alert and oriented × 4. Has history of generalized anxiety disorder, panic attacks, and depression. Currently not taking any medications. Since being fired, client has been unable to problem-solve, concentrate, or sleep. Is now frequently irritable and loses patience with children's behaviors. Feels fatigued most of the time; has frequent palpitations and nausea, especially when thinking about the family's financial situation. Currently shaky and diaphoretic. Skin moist and clammy. Pupils slightly dilated, but denies drug use. Reports started drinking heavily every night to help with sleep. VS: T 98.6°F (37°C), HR 115 beats/min and regular, RR 26 breaths/min, BP 168/92 mm Hg.

The nurse reviews the collected client data with the registered nurse. Select the **5** client findings that require immediate follow-up.

○ History of generalized anxiety disorder
○ Inability to concentrate and problem-solve
○ Difficulty sleeping
○ Irritability and lack of patience
○ Palpitations and nausea when anxious
○ Drinks excessive alcohol every night
○ Tachycardia
○ Elevated blood pressure

Thinking Exercise 10.1.2

The nurse is caring for a 40-year-old client at the mental health clinic.

History and Physical	Nurses' Notes	Orders	Progress Notes

1145: Client seeking health care due to worsening anxiety resulting from recent unexpected loss of job. Client is sole provider for family of 5, including 3 children younger than 6 years of age. Alert and oriented × 4. Has history of generalized anxiety disorder, panic attacks, and depression. Currently not taking any medications. Since being fired, client has been unable to problem-solve, concentrate, or sleep. Is now frequently irritable and loses patience with children's behaviors. Feels fatigued most of the time; has frequent palpitations and nausea, especially when thinking about the family's financial situation. Currently shaky and diaphoretic. Skin moist and clammy. Pupils slightly dilated, but denies drug use. Reports started drinking heavily every night to help with sleep. VS: T 98.6°F (37°C), HR 115 beats/min and regular, RR 26 breaths/min, BP 168/92 mm Hg.

The nurse reviews the collected data with the registered nurse. Complete the following sentence by selecting from the list of word choices below.

The nurse recognizes that the client is likely experiencing a [**Word Choice**].

WORD CHOICES
Panic attack
Situational crisis
Personality disorder
Psychotic disorder

Thinking Exercise 10.1.3

The nurse is caring for a 40-year-old client at the mental health clinic.

History and Physical	Nurses' Notes	Orders	Progress Notes

1145: Client seeking health care due to worsening anxiety resulting from recent unexpected loss of job. Client is sole provider for family of 5, including 3 children younger than 6 years of age. Alert and oriented × 4. Has history of generalized anxiety disorder, panic attacks, and depression. Currently not taking any medications. Since being fired, client has been unable to problem-solve, concentrate, or sleep. Is now frequently irritable and loses patience with children's behaviors. Feels fatigued most of the time; has frequent palpitations and nausea, especially when thinking about the family's financial situation. Currently shaky and diaphoretic. Skin moist and clammy. Pupils slightly dilated, but denies drug use. Reports started drinking heavily every night to help with sleep. VS: T 98.6°F (37°C), HR 115 beats/min and regular, RR 26 breaths/min, BP 168/92 mm Hg.

The nurse reviews the collected client data with the registered nurse. Complete the following sentence by selecting from the lists of options below.

The nurse determines the *priority* for care at this time is to ensure the client's **1 [Select]** because the client **2 [Select]** and **3 [Select]**.

OPTIONS FOR 1	OPTIONS FOR 2	OPTIONS FOR 3
Safety	Has tachycardia	Is drinking alcohol every night
Cardiovascular health	Is fatigued most of the time	Has frequent palpitations
Financial security	Is irritable and impatient	Experienced a job loss

Thinking Exercise 10.1.4

The nurse is caring for a 40-year-old client at the mental health clinic.

History and Physical	Nurses' Notes	Orders	Progress Notes

1145: Client seeking health care due to worsening anxiety resulting from recent unexpected loss of job. Client is sole provider for family of 5, including 3 children younger than 6 years of age. Alert and oriented × 4. Has history of generalized anxiety disorder, panic attacks, and depression. Currently not taking any medications. Since being fired, client has been unable to problem-solve, concentrate, or sleep. Is now frequently irritable and loses patience with children's behaviors. Feels fatigued most of the time; has frequent palpitations and nausea, especially when thinking about the family's financial situation. Currently shaky and diaphoretic. Skin moist and clammy. Pupils slightly dilated, but denies drug use. Reports started drinking heavily every night to help with sleep. VS: T 98.6°F (37°C), HR 115 beats/min and regular, RR 26 breaths/min, BP 168/92 mm Hg.

1155: Client reports having a large insurance policy that could support the family if the client was "gone." Safety assessment performed.

The nurse collaborates with the registered nurse and contributes to the client's plan of care. Which of the following questions would be appropriate for the nurse to ask the client at this time? **Select all that apply.**

○ "Are you considering killing or hurting yourself?"
○ "If you are thinking about suicide, do you have a plan?"
○ "Do you have a gun in your house or car?"
○ "Have you ever attempted suicide before?"
○ "Are you considering hurting any of your family members?"
○ "What do you have to live for now that you lost your job?"

Thinking Exercise 10.1.5

The nurse is caring for a 40-year-old client at the mental health clinic.

History and Physical	Nurses' Notes	Orders	Progress Notes

1145: Client seeking health care due to worsening anxiety resulting from recent unexpected loss of job. Client is sole provider for family of 5, including 3 children younger than 6 years of age. Alert and oriented × 4. Has history of generalized anxiety disorder, panic attacks, and depression. Currently not taking any medications. Since being fired, client has been unable to problem-solve, concentrate, or sleep. Is now frequently irritable and loses patience with children's behaviors. Feels fatigued most of the time; has frequent palpitations and nausea, especially when thinking about the family's financial situation. Currently shaky and diaphoretic. Skin moist and clammy. Pupils slightly dilated, but denies drug use. Reports started drinking heavily every night to help with sleep. VS: T 98.6°F (37°C), HR 115 beats/min and regular, RR 26 breaths/min, BP 168/92 mm Hg.

1155: Client reports having a large insurance policy that could support the family if the client was "gone." Safety assessment performed.

1210: Client determined not a high risk for suicide at this time. Began to cry, stating how much the client loves family and wants to find another job if anxiety can be controlled. Client will be managed in the community with support of clinic and case worker. Drug therapy prescribed for anxiety.

The nurse collaborates with the registered nurse and contributes to the client's plan of care. For each mental health need, select the potential nursing actions that are appropriate as part of the client's plan of care.

MENTAL HEALTH NEEDS	POTENTIAL NURSING ACTIONS
Coping	○ Identify the client's usual coping styles. ○ Teach the client about newly prescribed antianxiety drug therapy. ○ Teach the client about new ways to cope with crises.
Safety	○ Instruct the client to remove any weapons in the house or car, including guns. ○ Remind the client to report any thoughts of harm to self or others. ○ Identify any cultural or religious beliefs that may help the client experiencing crisis.
Support	○ Refer the client to community resources for substance use disorder. ○ Refer the client to a community vocational rehabilitation program. ○ Remind the client to regularly participate in outpatient group therapy for crisis stabilization and rehabilitation.

Thinking Exercise 10.1.6

The nurse is caring for a 40-year-old client at the mental health clinic.

History and Physical	Nurses' Notes	Orders	Progress Notes

Initial Clinic Visit

1145: Client seeking health care due to worsening anxiety resulting from recent unexpected loss of job. Client is sole provider for family of 5, including 3 children younger than 6 years of age. Alert and oriented × 4. Has history of generalized anxiety disorder, panic attacks, and depression. Currently not taking any medications. Since being fired, client has been unable to problem-solve, concentrate, or sleep. Is now frequently irritable and loses patience with children's behaviors. Feels fatigued most of the time; has frequent palpitations and nausea, especially when thinking about the family's financial situation. Currently shaky and diaphoretic. Skin moist and clammy. Pupils slightly dilated, but denies drug use. Reports starting drinking heavily every night to help with sleep. VS: T 98.6°F (37°C), HR 115 beats/min and regular, RR 26 breaths/min, BP 168/92 mm Hg.

1155: Client reports having a large insurance policy that could support the family if the client was "gone." Safety assessment performed.

1210: Client determined not a high risk for suicide at this time. Began to cry, stating how much the client loves family and wants to find another job if anxiety can be controlled. Client will be managed in the community with support of clinic and case worker. Drug therapy prescribed for anxiety.

Follow-up Clinic Visit 2 Weeks Later

1550: Client being followed up for evaluation of crisis management. Reports having several job interviews in the past week and feeling encouraged about finding a job soon. Was able to obtain a loan from parents to help during the job search. States being able to sleep better, usually 5 to 6 hours each night. Continues to drink at least two beers or glasses of wine at bedtime every night to relax. Feeling less irritable and more patient with family. Less frequent episodes of palpitations and nausea when compared with 2 weeks ago. VS: T 98.6°F (37°C), HR 88 beats/min and regular, RR 20 breaths/min, BP 170/90 mm Hg. Referred to primary health care provider to follow up on persistent high blood pressure.

The nurse reviews the most recent nurses' notes and is assisting to evaluate the client's current status with findings from 2 weeks ago. For each data collection finding, select whether the finding indicates that the client's status has improved or not improved.

DATA COLLECTION FINDING	IMPROVED	NOT IMPROVED
Heart rate		
Palpitations		
Sleep		
Substance use		

Unfolding Case Study 10.2

Thinking Exercise 10.2.1

The nurse is caring for a 37-year-old client in the emergency department (ED).

History and Physical	Nurses' Notes	Orders	Laboratory Results

0040: Client brought to ED by friends stating client drank more than 6 beers and multiple alcoholic cocktails at a party. Client started shaking and reported having chills and difficulty breathing about a half hour ago, but refused to seek medical care. Became confused, and skin turned bluish and clammy, allowing friends to get client into the car to go to the ED. Currently very drowsy, but able to arouse. Oriented to self only. Unable to follow conversation. No known significant medical history. Cranial nerves intact, but gag reflex diminished. Breath sounds clear in all lung fields, but respirations slow. S_1 and S_2 present and regular. Abdomen soft with bowel sounds present in all quadrants. Moves all extremities slowly. Reflexes diminished. VS: T 97.4°F (36.3°C), HR 58 beats/min, RR 10 breaths/min and irregular, BP 86/50 mm Hg, SpO_2 88% on RA.

0115: Stat blood work drawn. Vomited × 1. Positioned briefly on side.

The nurse reviews the collected client data with the registered nurse. Which of the following client findings require **immediate** follow-up? **Select all that apply**.

○ Level of consciousness (LOC)
○ Body temperature
○ Respiratory rate
○ Heart rate
○ Blood pressure
○ Oxygen saturation

Thinking Exercise 10.2.2

The nurse is caring for a 37-year-old client in the emergency department.

History and Physical	Nurses' Notes	Orders	Laboratory Results

0040: Client brought to ED by friends stating client drank more than 6 beers and multiple alcoholic cocktails at a party. Client started shaking and reported having chills and difficulty breathing about a half hour ago, but refused to seek medical care. Became confused, and skin turned bluish and clammy, allowing friends to get client into the car to go to the ED. Currently very drowsy, but able to arouse. Oriented to self only. Unable to follow conversation. No known significant medical history. Cranial nerves intact, but gag reflex diminished. Breath sounds clear in all lung fields, but respirations slow. S_1 and S_2 present and regular. Abdomen soft with bowel sounds present in all quadrants. Moves all extremities slowly. Reflexes diminished. VS: T 97.4°F (36.3°C), HR 58 beats/min, RR 10 breaths/min and irregular, BP 88/50 mm Hg, SpO_2 88% on RA.

0115: Stat blood work drawn. Vomited × 1. Positioned briefly on side.

0200: Stat lab results posted and reviewed.

History and Physical	Nurses' Notes	Orders	Laboratory Results
Laboratory Test and Reference Range		**0140 in ED**	
Blood alcohol content (BAC) (0.0 g/dL)		0.27 g/dL (270 mg/dL)	
Blood glucose (74–106 mg/dL [4.1–5.9 mmol/L])		60 mg/dL (3.3 mmol/L)	
Sodium (136–145 mEq/L [136–145 mmol/L])		128 mEq/L (128 mmol/L)	
Potassium (3.5–5.0 mEq/L [3.5–5.0 mmol/L])		3.1 mEq/L (3.1 mmol/L)	

The nurse reviews the collected client data and collaborates with the registered nurse. Complete the following sentence by selecting from the list of word choices below.

The nurse recognizes that the client is **most likely** experiencing **[Word Choice]**.

WORD CHOICES
Alcohol intoxication
Wernicke-Korsakoff syndrome
Alcohol withdrawal syndrome
Alcohol use relapse

Thinking Exercise 10.2.3

The nurse is caring for a 37-year-old client in the emergency department.

History and Physical	Nurses' Notes	Orders	Laboratory Results

0040: Client brought to ED by friends stating client drank more than 6 beers and multiple alcoholic cocktails at a party. Client started shaking and reported having chills and difficulty breathing about a half hour ago, but refused to seek medical care. Became confused, and skin turned bluish and clammy, allowing friends to get client into the car to go to the ED. Currently very drowsy but able to arouse. Oriented to self only. Unable to follow conversation. No known significant medical history. Cranial nerves intact, but gag reflex diminished. Breath sounds clear in all lung fields, but respirations slow. S_1 and S_2 present and regular. Abdomen soft with bowel sounds present in all quadrants. Moves all extremities slowly. Reflexes diminished. VS: T 97.4°F (36.3°C), HR 58 beats/min, RR 10 breaths/min and irregular, BP 88/50 mm Hg, SpO_2 88% on RA.

0115: Stat blood work drawn. Vomited × 1. Positioned briefly on side.

0200: Stat lab results posted and reviewed.

History and Physical	Nurses' Notes	Orders	Laboratory Results
Laboratory Test and Reference Range		**0140 in ED**	
Blood alcohol content (BAC) (0.0 g/dL)		0.27 g/dL (270 mg/dL)	
Blood glucose (74–106 mg/dL [4.1–5.9 mmol/L])		60 mg/dL (3.3 mmol/L)	
Sodium (136–145 mEq/L [136–145 mmol/L])		128 mEq/L (128 mmol/L)	
Potassium (3.5–5.0 mEq/L [3.5–5.0 mmol/L])		3.1 mEq/L (3.1 mmol/L)	

The nurse reviews the collected client data with the registered nurse. Complete the following sentence by selecting from the lists of options below.

The *priority* for care at this time is to manage the client's **1 [Select]** because alcohol is a/an **2 [Select]**.

OPTIONS FOR 1	OPTIONS FOR 2
Airway and breathing	Stimulant
Bradycardia	Depressant
Level of consciousness	Acid

Thinking Exercise 10.2.4

The nurse is caring for a 37-year-old client in the emergency department.

History and Physical	Nurses' Notes	Orders	Laboratory Results

0040: Client brought to ED by friends stating client drank more than 6 beers and multiple alcoholic cocktails at a party. Client started shaking and reported having chills and difficulty breathing about a half hour ago, but refused to seek medical care. Became confused, and skin turned bluish and clammy, allowing friends to get client into the car to go to the ED. Currently very drowsy, but able to arouse. Oriented to self only. Unable to follow conversation. No known significant medical history. Cranial nerves intact, but gag reflex diminished. Breath sounds clear in all lung fields, but respirations slow. S_1 and S_2 present and regular. Abdomen soft with bowel sounds present in all quadrants. Moves all extremities slowly. Reflexes diminished. VS: T 97.4°F (36.3°C), HR 58 beats/min, RR 10 breaths/min and irregular, BP 88/50 mm Hg, SpO_2 88% on RA.

0115: Stat blood work drawn. Vomited × 1. Positioned on side.

0200: Stat lab results posted and reviewed.

History and Physical	Nurses' Notes	Orders	Laboratory Results

Laboratory Test and Reference Range	**0140 in ED**
Blood alcohol content (BAC) (0.0 g/dL)	0.27 g/dL (270 mg/dL)
Blood glucose (74–106 mg/dL [4.1–5.9 mmol/L])	60 mg/dL (3.3 mmol/L)
Sodium (136–145 mEq/L [136–145 mmol/L])	128 mEq/L (128 mmol/L)
Potassium (3.5–5.0 mEq/L [3.5–5.0 mmol/L])	3.1 mEq/L (3.1 mmol/L)

The nurse collaborates with the registered nurse and contributes to the client's plan of care. Select whether the following potential nursing actions are indicated or not indicated for the client at this time.

POTENTIAL NURSING ACTIONS	INDICATED	NOT INDICATED
Maintain the client in an upright sitting position.		
Administer naloxone per agency protocol.		
Establish peripheral access for IV fluid and electrolyte replacement.		
Assess vital signs, including LOC, every 15 to 30 minutes.		
Administer supplemental oxygen.		

Thinking Exercise 10.2.5

The nurse is caring for a 37-year-old client in the emergency department.

History and Physical	Nurses' Notes	Orders	Laboratory Results

0040: Client brought to ED by friends stating client drank more than 6 beers and multiple alcoholic cocktails at a party. Client started shaking and reported having chills and difficulty breathing about a half hour ago, but refused to seek medical care. Became confused, and skin turned bluish and clammy, allowing friends to get client into the car to go to the ED. Currently very drowsy, but able to arouse. Oriented to self only. Unable to follow conversation. No known significant medical history. Cranial nerves intact, but gag reflex diminished. Breath sounds clear in all lung fields, but respirations slow. S_1 and S_2 present and regular. Abdomen soft with bowel sounds present in all quadrants. Moves all extremities slowly. Reflexes diminished. VS: T 97.4°F (36.3°C), HR 58 beats/min, RR 10 breaths/min and irregular, BP 88/50 mm Hg, SpO_2 88% on RA.

0115: Stat blood work drawn. Vomited $\times$ 1. Positioned on side.

0200: Stat lab results posted and reviewed.

0210: Peripheral access established, and IV fluids initiated per orders. 6 L/min O_2 via NC. Client more alert and talking slowly with slurred speech. Asking what led to the ED visit. VS: 97.8°F (36.5°C), HR 64 beats/min and irregular, RR 10 breaths/min and regular, BP 96/58 mm Hg, SpO_2 94% on oxygen.

History and Physical	Nurses' Notes	Orders	Laboratory Results

Laboratory Test and Reference Range	**0140 in ED**
Blood alcohol content (BAC) (0.0 g/dL)	0.27 g/dL (270 mg/dL)
Blood glucose (74–106 mg/dL [4.1–5.9 mmol/L])	60 mg/dL (3.3 mmol/L)
Sodium (136–145 mEq/L [136–145 mmol/L])	128 mEq/L (128 mmol/L)
Potassium (3.5–5.0 mEq/L [3.5–5.0 mmol/L])	3.1 mEq/L (3.1 mmol/L)

The nurse assists with implementation of the client's plan of care. Select the **4** actions that would be appropriate for the nurse to implement at this time.

○ Reorient the client frequently, including explaining what led up to the ED visit.
○ Schedule the client for a cranial CT scan.
○ Observe the client carefully for psychotic behaviors such as hallucinations.
○ Initiate continuous cardiac monitoring.
○ Plan to discharge the client to home with a friend.
○ Continue to monitor vital signs and neurologic status every 15 to 30 minutes.

Thinking Exercise 10.2.6

The nurse is caring for a 37-year-old client in the emergency department.

History and Physical	Nurses' Notes	Orders	Laboratory Results

0040: Client brought to ED by friends stating client drank more than 6 beers and multiple alcoholic cocktails at a party. Client started shaking and reported having chills and difficulty breathing about a half hour ago, but refused to seek medical care. Became confused, and skin turned bluish and clammy, allowing friends to get client into the car to go to the ED. Currently very drowsy, but able to arouse. Oriented to self only. Unable to follow conversation. No known significant medical history. Cranial nerves intact, but gag reflex diminished. Breath sounds clear in all lung fields, but respirations slow. S_1 and S_2 present and regular. Abdomen soft with bowel sounds present in all quadrants. Moves all extremities slowly. Reflexes diminished. VS: T 97.4°F (36.3°C), HR 58 beats/min, RR 10 breaths/min and irregular, BP 88/50 mm Hg, SpO_2 88% on RA.

0115: Stat blood work drawn. Vomited $\times$ 1. Positioned on side.

0200: Stat lab results posted and reviewed.

0210: Peripheral access established, and IV fluids initiated per orders. 6 L/min O_2 via NC. Client more alert and talking slowly with slurred speech. Asking what led to the ED visit. VS: 97.8°F (36.5°C), HR 64 beats/min and irregular, RR 10 breaths/min and regular, BP 96/58 mm Hg, SpO_2 94% on oxygen.

0225: Client experienced generalized seizure lasting 45 seconds. After seizure, stated feeling "foggy" and asking why the client is in the ED. Alert, but only oriented to self. VS: 97.8°F (36.5°C), HR 68 beats/min and regular, RR 12 breaths/min and regular, BP 106/66 mm Hg, SpO_2 92% on 6 L/min O_2 via NC.

The nurse collaborates with the registered nurse to evaluate client outcomes. For each current client finding, select whether the client has improved or not improved when compared with admission findings.

CURRENT CLIENT FINDING	IMPROVED	NOT IMPROVED
LOC		
Seizure activity		
Blood pressure		
SpO_2		

Unfolding Case Study 10.3

Thinking Exercise 10.3.1

The nurse is caring for a 20-year-old client at the mental health clinic.

History and Physical	Nurses' Notes	Orders	Progress Notes

1010: Client with history of major depressive disorder and self-mutilation (cutting) brought to the clinic by family member. No significant medical history except for having frequent STIs during the past year. Alert and oriented × 4. Has been managed in the past with paroxetine and gabapentin. States is a full-time college student and cannot afford the medications. Has been very sad since grandfather died unexpectedly 18 months ago. Feeling more stressed than usual; has frequent nightmares and insomnia. Usually eats only one meal a day due to anorexia and finances. Recently "broke up with boyfriend" after they were caught shoplifting. Attended a "cutting" party last night. Two oozing wounds on right medial upper arm covered with gauze pads and tape: One cut is 3 in (7.6 cm); the other is 2.5 in (6.4 cm). Left upper arm has 3 new wounds (cuts) that are not currently oozing and are covered with gauze pads and tape. Redressed wounds on both upper arms. VS: T 98.6°F (37°C), HR 98 beats/min and regular, RR 20 breaths/min, BP 108/66 mm Hg, SpO$_2$ 99% on RA. Height reported at 5 ft 10 in (177.8 cm); current weight 112 lb (50.8 kg); BMI 16.1.

The nurse reviews the collected client data with the registered nurse. Select the **4** client findings that require **immediate** follow-up.

O History of clinical depression
O History of frequent STIs
O Nonadherence with prescribed drug therapy
O Recent deep wounds from cuts
O Nutritional status
O Feeling more stressed than usual
O Frequent insomnia
O Heart rate

Thinking Exercise 10.3.2

The nurse is caring for a 20-year-old client at the mental health clinic.

History and Physical	Nurses' Notes	Orders	Progress Notes

1010: Client with history of major depressive disorder and self-mutilation (cutting) brought to the clinic by family member. No significant medical history except for having frequent STIs during the past year. Alert and oriented × 4. Has been managed in the past with paroxetine and gabapentin. States is a full-time college student and cannot afford the medications. Has been very sad since grandfather died unexpectedly 18 months ago. Feeling more stressed than usual; has frequent nightmares and insomnia. Usually eats only one meal a day due to anorexia and finances. Recently "broke up with boyfriend" after they were caught shoplifting. Attended a "cutting" party last night. Two oozing wounds on right medial upper arm covered with gauze pads and tape: One cut is 3 in (7.6 cm); the other is 2.5 in (6.4 cm). Left upper arm has 3 new wounds (cuts) that are not currently oozing and are covered with gauze pads and tape. Redressed wounds on both upper arms. VS: T 98.6°F (37°C), HR 98 beats/min and regular, RR 20 breaths/min, BP 108/66 mm Hg, SpO$_2$ 99% on RA. Height reported at 5 ft 10 in (177.8 cm); current weight 112 lb (50.8 kg); BMI 16.1.

The nurse reviews the collected client data with the registered nurse. For each client finding, select whether it is consistent with the health condition of major depressive disorder or dysfunctional grief. Some findings may be consistent with more than one condition.

DATA COLLECTION FINDINGS	MAJOR DEPRESSIVE DISORDER	DYSFUNCTIONAL GRIEF
Sadness due to grandfather's death 18 months ago		
Anorexia and insomnia		
Self-injury (cutting)		
Frequent nightmares		

Thinking Exercise 10.3.3

The nurse is caring for a 20-year-old client at the mental health clinic.

History and Physical	Nurses' Notes	Orders	Progress Notes

1010: Client with history of major depressive disorder and self-mutilation (cutting) brought to the clinic by family member. No significant medical history except for having frequent STIs during the past year. Alert and oriented × 4. Has been managed in the past with paroxetine and gabapentin. States is a full-time college student and cannot afford the medications. Has been very sad since grandfather died unexpectedly 18 months ago. Feeling more stressed than usual; has frequent nightmares and insomnia. Usually eats only one meal a day due to anorexia and finances. Recently "broke up with boyfriend" after they were caught shoplifting. Attended a "cutting" party last night. Two oozing wounds on right medial upper covered with gauze pads and tape: One cut is 3 in (7.6 cm); the other is 2.5 in (6.4 cm). Left upper arm has 3 new wounds (cuts) that are not currently oozing and are covered with gauze pads and tape. Redressed wounds on both upper arms. VS: T 98.6°F (37°C), HR 98 beats/min and regular, RR 20 breaths/min, BP 108/66 mm Hg, SpO$_2$ 99% on RA. Height reported at 5 ft 10 in (177.8 cm); current weight 112 lb (50.8 kg); BMI 16.1.

The nurse reviews the collected client data with the registered nurse. Complete the following sentence by selecting from the lists of options below.

The nurse determines the *priority* for care at this time is to ensure the client's **1 [Select]** because the client **2 [Select]** and **3 [Select]**.

OPTION 1	OPTION 2	OPTION 3
Nutrition	Is nonadherent with drug therapy	Continues to feel very sad
Skin integrity	Continues cutting	Has a low BMI
Safety	Eats only once a day	Has insomnia

Thinking Exercise 10.3.4

The nurse is caring for a 20-year-old client at the mental health clinic.

History and Physical	Nurses' Notes	Orders	Progress Notes

1010: Client with history of major depressive disorder and self-mutilation (cutting) brought to the clinic by family member. No significant medical history except for having frequent STIs during the past year. Alert and oriented × 4. Has been managed in the past with paroxetine and gabapentin. States is a full-time college student and cannot afford the medications. Has been very sad since grandfather died unexpectedly 18 months ago. Feeling more stressed than usual; has frequent nightmares and insomnia. Usually eats only one meal a day due to anorexia and finances. Recently "broke up with boyfriend" after they were caught shoplifting. Attended a "cutting" party last night. Two oozing wounds on right medial upper arm covered with gauze pads and tape: One cut is 3 in (7.6 cm); the other is 2.5 in (6.4 cm). Left upper arm has 3 new wounds (cuts) that are not currently oozing and are covered with gauze pads and tape. Redressed wounds on both upper arms. VS: T 98.6°F (37°C), HR 98 beats/min and regular, RR 20 breaths/min, BP 108/66 mm Hg, SpO$_2$ 99% on RA. Height reported at 5 ft 10 in (177.8 cm); current weight 112 lb (50.8 kg), BMI 16.1.

1030: Psychiatric clinical nurse specialist in to talk with client. Requested that family member not be present during interview.

The nurse anticipates interventions that would be required for the client. Which of the following nursing actions would be appropriate regarding the client's loss of a grandfather? **Select all that apply.**
O Encourage the client to express feelings about the loss.
O Provide a reminder that the client will get over the loss with time.
O Refer the client to comprehensive grief and bereavement services.
O Assess the client for suicidal thoughts or ideation.
O If the client does not wish to talk about the loss, suggest journaling or drawing.
O Encourage the client to recall positive memories of the grandfather.

Thinking Exercise 10.3.5

The nurse is caring for a 20-year-old client at the mental health clinic.

History and Physical	Nurses' Notes	Orders	Progress Notes

1010: Client with history of major depressive disorder and self-mutilation (cutting) brought to the clinic by family member. No significant medical history except for having frequent STIs during the past year. Alert and oriented × 4. Has been managed in the past with paroxetine and gabapentin. States is a full-time college student and cannot afford the medications. Has been very sad since grandfather died unexpectedly 18 months ago. Feeling more stressed than usual; has frequent nightmares and insomnia. Usually eats only one meal a day due to anorexia and finances. Recently "broke up with boyfriend" after they were caught shoplifting. Attended a "cutting" party last night. Two oozing wounds on right medial upper arm covered with gauze pads and tape: One cut is 3 in (7.6 cm); the other is 2.5 in (6.4 cm). Left upper arm has 3 new wounds (cuts) that are not currently oozing and are covered with gauze pads and tape. Redressed wounds on both upper arms. VS: T 98.6°F (37°C), HR 98 beats/min and regular, RR 20 breaths/min, BP 108/66 mm Hg, SpO_2 99% on RA. Height reported at 5 ft 10 in (177.8 cm); current weight 112 lb (50.8 kg), BMI 16.1.

1030: Psychiatric clinical nurse specialist in to talk with client. Requested that family member not be present during interview.

1105: Client states not having suicidal thoughts or ideation. Reviewed guidelines for helping client care for self while coping with overwhelming grief. Drug therapy prescribed for depression. Discount drug price app available to reduce cost to client.

The nurse assists with implementation of the client's plan of care. Select the **4** statements that would be appropriate for the nurse to include in the guidelines for helping the client overcome the grief of losing a family member.

O "It is very important that you take your antidepressant as prescribed to help you cope with this loss."

O "Take care of yourself by eating regularly, exercising as often as possible, and getting at least 7 hours of sleep each night."

O "Avoid any printed material about death and grieving to prevent you from getting more upset."

O "Seek support from friends, family, or others, and discuss your feelings about the loss with them."

O "Let's talk about other ways you might be able to cope with your emotional pain instead of cutting."

O "You might want to consider changing to being a part-time college student to help lessen your stress level."

Thinking Exercise 10.3.6

The nurse is caring for a 20-year-old client at the mental health clinic.

History and Physical	Nurses' Notes	Orders	Progress Notes

Initial Clinic Visit

1010: Client with history of major depressive disorder and self-mutilation (cutting) brought to the clinic by family member. No significant medical history except for having frequent STIs during the past year. Alert and oriented × 4. Has been managed in the past with paroxetine and gabapentin. States is a full-time college student and cannot afford the medications. Has been very sad since grandfather died unexpectedly 18 months ago. Feeling more stressed than usual; has frequent nightmares and insomnia. Usually eats only one meal a day due to anorexia and finances. Recently "broke up with boyfriend" after they were caught shoplifting. Attended a "cutting" party last night. Two oozing wounds on right medial upper arm covered with gauze pads and tape: One cut is 3 in (7.6 cm); the other is 2.5 in (6.4 cm). Left upper arm has 3 new wounds (cuts) that are not currently oozing and are covered with gauze pads and tape. Redressed wounds on both upper arms. VS: T 98.6°F (37°C), HR 98 beats/min and regular, RR 20 breaths/min, BP 108/66 mm Hg, SpO$_2$ 99% on RA. Height reported at 5 ft 10 in (177.8 cm); current weight 112 lb (50.8 kg), BMI 16.1.

1030: Psychiatric clinical nurse specialist in to talk with client. Requested that family member not be present during interview.

1105: Client states not having suicidal thoughts or ideation. Reviewed guidelines for helping client care for self while coping with overwhelming grief. Drug therapy prescribed for depression. Discount drug price app available to reduce cost to client.

Follow-up Clinic Visit in 4 Weeks

1555: Client came to clinic alone. Alert and oriented × 4. States feeling much better and has not been cutting for 4 weeks. Old wounds on arms healed. Is eating and sleeping better, but continues to have nightmares. Started journaling about feelings related to loss about 3 weeks ago. Finds this activity helpful in coping with loss. Has been adherent with drug therapy as prescribed. VS: T 98.6°F (37°C), HR 86 beats/min and regular, RR 18 breaths/min, BP 112/68 mm Hg, SpO$_2$ 99% on RA. Height reported at 5 ft 10 in (177.8 cm); current weight 114 lb (51.7 kg).

The nurse collaborates with the registered nurse to review the client findings and evaluate outcomes. Complete the following sentence by selecting from the list of word choices below.

The nurse determines that the client has not improved regarding **[Word Choice]**.

WORD CHOICES
Cutting behaviors
Coping
Nightmares
Nutrition
Sleep

Stand-Alone Thinking Exercise 10.1

The nurse is caring for a 55-year-old client at the psychiatrist office.

History and Physical	Nurses' Notes	Orders	Progress Notes

0040: Client seeking care related to recent excessive "worry about everything." Was hospitalized for emergency surgery 3 months ago, and has felt very vulnerable since discharge. Works full-time for a local car dealership that pays based on the number of cars sold; car sales have decreased in the past 6 months. Shares child care with divorced spouse; two adolescent children are enrolled in private schools. Client concerned that financial situation will result in a change of schools. Client having difficulty sleeping most nights, which is causing the client to feel very fatigued. Almost fell asleep yesterday while at work. Has had episodes of palpitations and diaphoresis during the past few weeks. Denies use of illicit drugs, but typically drinks a glass of wine each night to help with relaxation.

The nurse reviews the collected client data with the registered nurse. Complete the diagram by selecting from the choices below to specify what potential condition the client is likely experiencing, **2** nursing actions that are appropriate to take, and **2** parameters the nurse would monitor to assess the client's progress.

Action to Take		Potential Complication		Parameter to Monitor
Action to Take				Parameter to Monitor

Actions to Take	Potential Conditions	Parameters To Monitor
Teach deep breathing and relaxation techniques	Substance use disorder	Use of positive coping skills
Draw blood for blood alcohol level	Generalized anxiety disorder	Incidence of panic attacks
Notify child protective services	Major depressive disorder	Sleep pattern
Recommend support services such as groups and counseling	Posttraumatic stress disorder	Financial status
Assess the client for suicidal ideation		Additional visits to care provider

Client Conditions Affecting Perfusion

Unfolding Case Study 11.1

Thinking Exercise 11.1.1

The nurse is caring for a 72-year-old client at a skilled nursing and rehabilitation facility. Highlight the client findings that require **immediate** follow-up.

History and Physical	Nurses' Notes	Orders	Laboratory Results

0740: Client alert and oriented × 4. Ingested 100% of breakfast with 600 mL fluids. Health history includes atrial fibrillation, coronary artery disease, heart failure, and dyslipidemia. Morning medications administered: aspirin, atorvastatin, digoxin, and warfarin. Client transported off unit for PT as part of inpatient cardiac rehabilitation after recent hospitalization for myocardial infarction.

0910: Client returns to nursing unit after PT session. Alert and oriented × 4. Follows commands, and moves all extremities with equal strength. Client positioned in bedside chair in preparation for lunch. Respirations labored with use of accessory muscles. Chest rises and falls symmetrically. Crackles auscultated in lung fields. Skin warm and intact except for type 2 skin tear on right forearm with foam dressing. No bleeding or drainage noted; hyperpigmentation present around wound site. Dependent nonpitting edema present in bilateral lower extremities. VS: T 100.3°F (37.9°C), HR 122 beats/min and irregular, RR 28 breaths/min, BP 140/68 mm Hg, SpO$_2$ 88% on RA. Denies pain but reports dyspnea. Client states "I can't seem to catch my breath, even after resting for a few minutes."

Thinking Exercise 11.1.2

The nurse is caring for a 72-year-old client at a skilled nursing and rehabilitation facility.

History and Physical	Nurses' Notes	Orders	Laboratory Results

0740: Client alert and oriented × 4. Ingested 100% of breakfast with 600 mL fluids. Health history includes atrial fibrillation, coronary artery disease, heart failure, and dyslipidemia. Morning medications administered: aspirin, atorvastatin, digoxin, and warfarin. Client transported off unit for PT as part of inpatient cardiac rehabilitation after recent hospitalization for myocardial infarction.

0910: Client returns to nursing unit after PT session. Alert and oriented × 4. Follows commands, and moves all extremities with equal strength. Client positioned in bedside chair in preparation for lunch. Respirations labored with use of accessory muscles. Chest rises and falls symmetrically. Crackles auscultated in lung fields. Skin warm and intact except for type 2 skin tear on right forearm with foam dressing. No bleeding or drainage noted; hyperpigmentation present around wound site. Dependent nonpitting edema present in bilateral lower extremities. VS: T 100.3°F (37.9°C), HR 122 beats/min and irregular, RR 28 breaths/min, BP 140/68 mm Hg, SpO$_2$ 88% on RA. Denies pain but reports dyspnea. Client states "I can't seem to catch my breath, even after resting for a few minutes."

The nurse reviews the collected client data with the registered nurse. Which of the following conditions is the client potentially experiencing? **Select all that apply.**

O Atrial fibrillation with rapid ventricular response
O Heart failure exacerbation
O Lung cancer
O Myocardial infarction
O Pneumothorax

Thinking Exercise 11.1.3

The nurse is caring for a 72-year-old client at a skilled nursing and rehabilitation facility.

History and Physical	Nurses' Notes	Orders	Laboratory Results

0740: Client alert and oriented × 4. Ingested 100% of breakfast with 600 mL fluids. Health history includes atrial fibrillation, coronary artery disease, heart failure, and dyslipidemia. Morning medications administered: aspirin, atorvastatin, digoxin, and warfarin. Client transported off unit for PT as part of inpatient cardiac rehabilitation after recent hospitalization for myocardial infarction.

0910: Client returns to nursing unit after PT session. Alert and oriented × 4. Follows commands, and moves all extremities with equal strength. Client positioned in bedside chair in preparation for lunch. Respirations labored with use of accessory muscles. Chest rises and falls symmetrically. Crackles auscultated in lung fields. Skin warm and intact except for type 2 skin tear on right forearm with foam dressing. No bleeding or drainage noted; hyperpigmentation present around wound site. Dependent nonpitting edema present in bilateral lower extremities. VS: T 100.3°F (37.9°C), HR 122 beats/min and irregular, RR 28 breaths/min, BP 140/68 mm Hg, SpO$_2$ 88% on RA. Denies pain but reports dyspnea. Client states "I can't seem to catch my breath, even after resting for a few minutes."

0930: Registered nurse at bedside. Client remains in the chair. Frequently transitions from tripod position to sitting upright as if unable to find a comfortable position. Client states, "Something is very wrong. I am having difficulty breathing." Respirations labored, and crackles auscultated in lung fields. Nonproductive cough present. Chest x-ray completed, showing enlarged heart and hazy lung fields. Extremities cool and ashen. Peripheral pulses 1+ throughout. ECG reveals Afib with normal ST segment and T waves. Client denies nausea and reports no urine output since before breakfast. VS: T 100.8°F (38.2°C), HR 101 beats/min and irregular, RR 23 breaths/min, BP 136/65 mm Hg, SpO$_2$ 94% on 4 L/min O$_2$ via NC. Denies chest pain. Reports general discomfort rated 3/10.

History and Physical	Nurses' Notes	Orders	Laboratory Results
Serum Laboratory Test and Reference Range		**Today**	**Yesterday**
B-type natriuretic peptide (BNP) (<100 mcg/L [<100 pg/mL])		455 mcg/L (455 pg/mL)	230 mcg/L (230 pg/mL)
Hemoglobin (M: 14–18 g/dL [8.7–11.2 mmol/L]; F: 12–16 g/dL [7.4–9.9 mmol/L])		15 g/dL (150 g/L)	16 g/dL (160 g/L)
Hematocrit (M: 42%–52% [0.42–0.52 volume fraction]; F: 37%–47% [0.37–0.47 volume fraction])		44% (0.44 volume fraction)	47% (0.47 volume fraction)
International normalized ratio (INR) (0.8–1.1)		2.5	2.6
Prothrombin time (11–12.5 seconds)		18 seconds	17 seconds

The nurse reviews collected data with the registered nurse. Complete the following sentence by selecting from the list of word choices below.

The nurse recognizes that the client is *most likely* experiencing [**Word Choice**] and [**Word Choice**] from [**Word Choice**].

WORD CHOICES
Anemia
Cardiac ischemia
Inadequate cardiac output
Insufficient clotting
Left-sided heart failure
Pulmonary edema
Inappropriate warfarin dose

Thinking Exercise 11.1.4

The nurse is caring for a 72-year-old client at a skilled nursing and rehabilitation facility.

History and Physical	Nurses' Notes	Orders	Laboratory Results

0740: Client alert and oriented × 4. Ingested 100% of breakfast with 600 mL fluids. Health history includes atrial fibrillation, coronary artery disease, heart failure, and dyslipidemia. Morning medications administered: aspirin, atorvastatin, digoxin, and warfarin. Client transported off unit for PT as part of inpatient cardiac rehabilitation after recent hospitalization for myocardial infarction.

0910: Client returns to nursing unit after PT session. Alert and oriented × 4. Follows commands, and moves all extremities with equal strength. Client positioned in bedside chair in preparation for lunch. Respirations labored with use of accessory muscles. Chest rises and falls symmetrically. Crackles auscultated in lung fields. Skin warm and intact except for type 2 skin tear on right forearm with foam dressing. No bleeding or drainage noted; hyperpigmentation present around wound site. Dependent nonpitting edema present in bilateral lower extremities. VS: T 100.3°F (37.9°C), HR 122 beats/min and irregular, RR 28 breaths/min, BP 140/68 mm Hg, SpO$_2$ 88% on RA. Denies pain but reports dyspnea. Client states "I can't seem to catch my breath, even after resting for a few minutes."

0930: Registered nurse at bedside. Client remains in the chair. Frequently transitions from tripod position to sitting upright as if unable to find a comfortable position. Client states, "Something is very wrong. I am having difficulty breathing." Respirations labored, and crackles auscultated in lung fields. Nonproductive cough present. Chest x-ray completed, showing enlarged heart and hazy lung fields. Extremities cool and ashen. Peripheral pulses 1+ throughout. ECG reveals Afib with normal ST segment and T waves. Client denies nausea and reports no urine output since before breakfast. VS: T 100.8°F (38.2°C), HR 101 beats/min and irregular, RR 23 breaths/min, BP 136/65 mm Hg, SpO$_2$ 94% on 4 L/min O$_2$ via NC. Denies chest pain. Reports general discomfort rated 3/10.

The nurse collaborates with the registered nurse and contributes to the client's plan of care. Select whether the following potential nursing actions are indicated or not indicated for the client at this time.

POTENTIAL NURSING ACTIONS	INDICATED	NOT INDICATED
Collaborate with a registered dietitian nutritionist to provide a low-sodium diet.		
Promote rest by eliminating unnecessary activities including visitors.		
Schedule essential activities with frequent periods of rest.		
Teach the client to utilize pursed-lip breathing techniques.		
Weigh the client each morning at the same time on the same scale.		

Thinking Exercise 11.1.5—Pharmacology

The nurse is caring for a 72-year-old client at a skilled nursing and rehabilitation facility.

History and Physical	Nurses' Notes	Orders	Laboratory Results

0740: Client alert and oriented × 4. Ingested 100% of breakfast with 600 mL fluids. Health history includes atrial fibrillation, coronary artery disease, heart failure, and dyslipidemia. Morning medications administered: aspirin, atorvastatin, digoxin, and warfarin. Client transported off unit for PT as part of inpatient cardiac rehabilitation after recent hospitalization for myocardial infarction.

0910: Client returns to nursing unit after PT session. Alert and oriented × 4. Follows commands, and moves all extremities with equal strength. Client positioned in bedside chair in preparation for lunch. Respirations labored with use of accessory muscles. Chest rises and falls symmetrically. Crackles auscultated in lung fields. Skin warm and intact except for type 2 skin tear on right forearm with foam dressing. No bleeding or drainage noted; hyperpigmentation present around wound site. Dependent nonpitting edema present in bilateral lower extremities. VS: T 100.3°F (37.9°C), HR 122 beats/min and irregular, RR 28 breaths/min, BP 140/68 mm Hg, SpO$_2$ 88% on RA. Denies pain but reports dyspnea. Client states "I can't seem to catch my breath, even after resting for a few minutes."

0930: Registered nurse at bedside. Client remains in the chair. Frequently transitions from tripod position to sitting upright as if unable to find a comfortable position. Client states, "Something is very wrong. I am having difficulty breathing." Respirations labored, and crackles auscultated in lung fields. Nonproductive cough present. Chest x-ray completed, showing enlarged heart and hazy lung fields. Extremities cool and ashen. Peripheral pulses 1+ throughout. ECG reveals Afib with normal ST segment and T waves. Client denies nausea and reports no urine output since before breakfast. VS: T 100.8°F (38.2°C), HR 101 beats/min and irregular, RR 23 breaths/min, BP 136/65 mm Hg, SpO$_2$ 94% on 4 L/min O$_2$ via NC. Denies chest pain. Reports general discomfort rated 3/10.

1020: Client positioned to comfort in bed with adult children sitting at bedside. Client's condition and plan of care discussed. Orders reviewed, and furosemide IV administered.

History and Physical	Nurses' Notes	Orders	Laboratory Results

Admission:
- Aspirin 325 mg orally every day
- Atorvastatin 20 mg orally every day
- Digoxin 0.125 mg orally every day
- Warfarin 5 mg orally every day

Today 1015:
- Furosemide 20 mg IV × 1 dose
- Valsartan 40 mg orally 2 times a day
- Morphine 2 mg IV every 4 hours PRN, pain

The nurse assists with implementation of the client's plan of care. Select the **4** nursing actions that would be appropriate for the nurse to implement at this time.

○ Advise the client to eat foods low in potassium such as apples, carrots, and berries.
○ Assist the client with frequent oral hygiene to prevent dry mouth.
○ Assess the client for signs of acute confusion and dizziness.
○ Check the client's finger stick blood glucose (FSBG) level before meals and at bedtime.
○ Collaborate with unlicensed assistive personnel to routinely toilet the client.
○ Evaluate laboratory results for potential electrolyte imbalances.
○ Monitor the client's apical pulse rate and heart rhythm.

Thinking Exercise 11.1.6

The nurse is caring for a 72-year-old client at a skilled nursing and rehabilitation facility.

History and Physical	Nurses' Notes	Orders	Laboratory Results

0740: Client alert and oriented × 4. Ingested 100% of breakfast with 600 mL fluids. Health history includes atrial fibrillation, coronary artery disease, heart failure, and dyslipidemia. Morning medications administered: aspirin, atorvastatin, digoxin, and warfarin. Client transported off unit for PT as part of inpatient cardiac rehabilitation after recent hospitalization for myocardial infarction.

0910: Client returns to nursing unit after PT session. Alert and oriented × 4. Follows commands, and moves all extremities with equal strength. Client positioned in bedside chair in preparation for lunch. Respirations labored with use of accessory muscles. Chest rises and falls symmetrically. Crackles auscultated in lung fields. Skin warm and intact except for type 2 skin tear on right forearm with foam dressing. No bleeding or drainage noted; hyperpigmentation present around wound site. Dependent nonpitting edema present in bilateral lower extremities. VS: T 100.3°F (37.9°C), HR 122 beats/min and irregular, RR 28 breaths/min, BP 140/68 mm Hg, SpO$_2$ 88% on RA. Denies pain but reports dyspnea. Client states "I can't seem to catch my breath, even after resting for a few minutes."

0930: Registered nurse at bedside. Client remains in the chair. Frequently transitions from tripod position to sitting upright as if unable to find a comfortable position. Client states, "Something is very wrong. I am having difficulty breathing." Respirations labored, and crackles auscultated in lung fields. Nonproductive cough present. Chest x-ray completed, showing enlarged heart and hazy lung fields. Extremities cool and ashen. Peripheral pulses 1+ throughout. ECG reveals Afib with normal ST segment and T waves. Client denies nausea and reports no urine output since before breakfast. VS: T 100.8°F (38.2°C), HR 101 beats/min and irregular, RR 23 breaths/min, BP 136/65 mm Hg, SpO$_2$ 94% on 4 L/min O$_2$ via NC. Denies chest pain. Reports general discomfort rated 3/10.

1020: Client positioned to comfort in bed with adult children sitting at bedside. Client's condition and plan of care discussed. Orders reviewed, and furosemide IV administered.

1600: Client sleeping and easily aroused. Oriented × 4, and follows commands. Respirations equal and unlabored. Client states, "I am feeling better now, but I became breathless when I used the bedside commode." Crackles auscultated in lung fields. Productive cough with scant white, frothy sputum. Cardiac rhythm: Afib with frequent PVCs. Extremities warm, and peripheral pulses 2+ throughout. VS: T 99.9°F (37.7°C), HR 76 beats/min and irregular, RR 14 breaths/min, BP 122/45 mm Hg, SpO$_2$ 94% on 4 L/min O$_2$ via NC. Denies pain.

The nurse reviews the client findings with the registered nurse. For each data collection finding, select whether the finding indicates that the client's status has improved or not improved.

CLIENT FINDINGS	IMPROVED	NOT IMPROVED
Auscultated crackles in lung fields		
Cardiac rhythm: Afib with frequent PVCs		
Experiences breathlessness with activity		
Extremities warm with 2+ peripheral pulses throughout		
Productive cough with scant white, frothy sputum		
Sleeping when undisturbed		

Unfolding Case Study 11.2

Thinking Exercise 11.2.1

The nurse is caring for an 82-year-old client on a medical-surgical unit.

History and Physical	Nurses' Notes	Orders	Laboratory Results

Current Conditions:
- Left hip fracture
- Postoperative open reduction and internal fixation (ORIF)

Medical History:
- Type 2 diabetes mellitus
- Hypertension

Allergies: NKDA

Medications:
- Amlodipine
- Exenatide
- Glipizide
- Hydrochlorothiazide

Social History: Client is retired and lives with spouse of 52 years.

History and Physical	Nurses' Notes	Orders	Laboratory Results

Postoperative Day 3

0730: Bedside hand-off report provided to oncoming nurse. Client is alert and oriented × 4. Denies pain and shares, "I am looking forward to getting out of the hospital and going to the rehabilitation facility."

0800: Client is drowsy, and physical touch is required to arouse. Oriented to self only. Speech is slurred. Left facial weakness with drooling from side of mouth. VS: HR 98 beats/min and regular, RR 18 breaths/min, BP 177/92 mm Hg, SpO_2 95% on RA.

The nurse reviews the collected client data with the registered nurse. Which of the following client findings require **immediate** follow-up? **Select all that apply.**

○ Blood pressure
○ Dysarthria
○ Heart rate
○ Level of consciousness
○ Orientation status
○ SpO_2 level

Thinking Exercise 11.2.2

The nurse is caring for an 82-year-old client on a medical-surgical unit.

History and Physical	Nurses' Notes	Orders	Laboratory Results

Current Conditions:
- Left hip fracture
- Postoperative open reduction and internal fixation (ORIF)

Medical History:
- Type 2 diabetes mellitus
- Hypertension

Allergies: NKDA

Medications:
- Amlodipine
- Exenatide
- Glipizide
- Hydrochlorothiazide

Social History: Client is retired and lives with spouse of 52 years.

History and Physical	Nurses' Notes	Orders	Laboratory Results

Postoperative Day 3
0730: Bedside hand-off report provided to oncoming nurse. Client is alert and oriented × 4. Denies pain and shares, "I am looking forward to getting out of the hospital and going to the rehabilitation facility."

0800: Client is drowsy, and physical touch is required to arouse. Oriented to self only. Speech is slurred. Left facial weakness with drooling from side of mouth. VS: HR 98 beats/min and regular, RR 18 breaths/min, BP 177/92 mm Hg, SpO$_2$ 95% on RA.

The nurse reviews the collected client data with the registered nurse. For each data collection finding, select whether the finding is consistent with the health conditions of Bell's palsy, hypoglycemia, or stroke. Some findings may be consistent with more than one condition.

CLIENT FINDING	BELL'S PALSY	HYPOGLYCEMIA	STROKE
Acute confusion			
Drooling			
Drowsiness			
Facial weakness			
Slurred speech			

Thinking Exercise 11.2.3

The nurse is caring for an 82-year-old client on a medical-surgical unit.

History and Physical	Nurses' Notes	Orders	Laboratory Results

Current Conditions:
- Left hip fracture
- Postoperative open reduction and internal fixation (ORIF)

Medical History:
- Type 2 diabetes mellitus
- Hypertension

Allergies: NKDA

Medications:
- Amlodipine
- Exenatide
- Glipizide
- Hydrochlorothiazide

Social History: Client is retired and lives with spouse of 52 years.

History and Physical	Nurses' Notes	Orders	Laboratory Results

Postoperative Day 3
0730: Bedside hand-off report provided to oncoming nurse. Client is alert and oriented × 4. Denies pain and shares, "I am looking forward to getting out of the hospital and going to the rehabilitation facility."

0800: Client is drowsy, and physical touch is required to arouse. Oriented to self only. Speech is slurred. Left facial weakness with drooling from side of mouth. VS: HR 98 beats/min and regular, RR 18 breaths/min, BP 177/92 mm Hg, SpO$_2$ 95% on RA.

0815: Client nods appropriately and follows simple commands. Speech is undiscernible. Left-sided hemiplegia present. Respirations equal and unlabored. Peripheral pulses equal at 2+ throughout. Client denies chest pain or shortness of breath. Pallor present; no diaphoresis. Bowel sounds present in all quadrants. Client having difficulty clearing secretions; suctioned large amount of thin, clear secretions from oral cavity. FSBG 188 mg/dL (10.4 mmol/L).

The nurse reviews the collected client data with the registered nurse. Complete the following sentence by selecting from the lists of options below.

The client is *most likely* experiencing [**Word Choice**] and is at *high risk* for developing [**Word Choice**].

WORD CHOICES
Aspiration pneumonia
Bell's palsy
Contractures
Hypoglycemia
Pressure injury
Stroke
Urinary tract infection

Thinking Exercise 11.2.4

The nurse is caring for an 82-year-old client on a medical-surgical unit.

History and Physical	Nurses' Notes	Orders	Laboratory Results

Current Conditions:
- Left hip fracture
- Postoperative open reduction and internal fixation (ORIF)

Medical History:
- Type 2 diabetes mellitus
- Hypertension

Allergies: NKDA

Medications:
- Amlodipine
- Exenatide
- Glipizide
- Hydrochlorothiazide

Social History: Client is retired and lives with spouse of 52 years.

History and Physical	Nurses' Notes	Orders	Laboratory Results

Postoperative Day 3

0730: Bedside hand-off report provided to oncoming nurse. Client is alert and oriented × 4. Denies pain and shares, "I am looking forward to getting out of the hospital and going to the rehabilitation facility."

0800: Client is drowsy, and physical touch is required to arouse. Oriented to self only. Speech is slurred. Left facial palsy with drooling from side of mouth. VS: HR 98 beats/min and regular, RR 18 breaths/min, BP 177/92 mm Hg, SpO$_2$ 95% on RA.

0815: Client nods appropriately and follows simple commands. Speech is undiscernible. Left-sided hemiplegia present. Respirations equal and unlabored. Peripheral pulses equal at 2+ throughout. Client denies chest pain or shortness of breath. Pallor present; no diaphoresis. Bowel sounds present in all quadrants. Client having difficulty clearing secretions; suctioned large amount of thin, clear secretions from oral cavity. FSBG 188 mg/dL (10.4 mmol/L).

The nurse collaborates with the registered nurse and contributes to the client's plan of care. Select whether the following potential nursing actions are indicated or not indicated for the client at this time.

POTENTIAL NURSING ACTIONS	INDICATED	NOT INDICATED
Administer scheduled antihypertensive medications.		
Assist in completing the facility's approved stroke scale.		
Position the client to comfort with the head of the bed flat.		
Provide a variety of tools to help the client communicate.		
Report and document the time the symptoms began.		
Use a gait belt to ambulate the client to the bathroom.		

Thinking Exercise 11.2.5

The nurse is caring for an 82-year-old client on a medical-surgical unit.

History and Physical	Nurses' Notes	Orders	Laboratory Results

Current Conditions:
- Left hip fracture
- Postoperative open reduction and internal fixation (ORIF)

Medical History:
- Type 2 diabetes mellitus
- Hypertension

Allergies: NKDA

Medications:
- Amlodipine
- Exenatide
- Glipizide
- Hydrochlorothiazide

Social History: Client is retired and lives with spouse of 52 years.

History and Physical	Nurses' Notes	Orders	Laboratory Results

Postoperative Day 3

0730: Bedside hand-off report provided to oncoming nurse. Client is alert and oriented × 4. Denies pain and shares, "I am looking forward to getting out of the hospital and going to the rehabilitation facility."

0800: Client is drowsy, and physical touch is required to arouse. Oriented to self only. Speech is slurred. Left facial palsy with drooling from side of mouth. VS: HR 98 beats/min and regular, RR 18 breaths/min, BP 177/92 mm Hg, SpO$_2$ 95% on RA.

0815: Client nods appropriately and follows simple commands. Speech is undiscernible. Left-sided hemiplegia present. Respirations equal and unlabored. Peripheral pulses equal at 2+ throughout. Client denies chest pain or shortness of breath. Pallor present; no diaphoresis. Bowel sounds present in all quadrants. Client having difficulty clearing secretions; suctioned large amount of thin, clear secretions from oral cavity. FSBG 188 mg/dL (10.4 mmol/L).

0820: Stroke team at bedside.

The nurse assists with implementation of the client's plan of care. Complete the following sentence by selecting from the lists of options below.

The nurse determines the *priority* action at this time is to assess the client for **1 [Select]** in preparation for **2 [Select]**.

OPTIONS FOR 1	OPTIONS FOR 2
Adventitious breath sounds	Head computerized tomography (CT) scan
Bleeding	Nasotracheal suctioning
Contrast media allergy	Thrombolytic therapy

Thinking Exercise 11.2.6

The nurse is caring for an 82-year-old client on a medical-surgical unit.

History and Physical	Nurses' Notes	Orders	Laboratory Results

Current Conditions:
- Left hip fracture
- Postoperative open reduction and internal fixation (ORIF)

Medical History:
- Type 2 diabetes mellitus
- Hypertension

Allergies: NKDA

Medications:
- Amlodipine
- Exenatide
- Glipizide
- Hydrochlorothiazide

Social History: Client is retired and lives with spouse of 52 years.

History and Physical	Nurses' Notes	Orders	Laboratory Results

Postoperative Day 3

0730: Bedside hand-off report provided to oncoming nurse. Client is alert and oriented × 4. Denies pain and shares, "I am looking forward to getting out of the hospital and going to the rehabilitation facility."

0800: Client is drowsy, and physical touch is required to arouse. Oriented to self only. Speech is slurred. Left facial palsy with drooling from side of mouth. VS: HR 98 beats/min and regular, RR 18 breaths/min, BP 177/92 mm Hg, SpO$_2$ 95% on RA.

0815: Client nods appropriately and follows simple commands. Speech is undiscernible. Left-sided hemiplegia present. Respirations equal and unlabored. Peripheral pulses equal at 2+ throughout. Client denies chest pain or shortness of breath. Pallor present; no diaphoresis. Bowel sounds present in all quadrants. Client having difficulty clearing secretions; suctioned large amount of thin, clear secretions from oral cavity. FSBG 188 mg/dL (10.4 mmol/L).

0820: Stroke team at bedside.

0840: Care transitioned to registered nurse. Client transported to radiology.

Postoperative Day 6

1410: Client is alert and oriented × 4. Facial features and expressions symmetrical. Speech undiscernible; picture board used to communicate effectively. Follows commands, and moves right extremities with normal strength. Left upper extremity moves against gravity but not resistance. Wiggles left toes, but unable to move left lower extremity against gravity. Respirations equal and unlabored. Rhonchi auscultated in lung fields. Productive cough present. Client uses oral suctioning tool to clear secretions. Skin warm, dry, and normal coloration. Peripheral pulses equal throughout. 2+ edema in left lower extremity. Client denies chest pain or shortness of breath. Bowel sounds present in all quadrants. Ate 75% of lunch meal (chopped diet with nectar-thickened fluids). Uses bedside commode with assistance. VS: T 98.8°F (37.1°C), HR 72 beats/min and regular, RR 14 breaths/min, BP 136/52 mm Hg, SpO$_2$ 99% on 2 L/min O$_2$ via NC.

The nurse reviews the collected client data with the registered nurse. For each body system, select whether the finding indicates the client's status has improved.

BODY SYSTEMS	CLIENT FINDINGS
Respiratory	○ Productive cough present ○ RR 14 breaths/min ○ Rhonchi auscultated in lung fields
Cardiovascular	○ BP 136/52 mm Hg ○ 2+ edema in left lower extremity ○ Skin warm, dry, and normal coloration
Neurologic	○ Symmetrical facial features and expressions ○ Left upper extremity moves against gravity ○ Requires a picture board to communicate effectively

Stand-Alone Thinking Exercise 11.1

The nurse is caring for a 78-year-old client on a medical-surgical unit.

History and Physical	Nurses' Notes	Orders	Laboratory Results

1520: Client uses call bell to contact the nurse. Reports muscle pain and spasms in the right lower extremity. Pain is worsened with pressure and movement. Respirations equal and unlabored. Heart tones regular. Snapping sound from prosthetic mitral valve noted. Upper extremities and left lower extremity are warm with usual pigmentation and with 2+ palpable pulses. Right lower extremity is ashen and cool; pulses present with Doppler only. Abdomen soft and round with hyperactive bowel sounds. VS: T 99.1°F (37.2°C), HR 88 beats/min, RR 14 breaths/min, BP 99/26 mm Hg, SpO$_2$ 98% on RA.

The nurse reviews the collected client data with the registered nurse. Complete the diagram by selecting from the choices below to specify what potential condition the client is likely experiencing, **2** nursing actions that are appropriate to take, and **2** parameters the nurse would monitor to assess the client's progress.

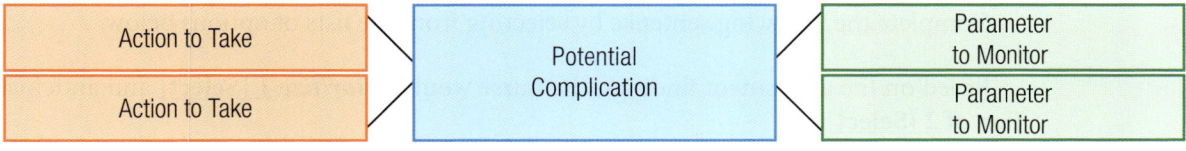

Actions to Take	Potential Conditions	Parameters to Monitor
Administer 0.9% normal saline IV fluid bolus	Peripheral arterial embolism	Color and sensation of affected limb
Collaborate with a registered dietitian nutritionist to provide a diet low in vitamin K	Dehydration	Daily weights
Maintain the client on bedrest with the leg immobilized	Deep vein thrombosis	Distal pulse strength
Obtain baseline laboratory results for hemoglobin, hematocrit, platelets, and aPTT	Hypercalcemia	Electrolytes
Request an order for subcutaneous calcitonin		Intake and output

Stand-Alone Thinking Exercise 11.2

The nurse is caring for an 85-year-old client in a long-term skilled nursing facility. To plan the most appropriate care, the nurse reviews the collected client data with the registered nurse.

History and Physical	Nurses' Notes	Nursing Flow Sheet	Laboratory Results	
Vital Signs	**0600**	**1200**	**1800**	**2000**
T	98.6°F (37°C)	100.8°F (38.2°C)	101.3°F (38.5°C)	101.8°F (38.8°C)
HR	76 beats/min	101 beats/min	110 beats/min	115 beats/min
RR	12 breaths/min	15 breaths/min	19 breaths/min	24 breaths/min
BP	128/36 mm Hg	130/38 mm Hg	135/46 mm Hg	99/43 mm Hg
SpO$_2$	98% on RA	97% on RA	96% on RA	92% on RA
Pain	Client denies pain, 0/10	Client denies pain but appears restless	Client confused, reoriented to person and situation, denies pain	Client confused and agitated, unable to reorient
Urine output	100 mL/h	80 mL/h	35 mL/h	20 mL/h

History and Physical	Nurses' Notes	Orders	Laboratory Results
Serum Laboratory Test and Reference Range	**0600**	**1800**	
Red blood cell (RBC) count (4.7–6.1 $\times$ 10^6/mm^3 [4.7–6.1 $\times$ 10^{12}/L])	5.6 $\times$ 10^6/mm^3 (5.6 $\times$ 10^{12}/L)	5.8 $\times$ 10^6/mm^3 (5.8 $\times$ 10^{12}/L)	
White blood cell (WBC) count (5000–10,000/mm^3 [5–10 $\times$ 10^9/L])	8000/mm^3 (8 $\times$ 10^9/L)	12,000/mm^3 (12 $\times$ 10^9/L)	
Glucose (74–106 mg/dL [4.1–5.9 mmol/L])	88 mg/dL (4.9 mmol/L)	195 mg/dL (10.8 mmol/L)	
Lactic acid (5–20 mg/dL [0.6–2.2 mmol/L])	20 mg/dL (2.2 mmol/L)	22.5 mg/dL (2.5 mmol/L)	

Complete the following sentence by selecting from the lists of options below.

Based on the assessment findings, the nurse would *prioritize* **1 [Select]** and anticipate administration of **2 [Select]**.

OPTIONS FOR 1	OPTIONS FOR 2
Blood cultures	Antibiotics
FSBG tests	IV fluids
Supplemental O$_2$	Subcutaneous insulin

Client Conditions Affecting Gas Exchange

Unfolding Case Study 12.1

Thinking Exercise 12.1.1

The nurse is caring for a 79-year-old client in the emergency department (ED).

History and Physical	Nurses' Notes	Orders	Progress Notes

0945: Client brought to ED by family due to new-onset confusion and fatigue. Health history of COPD and 30-pack-year history of cigarette smoking; quit 20 years ago. Client is a widow and lives independently. Currently visiting from out of state and staying with an adult grandchild who has a spouse and three children 3, 5, and 8 years of age. Client is alert and oriented to self and family members only. Speech is clear, facial features are symmetrical, and extremities move with equal strength to command. Rests comfortably in the semi-Fowler position. Family shares that the client reported a sore throat and congestion a couple days ago and has an intermittent, hacking cough that began last night. This morning, the client fell asleep at the breakfast table and could not recall where they were when awakened. Respirations equal, shallow, and assisted by accessory muscles. Diffuse course crackles and wheezing present upon auscultation. Skin cool and dry with dependent edema present in bilateral lower extremities. Pulses palpable throughout. Cough present and producing small amount of dark-red sputum. VS: T 102.1°F (38.9°C), HR 102 beats/min and regular, RR 24 breaths/min, BP 128/63 mm Hg, SpO_2 86% on RA. Height reported at 5 ft 2 in (157.5 cm); current weight 104 lb (47.1 kg); BMI 19. Client reports right lateral chest pain that hurts more when coughing.

The nurse reviews the collected client data with the registered nurse. Select the **3** client findings that require **immediate** follow-up.

○ BMI 19
○ Lateral chest pain
○ Cool, dry skin
○ Course crackles
○ Oriented to self and family
○ Dependent edema
○ SpO_2 86% on RA

Thinking Exercise 12.1.2

The nurse is caring for a 79-year-old client in the emergency department.

History and Physical	Nurses' Notes	Orders	Progress Notes

0945: Client brought to ED by family due to new-onset confusion and fatigue. Health history of COPD and 30-pack-year history of cigarette smoking; quit 20 years ago. Client is a widow and lives independently. Currently visiting from out of state and staying with an adult grandchild who has a spouse and three children 3, 5, and 8 years of age. Client is alert and oriented to self and family members only. Speech is clear, facial features are symmetrical, and extremities move with equal strength to command. Rests comfortably in the semi-Fowler position. Family shares that the client reported a sore throat and congestion a couple days ago and has an intermittent, hacking cough that began last night. This morning, the client fell asleep at the breakfast table and could not recall where they were when awakened. Respirations equal, shallow, and assisted by accessory muscles. Diffuse course crackles and wheezing present upon auscultation. Skin cool and dry with dependent edema present in bilateral lower extremities. Pulses palpable throughout. Cough present and producing small amount of dark-red sputum. VS: T 102.1°F (38.9°C), HR 102 beats/min and regular, RR 24 breaths/min, BP 128/63 mm Hg, SpO_2 86% on RA. Height reported at 5 ft 2 in (157.5 cm); current weight 104 lb (47.1 kg); BMI 19. Client reports right lateral chest pain that hurts more when coughing.

The nurse reviews the collected client data with the registered nurse. For each client finding, select whether the finding is consistent with the health conditions of COPD exacerbation, lung cancer, or pneumonia. Some findings may be consistent with more than one condition.

CLIENT FINDING	COPD EXACERBATION	LUNG CANCER	PNEUMONIA
Productive cough			
Chest pain			
Acute confusion			
Wheezing			
Fatigue			

Thinking Exercise 12.1.3

The nurse is caring for a 79-year-old client in the emergency department.

History and Physical	Nurses' Notes	Orders	Progress Notes

0945: Client brought to ED by family due to new onset-confusion and fatigue. Health history of COPD and 30-pack-year history of cigarette smoking; quit 20 years ago. Client is a widow and lives independently. Currently visiting from out of state and staying with an adult grandchild who has a spouse and three children 3, 5, and 8 years of age. Client is alert and oriented to self and family members only. Speech is clear, facial features are symmetrical, and extremities move with equal strength to command. Rests comfortably in the semi-Fowler position. Family shares that the client reported a sore throat and congestion a couple days ago and has an intermittent, hacking cough that began last night. This morning, the client fell asleep at the breakfast table and could not recall where they were when awakened. Respirations equal, shallow, and assisted by accessory muscles. Diffuse course crackles and wheezing present upon auscultation. Skin cool and dry with dependent edema present in bilateral lower extremities. Pulses palpable throughout. Cough present and producing small amount of dark-red sputum. VS: T 102.1°F (38.9°C), HR 102 beats/min and regular, RR 24 breaths/min, BP 128/63 mm Hg, SpO$_2$ 86% on RA. Height reported at 5 ft 2 in (157.5 cm); current weight 104 lb (47.1 kg); BMI 19. Client reports right lateral chest pain that hurts more when coughing.

The nurse reviews the collected client data with the registered nurse. Complete the following sentence by selecting from the lists of options below.

The nurse determines the ***priority*** for care at this time is to manage the client's **1 [Select]**. The nurse's ***first*** action would be to **2 [Select]**.

OPTIONS FOR 1	OPTIONS FOR 2
Acute pain	Administer oxygen to keep the SpO$_2$ between 88% and 92%.
Confusion	Complete a stroke scale assessment.
Hypoxemia	Collaborate with respiratory therapy for a nebulizer treatment.
Tachycardia	Place the client in the high-Fowler position.

Thinking Exercise 12.1.4

The nurse is caring for a 79-year-old client in the emergency department.

History and Physical	Nurses' Notes	Orders	Progress Notes

0945: Client brought to ED by family due to new-onset confusion and fatigue. Health history of COPD and 30-pack-year history of cigarette smoking; quit 20 years ago. Client is a widow and lives independently. Currently visiting from out of state and staying with an adult grandchild who has a spouse and three children 3, 5, and 8 years of age. Client is alert and oriented to self and family members only. Speech is clear, facial features are symmetrical, and extremities move with equal strength to command. Rests comfortably in the semi-Fowler position. Family shares that the client reported a sore throat and congestion a couple days ago and has an intermittent, hacking cough that began last night. This morning, the client fell asleep at the breakfast table and could not recall where they were when awakened. Respirations equal, shallow, and assisted by accessory muscles. Diffuse course crackles and wheezing present upon auscultation. Skin cool and dry with dependent edema present in bilateral lower extremities. Pulses palpable throughout. Cough present and producing small amount of dark-red sputum. VS: T 102.1°F (38.9°C), HR 102 beats/min and regular, RR 24 breaths/min, BP 128/63 mm Hg, SpO_2 86% on RA. Height reported at 5 ft 2 in (157.5 cm); current weight 104 lb (47.1 kg); BMI 19. Client reports right lateral chest pain that hurts more when coughing.

0950: Initiated supplemental oxygen at 4 L/min O_2 via NC. Placed peripheral IV in right forearm.

1000: Physician at bedside. Client diagnosed with community-acquired pneumonia, and orders received for inpatient care. VS: HR 98 beats/min and regular, RR 22 breaths/min, BP 130/62 mm Hg, SpO_2 90% on 4 L/min O_2 via NC.

Medical-Surgical Unit

1030: Client arrived at medical-surgical unit. Report received from ER nurse. Client alert and oriented to person and place. VS: HR 96 beats/min and regular, RR 20 breaths/min, BP 126/58 mm Hg, SpO_2 90% on 4 L/min O_2 via NC. Reports right lateral chest pain rated 4/10, and verbalizes acceptable pain level at <5/10. Family at bedside.

History and Physical	Nurses' Notes	Orders	Progress Notes

0900:
- Admit to medical-surgical unit
- Blood cultures × 2
- Chest physiotherapy
- Ciprofloxacin 400 mg IV every 12 hours
- Nutritional consultation
- Oxycodone hydrochloride 2.5 mg/acetaminophen 325 mg 1 tablet every 6 hours PRN, pain
- Sputum culture
- Strict monitoring of intake and output
- Titrate supplemental oxygen to keep SpO_2 between 88% and 92%

The unit nurse reviews orders and nurses' notes from the emergency department, then collaborates with the registered nurse and contributes to the client's plan of care. Select whether the following potential nursing actions are indicated or not indicated for the client at this time.

POTENTIAL NURSING ACTIONS	INDICATED	NOT INDICATED
Assist the client to perform deep-breathing and coughing exercises.		
Encourage the client to ambulate in the hallway at least twice each day.		
Insert an indwelling urinary catheter to gravity drainage.		
Organize patient care activities to allow periods of uninterrupted rest.		
Arrange for food options that are high in protein and preferred by the client.		
Place the client in a negative-airflow room, and provide surgical masks for all visitors and health care providers.		

Thinking Exercise 12.1.5

The nurse is caring for a 79-year-old client in the emergency department.

History and Physical	Nurses' Notes	Orders	Progress Notes

0945: Client brought to ED by family due to new-onset confusion and fatigue. Health history of COPD and 30-pack-year history of cigarette smoking; quit 20 years ago. Client is a widow and lives independently. Currently visiting from out of state and staying with an adult grandchild who has a spouse and three children 3, 5, and 8 years of age. Client is alert and oriented to self and family members only. Speech is clear, facial features are symmetrical, and extremities move with equal strength to command. Rests comfortably in the semi-Fowler position. Family shares that the client reported a sore throat and congestion a couple days ago and has an intermittent, hacking cough that began last night. This morning, the client fell asleep at the breakfast table and could not recall where they were when awakened. Respirations equal, shallow, and assisted by accessory muscles. Diffuse course crackles and wheezing present upon auscultation. Skin cool and dry with dependent edema present in bilateral lower extremities. Pulses palpable throughout. Cough present and producing small amount of dark-red sputum. VS: T 102.1°F (38.9°C), HR 102 beats/min and regular, RR 24 breaths/min, BP 128/63 mm Hg, SpO_2 86% on RA. Height reported at 5 ft 2 in (157.5 cm); current weight 104 lb (47.1 kg); BMI 19. Client reports right lateral chest pain that hurts more when coughing.

0950: Initiated supplemental oxygen at 4 L/min O_2 via NC. Placed peripheral IV in right forearm.

1000: Physician at bedside. Client diagnosed with community-acquired pneumonia, and orders received for inpatient care. VS: HR 98 beats/min and regular, RR 22 breaths/min, BP 130/62 mm Hg, SpO_2 90% on 4 L/min O_2 via NC.

Medical-Surgical Unit
1030: Client arrived at medical-surgical unit. Report received from ER nurse. Client alert and oriented to person and place. VS: HR 96 beats/min and regular, RR 20 breaths/min, BP 126/58 mm Hg, SpO_2 90% on 4 L/min O_2 via NC. Reports right lateral chest pain rated 4/10, and verbalizes acceptable pain level at <5/10. Family at bedside.

History and Physical	Nurses' Notes	Orders	Progress Notes

0900:
- Admit to medical-surgical unit
- Blood cultures × 2
- Chest physiotherapy
- Ciprofloxacin 400 mg IV every 12 hours
- Nutritional consultation
- Oxycodone hydrochloride 2.5 mg/acetaminophen 325 mg 1 tablet every 6 hours PRN, pain
- Sputum culture
- Strict monitoring of intake and output
- Titrate supplemental oxygen to keep SpO_2 between 88% and 92%

The nurse collaborates with the registered nurse to implement the plan of care for the client. Select the **2** orders the nurse would **prioritize** at this time.
○ Blood cultures × 2
○ Chest physiotherapy
○ Ciprofloxacin 400 mg IV every 12 hours
○ Nutritional consultation
○ Oxycodone hydrochloride 2.5 mg/acetaminophen 325 mg 1 tablet every 6 hours PRN, pain
○ Sputum culture
○ Strict monitoring of intake and output
○ Titrate supplemental oxygen to keep SpO_2 between 88% and 92%

Thinking Exercise 12.1.6

The nurse is caring for a 79-year-old client in the emergency department.

History and Physical	Nurses' Notes	Orders	Progress Notes

0945: Client brought to ED by family due to new-onset confusion and fatigue. Health history of COPD and 30-pack-year history of cigarette smoking; quit 20 years ago. Client is a widow and lives independently. Currently visiting from out of state and staying with an adult grandchild who has a spouse and three children 3, 5, and 8 years of age. Client is alert and oriented to self and family members only. Speech is clear, facial features are symmetrical, and extremities move with equal strength to command. Rests comfortably in the semi-Fowler position. Family shares that the client reported a sore throat and congestion a couple days ago and has an intermittent, hacking cough that began last night. This morning, the client fell asleep at the breakfast table and could not recall where they were when awakened. Respirations equal, shallow, and assisted by accessory muscles. Diffuse course crackles and wheezing present upon auscultation. Skin cool and dry with dependent edema present in bilateral lower extremities. Pulses palpable throughout. Cough present and producing small amount of dark-red sputum. VS: T 102.1°F (38.9°C), HR 102 beats/min and regular, RR 24 breaths/min, BP 128/63 mm Hg, SpO_2 86% on RA. Height reported at 5 ft 2 in (157.5 cm); current weight 104 lb (47.1 kg); BMI 19. Client reports right lateral chest pain that hurts more when coughing.

0950: Initiated supplemental oxygen at 4 L/min O_2 via NC. Placed peripheral IV in right forearm.

1020: Physician at bedside. Client diagnosed with community-acquired pneumonia, and orders received for inpatient care. VS: HR 98 beats/min and regular, RR 22 breaths/min, BP 130/62 mm Hg, SpO_2 90% on 4 L/min O_2 via NC.

Medical-Surgical Unit: Admission

1130: Client arrived at medical-surgical unit. Report received from ER nurse. Client alert and oriented to person and place. VS: HR 96 beats/min and regular, RR 20 breaths/min, BP 126/58 mm Hg, SpO_2 90% on 4 L/min O_2 via NC. Reports right lateral chest pain rated 4/10, and verbalizes acceptable pain level at <5/10. Family at bedside.

Medical-Surgical Unit: 2 Days Later

0900: Client alert and oriented × 4. Speech is clear, and facial features are symmetrical. Transfers with assistance to the chair for meals. Reports dyspnea with activity and at rest. Heart tones regular, and pulses palpable throughout. Skin warm and dry with dependent edema present in bilateral lower extremities. Left lung fields clear, and right lung fields diminished upon auscultation. Dry, nonproductive cough present. Abdomen soft and round with bowel sounds present in all quadrants. Client eats 60% to 75% of meals and drinks 1 protein shake between each meal. VS: T 98.1°F (36.7°C), HR 76 beats/min, RR 18 breaths/min, BP 122/60 mm Hg, SpO_2 93% on 4 L/min O_2 via NC. Denies pain.

The nurse reviews the most recent nurses' notes and is assisting to evaluate the client's current status with findings from 2 days ago. For each current client finding, select whether the client's status has improved or not improved.

CLIENT FINDING	IMPROVED	NOT IMPROVED
Alert and oriented × 4		
SpO_2 93% on 4 L/min O_2 via NC		
Dyspnea with activity and at rest		
Diminished right lobe breath sounds		
Drinks 1 protein shake between each meal		

Unfolding Case Study 12.2

Thinking Exercise 12.2.1

The nurse is caring for a 72-year-old client on an acute medical-surgical unit. Highlight the client findings that require **immediate** follow-up.

History and Physical	Nurses' Notes	Orders	Progress Notes

1320: Client admitted from surgical suite after an uncomplicated right total hip arthroplasty. Health history includes atrial fibrillation and osteoarthritis. Client is drowsy but easily aroused to voice and oriented × 4. Speech is clear, and simple commands followed appropriately. Skin cool and dry with palpable pulses throughout. Right hip dressing dry, wound drain intact, and 50 mL sanguineous drainage emptied. Respirations equal, unlabored, and without adventitious lung sounds. Abdomen soft with hypoactive bowel sounds. Denies nausea. Indwelling urinary catheter in place draining clear yellow urine to gravity. Urinary drainage bag emptied, 1500 mL output. Left forearm peripheral IV infusing 0.9% NS at 100 mL/h and morphine PCA with basal rate of 1 mg/h and demand rate of 0.5 mg every 8 minutes. VS: T 97.2°F (36.2°C), HR 102 beats/min and irregular, RR 13 beats/min, BP 120/58 mm Hg, SpO$_2$ 98% on 4 L/min O$_2$ via NC. Surgical site pain rated 7/10. PCA teaching reinforced, and client demonstrates appropriate use of demand feature. Client's adult child at bedside; all questions answered.

1430: Client sleeping. Unable to awaken with verbal stimuli, but arouses with moderate stimuli and then drifts back to sleep quickly. VS: HR 105 beats/min and irregular, RR 11 breaths/min, BP 109/52 mm Hg, SpO$_2$ 90% on 4 L/min O$_2$ via NC. Incisional dressing dry, and 20 mL sanguineous drainage in wound drain. Urinary drainage bag with 75 mL yellow urine. PCA reports 5 mg morphine infused. Adult child at bedside holding client's hand.

Thinking Exercise 12.2.2

The nurse is caring for a 72-year-old client on an acute medical-surgical unit.

History and Physical	Nurses' Notes	Orders	Progress Notes

1320: Client admitted from surgical suite after an uncomplicated right total hip arthroplasty. Health history includes atrial fibrillation and osteoarthritis. Client is drowsy but easily aroused to voice and oriented × 4. Speech is clear, and simple commands followed appropriately. Skin cool and dry with palpable pulses throughout. Right hip dressing dry, wound drain intact, and 50 mL sanguineous drainage emptied. Respirations equal, unlabored, and without adventitious lung sounds. Abdomen soft with hypoactive bowel sounds. Denies nausea. Indwelling urinary catheter in place draining clear yellow urine to gravity. Urinary drainage bag emptied, 1500 mL output. Left forearm peripheral IV infusing 0.9% NS at 100 mL/h and morphine PCA with basal rate of 1 mg/h and demand rate of 0.5 mg every 8 minutes. VS: T 97.2°F (36.2°C), HR 102 beats/min and irregular, RR 13 beats/min, BP 120/58 mm Hg, SpO$_2$ 98% on 4 L/min O$_2$ via NC. Surgical site pain rated 7/10. PCA teaching reinforced, and client demonstrates appropriate use of demand feature. Client's adult child at bedside; all questions answered.

1430: Client sleeping. Unable to awaken with verbal stimuli, but arouses with moderate stimuli and then drifts back to sleep quickly. VS: HR 105 beats/min and irregular, RR 11 breaths/min, BP 109/52 mm Hg, SpO$_2$ 90% on 4 L/min O$_2$ via NC. Incisional dressing dry, and 20 mL sanguineous drainage in wound drain. Urinary drainage bag with 75 mL yellow urine. PCA reports 5 mg morphine infused. Adult child at bedside holding client's hand.

The nurse reviews the collected client data with the registered nurse. Complete the following sentence by selecting from the list of word choices below.

The nurse recognizes that the client is *most likely* experiencing [**Word Choice**].

WORD CHOICES
Anaphylactic reaction
Hypovolemic shock
Opioid overdose
Pulmonary embolism

Thinking Exercise 12.2.3

The nurse is caring for a 72-year-old client on an acute medical-surgical unit.

History and Physical	Nurses' Notes	Orders	Progress Notes

1320: Client admitted from surgical suite after an uncomplicated right total hip arthroplasty. Health history includes atrial fibrillation and osteoarthritis. Client is drowsy but easily aroused to voice and oriented × 4. Speech is clear, and simple commands followed appropriately. Skin cool and dry with palpable pulses throughout. Right hip dressing dry, wound drain intact, and 50 mL sanguineous drainage emptied. Respirations equal, unlabored, and without adventitious lung sounds. Abdomen soft with hypoactive bowel sounds. Denies nausea. Indwelling urinary catheter in place draining clear yellow urine to gravity. Urinary drainage bag emptied, 1500 mL output. Left forearm peripheral IV infusing 0.9% NS at 100 mL/h and morphine PCA with basal rate of 1 mg/h and demand rate of 0.5 mg every 8 minutes. VS: T 97.2°F (36.2°C), HR 102 beats/min and irregular, RR 13 beats/min, BP 120/58 mm Hg, SpO_2 98% on 4 L/min O_2 via NC. Surgical site pain rated 7/10. PCA teaching reinforced, and client demonstrates appropriate use of demand feature. Client's adult child at bedside; all questions answered.

1430: Client sleeping. Unable to awaken with verbal stimuli, but arouses with moderate stimuli and then drifts back to sleep quickly. VS: HR 105 beats/min and irregular, RR 11 breaths/min, BP 109/52 mm Hg, SpO_2 90% on 4 L/min O_2 via NC. Incisional dressing dry, and 20 mL sanguineous drainage in wound drain. Urinary drainage bag with 75 mL yellow urine. PCA reports 5 mg morphine infused. Adult child at bedside holding client's hand.

The nurse reviews the relevant client data with the registered nurse. Complete the following sentence by selecting from the lists of options below.

The nurse determines the **priority** for care at this time is **1 [Select]** because the client is experiencing **2 [Select]** and **3 [Select]**.

OPTIONS FOR 1	OPTIONS FOR 2	OPTIONS FOR 3
Continuous cardiac monitoring	Cardiac arrhythmia	Cool, dry skin
Fluid replacement	Hypothermia	Hypoxemia
Ventilation support	Respiratory depression	Tachycardia

Thinking Exercise 12.2.4

The nurse is caring for a 72-year-old client on an acute medical-surgical unit.

History and Physical	Nurses' Notes	Orders	Progress Notes

1320: Client admitted from surgical suite after an uncomplicated right total hip arthroplasty. Health history includes atrial fibrillation and osteoarthritis. Client is drowsy but easily aroused to voice and oriented × 4. Speech is clear, and simple commands followed appropriately. Skin cool and dry with palpable pulses throughout. Right hip dressing dry, wound drain intact, and 50 mL sanguineous drainage emptied. Respirations equal, unlabored, and without adventitious lung sounds. Abdomen soft with hypoactive bowel sounds. Denies nausea. Indwelling urinary catheter in place draining clear yellow urine to gravity. Urinary drainage bag emptied, 1500 mL output. Left forearm peripheral IV infusing 0.9% NS at 100 mL/h and morphine PCA with basal rate of 1 mg/h and demand rate of 0.5 mg every 8 minutes. VS: T 97.2°F (36.2°C), HR 102 beats/min and irregular, RR 13 beats/min, BP 120/58 mm Hg, SpO_2 98% on 4 L/min O_2 via NC. Surgical site pain rated 7/10. PCA teaching reinforced, and client demonstrates appropriate use of demand feature. Client's adult child at bedside; all questions answered.

1430: Client sleeping. Unable to awaken with verbal stimuli, but arouses with moderate stimuli and then drifts back to sleep quickly. VS: HR 105 beats/min and irregular, RR 11 breaths/min, BP 109/52 mm Hg, SpO_2 90% on 4 L/min O_2 via NC. Incisional dressing dry, and 20 mL sanguineous drainage in wound drain. Urinary drainage bag with 75 mL yellow urine. PCA reports 5 mg morphine infused. Adult child at bedside holding client's hand.

The nurse collaborates with the registered nurse and contributes to the client's plan of care. Which of the following interventions would the nurse include in this client's plan of care? **Select all that apply.**
○ Ensure that bag-valve-mask ventilation equipment is at the bedside.
○ Notify the health care provider.
○ Position the client to maintain airway patency.
○ Recommend discontinuing the PCA.
○ Request an order for naloxone.
○ Titrate supplemental oxygen until the SpO_2 is greater than 94%.

Thinking Exercise 12.2.5

The nurse is caring for a 72-year-old client on an acute medical-surgical unit.

History and Physical	Nurses' Notes	Orders	Progress Notes

1320: Client admitted from surgical suite after an uncomplicated right total hip arthroplasty. Health history includes atrial fibrillation and osteoarthritis. Client is drowsy but easily aroused to voice and oriented × 4. Speech is clear, and simple commands followed appropriately. Skin cool and dry with palpable pulses throughout. Right hip dressing dry, wound drain intact, and 50 mL sanguineous drainage emptied. Respirations equal, unlabored, and without adventitious lung sounds. Abdomen soft with hypoactive bowel sounds. Denies nausea. Indwelling urinary catheter in place draining clear yellow urine to gravity. Urinary drainage bag emptied, 1500 mL output. Left forearm peripheral IV infusing 0.9% NS at 100 mL/h and morphine PCA with basal rate of 1 mg/h and demand rate of 0.5 mg every 8 minutes. VS: T 97.2°F (36.2°C), HR 102 beats/min and irregular, RR 13 beats/min, BP 120/58 mm Hg, SpO_2 98% on 4 L/min O_2 via NC. Surgical site pain rated 7/10. PCA teaching reinforced, and client demonstrates appropriate use of demand feature. Client's adult child at bedside; all questions answered.

1430: Client sleeping. Unable to awaken with verbal stimuli, but arouses with moderate stimuli and then drifts back to sleep quickly. VS: HR 105 beats/min and irregular, RR 11 breaths/min, BP 109/52 mm Hg, SpO_2 90% on 4 L/min O_2 via NC. Incisional dressing dry, and 20 mL sanguineous drainage in wound drain. Urinary drainage bag with 75 mL yellow urine. PCA reports 5 mg morphine infused. Adult child at bedside holding client's hand.

1435: Supplemental oxygen applied. Surgeon notified, and orders received.

1440: Naloxone 0.4 mg IV administered by the registered nurse. Morphine PCA discontinued.

1445: Client is drowsy but easily aroused and oriented to person and place. VS: HR 112 beats/min and irregular, RR 13 breaths/min, BP 128/55 mm Hg, SpO_2 94% on 40% FiO_2 via facemask.

1500: Client is lethargic, unable to arouse by voice but awakes with continuous physical stimulation. Oriented to self only. RR 10 breaths/min, SpO_2 91% on 40% FiO_2 via facemask.

The nurse collaborates with the registered nurse and contributes to the client's plan of care. Select the **2** actions the nurse would **prioritize** at this time.
○ Administer an additional dose of naloxone.
○ Alert the Rapid Response Team.
○ Increase the intravenous infusion rate to 150 mL/h.
○ Initiate bag-valve-mask manual breathing.
○ Place the client in the high-Fowler position.

Thinking Exercise 12.2.6

The nurse is caring for a 72-year-old client on an acute medical-surgical unit.

History and Physical	Nurses' Notes	Orders	Progress Notes

1320: Client admitted from surgical suite after an uncomplicated right total hip arthroplasty. Health history includes atrial fibrillation and osteoarthritis. Client is drowsy but easily aroused to voice and oriented × 4. Speech is clear, and simple commands followed appropriately. Skin cool and dry with palpable pulses throughout. Right hip dressing dry, wound drain intact, and 50 mL sanguineous drainage emptied. Respirations equal, unlabored, and without adventitious lung sounds. Abdomen soft with hypoactive bowel sounds. Denies nausea. Indwelling urinary catheter in place draining clear yellow urine to gravity. Urinary drainage bag emptied, 1500 mL output. Left forearm peripheral IV infusing 0.9% NS at 100 mL/h and morphine PCA with basal rate of 1 mg/h and demand rate of 0.5 mg every 8 minutes. VS: T 97.2°F (36.2°C), HR 102 beats/min and irregular, RR 13 beats/min, BP 120/58 mm Hg, SpO_2 98% on 4 L/min O_2 via NC. Surgical site pain rated 7/10. PCA teaching reinforced, and client demonstrates appropriate use of demand feature. Client's adult child at bedside; all questions answered.

1430: Client sleeping. Unable to awaken with verbal stimuli, but arouses with moderate stimuli and then drifts back to sleep quickly. VS: HR 105 beats/min and irregular, RR 11 breaths/min, BP 109/52 mm Hg, SpO2 90% on 4 L/min O_2 via NC. Incisional dressing dry, and 20 mL sanguineous drainage in wound drain. Urinary drainage bag with 75 mL yellow urine. PCA reports 5 mg morphine infused. Adult child at bedside holding client's hand.

1435: Supplemental oxygen applied. Physician notified and orders received.

1440: Naloxone 0.4 mg IV administered by the Registered Nurse. Morphine PCA discontinued.

1445: Client is drowsy but easily aroused and oriented to person and place. VS: HR 112 beats/min and irregular, RR 13 breaths/min, BP 128/55 mm Hg, SpO_2 94% on 40% FiO_2 via facemask.

1500: Client is lethargic, unable to arouse by voice but awakes with continuous physical stimulation. Oriented to self only. RR 10 breaths/min, SpO_2 91% on 40% FiO_2 via facemask.

1505: Naloxone 0.4 mg IV administered by the Registered Nurse.

1515: Rapid Response Team at bedside. Client is alert, oriented to person and place, and follows simple commands. Client reoriented to place and situation. Family at bedside, updated on patient status. VS: HR 120 beats/min and irregular, RR 16 breaths/min, BP 132/65 mm Hg, SpO_2 96% on 40% FiO_2 via facemask. Reports incisional pain rated 8/10. Denies nausea.

1530: Client alert and oriented × 4. RR 18 breaths/min, SpO_2 98% on 40% FiO_2 via facemask. Ibuprofen 800 mg IV administered.

1700: Sleeping but easily aroused and oriented × 4. Speech is clear, and simple commands followed appropriately. Respirations equal, unlabored, and without adventitious lung sounds. Right hip dressing dry, wound drain intact, and 40 mL serosanguineous drainage emptied. Abdomen soft with active bowel sounds in all quadrants. Denies nausea. Indwelling urinary catheter to gravity with 500 mL clear yellow urine. VS: T 98.6°F (37°C), HR 98 beats/min and irregular, RR 14 breaths/min, BP 128/56 mm Hg, SpO_2 98% on 4 L/min O_2 via NC. Surgical site pain rated 2/10.

The nurse collaborates with the registered nurse to evaluate client outcomes. Complete the following sentence by selecting from the list of word choices below.

The nurse determines the client's status has ***improved*** based on the client's [**Word Choice**] and [**Word Choice**].

WORD CHOICES
Bowel sounds
Orientation status
Oxygenation saturation
Urine output
Wound drainage

Stand-Alone Thinking Exercise 12.1

The nurse is caring for a 65-year-old client at a long-term acute care facility.

Progress Notes	Nurses' Notes	Orders	Laboratory Results

0645: Direct admission yesterday from hospital for acute care nursing and rehabilitation services. Health history includes COPD, substance use disorder with 10 years of sobriety, laryngeal cancer, and total laryngectomy with tracheostomy and percutaneous endoscopic gastrostomy tube placement 3 days ago. Mechanical ventilation discontinued this morning. Client's RR and SpO_2 within normal limits on 50% FiO_2 via tracheostomy collar. Client tolerating tube feedings, residuals <30 mL. Vital signs stable. Continue physical and occupational therapies. Speech therapy initiated.

Progress Notes	Nurses' Notes	Orders	Laboratory Results

0730: Client alert and oriented × 4. Uses white board to communicate. Respirations equal and unlabored. Course crackles present in bilateral lower extremities. Weak, unproductive cough present. Tracheal suctioning produces thick, pale secretions. Oral care provided. Bowel sounds present. PEG tube with continuous feedings at goal rate; residual of 20 mL. Free water flush administered. No bowel movement since admission. Voids 350 mL clear yellow urine. VS: T 98.8°F (37.1°C), HR 69 beats/min and regular; RR 14 breaths/min, BP 139/66 mm Hg, SpO_2 96% on 50% FiO_2 via tracheostomy collar. Repositioned and encouraged to perform deep-breathing and coughing exercises. Denies pain.

0820: Client anxious with eyes wide and arms waving in air. VS: HR 99 beats/min, RR 24 breaths/min, BP 141/68 mm Hg, SpO_2 91% on 50% FiO_2 via tracheostomy collar.

The nurse reviews the collected client data with the registered nurse. Complete the diagram by selecting from the choices below to specify what potential condition the client is likely experiencing, **2** nursing actions that are appropriate to take, and **2** parameters the nurse would monitor to assess the client's progress.

Actions to Take		Potential Condition		Parameters to Monitor
Actions to Take				Parameters to Monitor

Actions to Take	Potential Conditions	Parameters to Monitor
Administer prescribed lorazepam	Airway occlusion	Bowel sounds
Discontinue tube feedings	Autonomic dysreflexia	Noxious stimuli
Place the client in the high-Fowler position	Substance withdrawal	Oxygen saturation
Suction tracheostomy secretions	Tube feeding aspiration	Respiratory effort
Request a stool softener		Tube feeding residuals

Stand-Alone Thinking Exercise 12.2

A nurse is caring for an 84-year-old client at a rehabilitation facility after a recent left-hemisphere stroke.

History and Physical	Nurses' Notes	Orders	Nursing Flow Sheet

Admission Orders

- Routine vital signs and nursing care
- Supplemental oxygen to keep SpO_2 94%
- Consultations
  - Physical therapy
  - Occupational therapy
  - Speech therapy
- Chopped diet with nectar thick liquids
- Medications
  - Amlodipine 5 mg orally each day
  - Aspirin 325 mg orally each day
  - Docusate 50 mg orally every evening
  - Enoxaparin 40 mg SC every 12 hours

History and Physical	Nurses' Notes	Orders	Nursing Flow Sheet

2230: Admitted to facility. Orders received. Client alert and oriented $\times$ 4. Right-sided weakness and aphasia present. Respirations equal and unlabored. Heart tones regular. Picture board provided to facilitate communication. Client denies pain.

0800: Client alert and oriented $\times$ 4. Right-sided weakness and aphasia present. Uses a picture board to communicate. Respirations equal and unlabored. Lung fields clear throughout. Denies cough or shortness of breath. Demonstrates appropriate use of oral suction to clear secretions from mouth. Heart tones regular. Skin warm and dry with palpable pulses throughout. Abdomen soft and round with bowel sounds present in all quadrants. Client transferred to chair with two-person assist for breakfast and morning care. Denies pain.

1030: Nurse's presence requested by family at client's bedside. Client alert and sitting upright in a chair attempting to communicate. Speech is difficult to understand. Using a picture board, client reports upper chest discomfort rated 6/10. Respirations equal but slightly labored. Facial flushness and cough present. Fine crackles auscultated in lung fields. A partially consumed carbonated beverage present on client's bedside tray. The family shares that the client likes drinking a soda in the afternoon, so they brought one for the client.

History and Physical	Nurses' Notes	Orders	Nursing Flow Sheet
	1800	**0800**	**1030**
Vital Signs			
Temperature	98.5°F (36.9°C)	98.9°F (37.1°C)	–
HR	69 beats/min	71 beats/min	95 beats/min
BP	108/56 mm Hg	110/58 mm Hg	138/79 mm Hg
RR	12 breaths/min	13 breaths/min	19 breaths/min
SpO_2	97% on RA	98% on RA	94% on RA
Intake			
Oral fluids	540 mL Nectar thick	360 mL Nectar thick	100 mL Carbonated soda
Dietary	95% breakfast	80% lunch	
Output			
Urine	350 mL Clear, amber	400 mL Clear, yellow	
Stool	Soft brown		

The nurse collaborates with the registered nurse and contributes to the client's plan of care. Complete the following sentence by selecting from the list of word choices below.

The nurse determines that *priority* actions for the client at this time are [**Word Choice**] and [**Word Choice**].

WORD CHOICES
Completing a stroke scale assessment
Encouraging deep-breathing and coughing exercises
Monitoring oxygenation saturation
Reinforcing teaching related to nectar thick fluids
Transferring the client back to the bed

Client Conditions Affecting Mobility

CHAPTER 13

Unfolding Case Study 13.1

Thinking Exercise 13.1.1

The nurse is caring for a 78-year-old client at an assisted-living facility. Highlight the client findings that require **immediate** follow-up.

History and Physical	Nurses' Notes	Orders	Laboratory Results

0410: Client found slumped forward, moaning, and wedged between toilet and wall. Apparently fell while using the bathroom. Alert, but orientation difficult to assess due to severe pain. Usually ambulates with a rollator or cane, but no ambulatory device noted in bathroom. Crying out and grabbing right hip. Right leg shorter than left leg and externally rotated. Pedal pulses equal, and cap refill <3 sec. Client has long history of osteoporosis managed with risedronate. Skin intact except for large skin tear on right forearm oozing serosanguinous fluid. Bruising beginning to develop near skin tear. VS: T 98.6°F (37°C), HR 110 beats/min and regular, BP 154/88 mm Hg, RR 24 breaths/min, SpO$_2$ 93% on RA.

Thinking Exercise 13.1.2

The nurse is caring for a 78-year-old client at an assisted-living facility.

History and Physical	Nurses' Notes	Orders	Laboratory Results

0410: Client found slumped forward, moaning, and wedged between toilet and wall. Apparently fell while using the bathroom. Alert, but orientation difficult to assess orientation due to severe pain. Usually ambulates with a rollator or cane, but no ambulatory device noted in bathroom. Crying out and grabbing right hip. Right leg shorter than left leg and externally rotated. Pedal pulses equal, and cap refill <3 sec. Client has long history of osteoporosis managed with risedronate. Skin intact except for large skin tear on right forearm oozing serosanguinous fluid. Bruising beginning to develop near skin tear. VS: T 98.6°F (37°C), HR 110 beats/min and regular, BP 154/88 mm Hg, RR 24 breaths/min, SpO$_2$ 93% on RA.

0425: 911 and emergency family contact notified.

0515: Client transferred to local hospital ED; family meeting client at hospital.

The nurse reviews the collected client data with the registered nurse. Complete the following sentence by selecting from the lists of options below.

The client *most likely* has a **1 [Select]** as evidenced by **2 [Select]** and **3 [Select]**.

OPTIONS FOR 1	OPTIONS FOR 2	OPTIONS FOR 3
Fractured pelvis	Hip pain	Shortened leg
Fractured radius	History of osteoporosis	Skin tear
Fractured hip	Bruised forearm	Tachycardia

Thinking Exercise 13.1.3

The nurse is caring for a 78-year-old client in the emergency department (ED).

History and Physical	Nurses' Notes	Orders	Laboratory Results

Assisted Living

0410: Found client slumped forward, moaning, and wedged between toilet and wall. Apparently fell while using the bathroom. Alert, but orientation difficult to assess due to severe pain. Usually ambulates with a rollator or cane, but no ambulatory device noted in bathroom. Crying out and grabbing right hip. Right leg shorter than left leg and externally rotated. Pedal pulses equal, and cap refill <3 sec. Client has long history of osteoporosis managed with risedronate. Skin intact except for large skin tear on right forearm oozing serosanguinous fluid. Bruising beginning to develop near skin tear. VS: T 98.6°F (37°C), HR 110 beats/min and regular, BP 154/88 mm Hg, RR 24 breaths/min, SpO$_2$ 93% on RA.

0425: 911 and emergency family contact notified.

0515: Client transferred to local hospital ED; family meeting client at hospital.

Emergency Department

0540: Admitted to ED following fall at assisted living facility. Moaning and not responding to questions. Right hip x-ray confirms displaced femoral neck fracture with bleeding. Orthopedic consult for surgery to repair right hip. Client acutely confused as validated by delirium cognitive screening tool. Surgeon discussed surgical procedure with family, who signed operative consent for right hip open reduction and internal fixation (ORIF).

The nurse reviews the collected client data with the registered nurse. Complete the following sentence by selecting from the list of word choices below.

The nurse determines that the *priority* for client care is to surgically repair the fracture to prevent **[Word Choice]** and **[Word Choice]**.

WORD CHOICES
Severe pain
Hip contracture
Impaired blood flow to the hip
Worsening osteoporosis
Complications of immobility

Thinking Exercise 13.1.4

The nurse is caring for a 78-year-old client on an orthopedic acute care unit.

History and Physical	Nurses' Notes	Orders	Laboratory Results

Assisted Living

0410: Found client slumped forward, moaning, and wedged between toilet and wall. Apparently fell while using the bathroom. Alert, but orientation difficult to assess due to severe pain. Usually ambulates with a rollator or cane, but no ambulatory device noted in bathroom. Crying out and grabbing right hip. Right leg shorter than left leg and externally rotated. Pedal pulses equal, and cap refill <3 sec. Client has long history of osteoporosis managed with risedronate. Skin intact except for large skin tear on right forearm oozing serosanguinous fluid. Bruising beginning to develop near skin tear. VS: T 98.6°F (37°C), HR 110 beats/min and regular, BP 154/88 mm Hg, RR 24 breaths/min, SpO$_2$ 93% on RA.

0425: 911 and emergency family contact notified.

0515: Client transferred to local hospital ED; family meeting client at hospital.

Emergency Department

0540: Admitted to ED following fall at assisted living facility. Moaning and not responding to questions. Right hip x-ray confirmed displaced femoral neck fracture with bleeding. Orthopedic consult for surgery to repair right hip. Client acutely confused as validated by delirium cognitive screening tool. Surgeon discussed surgical procedure with family, who signed operative consent for right hip open reduction and internal fixation (ORIF).

Orthopedic Acute Care Unit (Surgical Day)

1345: Admitted to unit from PACU with right hip ORIF. Abduction pillow in place, and client sitting in semireclined position. Family member in room. Client drowsy but easily awakened; disoriented and unable to follow conversation. Lung sounds clear; S$_1$ and S$_2$ present and regular. Abdomen soft; bowel sounds diminished in all quadrants. Right hip dressing dry and intact. Pulses present in all extremities. Cap refill <3 sec. IV infusing at 100 mL/h; site intact without redness and covered with clear transparent dressing. Urinary catheter draining clear yellow urine. VS: T 98.6°F (37°C), HR 86 beats/min, RR 18 breaths/min, BP 106/64 mm Hg, SpO$_2$ 97% on 3 L/min O$_2$ via NC.

The nurse collaborates with the registered nurse to plan the client's care. Which of the following potential actions would the nurse likely implement to help prevent complications of immobility? **Select all that apply.**

O Reposition the client at least once every 8 hours.
O Apply sequential compression devices to both legs.
O Encourage the client to use the incentive spirometer.
O Administer an IV antibiotic per surgeon protocol.
O Administer an anticoagulant per surgeon protocol.
O Initiate physical and occupational therapy consults.

Thinking Exercise 13.1.5

The nurse is caring for a 78-year-old client on an orthopedic acute care unit.

History and Physical	Nurses' Notes	Orders	Laboratory Results

Assisted Living

0410: Found client slumped forward, moaning, and wedged between toilet and wall. Apparently fell while using the bathroom. Alert, but orientation difficult to assess due to severe pain. Usually ambulates with a rollator or cane, but no ambulatory device noted in bathroom. Crying out and grabbing right hip. Right leg shorter than left leg and externally rotated. Pedal pulses equal, and cap refill <3 sec. Client has long history of osteoporosis managed with risedronate. Skin intact except for large skin tear on right forearm oozing serosanguinous fluid. Bruising beginning to develop near skin tear. VS: T 98.6°F (37°C), HR 110 beats/min and regular, BP 154/88 mm Hg, RR 24 breaths/min, SpO_2 93% on RA.

0425: 911 and emergency family contact notified.

0515: Client transferred to local hospital ED; family meeting client at hospital.

Emergency Department

0540: Admitted to ED following fall at assisted living facility. Moaning and not responding to questions. Right hip x-ray confirmed displaced femoral neck fracture with bleeding. Orthopedic consult for surgery to repair right hip. Client acutely confused as validated by delirium cognitive screening tool. Surgeon discussed surgical procedure with family, who signed operative consent for right hip open reduction and internal fixation (ORIF).

Orthopedic Acute Care Unit (Surgical Day)

1345: Admitted to unit from PACU with right hip ORIF. Abduction pillow in place, and client sitting in semireclined position. Family member in room. Client drowsy but easily awakened; disoriented and unable to follow conversation. Lung sounds clear; S_1 and S_2 present and regular. Abdomen soft and round; bowel sounds diminished in all quadrants. Right hip dressing dry and intact. Pulses present in all extremities. Cap refill <3 sec. IV infusing at 100 mL/h; site intact without redness and covered with clear transparent dressing. Urinary catheter draining clear yellow urine. VS: T 98.6°F (37°C), HR 86 beats/min, RR 18 breaths/min, BP 106/64 mm Hg, SpO_2 97% on 3 L/min O_2 via NC.

Orthopedic Acute Care Unit (Postoperative Day 2)

1955: While helping client get back into bed, noted left calf redness and swelling. Client alert and oriented × 4. States left calf feels sore with a burning sensation. Lung sounds clear; S_1 and S_2 present and regular. Abdomen soft; bowel sounds present in all quadrants. Pulses present in all extremities. Cap refill <3 sec. Right hip incision closed and dry with staples intact. Reports hip pain currently rated 3/10. Voiding in bedside commode most of the time. Occasional urinary incontinence. No BM yet. VS: T 98.4°F (36.8°C), HR 80 beats/min, RR 16 breaths/min, BP 118/70 mm Hg, SpO_2 94% on RA.

The nurse assists with implementation of the client's plan of care. Select the **3** actions that would be appropriate for the nurse to implement at this time.

○ Notify the Rapid Response Team (RRT) immediately.
○ Anticipate an order for an oral anticoagulant such as dabigatran.
○ Elevate the client's left leg on a pillow.
○ Draw blood to test the client's platelet count.
○ Monitor the client for shortness of breath, chest pain, and acute confusion.

Thinking Exercise 13.1.6—Pharmacology

The nurse is caring for a 78-year-old client on an orthopedic acute care unit.

History and Physical	Nurses' Notes	Orders	Laboratory Results

Assisted Living

0410: Found client slumped forward, moaning, and wedged between toilet and wall. Apparently fell while using the bathroom. Alert, but orientation difficult to assess due to severe pain. Usually ambulates with a rollator or cane, but no ambulatory device noted in bathroom. Crying out and grabbing right hip. Right leg shorter than left leg and externally rotated. Pedal pulses equal, and cap refill <3 sec. Client has long history of osteoporosis managed with risedronate. Skin intact except for large skin tear on right forearm oozing serosanguinous fluid. Bruising beginning to develop near skin tear. VS: T 98.6°F (37°C), HR 110 beats/min and regular, BP 154/88 mm Hg, RR 24 breaths/min, SpO$_2$ 93% on RA.

0425: 911 and emergency family contact notified.

0515: Client transferred to local hospital ED; family meeting client at hospital.

Emergency Department

0540: Admitted to ED following fall at assisted living facility. Moaning and not responding to questions. Right hip x-ray confirmed displaced femoral neck fracture with bleeding. Orthopedic consult for surgery to repair right hip. Client acutely confused as validated by delirium cognitive screening tool. Surgeon discussed surgical procedure with family, who signed operative consent for right hip open reduction and internal fixation (ORIF).

Orthopedic Acute Care Unit (Surgical Day)

1345: Admitted to unit from PACU with right hip ORIF. Abduction pillow in place, and client sitting in semireclined position. Family member in room. Client drowsy but easily awakened; disoriented and unable to follow conversation. Lung sounds clear; S$_1$ and S$_2$ present and regular. Abdomen soft; bowel sounds diminished in all quadrants. Right hip dressing dry and intact. Pulses present in all extremities. Cap refill <3 sec. IV infusing at 100 mL/h; site intact without redness and covered with clear transparent dressing. Urinary catheter draining clear yellow urine. VS: T 98.6°F (37°C), HR 86 beats/min, RR 18 breaths/min, BP 106/64 mm Hg, SpO$_2$ 97% on 3 L/min O$_2$ via NC.

Orthopedic Acute Care Unit (Postoperative Day 2)

1955: While helping client get back into bed, noted left calf redness and swelling. Client alert and oriented × 4. States left calf feels sore with a burning sensation. Lung sounds clear; S$_1$ and S$_2$ present and regular. Abdomen soft; bowel sounds present in all quadrants. Pulses present in all extremities. Cap refill <3 sec. Right hip incision closed and dry with staples intact. Reports hip pain currently rated 3/10. Voiding in bedside commode most of the time. Occasional urinary incontinence. No BM yet. VS: T 98.4°F (36.8°C), HR 80 beats/min, RR 16 breaths/min, BP 118/70 mm Hg, SpO$_2$ 94% on RA.

2110: Surgeon in to examine client. Family member states that client had a lower extremity blood clot about 6 years ago after a total knee replacement. Client to start on dabigatran with limited ambulation. RN provided client and family education about the new drug.

The nurse reviews the collected client data with the registered nurse and reinforces teaching about dabigatran, which the client will continue after discharge. Select whether the following client statements indicate understanding or no understanding of the discharge teaching provided.

CLIENT STATEMENT	UNDERSTANDING	NO UNDERSTANDING
"When the redness and soreness in my calf goes away, I still need to take this drug."		
"I should contact my provider if I have any unexpected bleeding, chest pain, or dyspnea."		
"I will be sure to go to the lab for frequent blood tests needed while I'm on this drug."		
"I will take this capsule as prescribed and follow up with my provider."		

Unfolding Case Study 13.2

Thinking Exercise 13.2.1

The nurse is caring for a 69-year-old client at the neurologist office.

History and Physical	Nurses' Notes	Orders	Laboratory Results

1330: Family made follow-up appointment for client's Parkinson disease (PD). Client has been on the maximum dose of carbidopa/levodopa for the past 2 years and recently experienced several visual hallucinations. Medication has enabled client to be independent in ADLs since PD diagnosis. For the past few weeks, client has noticed increased rigidity and slowing gait. Client reports two episodes of dizziness and light-headedness yesterday that almost resulted in falling down the basement steps. Missed yesterday's Tai Chi class, which has helped with balance and coordination. Denies shortness of breath or chest pain. Reports occasional foot and ankle edema; currently 1+ nonpitting edema bilaterally. VS: T 97.8°F (36.6°C), HR 92 beats/min and irregular, BP 98/50 mm Hg (sitting), RR 16 breaths/min, SpO$_2$ 94% on RA.

Select the **3** client findings that require **immediate** follow-up.

○ SpO$_2$
○ Increased rigidity
○ Slowed gait
○ Blood pressure
○ Visual hallucinations
○ Bilateral foot and ankle edema
○ Dizziness and light-headedness

Thinking Exercise 13.2.2

The nurse is caring for a 69-year-old client at the neurologist office.

History and Physical	Nurses' Notes	Orders	Laboratory Results

1330: Family made follow-up appointment for client's Parkinson disease (PD). Client has been on the maximum dose of carbidopa/levodopa for the past 2 years and recently experienced several visual hallucinations. Medication has enabled client to be independent in ADLs since PD diagnosis. For the past few weeks, client has noticed increased rigidity and slowing gait. Client reports two episodes of dizziness and light-headedness yesterday that almost resulted in falling down the basement steps. Missed yesterday's Tai Chi class, which has helped with balance and coordination. Denies shortness of breath or chest pain. Reports occasional foot and ankle edema; currently 1+ nonpitting edema bilaterally. VS: T 97.8°F (36.6°C), HR 92 beats/min and irregular, BP 98/50 mm Hg (sitting), RR 16 breaths/min, SpO$_2$ 94% on RA.

1350: BP 110/62 mm Hg (lying down), BP 98/52 mm Hg (sitting), BP 88/50 mm Hg (standing). States feeling light-headed when moving from a sitting to standing position.

The nurse reviews the collected client data and collaborates with the neurologist. Complete the following sentence by selecting from the list of word choices below.

The nurse would recognize that the client is *most likely* experiencing [**Word Choice**] and [**Word Choice**].

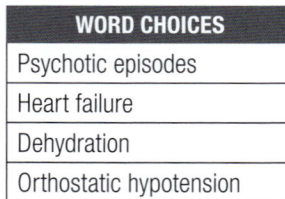

WORD CHOICES
Psychotic episodes
Heart failure
Dehydration
Orthostatic hypotension

Thinking Exercise 13.2.3

The nurse is caring for a 69-year-old client at the neurologist office.

History and Physical	Nurses' Notes	Orders	Laboratory Results

1330: Family made follow-up appointment for client's Parkinson disease (PD). Client has been on the maximum dose of carbidopa/levodopa for the past 2 years and recently experienced several visual hallucinations. Medication has enabled client to be independent in ADLs since PD diagnosis. For the past few weeks, client has noticed increased rigidity and slowing gait. Client reports two episodes of dizziness and light-headedness yesterday that almost resulted in falling down the basement steps. Missed yesterday's Tai Chi class, which has helped with balance and coordination. Denies shortness of breath or chest pain. Reports occasional foot and ankle edema; currently 1+ nonpitting edema bilaterally. VS: T 97.8°F (36.6°C), HR 92 beats/min and irregular, BP 98/50 mm Hg (sitting), RR 16 breaths/min, SpO_2 94% on RA.

1350: BP 110/62 mm Hg (lying down), BP 98/52 mm Hg (sitting), BP 88/50 mm Hg (standing). States feeling light-headed when moving from a sitting to standing position.

The nurse reviews the collected client data and collaborates with the neurologist. Complete the following sentence by selecting from the lists of options below.

The nurse determines that the **_priority_** for care at this time is to manage the client's **1 [Select]** because the client is at high risk for **2 [Select]**.

OPTIONS FOR 1	OPTIONS FOR 2
Hallucinations	Suicide
Foot and ankle edema	Contractures
Orthostatic hypotension	Heart failure
Immobility	Falls

Thinking Exercise 13.2.4

The nurse is caring for a 69-year-old client at the neurologist office.

History and Physical	Nurses' Notes	Orders	Laboratory Results

1330: Family made follow-up appointment for client's Parkinson disease (PD). Client has been on the maximum dose of carbidopa/levodopa for the past 2 years and recently experienced several visual hallucinations. Medication has enabled client to be independent in ADLs since PD diagnosis. For the past few weeks, client has noticed increased rigidity and slowing gait. Client reports two episodes of dizziness and light-headedness yesterday that almost resulted in falling down the basement steps. Missed yesterday's Tai Chi class, which has helped with balance and coordination. Denies shortness of breath or chest pain. Reports occasional foot and ankle edema; currently 1+ nonpitting edema bilaterally. VS: T 97.8°F (36.6°C), HR 92 beats/min and irregular, BP 98/50 mm Hg (sitting), RR 16 breaths/min, SpO_2 94% on RA.

1350: BP 110/62 mm Hg (lying down), BP 98/52 mm Hg (sitting), BP 88/50 mm Hg (standing). States feeling light-headed when moving from a sitting to standing position.

The nurse collaborates with the family and neurologist and contributes to the client's plan of care. Which of the following potential orders would the nurse anticipate? **Select all that apply.**
O Send the client to the nearby lab to draw blood for multiple tests.
O Send the client to the nearby imaging center for a head CT.
O Plan for direct client admission to the acute care hospital.
O Prescribe an antipsychotic medication to manage hallucinations.
O Instruct the family member to purchase an automated blood pressure machine for home.
O Encourage the client to drink plenty of fluids.

Thinking Exercise 13.2.5

The nurse is caring for a 69-year-old client in the acute care unit.

History and Physical	Nurses' Notes	Orders	Laboratory Results

Neurologist Office

1330: Family made follow-up appointment for client's Parkinson disease (PD). Client has been on the maximum dose of carbidopa/levodopa for the past 2 years and recently experienced several visual hallucinations. Medication has enabled client to be independent in ADLs since PD diagnosis. For the past few weeks, client has noticed increased rigidity and slowing gait. Client reports two episodes of dizziness and light-headedness yesterday that almost resulted in falling down the basement steps. Missed yesterday's Tai Chi class, which has helped with balance and coordination. Denies shortness of breath or chest pain. Reports occasional foot and ankle edema; currently 1+ nonpitting edema bilaterally. VS: T 97.8°F (36.6°C), HR 92 beats/min and irregular, BP 98/50 mm Hg (sitting), RR 16 breaths/min, SpO$_2$ 94% on RA.

1350: BP 110/62 mm Hg (lying down), BP 98/52 mm Hg (sitting), BP 88/50 mm Hg (standing). States feeling light-headed when moving from a sitting to standing position.

Acute Care Unit: Day of Admission

1615: Client admitted directly from neurologist office for orthostatic hypotension and recent visual hallucinations. Medical history includes PD, chronic gout, and type 2 diabetes mellitus controlled by metformin and diet. Alert and oriented × 4. Cranial nerves intact. Able to move all extremities. Uses a cane at times for ambulation but lately has become stiffer with a slower gait. No resting tremors noted. No adventitious breath sounds. Denies shortness of breath or chest pain. S$_1$ and S$_2$ present but irregular. All pulses present; cap refill <3 sec. 1+ nonpitting edema in both feet and ankles. Abdomen soft and round; bowel sounds present in all quadrants. VS: T 97.8°F (36.6°C), HR 76 beats/min and irregular, BP 96/52 mm Hg (sitting), RR 18 breaths/min, SpO$_2$ 93% on RA.

The nurse collaborates with the registered nurse and contributes to the client's plan of care. Select whether the following potential nursing actions are indicated or not indicated for the client at this time.

POTENTIAL NURSING ACTIONS	INDICATED	NOT INDICATED
Document frequent orthostatic blood pressure checks		
Place the client on nothing by mouth (NPO) status		
Begin supplemental oxygen via NC		
Hold the client's carbidopa/levodopa		
Remind the client to use the call light for assistance to get out of bed		

Thinking Exercise 13.2.6

The nurse is caring for a 69-year-old client in the acute care unit.

History and Physical	Nurses' Notes	Orders	Laboratory Results

Neurologist Office

1330: Family made follow-up appointment for client's Parkinson disease (PD). Client has been on the maximum dose of carbidopa/levodopa for the past 2 years and recently experienced several visual hallucinations. Medication has enabled client to be independent in ADLs since PD diagnosis. For the past few weeks, client has noticed increased rigidity and slowing gait. Client reports two episodes of dizziness and light-headedness yesterday that almost resulted in falling down the basement steps. Missed yesterday's Tai Chi class, which has helped with balance and coordination. Denies shortness of breath or chest pain. Reports occasional foot and ankle edema; currently 1+ nonpitting edema bilaterally. VS: T 97.8°F (36.6°C), HR 92 beats/min and irregular, BP 98/50 mm Hg (sitting), RR 16 breaths/min, SpO$_2$ 94% on RA.

1350: BP 110/62 mm Hg (lying down), BP 98/52 mm Hg (sitting), BP 88/50 mm Hg (standing). States feeling light-headed when moving from a sitting to standing position.

Acute Care Unit: Day of Admission

1615: Client admitted directly from neurologist office for orthostatic hypotension and recent visual hallucinations. Medical history includes PD, chronic gout, and type 2 diabetes mellitus controlled by metformin and diet. Alert and oriented × 4. Cranial nerves intact. Able to move all extremities. Uses a cane at times for ambulation but lately has become stiffer with a slower gait. No resting tremors noted. No adventitious breath sounds. Denies shortness of breath or chest pain. S$_1$ and S$_2$ present but irregular. All pulses present; cap refill <3 sec. 1+ nonpitting edema in both feet and ankles. Abdomen soft and round; bowel sounds present in all quadrants. VS: T 97.8°F (36.6°C), HR 76 beats/min and irregular, BP 96/52 mm Hg (sitting), RR 18 breaths/min, SpO$_2$ 93% on RA.

Acute Care Unit: Day 3

0825: Planning for discharge tomorrow pending lab results. Most recent blood pressures: BP 116/73 mm Hg (lying down), BP 114/72 mm Hg (sitting), BP 110/69 mm Hg (standing). States no light-headedness when moving from a sitting to standing position. Reports occasional resting tremors; has increased stiffness when walking with cane to bathroom. Is being re-evaluated for new PD drug regimen. Has had no hallucinations or delusions since hospital admission. Reports has not had a bowel movement during hospital stay. Docusate sodium started this morning before breakfast.

The nurse reviews the collected client data with the registered nurse. For each data collection finding in the most recent note at 0825, select whether the client finding indicates that the client's status has improved or not improved.

CLIENT FINDINGS	IMPROVED	NOT IMPROVED
Standing BP 110/69 mm Hg		
No light-headedness when changing positions		
No bowel movement during hospital stay		
Occasional resting tremors and increased stiffness		
No hallucinations or delusions during hospital stay		

Stand-Alone Thinking Exercise 13.1

The nurse is caring for an 73-year-old client in the emergency department (ED).

History and Physical	Nurses' Notes	Orders	Diagnostic Tests

0930: Client brought to ED by family after experiencing sudden severe low back pain when vacuuming carpet. Medical history includes breast cancer, hypertension, hysterectomy for uterine fibroids, left wrist and rib fractures, and severe osteoporosis. Alert and oriented × 4. Reports resting back pain rated 7/10, but increases to 10/10 when changing position. Pain does not radiate down to buttocks or legs. No adventitious breath sounds. S_1 and S_2 present and regular. Abdomen soft and round; bowel sounds present in all quadrants. Able to move all extremities. All pulses present; cap refill <3 sec. 1+ pitting edema in both feet, but states swelling subsides during the night when sleeping. Denies blood in urine, and is voiding as usual. No urinary or bowel incontinence. VS: T 98°F (36.7°C), HR 84 beats/min and regular, BP 146/80 mm Hg, RR 18 breaths/min, SpO_2 95% on RA.

The nurse reviews the collected client data with the registered nurse. Complete the diagram by selecting from the choices below to specify what potential condition the client is likely experiencing, **2** nursing actions that are appropriate to take, and **2** parameters the nurse would monitor to assess the client's progress.

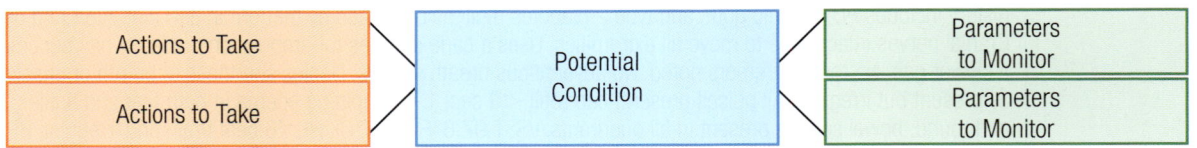

Actions to Take	Potential Conditions	Parameters to Monitor
Consult with physical therapy (PT)	Kidney stones	Pain level
Prepare client for vertebral x-rays and thoracolumbar MRI	Metastatic bone cancer	Presence of infection
Keep client NPO for a cystoscopy	Vertebral compression fracture(s)	Ability to ambulate independently
Request an order for an analgesic drug	Herniated lumbar disk	Serum calcium levels
Obtain consent for emergent surgery		Muscle strength

Stand-Alone Thinking Exercise 13.2

The nurse is caring for an 81-year-old client in the emergency department (ED).

History and Physical	Nurses' Notes	Orders	Diagnostic Tests

1100: Client brought to ED via ambulance following a motor vehicle accident. Alert and oriented × 4. Other than having two children, client has no significant health history. Reports abdominal pain rated 8/10 that worsens when changing position. States feeling "like bones in my lower abdomen are moving around." Large bruise in lower abdominal area near symphysis pubis. Abdomen distended; bowel sounds deferred due to pain. No adventitious breath sounds. S_1 and S_2 present and regular. Able to move all extremities. All pulses present; cap refill <3 sec. VS: T 98.6°F (37°C), HR 114 beats/min and regular, BP 102/58 mm Hg, RR 20 breaths/min, SpO_2 95% on RA.

The nurse reviews the collected client data with the registered nurse. Complete the diagram by selecting from the choices below to specify what potential condition the client is likely experiencing, **2** nursing actions that are appropriate to take, and **2** parameters the nurse would monitor to assess the client's progress.

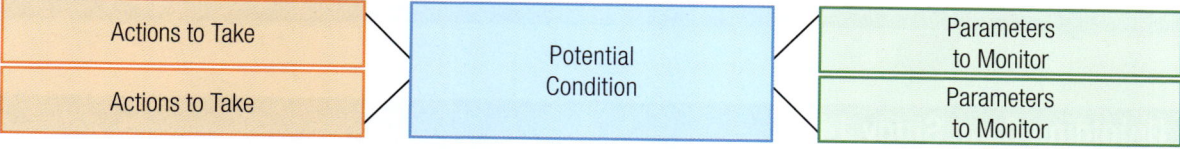

Actions to Take	Potential Conditions	Parameters to Monitor
Monitor urine quantity and quality	Small bowel obstruction	Pain level
Prepare client for pelvic x-rays and abdominal CT scan	Pelvic fracture(s)	Bowel sounds
Start supplemental oxygen via NC	Peritonitis	Blood pressure
Insert an indwelling urinary catheter	Hemothorax	Mobility status
Obtain consent for emergent surgery		SpO_2

Unfolding Case Study 14.1

Thinking Exercise 14.1.1

The nurse is caring for a 68-year-old client in the emergency department (ED).

History and Physical	Nurses' Notes	Orders	Laboratory Results

1545: Client brought to ED by family due to new-onset confusion and generalized weakness. Health history of type 2 diabetes mellitus, hypertension, and chronic kidney disease. Current medications include dulaglutide, losartan-hydrochlorothiazide, amlodipine, and furosemide. Client is drowsy, closing eyes when not directly addressed. Family reports that client has not been feeling well over the past few days and has had a decreased appetite due to nausea and vomiting small amounts of bile-colored emesis. Client is oriented to self and family only. Respirations shallow and labored with bilateral coarse crackles auscultated. Skin warm and dry with 3+ pitting edema, and paresthesia present in bilateral lower extremities. Pulses palpable throughout. Abdomen soft with active bowel sounds present in all quadrants. Reports diminishing urinary output over the past week with ongoing administration of prescribed diuretic therapy. VS: T 99.2°F (37.3°C), HR 76 beats/min, RR 21 breaths/min, BP 158/85 mm Hg, SpO$_2$ 94% on RA. Client denies pain. FSBG 128 mg/dL (7.1 mmol/L).

The nurse reviews the collected client data with the registered nurse. Select the **2** client findings that require *immediate* follow-up.

○ 3+ Pitting edema
○ Bile-colored emesis
○ Bilateral coarse crackles auscultated
○ Decreased appetite due to nausea
○ FSBG 128 mg/dL (7.1 mmol/L)
○ Oriented to self and family only
○ Paresthesia in bilateral lower extremities

Thinking Exercise 14.1.2

The nurse is caring for a 68-year-old client in the emergency department.

History and Physical	Nurses' Notes	Orders	Laboratory Results

1545: Client brought to ED by family due to new-onset confusion and generalized weakness. Health history of type 2 diabetes mellitus, hypertension, and chronic kidney disease. Current medications include dulaglutide, losartan-hydrochlorothiazide, amlodipine, and furosemide. Client is drowsy, closing eyes when not directly addressed. Family reports that client has not been feeling well over the past few days and has had a decreased appetite due to nausea and vomiting small amounts of bile-colored emesis. Client is oriented to self and family only. Respirations shallow and labored with bilateral coarse crackles auscultated. Skin warm and dry with 3+ pitting edema, and paresthesia present in bilateral lower extremities. Pulses palpable throughout. Abdomen soft with active bowel sounds present in all quadrants. Reports diminishing urinary output over the past week with ongoing administration of prescribed diuretic therapy. VS: T 99.2°F (37.3°C), HR 76 beats/min, RR 21 breaths/min, BP 158/85 mm Hg, SpO$_2$ 94% on RA. Client denies pain. FSBG 128 mg/dL (7.1 mmol/L).

The nurse reviews collected client data with the registered nurse. Complete the following sentence by selecting from the lists of options below.

The client is *most likely* experiencing **1 [Select]** as evidenced by **2 [Select]** and **3 [Select]**.

OPTIONS FOR 1	OPTIONS FOR 2	OPTIONS FOR 3
Deep vein thrombosis	Nausea	Bile-colored emesis
Pulmonary edema	Oliguria	Coarse crackles
Small bowel obstruction	Shallow, labored respirations	Pitting edema

Thinking Exercise 14.1.3

The nurse is caring for a 68-year-old client in the emergency department.

History and Physical	Nurses' Notes	Orders	Laboratory Results

1545: Client brought to ED by family due to new-onset confusion and generalized weakness. Health history of type 2 diabetes mellitus, hypertension, and chronic kidney disease. Current medications include dulaglutide, losartan-hydrochlorothiazide, amlodipine, and furosemide. Client is drowsy, closing eyes when not directly addressed. Family reports that client has not been feeling well over the past few days and has had a decreased appetite due to nausea and vomiting small amounts of bile-colored emesis. Client is oriented to self and family only. Respirations shallow and labored with bilateral coarse crackles auscultated. Skin warm and dry with 3+ pitting edema, and paresthesia present in bilateral lower extremities. Pulses palpable throughout. Abdomen soft with active bowel sounds present in all quadrants. Reports diminishing urinary output over the past week with ongoing administration of prescribed diuretic therapy. VS: T 99.2°F (37.3°C), HR 76 beats/min, RR 21 breaths/min, BP 158/85 mm Hg, SpO$_2$ 94% on RA. Client denies pain. FSBG 128 mg/dL (7.1 mmol/L).

1600: Phlebotomy for laboratory tests complete. Bedside 12-lead ECG: Sinus rhythm with peaked T waves and prolonged PR interval.

History and Physical	Nurses' Notes	Orders	Laboratory Results
Serum Laboratory Test and Reference Range		**1600**	
Hemoglobin (M: 14–18 g/dL [8.7–11.2 mmol/L]; F: 12–16 g/dL [7.4–9.9 mmol/L])		12.5 g/dL (7.76 mmol/L)	
Hematocrit (M: 42%–52% [0.42–0.52 volume fraction]; F: 37%–47% [0.37–0.47 volume fraction])		38% (0.38 volume fraction)	
Glucose (74–106 mg/dL [4.1–5.9 mmol/L])		130 mg/dL (7.2 mmol/L)	
Sodium (136–145 mEq/L [136–145mmol/L])		144 mEq/L (144 mmol/L)	
Potassium (3.5–5.0 mEq/L [3.5–5.0 mmol/L])		7.1 mEq/L (7.1 mmol/L)	
Calcium (9–10.5 mg/dL [2.25–2.62 mmol/L])		7.2 mg/dL (1.8 mmol/L)	
Phosphate (3–4.5 mg/dL [0.87–1.45 mmol/L])		5.4 mg/dL (1.74 mmol/L)	
Blood urea nitrogen (BUN) (10–20 mg/dL [3.6–7.1 mmol/L])		66 mg/dL (23.57 mmol/L)	
Creatinine (0.7–1.3 mg/dL [61.89–114.95 µmol/L])		3.2 mg/dL (282.9 µmol/L)	

The nurse reviews the collected client data and collaborates with the registered nurse. Complete the following sentence by selecting from the list of word choices below.

The nurse determines the **_priority_** for care at this time is emergent hemodialysis due to **[Word Choice]** and **[Word Choice]**.

WORD CHOICES
Bilateral pitting edema and oliguria
Decreased hemoglobin and hematocrit
Hyperkalemia with ECG changes
Elevated BUN and creatinine
Pulmonary edema with respiratory distress

Thinking Exercise 14.1.4

The nurse is caring for a 68-year-old client in the emergency department.

History and Physical	Nurses' Notes	Orders	Laboratory Findings

1545: Client brought to ED by family due to new-onset confusion and generalized weakness. Health history of type 2 diabetes mellitus, hypertension, and chronic kidney disease. Current medications include dulaglutide, losartan-hydrochlorothiazide, amlodipine, and furosemide. Client is drowsy, closing eyes when not directly addressed. Family reports that client has not been feeling well over the past few days and has had a decreased appetite due to nausea and vomiting small amounts of bile-colored emesis. Client is oriented to self and family only. Respirations shallow and labored with bilateral coarse crackles auscultated. Skin warm and dry with 3+ pitting edema, and paresthesia present in bilateral lower extremities. Pulses palpable throughout. Abdomen soft with active bowel sounds present in all quadrants. Reports diminishing urinary output over the past week with ongoing administration of prescribed diuretic therapy. VS: T 99.2°F (37.3°C), HR 76 beats/min, RR 21 breaths/min, BP 158/85 mm Hg, SpO$_2$ 94% on RA. Client denies pain. FSBG 128 mg/dL (7.1 mmol/L).

1600: Phlebotomy for laboratory tests complete. Bedside 12-lead ECG: Sinus rhythm with peaked T waves and prolonged PR interval.

1650: Physician at bedside discussing plan of care with client and family. Orders received for admission and emergent hemodialysis. VS: HR 78 beats/min, RR 22 breaths/min, BP 160/88 mm Hg, SpO$_2$ 97% on 2 L/min O$_2$ via NC. Current weight 165 lb (74.8 kg).

History and Physical	Nurses' Notes	Orders	Laboratory Results
Serum Laboratory Test and Reference Range		**1600**	
Hemoglobin (M: 14–18 g/dL [8.7–11.2 mmol/L]; F: 12–16 g/dL [7.4–9.9 mmol/L])		12.5 g/dL (7.76 mmol/L)	
Hematocrit (M: 42%–52% [0.42–0.52 volume fraction]; F: 37%–47% [0.37–0.47 volume fraction])		38% (0.38 volume fraction)	
Glucose (74–106 mg/dL [4.1–5.9 mmol/L])		130 mg/dL (7.2 mmol/L)	
Sodium (136–145 mEq/L [136–145 mmol/L])		144 mEq/L (144 mmol/L)	
Potassium (3.5–5.0 mEq/L [3.5–5.0 mmol/L])		7.1 mEq/L (7.1 mmol/L)	
Calcium (9–10.5 mg/dL [2.25–2.62 mmol/L])		7.2 mg/dL (1.8 mmol/L)	
Phosphate (3–4.5 mg/dL [0.87–1.45 mmol/L])		5.4 mg/dL (1.74 mmol/L)	
Blood urea nitrogen (BUN) (10–20 mg/dL [3.6–7.1 mmol/L])		66 mg/dL (23.57 mmol/L)	
Creatinine (0.7–1.3 mg/dL [61.89–114.95 μmol/L])		3.2 mg/dL (282.9 μmol/L)	

The nurse reviews the collected client data with the registered nurse and contributes to the client's plan of care. For each client condition listed below, select the potential nursing actions that are appropriate as part of the client's plan of care. More than one action may be selected for each problem.

CLIENT CONDITIONS	POTENTIAL NURSING ACTIONS
Fluid volume excess related to fluid retention because of kidney dysfunction.	○ Accurately calculate daily fluid intake from all sources. ○ Obtain daily weights at the same time using the same scale. ○ Assess vital signs, respiratory effort, and lung sounds every 4 hours.
Inadequate nutrition related to anorexia, nausea, vomiting, and dietary restrictions.	○ Collaborate with a registered dietary nutritionist to educate the client and family on nutritional needs and restrictions. ○ Provide the client with protein shakes between each meal. ○ Teach the client to use salt substitutes.
Potential for injury related to acute confusion, bone demineralization, and peripheral neuropathy.	○ Assess skin and bony areas for pressure wounds and unusual surface bumps or depressions. ○ Facilitate frequent client rounding to reorient and provide basic care needs. ○ Teach assistive nursing personnel the correct use of lift sheets to reposition the client in bed.

Thinking Exercise 14.1.5

The nurse is caring for a 68-year-old client on an acute medical-surgical unit.

History and Physical	Nurses' Notes	Orders	Laboratory Findings

1545: Client brought to ED by family due to new-onset confusion and generalized weakness. Health history of type 2 diabetes mellitus, hypertension, and chronic kidney disease. Current medications include dulaglutide, losartan-hydrochlorothiazide, amlodipine, and furosemide. Client is drowsy, closing eyes when not directly addressed. Family reports that client has not been feeling well over the past few days and has had a decreased appetite due to nausea and vomiting small amounts of bile-colored emesis. Client is oriented to self and family only. Respirations shallow and labored with bilateral coarse crackles auscultated. Skin warm and dry with 3+ pitting edema, and paresthesia present in bilateral lower extremities. Pulses palpable throughout. Abdomen soft with active bowel sounds present in all quadrants. Reports diminishing urinary output over the past week with ongoing administration of prescribed diuretic therapy. VS: T 99.2°F (37.3°C), HR 76 beats/min, RR 21 breaths/min, BP 158/85 mm Hg, SpO$_2$ 94% on RA. Client denies pain. FSBG 128 mg/dL (7.1 mmol/L).

1600: Phlebotomy for laboratory tests complete. Bedside 12-lead ECG: Sinus rhythm with peaked T waves and prolonged PR interval.

1650: Physician at bedside discussing plan of care with client and family. Orders received for admission and emergent hemodialysis. VS: HR 78 beats/min, RR 22 breaths/min, BP 160/88 mm Hg, SpO$_2$ 97% on 2 L/min O$_2$ via NC. Current weight 165 lb (74.8 kg).

1705: Client transferred to interventional radiology. Hand-off report given.

2 Days Later: Medical-Surgical Unit
1400: Hand-off report received. Client completed second hemodialysis treatment since admission. Remained stable with no complications during treatment. VS: HR 66 beats/min, RR 12 breaths/min, BP 130/55 mm Hg, SpO$_2$ 97% on RA. Current weight 154 lb (69.8 kg).

1415: Client arrived on unit. Alert and oriented × 4. Reports light-headedness when standing to transfer from the stretcher to the bed. Positioned to comfort in bed. Respirations equal and unlabored. Lung fields clear throughout. Heart rate normal. Temporary hemodialysis catheter site clean and dry with occlusive dressing. Skin warm and dry. Nonpitting dependent edema present. Abdomen soft with active bowel sounds in all quadrants. VS: HR 72 beats/min, RR 14 breaths/min, BP 128/52 mm Hg (supine), SpO$_2$ 97% on RA. Denies nausea, pain, and light-headedness when lying in bed.

The nurse collaborates with the registered nurse and contributes to the client's plan of care. Which of the following nursing actions would the nurse plan to implement? **Select all that apply.**

O Alert the Rapid Response Team.
O Assist the client when ambulating to the bathroom.
O Hold the next dose of losartan-hydrochlorothiazide.
O Obtain a bedside FSBG reading.
O Prepare to administer an IV bolus of 0.9% normal saline.
O Remind the client to use the call bell prior to rising from the bed.
O Request assistance to obtain orthostatic vital signs.

Thinking Exercise 14.1.6

The nurse is caring for a 68-year-old client on an acute medical-surgical unit.

History and Physical	Nurses' Notes	Orders	Laboratory Results

1545: Client brought to ED by family due to new-onset confusion and generalized weakness. Health history of type 2 diabetes mellitus, hypertension, and chronic kidney disease. Current medications include dulaglutide, losartan-hydrochlorothiazide, amlodipine, and furosemide. Client is drowsy, closing eyes when not directly addressed. Family reports that client has not been feeling well over the past few days and has had a decreased appetite due to nausea and vomiting small amounts of bile-colored emesis. Client is oriented to self and family only. Respirations shallow and labored with bilateral coarse crackles auscultated. Skin warm and dry with 3+ pitting edema, and paresthesia present in bilateral lower extremities. Pulses palpable throughout. Abdomen soft with active bowel sounds present in all quadrants. Reports diminishing urinary output over the past week with ongoing administration of prescribed diuretic therapy. VS: T 99.2°F (37.3°C), HR 76 beats/min, RR 21 breaths/min, BP 158/85 mm Hg, SpO$_2$ 94% on RA. Client denies pain. FSBG 128 mg/dL (7.1 mmol/L).

1600: Phlebotomy for laboratory tests complete. Bedside 12-lead ECG: Sinus rhythm with peaked T waves and prolonged PR interval.

1650: Physician at bedside discussing plan of care with client and family. Orders received for admission and emergent hemodialysis. VS: HR 78 beats/min, RR 22 breaths/min, BP 160/88 mm Hg, SpO$_2$ 97% on 2 L/min O$_2$ via NC. Current weight 165 lb (74.8 kg).

1705: Client transferred to interventional radiology. Hand-off report given.

2 Days Later: Medical-Surgical Unit
1400: Hand-off report received. Client completed second hemodialysis treatment since admission. Remained stable with no complications during treatment. VS: HR 66 beats/min, RR 12 breaths/min, BP 130/55 mm Hg, SpO$_2$ 97% on RA. Current weight 154 lb (69.8 kg).

1415: Client arrives on unit. Alert and oriented × 4. Reports light-headedness when standing to transfer from the stretcher to the bed. Positioned to comfort in bed. Respirations equal and unlabored. Lung fields clear throughout. Heart rate normal. Temporary hemodialysis catheter site clean and dry with occlusive dressing. Skin warm and dry. Nonpitting dependent edema present. Abdomen soft with active bowel sounds in all quadrants. VS: HR 72 beats/min, RR 14 breaths/min, BP 128/52 mm Hg (supine), SpO$_2$ 97% on RA. Denies nausea, pain, and light-headedness when lying in bed.

1650: Client transfers to chair for dinner. No dizziness or light-headedness present. Alert and oriented × 4. Denies nausea and expresses interest in eating dinner. VS: T 98.8°F (37.1°C), HR 69 beats/min, RR 12 breaths/min, BP 135/60 mm Hg, SpO$_2$ 96% on RA. Denies pain. FSBG 188 mg/dL (10.4 mmol/L).

The nurse reviews the most recent nurses' notes and is assisting to evaluate the client's current status with findings from 2 days ago. For each data collection finding, select whether the finding indicates that the client's status has improved or not improved.

DATA COLLECTION FINDING	IMPROVED	NOT IMPROVED
Alert and oriented × 4		
BP 135/60 mm Hg		
Denies nausea		
FSBG 188 mg/dL (10.4 mmol/L)		
No adventitious lung sounds		

Unfolding Case Study 14.2

Thinking Exercise 14.2.1

The nurse is caring for a 74-year-old male client at an ambulatory care clinic. Highlight the client findings that require **immediate** follow-up.

History and Physical	Nurses' Notes	Orders	Progress Notes

1000: Client made appointment due to new-onset urinary frequency and urgency. Client is alert and oriented × 4. Expresses embarrassment regarding urinary symptoms stating, "I have had trouble initiating urination for a while, but recently I have been voiding without warning, especially during the night." Client confirms postvoid dribbling and denies pain or burning with urination. Health history includes type 2 diabetes mellitus, hypertension, hyperlipidemia, and COPD. Current medications are metformin, losartan, amlodipine, and simvastatin. VS: T 98.5°F (36.9°C), HR 61 beats/min, RR 14 breaths/min, BP 138/66 mm Hg, SpO$_2$ 94% on RA. Denies pain. FSBG 132 mg/dL (7.3 mmol/L).

Thinking Exercise 14.2.2

The nurse is caring for a 74-year-old male client at an ambulatory care clinic.

History and Physical	Nurses' Notes	Orders	Progress Notes

1000: Client made appointment due to new-onset urinary frequency and urgency. Client is alert and oriented × 4. Expresses embarrassment regarding urinary symptoms stating, "I have had trouble initiating urination for a while, but recently I have been voiding without warning, especially during the night." Client confirms postvoid dribbling and denies pain or burning with urination. Health history includes type 2 diabetes mellitus, hypertension, hyperlipidemia, and COPD. Current medications are metformin, losartan, amlodipine, and simvastatin. VS: T 98.5°F (36.9°C), HR 61 beats/min, RR 14 breaths/min, BP 138/66 mm Hg, SpO$_2$ 94% on RA. Denies pain. FSBG 132 mg/dL (7.3 mmol/L).

The nurse reviews the collected client data with the registered nurse. Complete the following sentence by selecting from the list of word choices below.

The nurse recognizes that the client is ***most likely*** experiencing [**Word Choice**].

WORD CHOICES
Acute kidney disease
Benign prostatic hyperplasia
Bladder cancer
Renal calculi

Thinking Exercise 14.2.3

The nurse is caring for a 74-year-old male client at an ambulatory care clinic.

History and Physical	Nurses' Notes	Orders	Progress Notes

1000: Client made appointment due to new-onset urinary frequency and urgency. Client is alert and oriented × 4. Expresses embarrassment regarding urinary symptoms stating, "I have had trouble initiating urination for a while, but recently I have been voiding without warning, especially during the night." Client confirms postvoid dribbling and denies pain or burning with urination. Health history includes type 2 diabetes mellitus, hypertension, hyperlipidemia, and COPD. Current medications are metformin, losartan, amlodipine, and simvastatin. VS: T 98.5°F (36.9°C), HR 61 beats/min, RR 14 breaths/min, BP 138/66 mm Hg, SpO$_2$ 94% on RA. Denies pain. FSBG 132 mg/dL (7.3 mmol/L).

1020: Physician at bedside, updated on client findings. Physical and diagnostic examination completed. Client diagnosed with BPH.

The nurse reviews the collected client data with the registered nurse. Complete the following sentence by selecting from the lists of options below.

The nurse determines the *priority* for care at this time is improving **1 [Select]** to prevent complications such as **2 [Select]** and **3 [Select]**.

OPTIONS FOR 1	OPTIONS FOR 2	OPTIONS FOR 3
Detrusor muscle strength	Urinary retention	Bladder cancer
Fluid intake	Dehydration	Urinary tract infection
Urinary elimination	Urinary incontinence	Orthostatic hypotension

Thinking Exercise 14.2.4

The nurse is caring for a 74-year-old male client at an ambulatory care clinic.

History and Physical	Nurses' Notes	Orders	Progress Notes

1000: Client made appointment due to new-onset urinary frequency and urgency. Client is alert and oriented × 4. Expresses embarrassment regarding urinary symptoms stating, "I have had trouble initiating urination for a while, but recently I have been voiding without warning, especially during the night." Client confirms postvoid dribbling and denies pain or burning with urination. Health history includes type 2 diabetes mellitus, hypertension, hyperlipidemia, and COPD. Current medications are metformin, losartan, amlodipine, and simvastatin. VS: T 98.5°F (36.9°C), HR 61 beats/min, RR 14 breaths/min, BP 138/66 mm Hg, SpO$_2$ 94% on RA. Denies pain. FSBG 132 mg/dL (7.3 mmol/L).

1020: Physician at bedside, updated on client findings. Physical and diagnostic examination completed. Client diagnosed with BPH.

The nurse collaborates with the registered nurse and contributes to the client's plan of care. Select whether the following potential orders are indicated or not indicated for the client at this time.

POTENTIAL ORDERS	INDICATED	NOT INDICATED
Behavior modification to promote bladder emptying and minimize urge incontinence		
Daily urinary self-catheterization to prevent bladder distention		
Drug therapy with an alpha$_1$-adrenergic antagonist and/or a 5-alpha-reductase inhibitor		
Fluid restriction of less than 1200 mL per day		
Preoperative teaching for transurethral resection of the prostate (TURP)		

Thinking Exercise 14.2.5

The nurse is caring for a 74-year-old male client at an ambulatory care clinic.

History and Physical	Nurses' Notes	Orders	Progress Notes

1000: Client made appointment due to new-onset urinary frequency and urgency. Client is alert and oriented × 4. Expresses embarrassment regarding urinary symptoms stating, "I have had trouble initiating urination for a while, but recently I have been voiding without warning, especially during the night." Client confirms postvoid dribbling and denies pain or burning with urination. Health history includes type 2 diabetes mellitus, hypertension, hyperlipidemia, and COPD. Current medications are metformin, losartan, amlodipine, and simvastatin. VS: T 98.5°F (36.9°C), HR 61 beats/min, RR 14 breaths/min, BP 138/66 mm Hg, SpO$_2$ 94% on RA. Denies pain. FSBG 132 mg/dL (7.3 mmol/L).

1020: Physician at bedside, updated on client findings. Physical and diagnostic examination completed. Client diagnosed with BPH.

1100: Prescription for combination drug therapy with finasteride and doxazosin received. Client teaching provided.

The nurse assists with implementation of the client's plan of care. Which actions would be appropriate for the nurse to take? **Select all that apply.**

○ Assist the client to develop a schedule for voiding every 3 to 4 hours while awake.
○ Ask the client to keep a journal with fluid intake and urinary symptoms.
○ Have the client rise slowly from the bed and lie down if feeling dizzy.
○ Instruct the client to stop taking medications if impotence or sexual dysfunction occurs.
○ Obtain a baseline serum prostate-specific antigen (PSA) level.
○ Instruct the client to restrict fluids 2 hours before bedtime.
○ Teach the client to urinate as soon as the urge to void is felt.

Thinking Exercise 14.2.6

The nurse collaborates with the registered nurse to evaluate client outcomes for a 74-year-old male client. Highlight the client findings in the latest nurses' notes that indicate the client's current status has **improved** when compared with findings from 2 weeks ago.

History and Physical	Nurses' Notes	Orders	Progress Notes

1000: Client made appointment due to new-onset urinary frequency and urgency. Client is alert and oriented × 4. Expresses embarrassment regarding urinary symptoms stating, "I have had trouble initiating urination for a while, but recently I have been voiding without warning, especially during the night." Client confirms postvoid dribbling and denies pain or burning with urination. Health history includes type 2 diabetes mellitus, hypertension, hyperlipidemia, and COPD. Current medications are metformin, losartan, amlodipine, and simvastatin. VS: T 98.5°F (36.9°C), HR 61 beats/min, RR 14 breaths/min, BP 138/66 mm Hg, SpO$_2$ 94% on RA. Denies pain. FSBG 132 mg/dL (7.3 mmol/L).

1020: Physician at bedside, updated on client findings. Physical and diagnostic examination completed. Client diagnosed with BPH.

1100: Prescription for combination drug therapy with finasteride and doxazosin received. Client teaching provided.

2 Weeks Later
0910: Telemedicine follow-up call. Client alert and oriented. Reports drowsiness and light-headedness for a few days after starting drug therapy, but symptoms have subsided with no episodes of dizziness or orthostatic hypotension in the past few days. Client reports attempting to void every 90 minutes while awake and using the double-voiding technique with each attempt. Postmicturition dribble continues, but episodes of urge incontinence have stopped. Client also reports that limiting evening fluid intake has decreased nocturia, allowing for several hours of uninterrupted sleep every night. VS: T 98.6°F (37°C), HR 63 beats/min, RR 12 breaths/min, BP 132/65 mm Hg, SpO2 95% on RA. Denies bladder distention and burning or pain with urination. FSBG 144 mg/dL (8 mmol/L).

Stand-Alone Thinking Exercise 14.1

The nurse is caring for an 82-year-old client on an acute medical-surgical unit.

Progress Notes	Nurses' Notes	Orders	Laboratory Results

1830: Client arrived on medical-surgical unit after carotid endarterectomy procedure. Alert and oriented × 4. Follows commands and moves all extremities. Respirations equal and unlabored. Lung fields clear throughout and diminished in bases. Skin warm and dry. Pulses palpable throughout. Small neck incision well approximated, no drainage, Steri-Strips intact. Right forearm 20 g IV, saline locked. Abdomen soft and round. Bowel sounds present in all quadrants; no bowel movement for past 3 days. VS: T 99.1°F (37.2°C), HR 78 beats/min, RR 13 breaths/min, BP 145/58 mm Hg, SpO$_2$ 99% on 2 L/min O$_2$ via NC. Denies pain. Client is a widow and lives independently. Has one adult child who lives out of town and was delayed arriving before today's procedure. Adult child updated on client's status via phone and reports plans to arrive in the early morning hours.

1920: Client out of bed for dinner. Tolerates transfer without complications. Eats 80% of meal.

2010: Ambulates with standby assist to the bathroom. 680 mL of clear, dark-yellow urine and small amount of unformed brown stool.

2100: Client ambulates to bathroom independently. Contacts nursing staff after returning to bed. No urine voided. Expresses frustration stating, "Only a little bit of liquid stool came out."

2140: Client found on floor of bathroom by the toilet. Alert and oriented × 4. Reports becoming light-headed while attempting to move bowels. Denies hitting head. Moves all extremities without pain. No bumps or excoriation noted on head or limbs. Client assisted back to bed. Hard fecal mass palpated at rectal opening. VS: T 99.8°F (37.6°C), HR 85 beats/min, RR 15 breaths/min, BP 140/52 mm Hg, SpO$_2$ 95% on RA.

The nurse reviews the collected client data with the registered nurse. Complete the diagram by selecting from the choices below to specify what potential condition the client is likely experiencing, **2** nursing actions that are appropriate to take, and **2** parameters the nurse would monitor to assess the client's progress.

Actions to Take		Potential Condition		Parameters to Monitor
Actions to Take				Parameters to Monitor

Actions to Take	Potential Conditions	Parameters to Monitor
Administer an antidiarrheal	Diarrhea	Dietary fiber and fluid intake
Encourage oral fluids, especially water	Fecal impaction	Forceful pushing or straining when on the toilet
Maintain strict bedrest with use of a bedpan for elimination	Hemorrhoids	Rectal bleeding
Recommend a low-fiber diet	Orthostatic hypotension	Serum electrolyte levels
Prepare to instill a mineral oil enema		Vital signs while lying, sitting, and standing

Stand-Alone Thinking Exercise 14.2

A nurse is caring for an 86-year-old client at a long-term care facility. The client's health history includes dementia, osteoarthritis, hypertension, and congestive heart failure.

History and Physical	Nurses' Notes	Orders	Nursing Flow Sheet
Vital Signs	**2 Days Ago**	**Yesterday**	**Current Day**
Temperature	98.4°F (36.8°C)	98.7°F (37.1°C)	100.9°F (38.3°C)
HR	62 beats/min	66 beats/min	98 beats/min
BP	135/68 mm Hg	144/72 mm Hg	118/66 mm Hg
RR	14 breaths/min	13 breaths/min	14 breaths/min
SpO$_2$	95% on RA	95% on RA	94% on RA
Pain	Denies pain	Denies pain	Unable to assess
LOC	Alert, oriented to self and some persons and situations	Alert, oriented to self and some persons and situations	Lethargic, oriented to self only. Unable to reorient. Speech clear, but not appropriate to the situation
Activity	Ambulates with walker, gait steady. Participated in group activities	Ambulates with walker to and from dining hall. Visit from family members	Moves extremities equally but unable to follow simple commands
Intake Dietary	100% breakfast, 80% lunch, 45% dinner	90% breakfast, 65% lunch, 30% dinner	25% breakfast
Output Urine	Voids with standby assist, 6 times. Clear, yellow urine	Voids with standby assist, 8 times. Cloudy, amber urine	Incontinent, 3 times. Odorous urine
Stool	Soft brown	—	—

The nurse collaborates with the registered nurse and contributes to the client's plan of care. Which of the following actions would the nurse take? **Select all that apply**.

O Anticipate the need for straight catheterization to obtain a sterile urine sample.
O Cleanse the perineum and apply barrier cream after each incontinence episode.
O Collaborate with the interdisciplinary team to provide constant client supervision.
O Contact the stroke alert or Rapid Response Team.
O Keep the bed in the lowest position with the call bell within reach.
O Recommend a 1000-mL IV fluid bolus.
O Schedule client toileting every 60 to 90 minutes.

CHAPTER 15

Client Conditions Affecting Tissue Integrity

Unfolding Case Study 15.1

Thinking Exercise 15.1.1

The nurse is caring for a 75-year-old client in the emergency department (ED).

History and Physical	Nurses' Notes	Orders	Laboratory Results

2230: Client brought to ED by friend after trying to extinguish a fire caused by a propane heater in a tent encampment for unhoused individuals. Friend unable to provide health history or information about whether the client takes medications but states client is a veteran who served in Vietnam. Client appears unkempt with poor hygiene; alert and oriented $\times$ 2 (person and situation). Ragged, torn coat sleeves carefully removed to inspect skin. Palms of both hands blistered and swollen. 80% of lower arms from hands to elbows reddened and slightly swollen. Reports pain rated 7/10 and "waves of nausea." Smudges on face and soot around nares and mouth. No adventitious or abnormal lung sounds. Denies dyspnea or shortness of breath. Peripheral pulses 2+, except for pedal pulses, which are barely palpable. Cap refill >3 sec; 2+ nonpitting edema in both feet. Able to move all extremities. Abdomen soft and round with active bowel sounds present in all quadrants. VS: T 99°F (37.2°C), HR 92 beats/min and regular, RR 20 breaths/min, BP 135/82 mm Hg, SpO$_2$ 90% on RA.

The nurse reviews the collected client data with the registered nurse. Select the **2** client findings that require **immediate** follow-up.

○ 2+ nonpitting edema of feet
○ Pain rated 7/10
○ Blistered skin on both hands
○ Oriented $\times$ 2 (person and situation)
○ Soot around nares and mouth
○ BP 135/82 mm Hg
○ SpO$_2$ 90% on RA

Thinking Exercise 15.1.2

The nurse is caring for a 75-year-old client in the emergency department.

History and Physical	Nurses' Notes	Orders	Laboratory Results

2230: Client brought to ED by friend after trying to extinguish a fire caused by a propane heater in a tent encampment for unhoused individuals. Friend unable to provide health history or information about whether the client takes medications but states client is a veteran who served in Vietnam. Client appears unkempt with poor hygiene; alert and oriented $\times$ 2 (person and situation). Ragged, torn coat sleeves carefully removed to inspect skin. Palms of both hands blistered and swollen. 80% of lower arms from hands to elbows reddened and slightly swollen. Reports pain rated 7/10 and "waves of nausea." Smudges on face and soot around nares and mouth. No adventitious or abnormal lung sounds. Denies dyspnea or shortness of breath. Peripheral pulses 2+, except for pedal pulses, which are barely palpable. Cap refill >3 sec; 2+ nonpitting edema in both feet. Able to move all extremities. Abdomen soft and round with active bowel sounds present in all quadrants. VS: T 99°F (37.2°C), HR 92 beats/min and regular, RR 20 breaths/min, BP 135/82 mm Hg, SpO$_2$ 90% on RA.

The nurse reviews the collected client data with the registered nurse. Complete the following sentence by selecting from the lists of options below.

The client is most at risk for having **1 [Select]** because the client has **2 [Select]**.

OPTIONS FOR 1	OPTIONS FOR 2
Third-degree burns	Blistered skin
A hypertensive crisis	An elevated blood pressure
A smoke inhalation injury	Soot around the nares and mouth
Hypovolemic shock	Tachycardia

Thinking Exercise 15.1.3

The nurse is caring for a 75-year-old client in the emergency department.

History and Physical	Nurses' Notes	Orders	Laboratory Results

2230: Client brought to ED by friend after trying to extinguish a fire caused by a propane heater in a tent encampment for unhoused individuals. Friend unable to provide health history or information about whether the client takes medications but states client is a veteran who served in Vietnam. Client appears unkempt with poor hygiene; alert and oriented × 2 (person and situation). Ragged, torn coat sleeves carefully removed to inspect skin. Palms of both hands blistered and swollen. 80% of lower arms from hands to elbows reddened and slightly swollen. Reports pain rated 7/10 and "waves of nausea." Smudges on face and soot around nares and mouth. No adventitious or abnormal lung sounds. Denies dyspnea or shortness of breath. Peripheral pulses 2+, except for pedal pulses, which are barely palpable. Cap refill >3 sec; 2+ nonpitting edema in both feet. Able to move all extremities. Abdomen soft and round with active bowel sounds present in all quadrants. VS: T 99°F (37.2°C), HR 92 beats/min and regular, RR 20 breaths/min, BP 135/82 mm Hg, SpO$_2$ 90% on RA.

The nurse collaborates with the registered nurse to determine the client's priority for care. Complete the following sentence by selecting from the list of word choices below.

Based on the client's risk for complications, the **_priority_** for client care is to anticipate the need for potential **[Word Choice]** support.

WORD CHOICES
Cardiac
Respiratory
Gastrointestinal
Vascular

Thinking Exercise 15.1.4

The nurse is caring for a 75-year-old client in the emergency department.

History and Physical	Nurses' Notes	Orders	Laboratory Results

2230: Client brought to ED by friend after trying to extinguish a fire caused by a propane heater in a tent encampment for unhoused individuals. Friend unable to provide health history or information about whether the client takes medications but states client is a veteran who served in Vietnam. Client appears unkempt with poor hygiene; alert and oriented × 2 (person and situation). Ragged, torn coat sleeves carefully removed to inspect skin. Palms of both hands blistered and swollen. 80% of lower arms from hands to elbows reddened and slightly swollen. Reports pain rated 7/10 and "waves of nausea." Smudges on face and soot around nares and mouth. No adventitious or abnormal lung sounds. Denies dyspnea or shortness of breath. Peripheral pulses 2+, except for pedal pulses, which are barely palpable. Cap refill >3 sec; 2+ nonpitting edema in both feet. Able to move all extremities. Abdomen soft and round with active bowel sounds present in all quadrants. VS: T 99°F (37.2°C), HR 92 beats/min and regular, RR 20 breaths/min, BP 135/82 mm Hg, SpO$_2$ 90% on RA.

2310: Blood drawn for CMP and CBC. Peripheral IV access established in left forearm in nonburned area. NS infusing at 100 mL/h. Continues to be alert and oriented × 2. Pain medication administered. Reports feeling a "little short of breath" but has less nausea. Slight inspiratory wheezing auscultated throughout lung fields. Wound care provided. VS: T 99°F (37.2°C), HR 100 beats/min and regular, RR 22 breaths/min, BP 138/84 mm Hg, SpO$_2$ 88% on RA.

The nurse collaborates with the registered nurse and contributes to the client's plan of care. Which of the following potential nursing actions would be indicated for the client at this time? **Select all that apply.**

○ Administer supplemental oxygen therapy.
○ Place the client in an upright sitting position.
○ Administer acetaminophen for elevated temperature.
○ Monitor respiratory rate and SpO$_2$ at least every hour.
○ Administer an oral loop diuretic such as furosemide.
○ Observe burned areas for signs of infection.

Thinking Exercise 15.1.5

The nurse is caring for a 75-year-old client in the emergency department.

History and Physical	Nurses' Notes	Orders	Laboratory Results

2230: Client brought to ED by friend after trying to extinguish a fire caused by a propane heater in a tent encampment for unhoused individuals. Friend unable to provide health history or information about whether the client takes medications but states client is a veteran who served in Vietnam. Client appears unkempt with poor hygiene; alert and oriented × 2 (person and situation). Ragged, torn coat sleeves carefully removed to inspect skin. Palms of both hands blistered and swollen. Lower arms from hands to elbows reddened and slightly swollen. Reports pain rated 7/10 and "waves of nausea." Smudges on face and soot around nares and mouth. No adventitious or abnormal lung sounds. Denies dyspnea or shortness of breath. Peripheral pulses 2+, except for pedal pulses, which are barely palpable. Cap refill >3 sec; 2+ nonpitting edema in both feet. Able to move all extremities. Abdomen soft and round with active bowel sounds present in all quadrants. VS: T 99°F (37.2°C), HR 92 beats/min and regular, RR 20 breaths/min, BP 135/82 mm Hg, SpO$_2$ 90% on RA.

2310: Blood drawn for CMP and CBC. Peripheral IV access established in left forearm in nonburned area. NS infusing at 100 mL/h. Continues to be alert and oriented × 2. Pain medication administered. Reports feeling a "little short of breath" but has less nausea. Slight inspiratory wheezing auscultated throughout lung fields. Wound care provided. VS: T 99°F (37.2°C), HR 100 beats/min and regular, RR 22 breaths/min, BP 138/84 mm Hg, SpO$_2$ 88% on RA.

2355: Alert but disoriented and restless. Cannot follow conversation. Sitting in upright position. Occasional dry cough. Continues to have wheezing, which is worsening. VS: T 99°F (37.2°C), HR 108 beats/min and irregular, RR 30 breaths/min and shallow, BP 150/92 mm Hg, SpO$_2$ 89% on 4 L/min O$_2$ via NC.

The nurse reviews the most recent collected client data with the registered nurse to implement a revised plan of care. For each body system, select the nursing actions that are required at this time.

BODY SYSTEM	NURSING ACTIONS
Respiratory	○ Request a bedside chest x-ray. ○ Consult respiratory therapy. ○ Suction the client using a sterile catheter.
Neurologic	○ Request a carbon monoxide blood test. ○ Transfer client care to the registered nurse. ○ Monitor neurologic status every hour.
Integumentary	○ Apply an antimicrobial dressing to second-degree burn areas. ○ Elevate both arms above the heart. ○ Plan to admit the client to the acute burn unit.

Thinking Exercise 15.1.6

The nurse is caring for a 75-year-old client in the emergency department. Highlight the client findings in the 0045 Nurses' Note that indicate the client has **improved**.

History and Physical	Nurses' Notes	Orders	Laboratory Results

2230: Client brought to ED by friend after trying to extinguish a fire caused by a propane heater in a tent encampment for unhoused individuals. Friend unable to provide health history or information about whether the client takes medications but states client is a veteran who served in Vietnam. Client appears unkempt with poor hygiene; alert and oriented $\times$ 2 (person and situation). Ragged, torn coat sleeves carefully removed to inspect skin. Palms of both hands blistered and swollen. Lower arms from hands to elbows reddened and slightly swollen. Reports pain rated 7/10 and "waves of nausea." Smudges on face and soot around nares and mouth. No adventitious or abnormal lung sounds. Denies dyspnea or shortness of breath. Peripheral pulses 2+, except for pedal pulses, which are barely palpable. Cap refill >3 sec; 2+ nonpitting edema in both feet. Able to move all extremities. Abdomen soft and round with active bowel sounds present in all quadrants. VS: T 99°F (37.2°C), HR 92 beats/min and regular, RR 20 breaths/min, BP 135/82 mm Hg, SpO$_2$ 90% on RA.

2310: Blood drawn for CMP and CBC. Peripheral IV access established in left forearm in nonburned area. NS infusing at 100 mL/h. Continues to be alert and oriented $\times$ 2. Pain medication administered. Reports feeling a "little short of breath" but has less nausea. Slight inspiratory wheezing auscultated throughout lung fields. Wound care provided. VS: T 99°F (37.2°C), HR 100 beats/min and regular, RR 22 breaths/min, BP 138/84 mm Hg, SpO$_2$ 88% on RA.

2355: Alert but disoriented and restless. Cannot follow conversation. Continues to have wheezing, which is worsening. VS: T 99°F (37.2°C), HR 108 beats/min and irregular, RR 30 breaths/min and shallow, BP 150/92 mm Hg, SpO$_2$ 89% on 4 L/min O$_2$ via NC.

0010: Bedside chest x-ray performed. Bronchodilator via nebulizer administered by RT. Blood drawn for stat carbon monoxide level.

0045: Alert and oriented $\times$ 2. Able to follow conversation and respond appropriately. Wheezing improved. No smoke inhalation injury noted on chest x-ray. Antimicrobial dressings applied to both hands. VS: T 98.6°F (37°C), HR 88 beats/min and regular, RR 22 breaths/min, BP 148/88 mm Hg, SpO$_2$ 95% on 4 L/min O$_2$ via NC.

Unfolding Case Study 15.2

Thinking Exercise 15.2.1

The nurse is caring for an 80-year-old client at a skilled nursing facility (SNF).

History and Physical	Nurses' Notes	Orders	Laboratory Results

0730: Client admitted to SNF from acute care hospital 2 weeks ago with a stage 3 sacral pressure injury. History of type 2 diabetes mellitus, hypertension, and severe rheumatoid arthritis affecting client mobility. Received IV antibiotic therapy and debridement for sacral wound infection and cellulitis during hospital stay. When transferred to SNF, sacral wound drainage was minimal and cellulitis was resolved. Today client continues to be alert and oriented $\times$ 2 (person and place). Lung sounds clear. Abdomen soft and round; bowel sounds hypoactive but present in all quadrants. Reports pain rated 6/10 in sacral area. Has more pain when sitting in chair compared with lying in bed. States has not had much appetite for the past few days. Skin assessment shows sacral pressure injury has progressed to stage 4 with exposed muscle. Moderate amount of foul-smelling, purulent drainage on dressing. Wound 1.5 inches (3.8 cm) in diameter and 0.75 inches (1.9 cm) deep. Tissue around wound is warm and reddened, extending 1.2 inches (3 cm). VS: T 100.8°F (38.2°C), HR 102 beats/min and regular, RR 22 breaths/min, BP 98/54 mm Hg, SpO$_2$ 94% on RA. FSBG 286 mg/dL (15.9 mmol/L).

The nurse reviews the collected client data with the registered nurse. Which of the following client findings require **immediate** follow-up? **Select all that apply.**

○ 6/10 sacral area pain
○ Decreased appetite
○ Hypoactive bowel sounds
○ Elevated temperature
○ Tachycardia
○ Tachypnea
○ Low blood pressure
○ Elevated FSBG
○ Warm and reddened skin around wound

Thinking Exercise 15.2.2

The nurse is caring for an 80-year-old client at a SNF.

History and Physical	Nurses' Notes	Orders	Laboratory Results

0730: Client admitted to SNF from the acute care hospital 2 weeks ago with a stage 3 sacral pressure injury. History of type 2 diabetes mellitus, hypertension, and severe rheumatoid arthritis affecting client mobility. Received IV antibiotic therapy and debridement for sacral wound infection and cellulitis during hospital stay. When transferred to SNF, sacral wound drainage was minimal and cellulitis was resolved. Today client continues to be alert and oriented × 2 (person and place). Lung sounds clear. Abdomen soft and round; bowel sounds hypoactive but present in all quadrants. Reports pain rated 6/10 in sacral area. Has more pain when sitting in chair compared with lying in bed. States has not had much appetite for the past few days. Skin assessment shows sacral pressure injury has progressed to stage 4 with exposed muscle. Moderate amount of foul-smelling, purulent drainage on dressing. Wound 1.5 inches (3.8 cm) in diameter and .75 inches (1.9 cm) deep. Tissue around wound is warm and reddened, extending 1.2 inches (3 cm). VS: T 100.8°F (38.2°C), HR 102 beats/min and regular, RR 22 breaths/min, BP 98/54 mm Hg, SpO$_2$ 94% on RA. FSBG 286 mg/dL (15.9 mmol/L).

The nurse reviews the collected client data with the registered nurse. Select the **3 potential complications** for which this client is at high risk.

○ Sepsis
○ Heart failure
○ Bowel obstruction
○ Dehydration
○ Malnutrition
○ Hypoglycemia

Thinking Exercise 15.2.3

The nurse is caring for an 80-year-old client at a SNF.

History and Physical	Nurses' Notes	Orders	Laboratory Results

0730: Client admitted to SNF from the acute care hospital 2 weeks ago with a stage 3 sacral pressure injury. History of type 2 diabetes mellitus, hypertension, and severe rheumatoid arthritis affecting client mobility. Received IV antibiotic therapy and debridement for sacral wound infection and cellulitis during hospital stay. When transferred to SNF, sacral wound drainage was minimal and cellulitis was resolved. Today client continues to be alert and oriented × 2 (person and place). Lung sounds clear. Abdomen soft and round; bowel sounds hypoactive but present in all quadrants. Reports pain rated 6/10 in sacral area. Has more pain when sitting in chair compared with lying in bed. States has not had much appetite for the past few days. Skin assessment shows sacral pressure injury has progressed to stage 4 with exposed muscle. Moderate amount of foul-smelling, purulent drainage on dressing. Wound 1.5 inches (3.8 cm) in diameter and .75 inches (1.9 cm) deep. Tissue around wound is warm and reddened, extending 1.2 inches (3 cm). VS: T 100.8°F (38.2°C), HR 102 beats/min and regular, RR 22 breaths/min, BP 98/54 mm Hg, SpO$_2$ 94% on RA. FSBG 286 mg/dL (15.9 mmol/L).

The nurse reviews the collected client data with the registered nurse. Complete the following sentence by selecting from the list of word choices below.

The *priority* for the client's care is to prevent or monitor for [**Word Choice**].

WORD CHOICES
Sepsis
Osteomyelitis
Protein deficiency
Electrolyte imbalance

Thinking Exercise 15.2.4

The nurse is caring for an 80-year-old client at a SNF.

History and Physical	Nurses' Notes	Orders	Laboratory Results

0730: Client admitted to SNF from the acute care hospital 2 weeks ago with a stage 3 sacral pressure injury. History of type 2 diabetes mellitus, hypertension, and severe rheumatoid arthritis affecting client mobility. Received IV antibiotic therapy and debridement for sacral wound infection and cellulitis during hospital stay. When transferred to SNF, sacral wound drainage was minimal and cellulitis was resolved. Today client continues to be alert and oriented × 2 (person and place). Lung sounds clear. Abdomen soft and round; bowel sounds hypoactive but present in all quadrants. Reports pain rated 6/10 in sacral area. Has more pain when sitting in chair compared with lying in bed. States has not had much appetite for the past few days. Skin assessment shows sacral pressure injury has progressed to stage 4 with exposed muscle. Moderate amount of foul-smelling, purulent drainage on dressing. Wound 1.5 inches (3.8 cm) in diameter and .75 inches (1.9 cm) deep. Tissue around wound is warm and reddened, extending 1.2 inches (3 cm). VS: T 100.8°F (38.2°C), HR 102 beats/min and regular, RR 22 breaths/min, BP 98/54 mm Hg, SpO$_2$ 94% on RA. FSBG 286 mg/dL (15.9 mmol/L).

0835: Left phone message for nurse practitioner regarding change in client condition. Family also notified about client condition.

The nurse collaborates with the registered nurse and contributes to the client's plan of care. Select whether the following potential nursing actions are indicated or not indicated for the client at this time.

POTENTIAL NURSING ACTION	INDICATED	NOT INDICATED
Administer antibiotic therapy per agency protocol.		
Start IV fluids via peripheral IV access.		
Administer supplemental oxygen therapy via nasal cannula.		
Take and record vital signs every 4 hours.		
Request consults with a registered dietitian nutritionist and a certified wound specialist.		

Thinking Exercise 15.2.5

The nurse is caring for an 80-year-old client at a SNF.

History and Physical	Nurses' Notes	Orders	Laboratory Results

0730: Client admitted to SNF from the acute care hospital 2 weeks ago with a stage 3 sacral pressure injury. History of type 2 diabetes mellitus, hypertension, and severe rheumatoid arthritis affecting client mobility. Received IV antibiotic therapy and debridement for sacral wound infection and cellulitis during hospital stay. When transferred to SNF, sacral wound drainage was minimal and cellulitis was resolved. Today client continues to be alert and oriented × 2 (person and place). Lung sounds clear. Abdomen soft and round; bowel sounds hypoactive but present in all quadrants. Reports pain rated 6/10 in sacral area. Has more pain when sitting in chair compared with lying in bed. States has not had much appetite for the past few days. Skin assessment shows sacral pressure injury has progressed to stage 4 with exposed muscle. Moderate amount of foul-smelling, purulent drainage on dressing. Wound 1.5 inches (3.8 cm) in diameter and .75 inches (1.9 cm) deep. Tissue around wound is warm and reddened, extending 1.2 inches (3 cm). VS: T 100.8°F (38.2°C), HR 102 beats/min and regular, RR 22 breaths/min, BP 98/54 mm Hg, SpO$_2$ 94% on RA. FSBG 286 mg/dL (15.9 mmol/L).

0835: Left phone message for NP regarding change in client condition. Also notified family about client condition.

1010: Orders received from NP. Consults requested and scheduled for this afternoon. Peripheral IV started in left forearm with NS infusing at 100 mL/h.

1130: VS: T 101.4°F (38.6°C), HR 86 beats/min and regular, RR 20 breaths/min, BP 114/66 mm Hg, SpO$_2$ 94% on RA. FSBG 175 mg/dL (9.7 mmol/L). Acetaminophen given for fever.

1440: Wound specialist visit for consult. Plan for application of vacuum-assisted closure (wound VAC).

The nurse prepares to reinforce teaching for the client and family about the use of vacuum-assisted closure for the sacral pressure injury. Which health teaching statements would the nurse include? **Select all that apply.**

○ "A foam dressing that is covered with a clear adhesive layer will be used with the wound VAC device."

○ "The wound VAC device will be connected to a pump that removes drainage and air pressure from the wound and promotes healing."

○ "The foam dressing is changed once a month for most clients who have pressure injuries."

○ "An alarm will sound if the wound VAC system is not working properly."

○ "The nurse will monitor the amount and quality of the drainage from the wound frequently."

Thinking Exercise 15.2.6

The nurse is caring for an 80-year-old client at a SNF.

History and Physical	Nurses' Notes	Orders	Laboratory Results

0730: Client admitted to SNF from the acute care hospital 2 weeks ago with a stage 3 sacral pressure injury. History of type 2 diabetes mellitus, hypertension, and severe rheumatoid arthritis affecting client mobility. Received IV antibiotic therapy and debridement for sacral wound infection and cellulitis during hospital stay. When transferred to SNF, sacral wound drainage was minimal and cellulitis was resolved. Today client continues to be alert and oriented $\times$ 2 (person and place). Lung sounds clear. Abdomen soft and round; bowel sounds hypoactive but present in all quadrants. Reports pain rated 6/10 in sacral area. Has more pain when sitting in chair compared with lying in bed. States has not had much appetite for the past few days. Skin assessment shows sacral pressure injury has progressed to stage 4 with exposed muscle. Moderate amount of foul-smelling, purulent drainage on dressing. Wound 1.5 inches (3.8 cm) in diameter and .75 inches (1.9 cm) deep. Tissue around wound is warm and reddened, extending 1.2 inches (3 cm). VS: T 100.8°F (38.2°C), HR 102 beats/min and regular, RR 22 breaths/min, BP 98/54 mm Hg, SpO$_2$ 94% on RA. FSBG 286 mg/dL (15.9 mmol/L).

0835: Left phone message for nurse practitioner regarding change in client condition. Also notified family about client condition.

1010: Orders received from NP. Consults requested and scheduled for this afternoon. Peripheral IV started in left forearm with NS infusing at 100 mL/h.

1130: VS: T 101.4°F (38.6°C), HR 86 beats/min and regular, RR 20 breaths/min, BP 114/66 mm Hg, SpO$_2$ 94% on RA. FSBG 175 mg/dL (9.7 mmol/L). Acetaminophen given for fever.

1440: Wound specialist visit for consult. Vacuum-assisted closure (wound VAC) applied. IV antibiotics started.

10 Days Later
0755: Wound specialist visit to assess wound progress. Stage 4 sacral pressure injury draining decreasing amounts of serosanguineous drainage via wound VAC. Wound is 1.3 inches (3.3 cm) in diameter and 0.65 inches (1.6 cm) deep. Tissue around wound is slightly warm and pinkish, extending slightly less than ½ inch (1.3 cm). VS: T 98.6°F (37°C), HR 84 beats/min and regular, RR 20 breaths/min, BP 112/68 mm Hg, SpO$_2$ 94% on RA. FSBG 125 mg/dL (6.9 mmol/L).

The nurse reviews the most recent collected client data with the registered nurse. Complete the following sentence by selecting from the lists of options below.

The client's condition has **1 [Select]** as evidenced by **2 [Select]** and **3 [Select]**.

OPTIONS FOR 1	OPTIONS FOR 2	OPTIONS FOR 3
Improved	Elevated blood glucose	Decreased wound size
Not improved	Decreased body temperature	Continued drainage
Not changed	Blood pressure	Stage 4 pressure injury

Stand-Alone Thinking Exercise 15.1

The nurse is caring for a 71-year-old client in the emergency department (ED).

History and Physical	Nurses' Notes	Orders	Laboratory Results

0730: Client admitted to ED with new-onset acute confusion and exhaustion after shoveling snow for more than 30 minutes. Neighbor noticed client was not responding appropriately and was shivering while outside. Medical history and medications not known because client lives alone and is not a reliable historian at this time. Alert and disoriented. Is unable to follow directions; speech is slurred, and both pupils are dilated but react to light. Continues to strongly shiver, and unable to move extremities when asked. Skin is pale and cold. Lung sounds clear. S$_1$ and S$_2$ present but irregular. Abdomen soft and round; bowel sounds hypoactive but present in all quadrants. VS: T 91°F (32.8°C), HR 58 beats/min and irregular, RR 12 breaths/min, BP 88/50 mm Hg, SpO$_2$ 92% on RA.

The nurse reviews the collected client data with the registered nurse. Complete the diagram by selecting from the choices below to specify what potential condition the client is likely experiencing, **2** nursing actions that are appropriate to take, and **2** parameters the nurse would monitor to assess the client's progress.

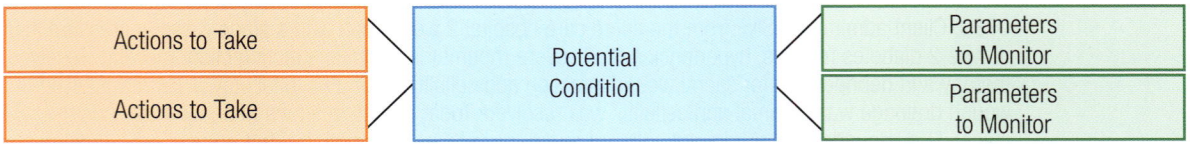

Actions to Take	Potential Conditions	Parameters to Monitor
Wrap the client in warm blankets	Frostbite	Vital signs
Warm the extremities before the torso	Hypothermia	Pain level
Initiate continuous cardiac monitoring	Bowel obstruction	Neurologic status
Start antibiotic therapy	Pulmonary embolus	Oxygen saturation
Prepare for debridement of hands and feet as needed		Prothrombin time/INR

Stand-Alone Thinking Exercise 15.2

The nurse is caring for an 82-year-old client at the urgent care center.

History and Physical	Progress Notes	Orders	Laboratory Results

1000: Client admitted to urgent care with report of new-onset, painful, blisterlike rash primarily on the back and chest that began to develop 2 days ago. Has not used any new skin products or laundry detergents in the past few months. Family states that client has been unable to sleep or function independently due to severe stabbing pain and itching at times. Client reports current pain rated 9/10. Medical history includes colorectal cancer, which is in remission, mild stroke with no residual deficits, hypertension, and gout. Was hospitalized 4 months ago with respiratory distress related to COVID-19 infection. Does not believe in the value of any type of vaccines or health supplements. Current prescribed medications include amlodipine 5 mg orally in the morning and HCTZ 25 mg orally in the morning.

VS: T 98.6°F (37°C), HR 74 beats/min and regular, RR 16 breaths/min, BP 146/90 mm Hg, SpO$_2$ 93% on RA.

The nurse reviews the collected client data with the registered nurse. Complete the diagram by selecting from the choices below to specify what potential condition the client is likely experiencing, **2** nursing actions that are appropriate to take, and **2** parameters the nurse would monitor to assess the client's progress.

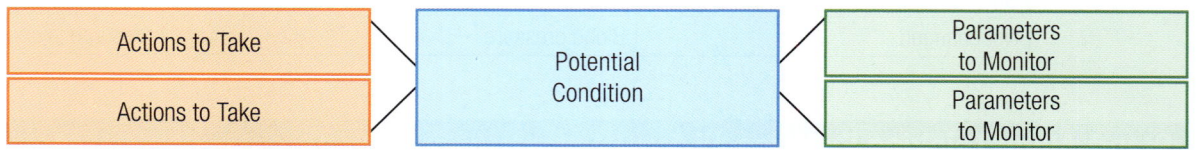

Actions to Take	Potential Conditions	Parameters to Monitor
Apply heat to the rash areas	Melanoma	Body temperature
Initiate oral antiviral drug therapy per agency protocol	Eczema	Pain level
Remind the client that this condition is not contagious	Contact dermatitis	Blood pressure
Document the distribution and appearance of the rash	Herpes zoster (shingles)	Rash response to treatment
Remove crusts when they form over the blisters		White blood cell count

Client Conditions Affecting Metabolism

Unfolding Case Study 16.1

Thinking Exercise 16.1.1

The nurse is caring for a 76-year-old client who was recently discharged from the hospital to home with home health services.

History and Physical	Nurses' Notes	Orders	Laboratory Results

Postoperative Day 4

1245: Initial home health visit after left hip arthroplasty. Client's health history includes osteoarthritis, hypertension, and a recent fall. Medications include acetaminophen, atenolol, and nifedipine. Client is lying on a couch covered in multiple blankets. Room is free from clutter, standard 4-point walker within client's reach, and cord for portable electric heater tucked under the couch. Client alert and oriented × 4. Reports feeling more fatigued than normal. Sits upright when asked and moves all extremities equally. Denies surgical pain but reports frequent headaches, joint stiffness, and extremity numbness. Heart tones regular. Pulses 2+ throughout. Nonpitting edema present in bilateral hands and feet. Respirations equal and unlabored with no adventitious breath sounds. Client denies chest pain or dyspnea. Skin warm and dry. Heberden nodes present on bilateral hands. Client reports feeling cold and asks spouse to turn up the heater. Left hip incision well approximated. No redness or swelling present. Client confirms active participation in home PT activities. VS: T 97.6°F (36.4°C), HR 58 beats/min and regular, RR 14 breaths/min, BP 129/66 mm Hg, SpO_2 96% on RA. Noted weight gain of 10 lb (4.5 kg) since annual physical 6 months ago.

The nurse reviews the collected client data with the registered nurse. Which of the following client findings require **immediate** follow-up? **Select all that apply.**

○ Approximated incision
○ Bradycardia
○ Extremity numbness
○ Heberden nodes
○ Increased fatigue
○ Portable electric heater
○ Report of feeling cold
○ Standard 4-point walker

Thinking Exercise 16.1.2

The nurse is caring for a 76-year-old client who was recently discharged from the hospital to home with home health services.

History and Physical	Nurses' Notes	Orders	Laboratory Results

Postoperative Day 4

1245: Initial home health visit after left hip arthroplasty. Client's health history includes osteoarthritis, hypertension, and a recent fall. Medications include acetaminophen, atenolol, and nifedipine. Client is lying on a couch covered in multiple blankets. Room is free from clutter, standard 4-point walker within client's reach, and cord for portable electric heater tucked under the couch. Client alert and oriented × 4. Reports feeling more fatigued than normal. Sits upright when asked and moves all extremities equally. Denies surgical pain but reports frequent headaches, joint stiffness, and extremity numbness. Heart tones regular. Pulses 2+ throughout. Nonpitting edema present in bilateral hands and feet. Respirations equal and unlabored with no adventitious breath sounds. Client denies chest pain or dyspnea. Skin warm and dry. Heberden nodes present on bilateral hands. Client reports feeling cold and asks spouse to turn up the heater. Left hip incision well approximated. No redness or swelling present. Client confirms active participation in home PT activities. VS: T 97.6°F (36.4°C), HR 58 beats/min and regular, RR 14 breaths/min, BP 129/66 mm Hg, SpO_2 96% on RA. Noted weight gain of 10 lb (4.5 kg) since annual physical 6 months ago.

The nurse reviews the collected client data with the registered nurse. For each client finding, select whether the finding is consistent with the health conditions of anemia, heart failure, or hypothyroidism. Some findings may be consistent with more than one condition.

CLIENT FINDINGS	ANEMIA	HEART FAILURE	HYPOTHYROIDISM
Fatigue			
Nonpitting edema			
Frequent headaches			
Weight gain			
Extremity numbness			

Thinking Exercise 16.1.3

The nurse is caring for a 76-year-old client who was recently discharged from the hospital to home with home health services.

History and Physical	Nurses' Notes	Orders	Laboratory Results

Postoperative Day 4

1245: Initial home health visit after left hip arthroplasty. Client's health history includes osteoarthritis, hypertension, and a recent fall. Medications include acetaminophen, atenolol, and nifedipine. Client is lying on a couch covered in multiple blankets. Room is free from clutter, standard 4-point walker within client's reach, and cord for portable electric heater tucked under the couch. Client alert and oriented × 4. Reports feeling more fatigued than normal. Sits upright when asked and moves all extremities equally. Denies surgical pain but reports frequent headaches, joint stiffness, and extremity numbness. Heart tones regular. Pulses 2+ throughout. Nonpitting edema present in bilateral hands and feet. Respirations equal and unlabored with no adventitious breath sounds. Client denies chest pain or dyspnea. Skin warm and dry. Heberden nodes present on bilateral hands. Client reports feeling cold and asks spouse to turn up the heater. Left hip incision well approximated. No redness or swelling present. Client confirms active participation in home PT activities. VS: T 97.6°F (36.4°C), HR 58 beats/min and regular, RR 14 breaths/min, BP 129/66 mm Hg, SpO$_2$ 96% on RA. Noted weight gain of 10 lb (4.5 kg) since annual physical 6 months ago.

1315: Provider notified. Laboratory tests ordered. Phlebotomy procedures completed, and samples prepared for transport to laboratory.

History and Physical	Nurses' Notes	Orders	Laboratory Results

Serum Laboratory Test and Reference Range	Postoperative Day 4
B-type natriuretic peptide (BNP) (<100 mcg/L [<100 pg/mL])	45 mcg/L (45 pg/mL)
Hemoglobin (M: 14–18 g/dL [8.7–11.2 mmol/L]; F: 12–16 g/dL [7.4–9.9 mmol/L])	14.2 g/dL (8.81 g/L)
Hematocrit (M: 42%–52% [0.42–0.52 volume fraction]; F: 37%–47% [0.37–0.47 volume fraction])	42% (0.42 volume fraction)
Free thyroxine (T$_4$) (0.8–2.8 ng/dL [10–26 pmol/L])	0.6 ng/dL (7.8 pmol/L)
Thyroid-stimulating hormone (TSH) (0.4–4.2 mIU/L)	5.4 mL mIU/L

The nurse reviews the client findings and laboratory test results from the home health visit with the registered nurse. Complete the following sentence by selecting from the list of options below.

The nurse recognizes that the client is *most likely* experiencing **1 [Select]**. The nurse would recommend **2 [Select]**.

OPTIONS FOR 1	OPTIONS FOR 2
Anemia	Fluid restrictions
Heart failure	Hormone replacement therapy
Hypothyroidism	Iron supplements

Thinking Exercise 16.1.4

The nurse is caring for a 76-year-old client who was recently discharged from the hospital to home with home health services.

History and Physical	Nurses' Notes	Orders	Laboratory Results

Postoperative Day 4

1245: Initial home health visit after left hip arthroplasty. Client's health history includes osteoarthritis, hypertension, and a recent fall. Medications include acetaminophen, atenolol, and nifedipine. Client is lying on a couch covered in multiple blankets. Room is free from clutter, standard 4-point walker within client's reach, and cord for portable electric heater tucked under the couch. Client alert and oriented × 4. Reports feeling more fatigued than normal. Sits upright when asked and moves all extremities equally. Denies surgical pain but reports frequent headaches, joint stiffness, and extremity numbness. Heart tones regular. Pulses 2+ throughout. Nonpitting edema present in bilateral hands and feet. Respirations equal and unlabored with no adventitious breath sounds. Client denies chest pain or dyspnea. Skin warm and dry. Heberden nodes present on bilateral hands. Client reports feeling cold and asks spouse to turn up the heater. Left hip incision well approximated. No redness or swelling present. Client confirms active participation in home PT activities. VS: T 97.6°F (36.4°C), HR 58 beats/min and regular, RR 14 breaths/min, BP 129/66 mm Hg, SpO$_2$ 96% on RA. Noted weight gain of 10 lb (4.5 kg) since annual physical 6 months ago.

1315: Provider notified. Laboratory tests ordered. Phlebotomy procedures completed, and samples prepared for transport to laboratory.

Postoperative Day 5

0900: Client prescribed levothyroxine 50 mcg orally every morning. Follow-up home visit scheduled.

History and Physical	Nurses' Notes	Orders	Laboratory Results

Serum Laboratory Test and Reference Range	Postoperative Day 4
B-type natriuretic peptide (BNP) (<100 mcg/L [<100 pg/mL])	45 mcg/L (45 pg/mL)
Hemoglobin (M: 14–18 g/dL [8.7–11.2 mmol/L]; F: 12–16 g/dL [7.4–9.9 mmol/L])	14.2 g/dL (8.81 g/L)
Hematocrit (M: 42%–52% [0.42–0.52 volume fraction]; F: 37%–47% [0.37–0.47 volume fraction])	42% (0.42 volume fraction)
Free thyroxine (T$_4$) (0.8–2.8 ng/dL [10–26 pmol/L])	0.6 ng/dL (7.8 pmol/L)
Thyroid-stimulating hormone (TSH) (0.4–4.2 mIU/L)	5.4 mL mIU/L

The nurse consults with the interprofessional team in preparation for a follow-up visit with the client. Select whether the following potential nursing actions are indicated or not indicated for the client at this time.

POTENTIAL NURSING ACTION	INDICATED	NOT INDICATED
Teach the client about hormone replacement therapy.		
Encourage the client to integrate periods of rest during activities of daily living.		
Assist the client in bathing twice a day to decrease skin drying.		
Consult a registered dietitian nutritionist for diet and food option recommendations.		
Wear a surgical mask during home health visits to minimize the risk of infection transmission.		

Thinking Exercise 16.1.5—Pharmacology

The nurse is caring for a 76-year-old client who was recently discharged from the hospital to home with home health services.

History and Physical	Nurses' Notes	Orders	Laboratory Results

Postoperative Day 4

1245: Initial home health visit after left hip arthroplasty. Client's health history includes osteoarthritis, hypertension, and a recent fall. Medications include acetaminophen, atenolol, and nifedipine. Client is lying on a couch covered in multiple blankets. Room is free from clutter, standard 4-point walker within client's reach, and cord for portable electric heater tucked under the couch. Client alert and oriented × 4. Reports feeling more fatigued than normal. Sits upright when asked and moves all extremities equally. Denies surgical pain but reports frequent headaches, joint stiffness, and extremity numbness. Heart tones regular. Pulses 2+ throughout. Nonpitting edema present in bilateral hands and feet. Respirations equal and unlabored with no adventitious breath sounds. Client denies chest pain or dyspnea. Skin warm and dry. Heberden nodes present on bilateral hands. Client reports feeling cold and asks spouse to turn up the heater. Left hip incision well approximated. No redness or swelling present. Client confirms active participation in home PT activities. VS: T 97.6°F (36.4°C), HR 58 beats/min and regular, BP 129/66 mm Hg, RR 14 breaths/min, SpO$_2$ 96% on RA. Noted weight gain of 10 lb (4.5 kg) since annual physical 6 months ago.

1315: Provider notified. Laboratory tests ordered. Phlebotomy procedures completed, and samples prepared for transport to laboratory.

Postoperative Day 5

0900: Client prescribed levothyroxine 50 mcg orally every morning. Follow-up home visit scheduled.

Postoperative Day 6

0920: Follow-up home health visit. Client alert and oriented × 4. Sitting at dining table finishing breakfast. Client states, "I had two cups of coffee and a glass of prune juice. I feel optimistic about a bowel movement today." VS: T 97.4°F (36.3°C), HR 57 beats/min and regular, BP 133/70 mm Hg, RR 15 breaths/min, SpO$_2$ 97% on RA. Denies pain. Incision well approximated, no redness or swelling noted. Client reports ambulating with walker to mailbox at front of house yesterday afternoon. Spouse present. Health teaching provided related to hypothyroidism and levothyroxine administration.

The nurse reviews the collected client data with the registered nurse and reinforces teaching with the client. Select the **3** statements the nurse would include in the client's health teaching.

○ "Constipation may result from hypothyroidism. Increasing your fluid and fiber intake may help with this condition."

○ "Fatigue and mental slowness are symptoms of hypothyroidism and should improve with treatment."

○ "If hormone replacement therapy is not successful, the health care provider may recommend surgical intervention."

○ "Laboratory tests need to be rechecked in 6 weeks, and you can stop taking levothyroxine if levels are normal."

○ "The best time to take your levothyroxine is 30 to 60 minutes before breakfast."

○ "You may take a sedative or tranquilizer if you are having difficulty sleeping through the night."

Thinking Exercise 16.1.6

The nurse is caring for a 76-year-old client who was recently discharged from the hospital to home with home health services.

The nurse collaborates with the registered nurse to evaluate client outcomes. Highlight the client findings in the latest nurses' notes that indicate client's current status has **improved** when compared with findings from 2 weeks ago.

History and Physical	Nurses' Notes	Orders	Laboratory Results

Postoperative Day 4

1245: Initial home health visit after left hip arthroplasty. Client's health history includes osteoarthritis, hypertension, and a recent fall. Medications include acetaminophen, atenolol, and nifedipine. Client is lying on a couch covered in multiple blankets. Room is free from clutter, standard 4-point walker within client's reach, and cord for portable electric heater tucked under the couch. Client alert and oriented × 4. Reports feeling more fatigued than normal. Sits upright when asked and moves all extremities equally. Denies surgical pain but reports frequent headaches, joint stiffness, and extremity numbness. Heart tones regular. Pulses 2+ throughout. Nonpitting edema present in bilateral hands and feet. Respirations equal and unlabored with no adventitious breath sounds. Client denies chest pain or dyspnea. Skin warm and dry. Heberden nodes present on bilateral hands. Client reports feeling cold and asks spouse to turn up the heater. Left hip incision well approximated. No redness or swelling present. Client confirms active participation in home PT activities. VS: T 97.6°F (36.4°C), HR 58 beats/min and regular, BP 129/66 mm Hg, RR 14 breaths/min, SpO$_2$ 96% on RA. Noted weight gain of 10 lb (4.5 kg) since annual physical 6 months ago.

1315: Provider notified. Laboratory tests ordered. Phlebotomy procedures completed, and samples prepared for transport to laboratory.

Postoperative Day 5

0900: Client prescribed levothyroxine 50 mcg orally every morning. Follow-up home visit scheduled.

Postoperative Day 6

0920: Follow-up home health visit. Client alert and oriented × 4. Sitting at dining table finishing breakfast. Client states, "I had two cups of coffee and a glass of prune juice. I feel optimistic about a bowel movement today." VS: T 97.4°F (36.3°C), HR 57 beats/min and regular, BP 133/70 mm Hg, RR 15 breaths/min, SpO$_2$ 97% on RA. Denies pain. Incision well approximated, no redness or swelling noted. Client reports ambulating with walker to mailbox at front of house yesterday afternoon. Spouse present. Health teaching provided related to hypothyroidism and levothyroxine administration.

3 Weeks After Surgery

1115: Follow-up clinic visit. Client alert and oriented × 4. Participates in PT three times weekly and reports needing to nap after each PT session. Respirations equal and unlabored. Lung fields clear throughout. Heart tones regular, pulses 2+ throughout, and no edema noted. Client denies paresthesia. Skin warm and dry. Reports eating well and having a bowel movement this morning. VS: T 98.6°F (37°C), HR 59 beats/min and regular, BP 134/62 mm Hg, RR 12 breaths/min, SpO$_2$ 96% on RA. Denies pain including headaches and surgical pain. No change in weight since surgery.

Unfolding Case Study 16.2

Thinking Exercise 16.2.1

The nurse is caring for an 82-year-old client at an assisted-living facility. Highlight the client findings that require **immediate** follow-up.

History and Physical	Nurses' Notes	Orders	Laboratory Results

1215: The nurse is requested by a visitor to the client's room. Upon arrival, the client is alert and observed wandering around the room without a shirt on. Oriented to self only. Skin warm and dry. Jaundice present. 2+ pitting edema present in bilateral lower extremities. Respirations labored. Abdomen distended with spider angiomas present. Client reorients to place and some situations, follows simple commands, and moves extremities equally. Facial features are symmetrical. Asterixis noted in bilateral hands. Client sits in a chair for a few minutes before rising and wandering again. Speaks loudly, "Get out of my house. I do not need your help." Equal movement in all extremities, but gait is unstable. VS: T 98.7°F (37°C), HR 92 beats/min, RR 18 breaths/min, BP 115/60 mm Hg, SpO$_2$ 94% on RA. Health history includes spinal disk herniation with diskectomy, chronic back pain, and hepatic cirrhosis.

Thinking Exercise 16.2.2

The nurse is caring for an 82-year-old client at an assisted-living facility.

History and Physical	Nurses' Notes	Orders	Laboratory Results

1215: The nurse is requested by a visitor to the client's room. Upon arrival, the client is alert and observed wandering around the room without a shirt on. Oriented to self only. Skin warm and dry. Jaundice present. 2+ pitting edema present in bilateral lower extremities. Respirations labored. Abdomen distended with spider angiomas present. Client reorients to place and some situations, follows simple commands, and moves extremities equally. Facial features are symmetrical. Asterixis noted in bilateral hands. Client sits in a chair for a few minutes before rising and wandering again. Speaks loudly, "Get out of my house. I do not need your help." Equal movement in all extremities, but gait is unstable. VS: T 98.7°F (37°C), HR 92 beats/min, RR 18 breaths/min, BP 115/60 mm Hg, SpO$_2$ 94% on RA. Health history includes spinal disk herniation with diskectomy, chronic back pain, and hepatic cirrhosis.

The nurse reviews collected client data with the registered nurse. Complete the following sentence by selecting from the list of word choices below.

The nurse recognizes that the client is *most likely* experiencing **[Word Choice]** as manifested by **[Word Choice]** and **[Word Choice]**.

WORD CHOICES
Alcohol-induced psychosis
Asterixis
Hemiparesis
Hepatic encephalopathy
Ischemic stroke
Mental confusion
Spider angioma

Thinking Exercise 16.2.3

The nurse is caring for an 82-year-old client at an assisted-living facility.

History and Physical	Nurses' Notes	Orders	Laboratory Results

Assisted-Living Facility

1215: The nurse is requested by a visitor to the client's room. Upon arrival, the client is alert and observed wandering around the room without a shirt on. Oriented to self only. Skin warm and dry. Jaundice present. 2+ pitting edema present in bilateral lower extremities. Respirations labored. Abdomen distended with spider angiomas present. Client reorients to place and some situations, follows simple commands, and moves extremities equally. Facial features are symmetrical. Asterixis noted in bilateral hands. Client sits in a chair for a few minutes before rising and wandering again. Speaks loudly, "Get out of my house. I do not need your help." Equal movement in all extremities, but gait is unstable. VS: T 98.7°F (37°C), HR 92 beats/min, RR 18 breaths/min, BP 115/60 mm Hg, SpO$_2$ 94% on RA. Health history includes spinal disk herniation with diskectomy, chronic back pain, and hepatic cirrhosis.

1240: Physician notified. Orders received for direct admission to acute care facility.

Acute Medical-Surgical Unit

1500: Client arrived on unit. Drowsy but easily aroused. Oriented to self only; unable to reorient. Facial features are symmetrical. Pupils equal and reactive to light. Heart tones regular. Skin dry and jaundiced. 2+ pitting edema present in bilateral lower extremities. Respirations labored with diminished breath sounds auscultated in bilateral bases. Client becomes anxious and refuses to lie in the supine position. Client more relaxed and seems comfortable in the high-Fowler position. Abdomen distended with spider angiomas present. Bowel sounds present throughout. Incontinent of urine; soiling bed with dark-yellow, odorous urine. VS: T 98.8°F (37.1°C), HR 110 beats/min, RR 15 breaths/min, BP 96/45 mm Hg, SpO$_2$ 90% on RA.

The medical-surgical nurse reviews preadmission and the most recent collected client data with the registered nurse. Select the **3** priorities for the client's care at this time.

○ Vital sign changes/abnormalities
○ Impaired skin integrity
○ Inadequate nutrition
○ Ineffective ventilation
○ Infection
○ Potential for injury

Thinking Exercise 16.2.4

The nurse is caring for an 82-year-old client on an acute medical-surgical unit.

History and Physical	Nurses' Notes	Orders	Laboratory Results

Assisted-Living Facility

1215: The nurse is requested by a visitor to the client's room. Upon arrival, the client is alert and observed wandering around the room without a shirt on. Oriented to self only. Skin warm and dry. Jaundice present. 2+ pitting edema present in bilateral lower extremities. Respirations labored. Abdomen distended with spider angiomas present. Client reorients to place and some situations, follows simple commands, and moves extremities equally. Facial features are symmetrical. Asterixis noted in bilateral hands. Client sits in a chair for a few minutes before rising and wandering again. Speaks loudly, "Get out of my house. I do not need your help." Equal movement in all extremities, but gait is unstable. VS: T 98.7°F (37°C), HR 92 beats/min, RR 18 breaths/min, BP 115/60 mm Hg, SpO$_2$ 94% on RA. Health history includes spinal disk herniation with diskectomy, chronic back pain, and hepatic cirrhosis.

1240: Physician notified. Orders received for direct admission to acute care facility.

Acute Medical-Surgical Unit

1500: Client arrived on unit. Drowsy but easily aroused. Oriented to self only; unable to reorient. Facial features are symmetrical. Pupils equal and reactive to light. Heart tones regular. Skin dry and jaundiced. 2+ pitting edema present in bilateral lower extremities. Respirations labored with diminished breath sounds auscultated in bilateral bases. Client becomes anxious and refuses to lie in the supine position. Client more relaxed and seems comfortable sitting in the high-Fowler position. Abdomen distended with spider angiomas present. Bowel sounds present throughout. Incontinent of urine; soiling bed with dark-yellow, odorous urine. VS: T 98.8°F (37.1°C), HR 110 beats/min, RR 15 breaths/min, BP 96/45 mm Hg, SpO$_2$ 90% on RA.

The nurse collaborates with the registered nurse and contributes to the client's plan of care. For each priority condition, select the appropriate nursing actions to be included in the plan of care. More than one nursing action may be selected for each priority condition.

PRIORITY CONDITIONS	POTENTIAL NURSING ACTIONS
Potential for injury	○ Collaborate with assistive nursing personnel to check on the client frequently. ○ Monitor changes in level of consciousness and orientation. ○ Obtain an order for soft wrist restraints to prevent client falls.
Hemodynamic instability	○ Accurately measure and record intake and output. ○ Frequently assess vital signs. ○ Monitor hemoglobin and hematocrit levels.
Respiratory distress	○ Initiate supplemental oxygen to keep SpO$_2$ >92%. ○ Measure abdominal girth daily. ○ Position the client in the supine position with the head of the bed elevated no more than 30 degrees.

Thinking Exercise 16.2.5—Pharmacology

The nurse is caring for an 82-year-old client on an acute medical-surgical unit.

History and Physical	Nurses' Notes	Orders	Laboratory Results

Assisted-Living Facility

1215: The nurse is requested by a visitor to the client's room. Upon arrival, the client is alert and observed wandering around the room without a shirt on. Oriented to self only. Skin warm and dry. Jaundice present. 2+ pitting edema present in bilateral lower extremities. Respirations labored. Abdomen distended with spider angiomas present. Client reorients to place and some situations, follows simple commands, and moves extremities equally. Facial features are symmetrical. Asterixis noted in bilateral hands. Client sits in a chair for a few minutes before rising and wandering again. Speaks loudly, "Get out of my house. I do not need your help." Equal movement in all extremities, but gait is unstable. VS: T 98.7°F (37°C), HR 92 beats/min, RR 18 breaths/min, BP 115/60 mm Hg, SpO$_2$ 94% on RA. Health history includes spinal disk herniation with diskectomy, chronic back pain, and hepatic cirrhosis.

1240: Physician notified. Orders received for direct admission to acute care facility.

Acute Medical-Surgical Unit

1500: Client arrives on unit. Drowsy but easily aroused. Oriented to self only, unable to reorient. Facial features are symmetrical. Pupils equal and reactive to light. Heart tones regular. Skin dry and jaundiced. 2+ pitting edema present in bilateral lower extremities. Respirations labored with diminished breath sounds auscultated in bilateral bases. Client becomes anxious and refuses to lie in the supine position. Client more relaxed and seems comfortable sitting in the high-Fowler position. Abdomen distended with spider angiomas present. Bowel sounds present throughout. Incontinent of urine, soiling bed with dark-yellow, odorous urine. VS: T 98.8°F (37.1°C), HR 110 beats/min, RR 15 breaths/min, BP 96/45 mm Hg, SpO$_2$ 90% on RA.

1520: Client alert and oriented to self only. Respirations shallow and labored. VS: HR 115 beats/min, RR 18 breaths/min, BP 102/47 mm Hg, SpO$_2$ 91% on 4 L/min O$_2$ via NC. Physician at bedside. Orders received.

History and Physical	Nurses' Notes	Orders	Laboratory Results

1620:
- Vital signs every 4 hours
- Oxygen to keep SpO$_2$ >92%
- Medications:
  - Lactulose 30 mL orally twice daily
  - Propranolol 20 mg orally twice daily
  - Furosemide 20 mg IV every 8 hours
- Consult
  - Registered dietitian nutritionist to meet client's dietary needs
  - Interventional radiologist for abdominal paracentesis

The nurse reviews the physician orders and collaborates with the registered nurse. Which actions would be appropriate for the nurse to implement at this time? **Select all that apply.**

○ Assist the physician to contact the client's medical power of attorney.
○ Collaborate with assistive nursing personnel to ensure safe access for toileting.
○ Hold oral medications until after the procedure.
○ Increase the flow of supplemental oxygen.
○ Monitor serum electrolyte levels.
○ Obtain the client's signature on a consent form for abdominal paracentesis.
○ Weigh the client prior to administering medications.

CHAPTER 16   Client Conditions Affecting Metabolism   189

Thinking Exercise 16.2.6

The nurse is caring for an 82-year-old client on an acute medical-surgical unit.

History and Physical	Nurses' Notes	Orders	Laboratory Results

Assisted-Living Facility

1215: The nurse is requested by a visitor to the client's apartment. Upon arrival, the client is alert and observed wandering around the room without a shirt on. Oriented to self only. Skin warm and dry. Jaundice present. 2+ pitting edema present in bilateral lower extremities. Respirations labored. Abdomen distended with spider angiomas present. Client reorients to place and some situations, follows simple commands, and moves extremities equally. Facial features are symmetrical. Asterixis noted in bilateral hands. Client sits in a chair for a few minutes before rising and wandering again. Speaks loudly, "Get out of my house. I do not need your help." Equal movement in all extremities, but gait is unstable. VS: T 98.7°F (37°C), HR 92 beats/min, RR 18 breaths/min, BP 115/60 mm Hg, SpO$_2$ 94% on RA. Health history includes spinal disk herniation with diskectomy, chronic back pain, and hepatic cirrhosis.

1240: Physician notified. Orders received for direct admission to acute care facility.

Acute Medical-Surgical Unit

1500: Client arrived on unit. Drowsy but easily aroused. Oriented to self only; unable to reorient. Facial features are symmetrical. Pupils equal and reactive to light. Heart tones regular. Skin dry and jaundiced. 2+ pitting edema present in bilateral lower extremities. Respirations labored with diminished breath sounds auscultated in bilateral bases. Client becomes anxious and refuses to lie in the supine position. Client more relaxed and seems comfortable sitting in the high-Fowler position. Abdomen distended with spider angiomas present. Bowel sounds present throughout. Incontinent of urine; soiling bed with dark-yellow, odorous urine. VS: T 98.8°F (37.1°C), HR 110 beats/min, RR 15 breaths/min, BP 96/45 mm Hg, SpO$_2$ 91% on RA.

1520: Client alert and oriented to self only. Respirations shallow and labored. VS: HR 115 beats/min, RR 18 breaths/min, BP 102/47 mm Hg, SpO$_2$ 92% on 4 L/min O$_2$ via NC. Physician at bedside. Orders received.

2 Days Later

1300: Client alert and oriented × 4. Out of bed in chair. Moves extremities equally, follows all commands, and actively participates in plan of care. Respirations equal and unlabored. Lung fields clear with diminished breath sounds auscultated in bilateral bases. Heart tones regular. Skin warm and dry. Jaundice present. Nonpitting edema in bilateral lower extremities. Abdomen soft and round with active bowel sounds in all quadrants. Client eats 35% of lunch. Bathroom privileges with one person, standby assist. Voids bright-yellow, clear urine. Last bowel movement this morning. Stool liquid brown. VS: T 98.8°F (37.1°C), HR 75 beats/min, RR 12 breaths/min, BP 126/65 mm Hg, SpO$_2$ 97% on 2 L/min O$_2$ via NC. Denies pain at this time.

The nurse reinforces discharge teaching with the client. Select whether the following client statements indicate understanding or no understanding of the discharge teaching provided.

CLIENT STATEMENTS	UNDERSTANDING	NO UNDERSTANDING
"I will ask the assistive care staff to help manage my medications."		
"I will bathe in tepid water, vigorously scrubbing with mild soap to manage dry skin."		
"I will consult the physician before taking any over-the-counter medications."		
"I will eat small but frequent, low-protein meals throughout each day."		
"I will sleep in my recliner because I am most comfortable there."		

Stand-Alone Thinking Exercise 16.1

The nurse is caring for a 71-year-old client at an ambulatory care clinic. To plan the most appropriate care, the nurse reviews the client findings recorded on the nursing flow sheet and laboratory results.

History and Physical	Nursing Flow Sheet	Orders	Laboratory Results
Parameters	Results: Today	Results: 1 Year Ago	
Heart rate	78 beats/min	76 beats/min	
Respiratory rate	14 breaths/min	12 breaths/min	
Blood pressure	160/110 mm Hg	138/80 mm Hg	
SpO$_2$	95% on RA	96% on RA	
Height	5 feet 4 inches (165 cm)	5 feet 4 inches (165 cm)	
Weight	181 lb (82.1 kg)	155 lb (70.3 kg)	
BMI	31	26.6	
Waist-to-hip ratio (Male: <0.95 low risk; 0.96–1 moderate risk; >1 high risk) (Female: <0.8 low risk; 0.81–0.85 moderate risk; >0.85 high risk)	0.98	0.83	

History and Physical	Nursing Flow Sheet	Orders	Laboratory Results
Serum Laboratory Test and Reference Range	Results: Today	Results: 1 Year Ago	
Fasting glucose (70–110 mg/dL [<6.1 mmol/L])	140 mg/dL (7.8 mmol/L)	105 mg/dL (5.8 mmol/L)	
Hemoglobin A1c (<7%)	8.5%	–	
LDL cholesterol (<130 mg/dL [<3.3 mmol/L])	215 mg/dL (5.6 mmol/L)	174 mg/dL (4.5 mmol/L)	
HDL cholesterol (Male: >45 mg/dL [>1.16 mmol/L]) (Female: >55 mg/dL [>1.42 mmol/L])	34.8 mg/dL (0.9 mmol/L)	40.2 mg/dL (1.03 mmol/L)	
Triglycerides (Male: 40–160 mg/dL [0.45–1.81 mmol/L]) (Female: 35–135 mg/dL [0.40–1.52 mmol/L])	195.5 mg/dL (2.2 mmol/L)	160.8 mg/dL (1.83 mmol/L)	

The nurse collaborates with the registered nurse and contributes to the client's plan of care. Complete the following sentences by selecting from the lists of options below.

The nurse recognizes that the client is *most likely* experiencing **1 [Select]**. The nurse would *prioritize* health teaching focused on **2 [Select]** and **3 [Select]**.

OPTIONS FOR 1	OPTIONS FOR 2	OPTIONS FOR 3
Cholestatic liver disease	Blood pressure monitoring	Fluid restriction
Type 1 diabetes mellitus	Dietary intake	Glucose monitoring
Metabolic syndrome	Emotional support	Physical activity

Stand-Alone Thinking Exercise 16.2

The nurse is caring for a 67-year-old female client at an ambulatory care clinic.

Progress Notes	Nurses' Notes	Orders	Laboratory Results

1000: Follow-up appointment after seeking emergency medical care 2 days ago. Client fell at home and fractured right wrist. Alert and oriented × 4. Speech clear and appropriate. Denies muscle weakness or balance issues. Client tripped over the dog when going to the bathroom in the middle of the night. Right arm in sling with hard cast over forearm and wrist. Right fingers pink and warm; cap refill <3 sec. Client begins to cry and states, "It is my fault. I worked so hard to get everything back to normal, but my body is simply falling apart." Further questioning reveals that the client experienced a significant emotional period in the early and mid-50s that almost caused an end to the client's marriage. Client shares that emotions have stabilized, but recently was diagnosed with hypertension and recognized the need for reading glasses. Client also reports stress incontinence that requires wearing a small urinary pad every day. Denies anorexia, weight loss, and bowel elimination issues. Is in a monogamous relationship but reports dreading sexual intercourse because it is painful. VS: T 98.6°F (37°C), HR 87 beats/min, RR 15 breaths/min, BP 136/68 mm Hg, SpO$_2$ 97% on RA. Denies pain at this time.

The nurse reviews the collected client data and collaborates with the registered nurse. Complete the diagram by selecting from the choices below to specify what potential condition the client is likely experiencing, **2** nursing actions that are appropriate to take, and **2** parameters the nurse would monitor to assess the client's progress.

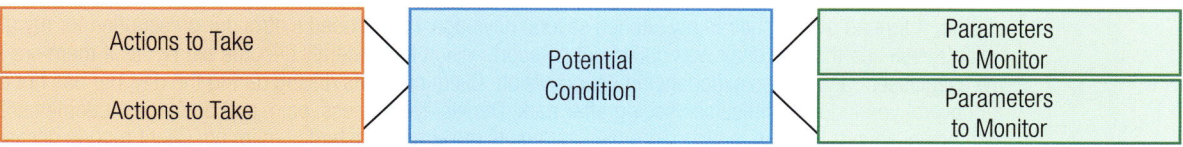

Actions to Take	Potential Conditions	Parameters to Monitor
Consult a case manager for home aid referral	Adrenal insufficiency	Orientation and cognition
Encourage weight-bearing exercises	Diabetes insipidus	Bone mineral density
Provide community resources for diabetes	Estrogen deficiency	Heart rate and rhythm
Restrict fluids to 1500 mL each day	Hypoparathyroidism	LDL cholesterol and triglyceride levels
Teach the client how to use water-soluble lubricants		Urine specific gravity

Unfolding Case Study 17.1

Thinking Exercise 17.1.1

The nurse is caring for a 78-year-old client at an ambulatory care clinic. Highlight the client findings that require **immediate** follow-up.

History and Physical	Nurses' Notes	Orders	Laboratory Results

1400: Client presents for a routine appointment to follow up on multiple medical conditions including hypertension, hyperlipidemia, and congestive heart failure. Current medications are carvedilol, digoxin, simvastatin, and furosemide. The client is a widower and lives independently. Alert and oriented × 4. Respirations equal and unlabored. Fine crackles auscultated in bilateral lower lobes of lungs. Productive cough present with scant pale secretions expectorated. Denies shortness of breath. Skin warm and dry with generalized nonpitting edema and 1+ pitting edema in bilateral feet and ankles. A scabbed wound is present on right knee and surrounded by yellowish-green bruising. Client reports a recent fall, stating, "I tripped over a chair in my kitchen several days ago. I must need a stronger prescription for my glasses because I didn't even see that the chair was pulled out." Reports vision has recently become blurry, "as if there are smudges on my eyeglasses" and is also experiencing double vision. Client confirms driving during the day, but has not driven at night for several years due to difficulties seeing after dark. Denies eye redness, pain, and drainage. Abdomen soft and round with bowel sounds present in all quadrants. Last bowel movement yesterday morning. Client reports occasional urinary incontinence, stating, "I have to stay close to a bathroom in the morning to prevent an accident." VS: T 98.4°F (36.8°C), HR 58 beats/min and regular, RR 13 breaths/min, BP 133/45 mm Hg, SpO$_2$ 95% on RA. Client denies pain.

Thinking Exercise 17.1.2

The nurse is caring for a 78-year-old client at an ambulatory care clinic.

History and Physical	Nurses' Notes	Orders	Laboratory Results

1400: Client presents for a routine appointment to follow up on multiple medical conditions including hypertension, hyperlipidemia, and congestive heart failure. Current medications are carvedilol, digoxin, simvastatin, and furosemide. The client is a widower and lives independently. Alert and oriented × 4. Respirations equal and unlabored. Fine crackles auscultated in bilateral lower lobes of lungs. Productive cough present with scant pale secretions expectorated. Denies shortness of breath. Skin warm and dry with generalized nonpitting edema and 1+ pitting edema in bilateral feet and ankles. A scabbed wound is present on right knee and surrounded by yellowish-green bruising. Client reports a recent fall, stating, "I tripped over a chair in my kitchen several days ago. I must need a stronger prescription for my glasses because I didn't even see that the chair was pulled out." Reports vision has recently become blurry, "as if there are smudges on my eyeglasses" and is also experiencing double vision. Client confirms driving during the day, but has not driven at night for several years due to difficulties seeing after dark. Denies eye redness, pain, and drainage. Abdomen soft and round with bowel sounds present in all quadrants. Last bowel movement yesterday morning. Client reports occasional urinary incontinence, stating, "I have to stay close to a bathroom in the morning to prevent an accident." VS: T 98.4°F (36.8°C), HR 58 beats/min and regular, RR 13 breaths/min, BP 133/45 mm Hg, SpO$_2$ 95% on RA. Client denies pain.

The nurse reviews the collected client data with the registered nurse. Complete the following sentence by selecting from the list of word choices below.

The nurse recognizes that the client's vision changes are *most likely* caused by a **[Word Choice].**

WORD CHOICES
Condition of the eye
Neurologic condition
Normal aging process

Thinking Exercise 17.1.3

The nurse is caring for a 78-year-old client at an ambulatory care clinic.

History and Physical	Nurses' Notes	Orders	Laboratory Results

1400: Client presents for a routine appointment to follow up on multiple medical conditions including hypertension, hyperlipidemia, and congestive heart failure. Current medications are carvedilol, digoxin, simvastatin, and furosemide. The client is a widower and lives independently. Alert and oriented × 4. Respirations equal and unlabored. Fine crackles auscultated in bilateral lower lobes of lungs. Productive cough present with scant pale secretions expectorated. Denies shortness of breath. Skin warm and dry with generalized nonpitting edema and 1+ pitting edema in bilateral feet and ankles. A scabbed wound is present on right knee and surrounded by yellowish-green bruising. Client reports a recent fall, stating, "I tripped over a chair in my kitchen several days ago. I must need a stronger prescription for my glasses because I didn't even see that the chair was pulled out." Reports vision has recently become blurry, "as if there are smudges on my eyeglasses" and is also experiencing double vision. Client confirms driving during the day, but has not driven at night for several years due to difficulties seeing after dark. Denies eye redness, pain, and drainage. Abdomen soft and round with bowel sounds present in all quadrants. Last bowel movement yesterday morning. Client reports occasional urinary incontinence, stating, "I have to stay close to a bathroom in the morning to prevent an accident." VS: T 98.4°F (36.8°C), HR 58 beats/min and regular, RR 13 breaths/min, BP 133/45 mm Hg, SpO$_2$ 95% on RA. Client denies pain.

The nurse reviews the client findings with the registered nurse. Complete the following sentence by selecting from the lists of options below.

The *priority* for the client's care at this time is to **1 [Select]** because the client is experiencing **2 [Select]**.

OPTIONS FOR 1	OPTIONS FOR 2
Assess safety risks	Impaired visual perception
Obtain a urine sample	Incontinence of urine
Promote skin integrity	Pitting edema

Thinking Exercise 17.1.4

The nurse is caring for a 78-year-old client at an ambulatory care clinic.

History and Physical	Nurses' Notes	Orders	Laboratory Results

1400: Client presents for a routine appointment to follow up on multiple medical conditions including hypertension, hyperlipidemia, and congestive heart failure. Current medications are carvedilol, digoxin, simvastatin, and furosemide. The client is a widower and lives independently. Alert and oriented × 4. Respirations equal and unlabored. Fine crackles auscultated in bilateral lower lobes of lungs. Productive cough present with scant pale secretions expectorated. Denies shortness of breath. Skin warm and dry with generalized nonpitting edema and 1+ pitting edema in bilateral feet and ankles. A scabbed wound is present on right knee and surrounded by yellowish-green bruising. Client reports a recent fall, stating, "I tripped over a chair in my kitchen several days ago. I must need a stronger prescription for my glasses because I didn't even see that the chair was pulled out." Reports vision has recently become blurry, "as if there are smudges on my eyeglasses" and is also experiencing double vision. Client confirms driving during the day, but has not driven at night for several years due to difficulties seeing after dark. Denies eye redness, pain, and drainage. Abdomen soft and round with bowel sounds present in all quadrants. Last bowel movement yesterday morning. Client reports occasional urinary incontinence, stating, "I have to stay close to a bathroom in the morning to prevent an accident." VS: T 98.4°F (36.8°C), HR 58 beats/min and regular, RR 13 breaths/min, BP 133/45 mm Hg, SpO$_2$ 95% on RA. Client denies pain.

The nurse collaborates with the registered nurse and contributes to the client's plan of care. Select whether the following potential nursing actions are indicated or not indicated for the client at this time.

POTENTIAL NURSING ACTIONS	INDICATED	NOT INDICATED
Assist with programming the client's phone with automatic dialing of emergency numbers.		
Collaborate with the case management nurse for admission to a skilled nursing facility.		
Encourage installation of handgrips in the bathroom and a nonskid surface on the shower floor.		
Identify a friend or family member who will assist to organize daily drugs in different shape containers.		
Provide information about food delivery services including groceries and prepared meals.		

Thinking Exercise 17.1.5

The nurse is caring for a 78-year-old client at an ambulatory surgical care clinic after cataract surgery.

History and Physical	Nurses' Notes	Orders	Laboratory Results

Ambulatory Care Clinic

1400: Client presents for a routine appointment to follow up on multiple medical conditions including hypertension, hyperlipidemia, and congestive heart failure. Current medications are carvedilol, digoxin, simvastatin, and furosemide. The client is a widower and lives independently. Alert and oriented × 4. Respirations equal and unlabored. Fine crackles auscultated in bilateral lower lobes of lungs. Productive cough present with scant pale secretions expectorated. Denies shortness of breath. Skin warm and dry with generalized nonpitting edema and 1+ pitting edema in bilateral feet and ankles. A scabbed wound is present on right knee and surrounded by yellowish-green bruising. Client reports a recent fall, stating, "I tripped over a chair in my kitchen several days ago. I must need a stronger prescription for my glasses because I didn't even see that the chair was pulled out." Reports vision has recently become blurry, "as if there are smudges on my eyeglasses" and is also experiencing double vision. Client confirms driving during the day, but has not driven at night for several years due to difficulties seeing after dark. Denies eye redness, pain, and drainage. Abdomen soft and round with bowel sounds present in all quadrants. Last bowel movement yesterday morning. Client reports occasional urinary incontinence, stating, "I have to stay close to a bathroom in the morning to prevent an accident." VS: T 98.4°F (36.8°C), HR 58 beats/min and regular, RR 13 breaths/min, BP 133/45 mm Hg, SpO$_2$ 95% on RA. Client denies pain.

1620: Eye exam performed; client diagnosed with cataracts and scheduled for surgery at a local ambulatory care clinic in 2 weeks.

Ambulatory Surgical Care Clinic

0830: Client arrives for surgical procedure. Alert and oriented × 4. Daughter at bedside and assigned to drive client home after procedure. Physician explains procedure and answers questions. Client signs surgical consent.

1000: Client arrived in PACU for recovery. Antibiotic and steroid surgical eye ointments instilled. VS: T 98.6°F (37°C), HR 62 beats/min and regular, RR 14 breaths/min, BP 124/42 mm Hg, SpO$_2$ 94% on RA. Client denies pain.

The ambulatory care nurse reviews the presurgical and newly collected client data with the registered nurse. Which **priority** nursing actions would the nurse plan to implement at this time? **Select all that apply.**
O Administer supplemental oxygen.
O Assess the client's pupil response and visual acuity.
O Assist the client to clear the airway by blowing the nose.
O Ensure that the client can properly instill eyedrops.
O Position the head of the bed lower than 30 degrees.
O Reinforce activity restrictions.
O Review prescribed eyedrops and administration schedule.

Thinking Exercise 17.1.6

The nurse is caring for a 78-year-old client during a follow-up telehealth visit.

History and Physical	Nurses' Notes	Orders	Laboratory Results

Ambulatory Care Clinic

1400: Client presents for a routine appointment to follow up on multiple medical conditions including hypertension, hyperlipidemia, and congestive heart failure. Current medications are carvedilol, digoxin, simvastatin, and furosemide. The client is a widower and lives independently. Alert and oriented $\times$ 4. Respirations equal and unlabored. Fine crackles auscultated in bilateral lower lobes of lungs. Productive cough present with scant pale secretions expectorated. Denies shortness of breath. Skin warm and dry with generalized nonpitting edema and 1+ pitting edema in bilateral feet and ankles. A scabbed wound is present on right knee and surrounded by yellowish-green bruising. Client reports a recent fall, stating, "I tripped over a chair in my kitchen several days ago. I must need a stronger prescription for my glasses because I didn't even see that the chair was pulled out." Reports vision has recently become blurry, "as if there are smudges on my eyeglasses" and is also experiencing double vision. Client confirms driving during the day, but has not driven at night for several years due to difficulties seeing after dark. Denies eye redness, pain, and drainage. Abdomen soft and round with bowel sounds present in all quadrants. Last bowel movement yesterday morning. Client reports occasional urinary incontinence, stating, "I have to stay close to a bathroom in the morning to prevent an accident." VS: T 98.4°F (36.8°C), HR 58 beats/min and regular, RR 13 breaths/min, BP 133/45 mm Hg, SpO$_2$ 95% on RA. Client denies pain.

1620: Eye exam performed; client is diagnosed with cataracts and scheduled for surgery at a local ambulatory care clinic in 2 weeks.

Ambulatory Surgical Care Clinic

0830: Client arrives for surgical procedure. Alert and oriented $\times$ 4. Daughter at bedside and assigned to drive client home after procedure. Physician explains procedure and answers questions. Client signs surgical consent.

1000: Surgery complete. Client in recovery area. Antibiotic and steroid ointments instilled. VS: T 98.6°F (37°C), HR 62 beats/min and regular, RR 14 breaths/min, BP 124/42 mm Hg, SpO$_2$ 94% on RA. Client denies pain.

Telehealth Visit—1 Day After Surgery

0900: Client alert and oriented $\times$ 4. Reports taking acetaminophen for eye discomfort and then sleeping well during the night. Eyelid is very swollen and does not fully open without assistance. Sclera bloodshot. No drainage noted. Client reports vision is better but remains slightly blurry, and the eye feels scratchy, "like sand in the eye." Denies seeing flashes of light or floating shapes. Daughter is present and reports administering eyedrops as prescribed. VS: T 98.5°F (36.9°C), HR 60 beats/min and regular, RR 13 breaths/min, BP 142/50 mm Hg, SpO$_2$ 95% on RA. Denies eye pain, but reports a headache and nausea, which prevented the client from eating breakfast this morning.

The nurse reviews the most recent nurses' notes and is assisting to evaluate the client's current status after surgery. Select the **2** client findings that indicate a potential complication after surgery.

○ Headache and nausea
○ Bloodshot sclera
○ Scratchy, sandlike feeling in eye
○ Swollen eyelid
○ Took acetaminophen for pain
○ Vision remains blurry

Unfolding Case Study 17.2

Thinking Exercise 17.2.1

The nurse is screening a 68-year-old client at a community health fair.

History and Physical	Nurses' Notes	Orders	Diagnostic Results

1020: Alert and oriented × 4; accompanied by spouse. Client shares health history including type 2 diabetes mellitus, hypertension, and early chronic kidney disease. Generalized edema in bilateral lower extremities. Pulses palpable throughout. Client reports performing daily diabetic foot care, but states it is getting more difficult due to "aging eyes." Round open lesion, 0.5-inch (1.3-cm) diameter, noted on interior edge of left first toe. Wound bed pink with surrounding tissues pink and blanchable. Client and spouse both claim to have been unaware of the wound. Client reports experiencing "blurriness around the edges" and "random dark spots" in visual fields as well as "rainbow-colored circles" around bright lights. Sclera reddened, but no drainage present. Pupils light brown, equal, and reactive to light. Visual acuity testing demonstrates limited distance and near vision. Client reports a loss of 20 lb (9.1 kg) during the past 4 months; current BMI 28. VS: T 98.9°F (37.1°C), HR 78 beats/min and regular, RR 15 breaths/min, BP 128/50 mm Hg, SpO$_2$ 96% on RA. Denies pain, but reports occasional headaches with mild eye discomfort. FSBG 133 mg/dL (7.4 mmol/L).

The nurse reviews collected client data with the registered nurse. Select the **2** client findings that require **immediate** follow-up.

○ Blood glucose level
○ Blood pressure
○ Diabetic foot ulcer
○ Lower extremity edema
○ Visual disturbances
○ Weight loss

Thinking Exercise 17.2.2

The nurse is screening a 68-year-old client at a community health fair.

History and Physical	Nurses' Notes	Orders	Diagnostic Results

1020: Alert and oriented × 4; accompanied by spouse. Client shares health history including type 2 diabetes mellitus, hypertension, and early renal insufficiency. Generalized edema in bilateral lower extremities. Pulses palpable throughout. Client reports performing daily diabetic foot care, but states it is getting more difficult due to "aging eyes." Round open lesion, 0.5-inch (1.3-cm) diameter, noted on interior edge of left first toe. Wound bed pink with surrounding tissues pink and blanchable. Client and spouse both claim to have been unaware of the wound. Client reports experiencing "blurriness around the edges" and "random dark spots" in visual fields as well as "rainbow-colored circles" around bright lights. Sclera reddened, but no drainage present. Pupils light brown, equal, and reactive to light. Visual acuity testing demonstrates limited distance and near vision. Client reports a loss of 20 lb (9.1 kg) during the past 4 months; current BMI 28. VS: T 98.9°F (37.1°C), HR 78 beats/min and regular, RR 15 breaths/min, BP 128/50 mm Hg, SpO$_2$ 96% on RA. Denies pain, but reports occasional headaches with mild eye discomfort. FSBG: 133 mg/dL (7.4 mmol/L).

The nurse reviews the collected client data with the registered nurse. For each client finding, select whether the finding is consistent with the health conditions of cataract, glaucoma, or retinopathy. Some findings may be consistent with more than one condition.

CLIENT FINDINGS	CATARACT	GLAUCOMA	RETINOPATHY
Blurry vision			
Spots in visual field			
Vision-impairing ADLs			
Halos around lights			

Thinking Exercise 17.2.3

The nurse is caring for a 68-year-old client at an ambulatory care clinic.

History and Physical	Nurses' Notes	Orders	Diagnostic Results

Community Health Fair

1020: Alert and oriented × 4; accompanied by spouse. Client shares health history including type 2 diabetes mellitus, hypertension, and early renal insufficiency. Generalized edema in bilateral lower extremities. Pulses palpable throughout. Client reports performing daily diabetic foot care, but states it is getting more difficult due to "aging eyes." Round open lesion, 0.5-inch (1.3-cm) diameter, noted on interior edge of left first toe. Wound bed pink with surrounding tissues pink and blanchable. Client and spouse both claim to have been unaware of the wound. Client reports experiencing "blurriness around the edges" and "random dark spots" in visual fields as well as "rainbow-colored circles" around bright lights. Sclera reddened, but no drainage present. Pupils light brown, equal, and reactive to light. Visual acuity testing demonstrates limited distance and near vision. Client reports a loss of 20 lb (9.1 kg) during the past 4 months; current BMI 28. VS: T 98.9°F (37.1°C), HR 78 beats/min and regular, RR 15 breaths/min, BP 128/50 mm Hg, SpO$_2$ 96% on RA. Denies pain, but reports occasional headaches with mild eye discomfort. FSBG: 133 mg/dL (7.4 mmol/L).

1045: Instructed to have comprehensive eye exam and visit primary provider for follow-up.

2 Weeks Later at Ambulatory Care Clinic

0840: Alert and oriented × 4. Expresses anxiety related to ophthalmology diagnostic results.

History and Physical	Nurses' Notes	Orders	Diagnostic Results

Ophthalmoscopic examination:

- Lens clear
- Retina visualized; no edema or bleeding present
- Positive red reflex
- Shallow anterior chamber with cloudy aqueous humor
- Intraocular pressure (Normal 10–20 mm Hg)
  - OD—28 mm Hg
  - OS—24 mm Hg

The nurse reviews the collected client data with the registered nurse and reinforces teaching with the client. Complete the following sentence by selecting from the lists of options below.

The nurse recognizes that the client is *most likely* experiencing **1 [Select]** and will *prioritize* health teaching regarding **2 [Select]** to **3 [Select]** of visual sensory perception.

OPTIONS FOR 1	OPTIONS FOR 2	OPTIONS FOR 3
Cataract	Lifestyle changes	Promote restoration
Glaucoma	Medication therapy	Prevent further loss
Retinopathy	Surgical interventions	Reverse deterioration

Thinking Exercise 17.2.4—Pharmacology

The nurse is caring for a 68-year-old client at an ambulatory care clinic.

History and Physical	Nurses' Notes	Orders	Diagnostic Results

1020: Alert and oriented × 4 and accompanied by spouse. Client shares health history including type 2 diabetes mellitus, hypertension, and early renal insufficiency. Generalized edema in bilateral lower extremities. Pulses palpable throughout. Client reports performing daily diabetic foot care, but states it is getting more difficult due to "aging eyes." Round open lesion, 0.5-inch (1.3-cm) diameter, noted on interior edge of left first toe. Wound bed pink with surrounding tissues pink and blanchable. Client and spouse both claim to have been unaware of the wound. Client reports experiencing "blurriness around the edges" and "random dark spots" in visual fields as well as "rainbow-colored circles" around bright lights. Sclera reddened, but no drainage present. Pupils light brown, equal, and reactive to light. Visual acuity testing demonstrates limited distance and near vision. Client reports a loss of 20 lb (9.1 kg) during the past 4 months; current BMI 28. VS: T 98.9°F (37.1°C), HR 78 beats/min and regular, RR 15 breaths/min, BP 128/50 mm Hg, SpO$_2$ 96% on RA. Denies pain, but reports occasional headaches with mild eye discomfort. FSBG: 133 mg/dL (7.4 mmol/L).

1045: Instructed to have comprehensive eye exam and visit primary provider for follow-up.

2 Weeks Later at Ambulatory Care Clinic

0840: Alert and oriented × 4. Expresses anxiety related to ophthalmology diagnostic results.

0900: Client diagnosed with glaucoma. Physician at bedside to explain diagnostic results and treatment plan.

History and Physical	Nurses' Notes	Orders	Diagnostic Results

New prescriptions:
- Bimatoprost ophthalmic solution 0.03% one drop in each eye every night
- Timolol maleate ophthalmic solution 0.5% one drop in each eye twice daily

The nurse reviews the collected client data and contributes to the client's plan of care. Which statements would the nurse plan to include to reinforce health teaching? **Select all that apply.**

O "Avoid touching the drug container tip to any part of the eye."

O "Contact the provider if you experience tearing and mild burning immediately after instillation."

O "Hold medications if you experience severe eye pain and/or headache."

O "Perform good handwashing before administering eyedrops."

O "Place pressure on the corner of the eye near the nose immediately after instillation."

O "These drugs decrease intraocular pressure by limiting the production and increasing the drainage of fluid within the eye."

O "Wait 5 to 10 minutes between administration of each medication."

Thinking Exercise 17.2.5

The nurse is caring for a 68-year-old client during a follow-up telehealth visit.

History and Physical	Nurses' Notes	Orders	Diagnostic Results

Community Health Fair

1020: Alert and oriented × 4 and accompanied by spouse. Client shares health history including type 2 diabetes mellitus, hypertension, and early renal insufficiency. Generalized edema in bilateral lower extremities. Pulses palpable throughout. Client reports performing daily diabetic foot care, but states it is getting more difficult due to "aging eyes." Round open lesion, 0.5-inch (1.3-cm) diameter, noted on interior edge of left first toe. Wound bed pink with surrounding tissues pink and blanchable. Client and spouse both claim to have been unaware of the wound. Client reports experiencing "blurriness around the edges" and "random dark spots" in visual fields as well as "rainbow-colored circles" around bright lights. Sclera reddened, but no drainage present. Pupils light brown, equal, and reactive to light. Visual acuity testing demonstrates limited distance and near vision. Client reports a loss of 20 lb (9.1 kg) during the past 4 months; current BMI 28. VS: T 98.9°F (37.1°C), HR 78 beats/min and regular, BP 128/50 mm Hg, RR 15 breaths/min, SpO$_2$ 96% on RA. Denies pain, but reports occasional headaches with mild eye discomfort. FSBG: 133 mg/dL (7.4 mmol/L).

1045: Instructed to have comprehensive eye exam and visit primary provider for follow-up.

2 Weeks Later at Ambulatory Care Clinic

0840: Alert and oriented × 4. Expresses anxiety related to ophthalmology diagnostic results.

0900: Client diagnosed with glaucoma. Physician at bedside to explain diagnostic results and treatment plan.

72 Hours Later at Follow-up Telehealth Visit

0830: Client alert and oriented × 4. Verbalizes appropriate administration, dosage, and schedule for prescribed eyedrops. Reports feeling lightheaded when rising from the bed or sitting positions. VS: HR 56 beats/min, RR 14 breaths/min, BP 94/56 mm Hg, SpO$_2$ 95% on RA. Denies pain.

History and Physical	Nurses' Notes	Orders	Diagnostic Results

New prescriptions:
- Bimatoprost ophthalmic solution 0.03% one drop in each eye every night
- Timolol maleate ophthalmic solution 0.5% one drop in each eye twice daily

The nurse reviews the collected client data with the registered nurse. Select the **4 priority** actions that would be appropriate for the nurse to implement at this time.

O Check finger stick blood glucose level.
O Complete medication reconciliation.
O Encourage rising and changing positions slowly.
O Recommend discontinuation of bimatoprost eyedrops.
O Recommend discontinuation of timolol eyedrops.
O Reinforce teaching related to punctual occlusion.
O Suggest the client wear dark glasses.

Thinking Exercise 17.2.6

The nurse is caring for a 68-year-old client at an ambulatory care clinic.

History and Physical	Nurses' Notes	Orders	Diagnostic Results

Community Health Fair

1020: Alert and oriented × 4; accompanied by spouse. Client shares health history including type 2 diabetes mellitus, hypertension, and early renal insufficiency. Generalized edema in bilateral lower extremities. Pulses palpable throughout. Client reports performing daily diabetic foot care, but states it is getting more difficult due to "aging eyes." Round open lesion, 0.5-inch (1.3-cm) diameter, noted on interior edge of left first toe. Wound bed pink with surrounding tissues pink and blanchable. Client and spouse both claim to have been unaware of the wound. Client reports experiencing "blurriness around the edges" and "random dark spots" in visual fields as well as "rainbow-colored circles" around bright lights. Sclera reddened, but no drainage present. Pupils light brown, equal, and reactive to light. Visual acuity testing demonstrates limited distance and near vision. Client reports a loss of 20 lb (9.1 kg) during the past 4 months; current BMI 28. VS: T 98.9°F (37.1°C), HR 78 beats/min and regular, RR 15 breaths/min, BP 128/50 mm Hg, SpO$_2$ 96% on RA. Denies pain, but reports occasional headaches with mild eye discomfort. FSBG: 133 mg/dL (7.4 mmol/L).

2 Weeks Later at Ambulatory Care Clinic

0840: Alert and oriented × 4. Expresses anxiety related to ophthalmology diagnostic results.

0900: Client diagnosed with glaucoma. Physician at bedside to explain diagnostic results and treatment plan.

72 Hours Later at Follow-up Telehealth Visit

0830: Client alert and oriented × 4. Verbalizes appropriate administration, dosage, and schedule for prescribed eyedrops. Reports feeling lightheaded when rising from bed or sitting positions. VS: HR 56 beats/min, RR 14 breaths/min, BP 48/56 mm Hg, SpO$_2$ 95% on RA. Denies pain.

3 Weeks Later at Ambulatory Care Clinic

1010: Spouse accommodates client for follow-up visit. Client alert and oriented × 4. Spouse expresses concern regarding client's health including insomnia, decreased appetite, and darkening of eye color. Client states, "My spouse takes good care of me. There is nothing for me to do for myself." Client has difficulty self-administering eyedrops and allows spouse to instill drops. Spouse verbalizes appropriate technique and schedule for eyedrops. No lightheadedness or issues with orthostatic hypotension have occurred since spouse took over administration. The spouse also assists with foot care. Left foot toe wound, <0.2-inch (<0.5-cm) diameter, with surrounding tissues warm and pink. Cap refill <3 sec. Client checks blood glucose frequently. No episodes of hypoglycemia experienced. VS: T 98.7°F (37°C), HR 68 beats/min and regular, RR 17 breaths/min, BP 132/54 mm Hg, SpO$_2$ 96% on RA. Denies pain. Report no headaches or eye discomfort. FSBG: 128 mg/dL (7.1 mmol/L).

The clinic nurse reviews the most recent collected client data with the registered nurse. Complete the following sentence by selecting from the list of word choices below.

The client's condition has **_worsened_** as evidenced by **[Word Choice]** and **[Word Choice]**.

WORD CHOICES
Blood glucose level
Darkened eye color
Decreased appetite
Insomnia
Wound diameter

Stand-Alone Thinking Exercise 17.1

The nurse is caring for a 78-year-old client at a skilled nursing facility.

Nursing Flow Sheet	Nurses' Notes	Orders	Laboratory Results
Parameters	**Results: Today at 0910**	**Results: Yesterday at 2150**	**Results: Yesterday at 1410**
Heart rate	86 beats/min	75 beats/min	82 beats/min
Respiratory rate	16 breaths/min	14 breaths/min	15 breaths/min
Blood pressure	145/60 mm Hg	138/55 mm Hg	142/58 mm Hg
SpO_2	95% on RA	96% on RA	95% on RA
Pain	0/10	5/10 generalized pain	0/10

Nursing Flow Sheet	Nurses' Notes	Orders	Diagnostic Results

Yesterday

1410: Client admitted from hospital post-hemicolectomy and temporary colostomy placement. Alert and oriented × 4. Follows commands and moves all extremities equally. Wears bifocal glasses for near and far sight. Asks nurse to frequently repeat questions when obtaining health history, which includes colon cancer, osteoarthritis, and benign prostatic hyperplasia. Respirations equal and unlabored with no adventitious lung sounds auscultated. Heart tones regular. Skin warm and dry with palpable pulses throughout. Abdomen flat and soft with positive bowel sounds in all quadrants. Ostomy moist and red. Peristomal skin within normal limits. Appliance intact with small amount of brown, loose stool. Client ambulates to bathroom with stand by assist. Gait steady. Difficulty initiating urination; weak stream. Urine clear and yellow. Returns to the bed and positioned to comfort. When asked, "Are you cold?," Client responds, "Why would you ask me if I am old?" Situation clarified, and client provided with an additional blanket.

1900: Case management nurse at bedside to initiate discharge planning. Client alert and oriented × 4. Leans in, and tilts head to the right. Reports living alone in a single-story home. Has an adult child with several grandchildren who live within a few miles of home, but states does not see them very often due to "liking my privacy." Drives during daylight only, and uses a delivery service for most meals, stating, "I don't like to cook for myself, nor do I like eating in a noisy restaurant." Reports ability to perform activities of daily living independently. Denies needing assistance at home.

2150: Alert and oriented × 4. Sitting in a chair and watching a movie on television at full volume. States, "I like it loud. It feels like I am at a theater." Client decides to turn movie off and go to bed since the volume is bothering others on the unit. Assisted to bed. Acetaminophen administered orally for pain.

Today

0930: Alert and oriented × 4. Participates in health teaching regarding ostomy appliance. Adult child and two grandchildren at bedside. Client taught to measure and cut new wafer, remove used pouch, cleanse skin around ostomy, and place new pouch. Client frequently interrupts and talks over directions. Adult child becomes frustrated and states, "You never listen to anyone," and leaves with grandchildren prior to completing the health teaching. Health teaching completed, and client demonstrates procedure appropriately with minimal assistance opening packages and peeling back from ostomy wafer.

The nurse reviews the collected client data with the registered nurse. Complete the following sentence by selecting from the lists of options below.

The **priority** interventions for the client's care at this time would focus on improving the client's ability to **1 [Select]** and **2 [Select]** due to **3 [Select]**.

OPTIONS FOR 1	OPTIONS FOR 2	OPTIONS FOR 3
Communicate effectively	Adapt to changes in social interactions	Early-stage dementia
Manage pain	Complete colostomy and appliance care	Impaired hearing
Maintain independence	Perform activities of daily living	Osteoarthritis

Stand-Alone Thinking Exercise 17.2

A nurse is caring for a 60-year-old client in the emergency department (ED).

Progress Notes	Nurses' Notes	Orders	Diagnostic Results

1620: Client presents to ED after an extended episode of vertigo lasting several hours. Alert and oriented × 4. States, "I used to have occasional dizzy spells, but recently episodes occur every day, last longer, and are more severe." Reports experiencing intermittent tinnitus, diaphoresis, nausea, and vomiting with vertigo attacks. Client also reports difficulty hearing and a feeling of fullness in the ear. Inspection of external ear within normal limits; no foreign bodies, cerumen, or excessive hair noticed in external ear canal. Health history includes chronic obstructive pulmonary disease, hypertension, and 44–pack-year smoking history. Client confirms quitting smoking 3 years ago. Respirations equal and unlabored. Client denies recent sinus or upper respiratory infection and reports no allergies. VS: T 98.9°F (37.1°C), HR 77 beats/min and regular, RR 16 breaths/min, BP 148/72 mm Hg, SpO$_2$ 95% on RA. Denies pain.

1830: Diagnostic tests completed. Audiogram confirms loss of ability to hear low-frequency sounds. Audiometry reveals improved hearing after oral glycerol administration. Head CT negative.

The nurse reviews the collected client data with the registered nurse. Complete the diagram by selecting from the choices below to specify what potential condition the client is likely experiencing, **2** nursing actions that are appropriate to take, and **2** parameters the nurse would monitor to assess the client's progress.

Action to Take		Potential Condition		Parameter to Monitor
Action to Take				Parameter to Monitor

Actions to Take	Potential Conditions	Parameters to Monitor
Position the client to comfort in the bed with the call bell within reach	External otitis	Blood glucose level
Prepare the client for surgical intervention	Mastoiditis	Cranial nerves
Recommend vestibular rehabilitation consultation	Meniere disease	Hearing acuity
Reduce fluid intake to less than 1000 mL/day	Presbycusis	Nausea and vomiting
Teach the client to eat a high-calorie, low-fat diet		Stimuli that trigger attacks

Thinking Exercise 18.1.1

The nurse is caring for a 78-year-old client in the acute orthopedic unit.

History and Physical	Nurses' Notes	Orders	Laboratory Results

1520: Client returned from PACU following a left hip open reduction and internal fixation (ORIF) for a fracture caused by falling down the stairs at home. According to family, prior to surgery client lived alone, was independent in ADLs, and was alert and oriented × 4. Currently drowsy and disoriented. Unable to follow conversation. When performing the admission assessment, client began screaming and crying; tried to get out of bed. Family holding client's hand and offering reassurance to help calm client. IV lactated Ringer's solution infusing at 100 mL/h in right forearm. Lungs clear throughout; abdomen soft and round with diminished bowel sounds in all quadrants. Left hip surgical dressing dry and intact. Indwelling urinary catheter draining clear yellow urine. Pedal pulses 1+ and equal. Both feet cool and move equally. SCDs in place. VS: T 98°F (36.7°C), HR 80 beats/min and regular, RR 16 breaths/min, BP 115/62 mm Hg, SpO$_2$ 95% on 3 L/min O$_2$ via NC.

The nurse reviews the collected data with the registered nurse. Select the **2** client findings that require **immediate** follow-up.

○ Both feet cool
○ Pedal pulses 1+ and equal
○ Trying to get out of bed
○ Diminished bowel sounds
○ Screaming and crying

Thinking Exercise 18.1.2

The nurse is caring for a 78-year-old client in the acute orthopedic unit.

History and Physical	Nurses' Notes	Orders	Laboratory Results

1520: Client returned from PACU following a left hip open reduction and internal fixation (ORIF) for a fracture caused by falling down the stairs at home. According to family, prior to surgery client lived alone, was independent in ADLs, and was alert and oriented × 4. Currently drowsy and disoriented. Unable to follow conversation. When performing the admission assessment, client began screaming and crying; tried to get out of bed. Family holding client's hand and offering reassurance to help calm client. IV lactated Ringer's solution infusing at 100 mL/h in right forearm. Lungs clear throughout; abdomen soft and round with diminished bowel sounds in all quadrants. Left hip surgical dressing dry and intact. Indwelling urinary catheter draining clear yellow urine. Pedal pulses 1+ and equal. Both feet cool and move equally. SCDs in place. VS: T 98°F (36.7°C), HR 80 beats/min and regular, RR 16 breaths/min, BP 115/62 mm Hg, SpO$_2$ 95% on 3 L/min O$_2$ via NC.

The nurse reviews the collected client data with the registered nurse to determine the client's condition. Complete the following sentence by selecting from the list of word choices below.

Based on the collected data, the client *most likely* has [Word Choice].

WORD CHOICES
Hypoxia
Delirium
Dementia
Depression

Thinking Exercise 18.1.3

The nurse is caring for a 78-year-old client in the acute orthopedic unit.

History and Physical	Nurses' Notes	Orders	Laboratory Results

1520: Client returned from PACU following a left hip open reduction and internal fixation (ORIF) for a fracture caused by falling down the stairs at home. According to family, prior to surgery client lived alone, was independent in ADLs, and was alert and oriented × 4. Currently drowsy and disoriented. Unable to follow conversation. When performing the admission assessment, client began screaming and crying; tried to get out of bed. Family holding client's hand and offering reassurance to help calm client. IV lactated Ringer's solution infusing at 100 mL/h in right forearm. Lungs clear throughout; abdomen soft and round with diminished bowel sounds in all quadrants. Left hip surgical dressing dry and intact. Indwelling urinary catheter draining clear yellow urine. Pedal pulses 1+ and equal. Both feet cool and move equally. SCDs in place. VS: T 98°F (36.7°C), HR 80 beats/min and regular, RR 16 breaths/min, BP 115/62 mm Hg, SpO$_2$ 95% on 3 L/min O$_2$ via NC.

The nurse reviews the collected client data with the registered nurse. Complete the following sentence by selecting from the lists of options below.

The *priority* for the client's care at this time is to ensure **1 [Select]** because the client is **2 [Select]**.

OPTIONS FOR 1	OPTIONS FOR 2
Adequate oxygen	Hypoxic
Safety	At risk for falls
Gastrointestinal function	Experiencing diminished bowel sounds

Thinking Exercise 18.1.4

The nurse is caring for a 78-year-old client in the acute orthopedic unit.

History and Physical	Nurses' Notes	Orders	Laboratory Results

1520: Client returned from PACU following a left hip open reduction and internal fixation (ORIF) for a fracture caused by falling down the stairs at home. According to family, prior to surgery client lived alone, was independent in ADLs, and was alert and oriented × 4. Currently drowsy and disoriented. Unable to follow conversation. When performing the admission assessment, client began screaming and crying; tried to get out of bed. Family holding client's hand and offering reassurance to help calm client. IV lactated Ringer's solution infusing at 100 mL/h in right forearm. Lungs clear throughout; abdomen soft and round with diminished bowel sounds in all quadrants. Left hip surgical dressing dry and intact. Indwelling urinary catheter draining clear yellow urine. Pedal pulses 1+ and equal. Both feet cool and move equally. SCDs in place. VS: T 98°F (36.7°C), HR 80 beats/min and regular, RR 16 breaths/min, BP 115/62 mm Hg, SpO$_2$ 95% on 3 L/min O$_2$ via NC.

1640: Client very restless and moaning; picking at covers and IV dressing. Family states client grimaces when staff turns and repositions the client.

The nurse reviews the most recent nurses' notes and prepares to contribute to the client's plan of care. Select whether the following potential nursing actions are indicated or not indicated for the client at this time.

POTENTIAL NURSING ACTIONS	INDICATED	NOT INDICATED
Darken the client's room to prevent overstimulation.		
Ask the family to stay with the client as long as possible.		
Use soft restraints to prevent IV catheter dislodgement.		
Frequently reorient the client to reality.		
Administer medication for pain per agency protocol.		

Thinking Exercise 18.1.5

The nurse is caring for a 78-year-old client in the acute orthopedic unit.

History and Physical	Nurses' Notes	Orders	Laboratory Results

1520: Client returned from PACU following a left hip open reduction and internal fixation (ORIF) for a fracture caused by falling down the stairs at home. According to family, prior to surgery client lived alone, was independent in ADLs, and was alert and oriented × 4. Currently drowsy and disoriented. Unable to follow conversation. When performing the admission assessment, client began screaming and crying; tried to get out of bed. Family holding client's hand and offering reassurance to help calm client. IV lactated Ringer's solution infusing at 100 mL/h in right forearm. Lungs clear throughout; abdomen soft and round with diminished bowel sounds in all quadrants. Left hip surgical dressing dry and intact. Indwelling urinary catheter draining clear yellow urine. Pedal pulses 1+ and equal. Both feet cool and move equally. SCDs in place. VS: T 98°F (36.7°C), HR 80 beats/min and regular, RR 16 breaths/min, BP 115/62 mm Hg, SpO$_2$ 95% on 3 L/min O$_2$ via NC.

1640: Client very restless and moaning; picking at covers and IV dressing. Family states client grimaces when staff repositions the client.

1705: Acetaminophen and gabapentin administered for pain. Family states they plan to stay overnight to prevent client from getting out of bed unsupervised. Client tolerating sips of water and juice. Refused dinner tray; swiped hand and knocked tray from overbed table.

The nurse reviews the most recent collected client data with the registered nurse and contributes to the client's plan of care. Which of the following nursing actions would be appropriate to help improve the client's cognition? **Select all that apply.**

○ Use simple and short sentences when communicating with the client.
○ Ensure that the client wears glasses and hearing aids, if appropriate.
○ Monitor the client for hallucinations or delusions.
○ Ensure that staff members introduce themselves at each encounter with the client.
○ Request an order for medication for agitation and confusion.

Thinking Exercise 18.1.6

The nurse is caring for a 78-year-old client in the acute orthopedic unit. Highlight the client findings in the most recent nurses' note that indicate the client's condition may be **worsening**

History and Physical	Nurses' Notes	Orders	Laboratory Results

Admission to Orthopedic Unit

1520: Client returned from PACU following a left hip open reduction and internal fixation (ORIF) for a fracture caused by falling down the stairs at home. According to family, prior to surgery client lived alone, was independent in ADLs, and was alert and oriented × 4. Currently drowsy and disoriented. Unable to follow conversation. When performing the admission assessment, client began screaming and crying; tried to get out of bed. Family holding client's hand and offering reassurance to help calm client. IV lactated Ringer's solution infusing at 100 mL/h in right forearm. Lungs clear throughout; abdomen soft and round with diminished bowel sounds in all quadrants. Left hip surgical dressing dry and intact. Indwelling urinary catheter draining clear yellow urine. Pedal pulses 1+ and equal. Both feet cool and move equally. SCDs in place. VS: T 98°F (36.7°C), HR 80 beats/min and regular, RR 16 breaths/min, BP 115/62 mm Hg, SpO$_2$ 95% on 3 L/min O$_2$ via NC.

1640: Client very restless and moaning; picking at covers and IV dressing. Family states client grimaces when staff repositions the client.

1705: Acetaminophen and gabapentin administered for pain with assistance of family. Family states they plan to stay overnight to prevent client from getting out of bed unsupervised. Client tolerating sips of water and juice. Refused dinner tray; swiped hand and knocked tray off of overbed table.

4 Days Later

0915: Client alert and oriented × 4. Able to follow conversation. Scheduled to be discharged today to rehabilitation unit. No adventitious or abnormal breath sounds throughout, but breath sounds in left lower lung diminished when compared with right lung. Abdomen soft and round with active bowel sounds in all quadrants. Ambulates with walker and supervision to bathroom, but states feeling "a little short of breath" after that activity; voiding clear yellow urine without difficulty. Pedal pulses 1+ and equal. Both feet cool and move equally. VS: T 100.6°F (38.1°C), HR 90 beats/min and regular, RR 20 breaths/min, BP 122/70 mm Hg, SpO$_2$ 93% on RA.

Unfolding Case Study 18.2

Thinking Exercise 18.2.1

The nurse is caring for a 65-year-old client at the physician's office.

History and Physical	Progress Notes	Nurses' Notes	Laboratory Results

1120: Client scheduled for annual physical examination today. Has long-term history of low back pain, osteoarthritis, clinical depression, and hypertension. Is widowed, and works full-time as a hairstylist. Reports having memory lapses that have increased in the past few months. Client concerned about sometimes having difficulty remembering words or names. Feels more disorganized lately. Remains independent in ADLs. Denies feeling sad, having sleep disturbances, or having a change in appetite. Denies suicidal ideation. Has been on a low-carbohydrate diet for several months, and lost 15 lb (6.8 kg). Currently weighs 184 lb (83.5 kg); height 64 inches (162.6 cm); BMI 31.6. Lungs clear throughout; abdomen soft and round with active bowel sounds in all quadrants. Peripheral pulses 2+ and equal. All extremities move freely. Strong hand grip. No tremors or weakness. VS: T 98.2°F (36.8°C), HR 72 beats/min and regular, RR 18 breaths/min, BP 135/82 mm Hg, SpO$_2$ 96% on RA.

The nurse reviews the collected client data with the registered nurse. Select the **2** client findings that require **immediate** follow-up.

○ Obesity
○ Blood pressure
○ Memory lapses
○ Weight loss
○ Forgetting words
○ Peripheral pulses

Thinking Exercise 18.2.2

The nurse is caring for a 65-year-old client at the physician's office.

History and Physical	Progress Notes	Nurses' Notes	Laboratory Results

> **1120:** Client scheduled for annual physical examination today. Has long-term history of low back pain, osteoarthritis, clinical depression, and hypertension. Is widowed, and works full-time as a hairstylist. Reports having memory lapses that have increased in the past few months. Client concerned about sometimes having difficulty remembering words or names. Feels more disorganized lately. Remains independent in ADLs. Denies feeling sad, having sleep disturbances, or having a change in appetite. Denies suicidal ideation. Has been on a low-carbohydrate diet for several months, and lost 15 lb (6.8 kg). Currently weighs 184 lb (83.5 kg); height 64 inches (162.6 cm); BMI 31.6. Lungs clear throughout; abdomen soft and round with active bowel sounds in all quadrants. Peripheral pulses 2+ and equal. All extremities move freely. Strong hand grip. No tremors or weakness. VS: T 98.2°F (36.8°C), HR 72 beats/min and regular, RR 18 breaths/min, BP 135/82 mm Hg, SpO$_2$ 96% on RA.

The nurse reviews the collected client data with the registered nurse. Complete the following sentence by selecting from the list of word choices below.

Based on the assessment findings, the client *most likely* has **[Word Choice]**.

WORD CHOICES
Acute delirium
Clinical depression
Early-stage dementia

Thinking Exercise 18.2.3

The nurse is caring for a 65-year-old client at the physician's office.

History and Physical	Progress Notes	Nurses' Notes	Laboratory Results

> **1120:** Client scheduled for annual physical examination today. Has long-term history of low back pain, osteoarthritis, clinical depression, and hypertension. Is widowed, and works full-time as a hairstylist. Reports having memory lapses that have increased in the past few months. Client concerned about sometimes having difficulty remembering words or names. Feels more disorganized lately. Remains independent in ADLs. Denies feeling sad, having sleep disturbances, or having a change in appetite. Denies suicidal ideation. Has been on a low-carbohydrate diet for several months, and lost 15 lb (6.8 kg). Currently weighs 184 lb (83.5 kg); height 64 inches (162.6 cm); BMI 31.6. Lungs clear throughout; abdomen soft and round with active bowel sounds in all quadrants. Peripheral pulses 2+ and equal. All extremities move freely. Strong hand grip. No tremors or weakness. VS: T 98.2°F (36.8°C), HR 72 beats/min and regular, RR 18 breaths/min, BP 135/82 mm Hg, SpO$_2$ 96% on RA.

The nurse reviews the collected client data with the registered nurse to identify the priority for client care. Complete the following sentence by selecting from the lists of options below.

The *priority* for the client's care at this time is **1 [Select]** to **2 [Select]**.

OPTIONS FOR 1	OPTIONS FOR 2
Preventing falls	Keep the client safe
Improving cognition	Prevent illness
Ensuring adequate nutrition	Help the client maintain employment

Thinking Exercise 18.2.4

The nurse is caring for a 65-year-old client at the physician's office.

History and Physical	Progress Notes	Nurses' Notes	Laboratory Results

1120: Client scheduled for annual physical examination today. Has long-term history of low back pain, osteoarthritis, clinical depression, and hypertension. Is widowed, and works full-time as a hairstylist. Reports having memory lapses that have increased in the past few months. Client concerned about sometimes having difficulty remembering words or names. Feels more disorganized lately. Remains independent in ADLs. Denies feeling sad, having sleep disturbances, or having a change in appetite. Denies suicidal ideation. Has been on a low-carbohydrate diet for several months, and lost 15 lb (6.8 kg). Currently weighs 184 lb (83.5 kg); height 64 inches (162.6 cm); BMI 31.6. Lungs clear throughout; abdomen soft and round with active bowel sounds in all quadrants. Peripheral pulses 2+ and equal. All extremities move freely. Strong hand grip. No tremors or weakness. VS: T 98.2°F (36.8°C), HR 72 beats/min and regular, RR 18 breaths/min, BP 135/82 mm Hg, SpO$_2$ 96% on RA.

The nurse collaborates with the registered nurse and contributes to the client's plan of care. Select whether the following potential nursing actions are indicated or not indicated for the client at this time.

POTENTIAL NURSING ACTIONS	INDICATED	NOT INDICATED
Use a reliable mental status tool to assess cognition.		
Reinforce teaching about cholinesterase inhibitors.		
Prepare the client for admission to an inpatient mental health unit or facility.		
Refer the client to a neuropsychologist or other qualified mental health care professional.		

Thinking Exercise 18.2.5—Pharmacology

The nurse is caring for a 65-year-old client at the physician's office.

History and Physical	Progress Notes	Nurses' Notes	Laboratory Results

1120: Client scheduled for annual physical examination today. Has long-term history of low back pain, osteoarthritis, clinical depression, and hypertension. Is widowed, and works full-time as a hairstylist. Reports having memory lapses that have increased in the past few months. Client concerned about sometimes having difficulty remembering words or names. Feels more disorganized lately. Remains independent in ADLs. Denies feeling sad, having sleep disturbances, or having a change in appetite. Denies suicidal ideation. Has been on a low-carbohydrate diet for several months, and lost 15 lb (6.8 kg). Currently weighs 184 lb (83.5 kg); height 64 inches (162.6 cm); BMI 31.6. Lungs clear throughout; abdomen soft and round with active bowel sounds in all quadrants. Peripheral pulses 2+ and equal. All extremities move freely. Strong hand grip. No tremors or weakness. VS: T 98.2°F (36.8°C), HR 72 beats/min and regular, RR 18 breaths/min, BP 135/82 mm Hg, SpO$_2$ 96% on RA.

1215: Referral to neuropsychologist. Prescription for donepezil to begin immediately.

The nurse reviews the collected client data with the registered nurse and reinforces teaching with the client about taking donepezil. Which of the following statements would be appropriate for the nurse to include in the health teaching? **Select all that apply.**

○ "Take this drug on an empty stomach first thing each morning."
○ "Do not take nonsteroidal anti-inflammatory drugs (NSAIDs) while taking donepezil."
○ "Report a pulse below 60 beats/min to the provider as soon as possible."
○ "This drug should help improve your memory, but it may not return to your usual level."
○ "Donepezil can only be taken during the early stage of Alzheimer dementia."

Thinking Exercise 18.2.6

The nurse is caring for a 65-year-old client at the physician's office. Highlight the client findings in the 2-month follow-up visit nurses' note that indicate the client is **improving**.

History and Physical	Progress Notes	Nurses' Notes	Laboratory Results

1120: Client scheduled for annual physical examination today. Has long-term history of low back pain, osteoarthritis, clinical depression, and hypertension. Is widowed, and works full-time as a hairstylist. Reports having memory lapses that have increased in the past few months. Client concerned about sometimes having difficulty remembering words or names. Feels more disorganized lately. Remains independent in ADLs. Denies feeling sad, having sleep disturbances, or having a change in appetite. Denies suicidal ideation. Has been on a low-carbohydrate diet for several months, and lost 15 lb (6.8 kg). Currently weighs 184 lb (83.5 kg); height 64 inches (162.6 cm); BMI 31.6. Lungs clear throughout; abdomen soft and round with active bowel sounds in all quadrants. Peripheral pulses 2+ and equal. All extremities move freely. Strong hand grip. No tremors or weakness. VS: T 98.2°F (36.8°C), HR 72 beats/min and regular, RR 18 breaths/min, BP 135/82 mm Hg, SpO$_2$ 96% on RA.

1215: Referral to neuropsychologist. Prescription for donepezil to begin immediately.

2-Month Follow-Up Visit

0830: Follow-up visit after client diagnosed with early-stage dementia, probably Alzheimer disease, and starting donepezil 2 months ago. Client states feeling that memory is better with fewer lapses and beginning to feel more organized at work and home. Fewer problems with remembering words and names since starting drug therapy. Continuing diet, but has lost only 3 lb (1.4 kg) during the past 2 months. Is frustrated that weight loss has slowed, and considering joining an established weight-loss program.

Stand-Alone Thinking Exercise 18.1

The nurse is caring for an 83-year-old client at the urgent care center.

History and Physical	Nurses' Notes	Orders	Laboratory Results

1520: Client visit to urgent care center for injured right wrist. Client alert and oriented × 4; reports being dependent in most ADLs for 3 years. Lives with daughter and son-in-law, who brought client to urgent care center. Family noticed swelling and bruising on right wrist when assisting client with a shower. Client appears clean and well-groomed. Pupils equal and reactive. Lungs clear throughout; no adventitious or abnormal breath sounds. Abdomen soft and round with active bowel sounds in all quadrants. Old bruises on back and buttocks in varying stages of healing. Peripheral pulses present bilaterally; cap refill >3 sec. Can move all extremities, but right arm more painful when moved. VS: T 98°F (36.7°C), HR 68 beats/min and irregular, RR 18 breaths/min, BP 146/84 mm Hg, SpO$_2$ 93% on RA. Has gained 3 lb (1.36 kg) since last visit to center 6 months ago for respiratory infection.

The nurse reviews the collected client data with the registered nurse. Complete the diagram by selecting from the choices below to specify what potential condition the client is likely experiencing, **2** nursing actions that are appropriate to take, and **2** parameters the nurse would monitor to assess the client's progress.

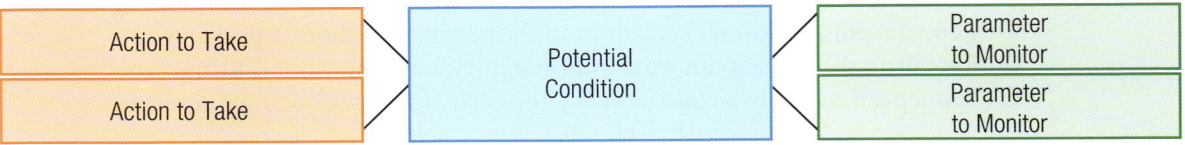

Actions to Take	Potential Conditions	Parameters to Monitor
Interview the client without the family present	Abuse	Pain level
Obtain consent for emergent surgery	Neglect	Blood pressure
Recommend community and caregiver services	Anxiety	New bruising or other new physical injury
Consult with respiratory therapy for SpO$_2$	Depression	SpO$_2$
Contact Adult Protective Services to report the client's condition		Body weight

Stand-Alone Thinking Exercise 18.2

The nurse is caring for a 69-year-old client in the emergency department (ED).

History and Physical	Nurses' Notes	Orders	Laboratory Results

1445: Client presents to ED for acute confusion and altered gait that began 2 days ago. According to spouse, client's medical history includes hypertension, GERD, generalized anxiety disorder, myocardial infarction, and irritable bowel syndrome. Has also had episodes of acute clinical depression, spousal abuse, and one suicide attempt last year. Does not smoke tobacco or cannabis, and does not use illicit drugs. However, the client has been a heavy alcohol drinker for 30 years, and drinking has increased during the past 5 years since the client's brother died. Client currently alert but totally disoriented. Unable to follow conversation. Pupils not equal with sluggish reaction to light. Lungs clear throughout; no adventitious or abnormal breath sounds. Abdomen soft and round with active bowel sounds in all quadrants. Peripheral pulses present bilaterally; cap refill <3 sec. Can move all extremities and has strong grip. VS: T 98.6°F (37°C), HR 72 beats/min and irregular, RR 18 breaths/min, BP 154/90 mm Hg, SpO$_2$ 97% on RA.

The nurse reviews the collected client data with the registered nurse. Complete the diagram by selecting from the choices below to specify what potential condition the client is likely experiencing, **2** nursing actions that are appropriate to take, and **2** parameters the nurse would monitor to assess the client's progress.

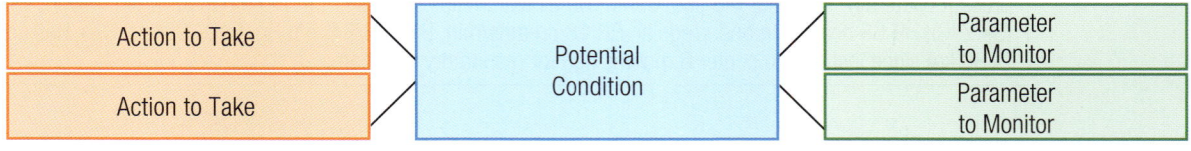

Actions to Take	Potential Conditions	Parameters to Monitor
Admit the client to an acute care hospital unit	Dementia	Cognitive status
Consult with the social worker or psychologist	Acute delirium	Blood pressure
Reorient the client frequently	Korsakoff syndrome	Alcohol intake
Begin administration of IV thiamine	Wernicke encephalopathy	Gait
Screen the client for clinical depression		Suicidal ideation or attempt

Stand-Alone Thinking Exercise 18.3

The nurse is caring for a 70-year-old client at the ambulatory mental health clinic.

History and Physical	Nurses' Notes	Orders	Laboratory Results

1130: Client presents to clinic for follow-up of long-term schizophrenia, which has been treated with drug therapy for many years. Client lives with family, who accompanied client today for visit; is independent in basic ADLs. Currently alert and oriented × 4. Client appears clean and well-groomed. Family states that client has had no hallucinations or delusions for several decades and that client's thinking is more organized. However, the client has difficulty making or maintaining friendships and has problems with processing new information or tasks. Client recently wanted to volunteer for a local food bank but could not comprehend the scope of the volunteer role based on the training and orientation. Has difficulty with memory and maintaining attention, which adds to the inability to volunteer, have a job, or develop social relationships. Is frustrated that mental health condition continues to interfere with quality of life.

The nurse reviews the collected client data with the registered nurse. Complete the diagram by selecting from the choices below to specify what type of symptoms the client is likely experiencing, **2** nursing actions that are appropriate to take, and **2** parameters the nurse would monitor to assess the client's progress.

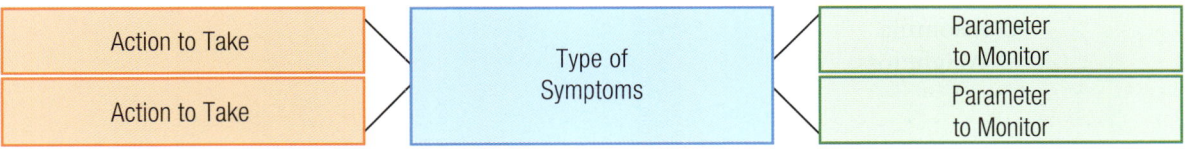

Actions to Take	Type of Symptoms	Parameters to Monitor
Prepare for admission to an acute mental health unit or facility	Positive symptoms	Presence of hallucinations or delusions
Request a change in the client's drug regimen	Negative symptoms	Increase in daily social interactions
Refer the client for social skills training	Cognitive symptoms	Substance use
Screen the client for suicidal ideation	Affective symptoms	Response to social situations
Encourage participation in community groups		Suicidal ideation or attempt

Unfolding Case Study 19.1

Thinking Exercise 19.1.1

The nurse is caring for a 66-year-old client in the acute rehabilitation unit.

History and Physical	Nurses' Notes	Orders	Laboratory Results

0845: Client very concerned about planned discharge to home with spouse later this week after being at acute rehabilitation facility for 4 weeks following a right cerebral ischemic stroke. Reports having trouble sleeping most nights and a declining appetite in the past 2 weeks resulting in an unintended 5-lb (2.3-kg) weight loss. Is worried about the future and retirement. Client is owner of a construction company, but currently has left-sided weakness and slurred speech. Walks independently with a walker, but has occasional dizziness. Feels sad most mornings, but is "moody" during the day. Spouse visiting later today.

1310: Spouse expresses concern about client's mental and emotional state. Client reports sadness and anger because of inability to provide for the family. Client has had several anger outbursts when spouse visits.

The nurse reviews the collected client data with the registered nurse. Select the **3** client findings that require **immediate** follow-up.

○ Left-sided weakness
○ Slurred speech
○ Occasional dizziness
○ Feeling sad and "moody"
○ Insomnia
○ Weight loss

Thinking Exercise 19.1.2

The nurse is caring for a 66-year-old client in the acute rehabilitation unit.

History and Physical	Nurses' Notes	Orders	Laboratory Results

0845: Client very concerned about planned discharge to home with spouse later this week after being at acute rehabilitation facility for 4 weeks following a right cerebral ischemic stroke. Reports having trouble sleeping most nights and a declining appetite in the past 2 weeks resulting in an unintended 5-lb (2.3-kg) weight loss. Is worried about the future and retirement. Client is owner of a construction company, but currently has left-sided weakness and slurred speech. Walks independently with a walker, but has occasional dizziness. Feels sad most mornings, but is "moody" during the day. Spouse visiting later today.

1310: Spouse expresses concern about client's mental and emotional state. Client reports sadness and anger because of inability to provide for the family. Client has had several anger outbursts when spouse visits.

The nurse reviews the collected client data with the registered nurse. Complete the following sentence by selecting from the lists of options below.

The client is likely experiencing secondary **1 [Select]** as a result of the client's **2 [Select]**.

OPTIONS FOR 1	OPTIONS FOR 2
Anxiety	Stroke
Depression	Weight loss
Bipolar disorder	Possible retirement

Thinking Exercise 19.1.3

The nurse is caring for a 66-year-old client in the acute rehabilitation unit.

History and Physical	Nurses' Notes	Orders	Laboratory Results

0845: Client very concerned about planned discharge to home with spouse later this week after being at acute rehabilitation facility for 4 weeks following a right cerebral ischemic stroke. Reports having trouble sleeping most nights and a declining appetite in the past 2 weeks resulting in an unintended 5-lb (2.3-kg) weight loss. Is worried about the future and retirement. Client is owner of a construction company, but currently has left-sided weakness and slurred speech. Walks independently with a walker, but has occasional dizziness. Feels sad most mornings, but is "moody" during the day. Spouse visiting later today.

1310: Spouse expresses concern about client's mental and emotional state. Client reports sadness and anger because of inability to provide for the family. Client has had several anger outbursts when spouse visits.

The nurse reviews the collected client data with the registered nurse to determine the priority for client care. Complete the following sentence by selecting from the list of word choices below.

The *priority* for the client's care at this time is to assess for **[Word Choice]**.

WORD CHOICES
Falls risk
Nutritional risk
Suicide risk

Thinking Exercise 19.1.4

The nurse is caring for a 66-year-old client in the acute rehabilitation unit.

History and Physical	Nurses' Notes	Orders	Laboratory Results

0845: Client very concerned about planned discharge to home with spouse later this week after being at acute rehabilitation facility for 4 weeks following a right cerebral ischemic stroke. Reports having trouble sleeping most nights and a declining appetite in the past 2 weeks resulting in an unintended 5-lb (2.3-kg) weight loss. Is worried about the future and retirement. Client is owner of a construction company, but currently has left-sided weakness and slurred speech. Walks independently with a walker, but has occasional dizziness. Feels sad most mornings, but is "moody" during the day. Spouse visiting later today.
1310: Spouse expresses concern about client's mental and emotional state. Client reports sadness and anger because of inability to provide for the family. Client has had several anger outbursts when spouse visits.

The nurse collaborates with the registered nurse and contributes to the client's plan of care. Select whether the following potential nursing actions are indicated or not indicated for the client at this time.

POTENTIAL NURSING ACTIONS	INDICATED	NOT INDICATED
Consult with the social worker for evaluation.		
Assess the client for suicide risk.		
Frequently reorient the client to reality.		
Request drug therapy for the client's condition.		
Remind the client and spouse that the client is independent in ambulation.		

Thinking Exercise 19.1.5—Pharmacology

The nurse is caring for a 66-year-old client in the acute rehabilitation unit.

History and Physical	Nurses' Notes	Orders	Laboratory Results

0845: Client very concerned about planned discharge to home with spouse later this week after being at acute rehabilitation facility for 4 weeks following a right cerebral ischemic stroke. Reports having trouble sleeping most nights and a declining appetite in the past 2 weeks resulting in an unintended 5-lb (2.3-kg) weight loss. Is worried about the future and retirement. Client is owner of a construction company, but currently has left-sided weakness and slurred speech. Walks independently with a walker, but has occasional dizziness. Feels sad most mornings, but is "moody" during the day. Spouse visiting later today.
1310: Spouse expresses concern about client's mental and emotional state. Client reports sadness and anger because of inability to provide for the family. Client has had several anger outbursts when spouse visits.
1625: Social worker in to visit spouse and family. Suicide risk assessment conducted; currently not at risk.
1800: Antidepressant drug therapy initiated. Health teaching about drug provided to both client and spouse.

The nurse reviews the collected client data with the registered nurse and reinforces health teaching about venlafaxine with the client. Which of the following statements related to this medication would be appropriate to include in the teaching? **Select all that apply.**

○ "This drug will be started at a low dose to determine the best dosage for you."
○ "When you feel better, you can discontinue this drug whenever you want."
○ "This drug is taken orally several times a day with food to help prevent nausea."
○ "While taking this drug, you won't need to see your counselor or therapist."
○ "Monitor your blood pressure and pulse, and contact your provider if they significantly increase."

Thinking Exercise 19.1.6

The nurse is collecting data for a 66-year-old client scheduled for a follow-up visit with the provider following discharge from an acute rehabilitation unit with a diagnosis of stroke with secondary depression. Highlight the client findings in the 0945 follow-up nurses' note that indicate the client's condition is **improving**.

History and Physical	Nurses' Notes	Orders	Laboratory Results

Acute Rehabilitation Unit

0845: Client very concerned about planned discharge to home with spouse later this week after being at acute rehabilitation facility for 4 weeks following a right cerebral ischemic stroke. Reports having trouble sleeping most nights and a declining appetite in the past 2 weeks resulting in an unintended 5-lb (2.3-kg) weight loss. Is worried about the future and retirement. Client is owner of a construction company, but currently has left-sided weakness and slurred speech. Walks independently with a walker, but has occasional dizziness. Feels sad most mornings, but is "moody" during the day. Spouse visiting later today.

1310: Spouse expresses concern about client's mental and emotional state. Client reports sadness and anger because of inability to provide for the family. Client has had several anger outbursts when spouse visits.

1625: Social worker in to visit spouse and family. Suicide risk assessment conducted; currently not at risk.

1800: Antidepressant drug therapy initiated. Health teaching about drug provided to both client and spouse.

Follow-up Provider Visit—4 Weeks After Discharge

0945: Client and spouse at provider's office for follow-up visit after discharge from acute rehabilitation facility. Client reports feeling less sad and less moody since being on venlafaxine. Had several episodes of nausea when first starting medication, but has had no nausea for the past 2 weeks. Spouse reports that client has worked in office 2 to 3 days a week, and construction business is "doing well." Client not able to drive yet, but has been using a cane independently for ambulation for the past week. Attends psychotherapy at least once a week.

Unfolding Case Study 19.2

Thinking Exercise 19.2.1

The nurse is caring for an 81-year-old client in the emergency department (ED). Highlight the client findings that require **immediate** follow-up.

History and Physical	Nurses' Notes	Orders	Laboratory Results

2145: Client admitted to ED via ambulance after family found client on floor. Was unresponsive at home when paramedics arrived. Family reported client may have taken a large number of oxycodone tablets because prescription bottle is empty. Increased level of consciousness noted after naloxone administration. On ED admission, client drowsy but oriented × 4. When asked about what happened, client started crying and repeated several times, "I don't want to be a burden to anyone. Please just let me die." Family explained that client has recently experienced worsening chronic pain from metastatic bone cancer. Client frequently expresses hopelessness and wonders if cancer treatment should continue because current "last resort" cancer drug causes extreme nausea and fatigue.

Thinking Exercise 19.2.2

The nurse is caring for an 81-year-old client in the emergency department.

History and Physical	Nurses' Notes	Orders	Laboratory Results

2145: Client admitted to ED via ambulance after family found client on floor. Was unresponsive at home when paramedics arrived. Family reported client may have taken a large number of oxycodone tablets because prescription bottle is empty. Increased level of consciousness noted after naloxone administration. On ED admission, client drowsy but oriented × 4. When asked about what happened, client started crying and repeated several times, "I don't want to be a burden to anyone. Please just let me die." Family explained that client has recently experienced worsening chronic pain from metastatic bone cancer. Client frequently expresses hopelessness and wonders if cancer treatment should continue because current "last resort" cancer drug causes extreme nausea and fatigue.

The nurse reviews the collected client data with the registered nurse. Complete the following sentence by selecting from the lists of options below.

The client is at highest risk for **1 [Select]** because the client **2 [Select]**.

OPTIONS FOR 1	OPTIONS FOR 2
Falling	Is an older adult
Suicide	Has opioid use disorder
Cognitive decline	Had a suicide attempt

Thinking Exercise 19.2.3

The nurse is caring for an 81-year-old client in the emergency department.

History and Physical	Nurses' Notes	Orders	Laboratory Results

2145: Client admitted to ED via ambulance after family found client on floor. Was unresponsive at home when paramedics arrived. Family reported client may have taken a large number of oxycodone tablets because prescription bottle is empty. Increased level of consciousness noted after naloxone administration. On ED admission, client drowsy but oriented × 4. When asked about what happened, client started crying and repeated several times, "I don't want to be a burden to anyone. Please just let me die." Family explained that client has recently experienced worsening chronic pain from metastatic bone cancer. Client frequently expresses hopelessness and wonders if cancer treatment should continue because current "last resort" cancer drug causes extreme nausea and fatigue.

The nurse reviews the collected client data with the registered nurse to determine the priority need for the client. Complete the following sentence by selecting from the list of word choices below.

The *priority* need for the client at this time is to **[Word Choice]**.

WORD CHOICES
Prevent cognitive impairment
Maintain safety
Manage pain

Thinking Exercise 19.2.4

The nurse is caring for an 81-year-old client in the emergency department.

History and Physical	Nurses' Notes	Orders	Laboratory Results

2145: Client admitted to ED via ambulance after family found client on floor. Was unresponsive at home when paramedics arrived. Family reported client may have taken a large number of oxycodone tablets because prescription bottle is empty. Increased level of consciousness noted after naloxone administration. On ED admission, client drowsy but oriented × 4. When asked about what happened, client started crying and repeated several times, "I don't want to be a burden to anyone. Just let me die." Family explained that client has recently experienced worsening chronic pain from metastatic bone cancer. Client frequently expresses hopelessness and wonders if cancer treatment should continue because current "last resort" cancer drug causes extreme nausea and fatigue.

2305: Consult with social worker. Family reports that client lives alone and has previously refused to move in with family for assistance as needed. Psychiatric consult requested.

The nurse collaborates with the registered nurse and contributes to the client's plan of care. Which of the following nursing actions would be appropriate as part of the client's plan of care? **Select all that apply.**

O Identify the client's risk for another suicide attempt.
O Determine the level of suicide precautions that are needed for the client at this time.
O Identify the client's support system and protective factors.
O Collaborate with the family to plan for possible client discharge to home with them.
O Prepare the family for possible admission to an inpatient acute psychiatric unit.
O Request psychoactive drug therapy to sedate the client to prevent another suicide attempt.

Thinking Exercise 19.2.5

The nurse is caring for an 81-year-old client in the emergency department.

History and Physical	Nurses' Notes	Orders	Laboratory Results

2145: Client admitted to ED via ambulance after family found client on floor. Was unresponsive at home when paramedics arrived. Family reported client may have taken a large number of oxycodone tablets because prescription bottle is empty. Increased level of consciousness noted after naloxone administration. On ED admission, client drowsy but oriented × 4. When asked about what happened, client started crying and repeated several times, "I don't want to be a burden to anyone. Just let me die." Family explained that client has recently experienced worsening chronic pain from metastatic bone cancer. Client frequently expresses hopelessness and wonders if cancer treatment should continue because current "last resort" cancer drug causes extreme nausea and fatigue.

2305: Consult with social worker. Family reports that client lives alone and has previously refused to move in with family for assistance as needed. Psychiatric consult requested.

2430: Client more alert and oriented × 4. After long discussion with family and social worker, client agreed to be managed at home and stay with family for observation and support.

The nurse assists with implementation of the client's discharge plan. Select the **5** actions that would be appropriate for the nurse to implement at this time.

O Teach the client and family about prescribed antidepressant drug therapy.
O Teach the family about behaviors associated with worsening depression or suicide risk.
O Schedule a follow-up visit for the client in 6 to 8 weeks.
O Provide the client and family with crisis or emergency hotline information.
O Identify social supports for client and the need to contact them.
O Teach the client and family the importance of professional counseling as soon as possible.

Thinking Exercise 19.2.6

The nurse is interviewing an 81-year-old client who attempted suicide last week.

History and Physical	Nurses' Notes	Orders	Laboratory Results

Emergency Department

2145: Client admitted to ED via ambulance after family found client on floor. Was unresponsive at home when paramedics arrived. Family reported client may have taken a large number of oxycodone tablets because prescription bottle is empty. Increased level of consciousness noted after naloxone administration. On ED admission, client drowsy but oriented × 4. When asked about what happened, client started crying and repeated several times, "I don't want to be a burden to anyone. Just let me die." Family explained that client has recently experienced worsening chronic pain from metastatic bone cancer. Client frequently expresses hopelessness and wonders if cancer treatment should continue because current "last resort" cancer drug causes extreme nausea and fatigue.

2305: Consult with social worker. Family reports that client lives alone and has previously refused to move in with family for assistance as needed. Psychiatric consult requested.

2430: Client more alert and oriented × 4. After long discussion with family and social worker, client agreed to be managed at home and stay with family for observation and support.

Psychiatric Follow-up Visit—1 Week Later

1515: Client alert and oriented × 4. Seems quiet, but states feeling less hopeless when compared with the previous week. Has decided to discontinue cancer treatment, and plans to move in with family on a permanent basis. Has started using fentanyl patches, which have lessened the client's pain. Taking antidepressant as prescribed, and meeting with licensed counselor twice a week. Has not had suicidal ideation since being discharged from ED. Appetite has been poor this past week; client sleeping more than usual. States that pain patch causes sleepiness, which should improve over time.

The nurse collaborates with the registered nurse to evaluate client outcomes. For each current client finding documented in the follow-up visit note, select whether the client has improved or not improved.

CLIENT FINDINGS	IMPROVED	NOT IMPROVED
Mood and affect		
Appetite		
Pain control		
Suicidal ideation		

Stand-Alone Thinking Exercise 19.1

The nurse is caring for a 65-year-old client in the emergency department (ED).

History and Physical	Nurses' Notes	Orders	Laboratory Results

1520: Client taken to ED by family with new-onset acute confusion, abdominal pain, diarrhea, diaphoresis, and mood change. Lying in a fetal position guarding abdomen; restless and "picking" at covers. Family reports client's medical history includes major depressive disorder, osteoarthritis, and hypothyroidism. Drugs include levothyroxine, ibuprofen, acetaminophen, and paroxetine. Client alert and oriented × 1 (person only). Pupils equal and reactive. Lungs clear throughout; no adventitious or abnormal breath sounds. Skin very warm and moist. Abdomen soft and round with hyperactive bowel sounds in all four quadrants. Peripheral pulses present bilaterally; cap refill < 3 sec. Can move all extremities. VS: T 102.8°F (39.3°C), HR 122 beats/min, RR 20 breaths/min, BP 176/104 mm Hg, SpO$_2$ 94% on RA.

The nurse reviews the collected client data with the registered nurse. Complete the diagram by selecting from the choices below to specify what potential condition the client is likely experiencing, **2** nursing actions that are appropriate to take, and **2** parameters the nurse would monitor to assess the client's progress.

Action to Take		
Action to Take	Potential Condition	Parameter to Monitor
		Parameter to Monitor

Actions to Take	Potential Conditions	Parameters to Monitor
Place the client on a cooling blanket	Dementia	SpO$_2$
Discontinue paroxetine immediately	Thyroid storm	Vital signs
Perform a mental status assessment	Gastroenteritis	Quality of stools
Begin continuous cardiac monitoring	Serotonin syndrome	Pain level
Draw labs for thyroid-stimulating hormone (TSH) level		Seizure activity

Stand-Alone Thinking Exercise 19.2

The nurse is caring for a 74-year-old client at the ambulatory care mental health clinic.

History and Physical	Nurses' Notes	Progress Notes	Laboratory Results

0815: Client visit for follow-up after medication change for mania associated with bipolar disorder. Client has been taking lithium for many years, but changed to valproic acid 2 months ago. Client alert and oriented × 4. States feeling better with less mania. Sleep has improved since being on new drug, but has been feeling more fatigued lately. Labs drawn last week for comparison with initial labs prior to valproic acid prescription.

History and Physical	Nurses' Notes	Orders	Laboratory Results
Serum Laboratory Test and Reference Range	**Results Last Week**	**Results 2 Months Ago**	
Red blood cell count (4.2–5.4 × 10^6/μL [4.2–5.4 × 10^{12}/L])	4.2 × 10^6/μL (4.2 × 10^{12}/L)	4.3 × 10^6/μL (4.3 × 10^{12}/L)	
Hemoglobin (14–18 g/dL)	13.8 g/dL	14.2 g/dL	
Hematocrit (37%–47% [0.37–0.47 volume fraction])	38% (0.38 volume fraction)	39% (0.39 volume fraction)	
Platelet count (150,000–400,000/mm^3 [150–400 × 10^9/L])	126,000/mm^3 (126 × 10^9/L)	235,000/mm^3 (235 × 10^9/L)	
Alkaline phosphatase (ALP) (30–120 U/L)	247 U/L	103 U/L	
Alanine aminotransferase (ALT) (4–36 U/L)	75 U/L	40 U/L	
Aspartate aminotransferase (AST) (0–35 U/L)	89 U/L	10 U/L	
Total bilirubin (0.3–1 mg/dL [5.13–17.1 μmol/L])	3.2 mg/dL (54.72 μmol/L)	0.3 mg/dL (5.13 μmol/L)	

The nurse reviews the collected client data with the registered nurse. Complete the following sentence by selecting from the list of word choices below.

Based on the collected data, the client is most likely experiencing [**Word Choice**].

WORD CHOICES
Depression
Hepatitis
Drug toxicity
Bleeding

Commonly Occurring Client Conditions Affecting Peripartum Care

Unfolding Case Study 20.1

Thinking Exercise 20.1.1

The nurse is caring for a 32-year-old client at an ambulatory obstetric clinic. The nurse reviews the collected client data with the registered nurse. Highlight the client findings that require **immediate** follow-up.

History and Physical	Nurses' Notes	Orders	Laboratory Results

1010: Client presents at 19 weeks' gestation for initial prenatal visit. Obstetric history: G4P3. Medical history: asthma, depression, and atopic dermatitis. Alert and oriented × 4. Reports feeling stressed, stating, "I didn't plan on getting pregnant again. I can't afford another child." Respirations equal and unlabored with mild expiratory wheezing noted on auscultation. Skin warm with dry, inflamed areas noted on bilateral hands and right lower arm. Bowel sounds present in all quadrants. Denies nausea, vomiting, excessive thirst, and dysuria. Reports urinary frequency. Fetal heart tones auscultated in lower abdomen with client in semi-Fowler's position. Fetal HR 116 beats/min. Fundal height 19 cm. Client reports signs of positive quickening. Client works 32 hours weekly as a retail clerk, lives with spouse and three children, and denies extended family or support systems outside of the home. VS: T 98.6°F (37°C), HR 84 beats/min and regular, RR 16 breaths/min, BP 124/74 mm Hg, SpO$_2$ 96% on RA.

Thinking Exercise 20.1.2

The nurse is caring for a 32-year-old client at an ambulatory obstetric clinic.

History and Physical	Nurses' Notes	Orders	Laboratory Results

1010: Client presents at 19 weeks' gestation for initial prenatal visit. Obstetric history: G4P3. Medical history: asthma, depression, and atopic dermatitis. Alert and oriented × 4. Reports feeling stressed, stating, "I didn't plan on getting pregnant again. I can't afford another child." Respirations equal and unlabored with mild expiratory wheezing noted on auscultation. Skin warm with dry, inflamed areas noted on bilateral hands and right lower arm. Bowel sounds present in all quadrants. Denies nausea, vomiting, excessive thirst, and dysuria. Reports urinary frequency. Fetal heart tones auscultated in lower abdomen with client in semi-Fowler's position. Fetal HR 116 beats/min. Fundal height 19 cm. Client reports signs of positive quickening. Client works 32 hours weekly as a retail clerk, lives with spouse and three children, and denies extended family or support systems outside of the home. VS: T 98.6°F (37°C), HR 84 beats/min and regular, RR 16 breaths/min, BP 124/74 mm Hg, SpO$_2$ 96% on RA.

1030: Client shares feelings of being overwhelmed with daily activities and care of children, who are 6, 8, and 9 years of age. States, "I live for my beautiful children, and all of my energy is spent caring for them. I have nothing left at the end of the day and frequently go to bed without eating or bathing because I am so tired." Client reports spouse works overtime hours to provide for financial needs, and family eats takeout for most meals. Denies taking daily prenatal vitamins. Current medications include budesonide, albuterol, sertraline, and over-the-counter topical corticosteroids.

The nurse reviews the collected client data with the registered nurse. Complete the following sentence by selecting from the lists of options below.

The nurse recognizes that the client is *most likely* experiencing **1 [Select]** as manifested by **2 [Select]** and **3 [Select]**.

OPTIONS FOR 1	OPTIONS FOR 2	OPTIONS FOR 3
Domestic violence	Delayed prenatal care	Blood glucose level
Self-care deficit	Eating takeout for most meals	Not bathing or eating
Suicidal ideation	Statement of "living for children"	Spouse working overtime

Thinking Exercise 20.1.3

The nurse is caring for a 32-year-old client at an ambulatory obstetric clinic.

History and Physical	Nurses' Notes	Orders	Laboratory Results

1010: Client presents at 19 weeks' gestation for initial prenatal visit. Obstetric history: G4P3. Medical history: asthma, depression, and atopic dermatitis. Alert and oriented × 4. Reports feeling stressed, stating, "I didn't plan on getting pregnant again. I can't afford another child." Respirations equal and unlabored with mild expiratory wheezing noted on auscultation. Skin warm with dry, inflamed areas noted on bilateral hands and right lower arm. Bowel sounds present in all quadrants. Denies nausea, vomiting, excessive thirst, and dysuria. Reports urinary frequency. Fetal heart tones auscultated in lower abdomen with client in semi-Fowler's position. Fetal HR 116 beats/min. Fundal height 19 cm. Client reports signs of positive quickening. Client works 32 hours weekly as a retail clerk, lives with spouse and three children, and denies extended family or support systems outside of the home. VS: T 98.6°F (37°C), HR 84 beats/min and regular, RR 16 breaths/min, BP 124/74 mm Hg, SpO$_2$ 96% on RA.

1030: Client shares feelings of being overwhelmed with daily activities and care of children, who are 6, 8, and 9 years of age. States, "I live for my beautiful children, and all of my energy is spent caring for them. I have nothing left at the end of the day and frequently go to bed without eating or bathing because I am so tired." Client reports spouse works overtime hours to provide for financial needs, and family eats takeout for most meals. Denies taking daily prenatal vitamins. Current medications include budesonide, albuterol, sertraline, and over-the-counter topical corticosteroids.

The nurse reviews the client findings with the registered nurse. Complete the following sentence by selecting from the list of word choices below.

The *priority* for the client's care at this time is **[Word Choice]** and **[Word Choice]** to address the physical, emotional, and psychological changes that occur with pregnancy.

WORD CHOICES
Anticipatory guidance
Antidepressants
Community resources
Transvaginal ultrasonography
Vocational rehabilitation

Thinking Exercise 20.1.4

The nurse is caring for a 32-year-old client at an ambulatory obstetric clinic.

History and Physical	Nurses' Notes	Orders	Laboratory Results

1010: Client presents at 19 weeks' gestation for initial prenatal visit. Obstetric history: G4P3. Medical history: asthma, depression, and atopic dermatitis. Alert and oriented $\times$ 4. Reports feeling stressed, stating, "I didn't plan on getting pregnant again. I can't afford another child." Respirations equal and unlabored with mild expiratory wheezing noted on auscultation. Skin warm with dry, inflamed areas noted on bilateral hands and right lower arm. Bowel sounds present in all quadrants. Denies nausea, vomiting, excessive thirst, and dysuria. Reports urinary frequency. Fetal heart tones auscultated in lower abdomen with client in semi-Fowler's position. Fetal HR 116 beats/min. Fundal height 19 cm. Client reports signs of positive quickening. Client works 32 hours weekly as a retail clerk, lives with spouse and three children, and denies extended family or support systems outside of the home. VS: T 98.6°F (37°C), HR 84 beats/min and regular, RR 16 breaths/min, BP 124/74 mm Hg, SpO$_2$ 96% on RA.

1030: Client shares feelings of being overwhelmed with daily activities and care of children, who are 6, 8, and 9 years of age. States, "I live for my beautiful children, and all of my energy is spent caring for them. I have nothing left at the end of the day and frequently go to bed without eating or bathing because I am so tired." Client reports spouse works overtime hours to provide for financial needs, and family eats takeout for most meals. Denies taking daily prenatal vitamins. Current medications include budesonide, albuterol, sertraline, and over-the-counter topical corticosteroids.

The nurse reviews the collected client data and reinforces teaching with the client. Which of the following statements would the nurse include in the anticipatory guidance to promote a healthy pregnancy? **Select all that apply.**

○ "Ask your doctor to discontinue sertraline during your pregnancy."
○ "Drink plenty of water between meals, but limit your fluid intake with meals."
○ "Keep a 24-hour intake diary to assess your current eating patterns."
○ "Participate in 30 minutes of mild to moderate exercise 5 days per week."
○ "Schedule an appointment to receive the varicella vaccination."
○ "Take a prenatal vitamin every day."
○ "Treat yourself to a spa day, and soak in a hot tub or sit in a sauna to relax."
○ "Use a food guide to plan two to three large daily meals that include iron and protein-rich foods."

Thinking Exercise 20.1.5

The nurse is caring for a 32-year-old client at an ambulatory obstetric clinic.

History and Physical	Nurses' Notes	Orders	Laboratory Results

1010: Client presents at 19 weeks' gestation for initial prenatal visit. Obstetric history: G4P3. Medical history: asthma, depression, and atopic dermatitis. Alert and oriented $\times$ 4. Reports feeling stressed, stating, "I didn't plan on getting pregnant again. I can't afford another child." Respirations equal and unlabored with mild expiratory wheezing noted on auscultation. Skin warm with dry, inflamed areas noted on bilateral hands and right lower arm. Bowel sounds present in all quadrants. Denies nausea, vomiting, excessive thirst, and dysuria. Reports urinary frequency. Fetal heart tones auscultated in lower abdomen with client in semi-Fowler's position. Fetal HR 116 beats/min. Fundal height 19 cm. Client reports signs of positive quickening. Client works 32 hours weekly as a retail clerk, lives with spouse and three children, and denies extended family or support systems outside of the home. VS: T 98.6°F (37°C), HR 84 beats/min and regular, RR 16 breaths/min, BP 124/74 mm Hg, SpO$_2$ 96% on RA.

1030: Client shares feelings of being overwhelmed with daily activities and care of children, who are 6, 8, and 9 years of age. States, "I live for my beautiful children, and all of my energy is spent caring for them. I have nothing left at the end of the day and frequently go to bed without eating or bathing because I am so tired." Client reports spouse works overtime hours to provide for financial needs, and family eats takeout for most meals. Denies taking daily prenatal vitamins. Current medications include budesonide, albuterol, sertraline, and over-the-counter topical corticosteroids.

4 Weeks Later

0900: Client presents at 23 weeks' gestation for follow-up prenatal visit. Alert and oriented $\times$ 4. Lying supine on the exam table. Denies feelings of depression or suicidal ideation. States meeting with a registered dietitian nutritionist, and has started eating small nutrient-packed snacks throughout the day. While obtaining vital signs, client reports sudden onset of nausea and dizziness. Skin pale and clammy. Respirations labored. VS: T 98.9°F (37.2°C), HR 104 beats/min and regular, BP 96/34 mm Hg, RR 18 breaths/min, SpO$_2$ 95% on RA.

The nurse reviews the collected client data with the registered nurse. Select the **2 priority** actions that would be appropriate for the nurse to implement at this time.

O Administer supplemental oxygen.
O Elevate the client's legs above the heart.
O Massage the client's lower back.
O Monitor vital signs until symptoms subside.
O Obtain a finger stick blood glucose (FSBG) level.
O Provide an emesis bag to collect any vomitus.
O Reposition the client to the lateral side-lying position.

Thinking Exercise 20.1.6

The nurse is caring for a 32-year-old client at an ambulatory obstetric clinic.

History and Physical	Nurses' Notes	Orders	Laboratory Results

1010: Client presents at 19 weeks' gestation for initial prenatal visit. Obstetric history: G4P3. Medical history: asthma, depression, and atopic dermatitis. Alert and oriented × 4. Reports feeling stressed, stating, "I didn't plan on getting pregnant again. I can't afford another child." Respirations equal and unlabored with mild expiratory wheezing noted on auscultation. Skin warm with dry, inflamed areas noted on bilateral hands and right lower arm. Bowel sounds present in all quadrants. Denies nausea, vomiting, excessive thirst, and dysuria. Reports urinary frequency. Fetal heart tones auscultated in lower abdomen with client in semi-Fowler's position. Fetal HR 116 beats/min. Fundal height 19 cm. Client reports signs of positive quickening. Client works 32 hours weekly as a retail clerk, lives with spouse and three children, and denies extended family or support systems outside of the home. VS: T 98.6°F (37°C), HR 84 beats/min and regular, RR 16 breaths/min, BP 124/74 mm Hg, SpO$_2$ 96% on RA.

1030: Client shares feelings of being overwhelmed with daily activities and care of children, who are 6, 8, and 9 years of age. States, "I live for my beautiful children, and all of my energy is spent caring for them. I have nothing left at the end of the day and frequently go to bed without eating or bathing because I am so tired." Client reports spouse works overtime hours to provide for financial needs, and family eats takeout for most meals. Denies taking daily prenatal vitamins. Current medications include budesonide, albuterol, sertraline, and over-the-counter topical corticosteroids.

4 Weeks Later

0900: Client presents at 23 weeks' gestation for follow-up prenatal visit. Alert and oriented × 4. Lying supine on the exam table. Denies feelings of depression or suicidal ideation. States meeting with a registered dietitian nutritionist and has started eating small nutrient-packed snacks throughout the day. While obtaining vital signs, the client reports sudden onset of nausea and dizziness. Skin pale and clammy. Respirations labored. VS: T 98.9°F (37.2°C), HR 104 beats/min and regular, RR 18 breaths/min, BP 96/34 mm Hg, SpO$_2$ 95% on RA.

0930: Client sitting upright. Denies dizziness or nausea. Skin warm and dry. Respirations equal and unlabored with mild expiratory wheezing noted on auscultation. Abdomen round. Fetal HR 126 beats/min. Fundal height 21 cm. Client states, "I'm still concerned about how we will afford this child, but I have arranged for my children to attend an after-school program so I have time to care for myself and ensure that the baby is healthy." VS: HR 89 beats/min and regular, RR 14 breaths/min, BP 128/78 mm Hg, SpO$_2$ 96% on RA.

The nurse collaborates with the registered nurse to determine if the client's plan of care has been effective. For each current client finding, select whether the client's condition has improved or not improved.

CLIENT FINDINGS	IMPROVED	NOT IMPROVED
Arranged time for self-care		
Collaborated with a registered dietitian nutritionist		
Expresses financial concerns		
Eats small, nutrient-dense meals and snacks		
Fundal height 21 cm		

Unfolding Case Study 20.2

Thinking Exercise 20.2.1

The nurse is caring for a 24-year-old postpartum client in a mother-newborn care unit.

History and Physical	Nurses' Notes	Orders	Laboratory Results

1010: G2P2 client delivered a viable male at 38 weeks' gestation via repeat cesarean section for breech presentation. Apgar scores 6, 8, and 9 at 1, 5, and 10 minutes, respectively. Weight 6 lb, 4 ounces (2.8 kg). Cord blood sent for typing. Estimated blood loss 1200 mL.

1130: Transferred to mother-newborn care unit. Client alert and oriented × 4. VS: T 99.3°F (37.3°C), HR 89 beats/min and regular, BP 112/65 mm Hg, RR 14 breaths/min, SpO$_2$ 96% on RA. Partner at bedside and exhibiting appropriate bonding with newborn.

1600: Client alert and oriented × 4. Cradling newborn with skin-to-skin contact. Respirations equal and unlabored with no adventitious breath sounds. Skin warm and dry with 1+ pitting edema in bilateral lower extremities. Abdomen round with bowel sounds present in all quadrants. Positive flatus and tenderness noted with light palpation. Abdominal incision well-approximated with staples intact. Erythema, swelling, and moderate amount of serosanguineous drainage present. Fundus soft at umbilicus. Moderate amount of lochia rubra noted; no clots. Client uses toilet with standby assist due to reports of light-headedness. Voids 775 mL dark-yellow urine; no burning or difficulty urinating. VS: T 100.6°F (38.1°C), HR 112 beats/min and regular, BP 94/52 mm Hg, RR 16 breaths/min, SpO$_2$ 95% on RA.

The nurse reviews the collected client data with the registered nurse. Select the **3** client findings that require **immediate** follow-up.

○ Apgar scores
○ Blood pressure
○ Erythematous and swollen incision
○ Heart rate
○ Soft fundus at umbilicus
○ Temperature

Thinking Exercise 20.2.2

The nurse is caring for a 24-year-old postpartum client in a mother-newborn care unit.

History and Physical	Nurses' Notes	Orders	Laboratory Results

1010: G3P2 client delivered a viable male at 38 weeks' gestation via repeat cesarean section for breech presentation. Apgar scores 6, 8, and 9 at 1, 5, and 10 minutes, respectively. Weight 6 lb, 4 ounces (2.8 kg). Cord blood sent for typing. Estimated blood loss 1200 mL.

1130: Transferred to mother-newborn care unit. Client alert and oriented × 4. VS: T 99.3°F (37.3°C), HR 89 beats/min and regular, RR 14 breaths/min, BP 112/62 mm Hg, SpO$_2$ 96% on RA. Partner at bedside and exhibiting appropriate bonding with newborn.

1600: Client alert and oriented × 4. Cradling newborn with skin-to-skin contact. Respirations equal and unlabored with no adventitious breath sounds. Skin warm and dry with 1+ pitting edema in bilateral lower extremities. Abdomen round with bowel sounds present in all quadrants. Positive flatus and tenderness noted with light palpation. Abdominal incision well-approximated with staples intact. Erythema, swelling, and moderate amount of serosanguineous drainage present. Fundus soft at umbilicus. Moderate amount of lochia rubra noted; no clots. Client uses toilet with standby assist due to reports of light-headedness. Voids 775 mL dark-yellow urine; no burning or difficulty urinating. VS: T 100.6°F (38.1°C), HR 112 beats/min and regular, RR 16 breaths/min, BP 94/69 mm Hg, SpO$_2$ 95% on RA.

The nurse reviews the collected client data with the registered nurse. For each client finding, select whether the finding is consistent with the health conditions of postpartum infection or postpartum hemorrhage. Some findings may be consistent with more than one condition.

CLIENT FINDINGS	POSTPARTUM INFECTION	POSTPARTUM HEMORRHAGE
Red and swollen incision		
Fever		
Narrowing pulse pressure		
Soft fundus		
Tachycardia		

Thinking Exercise 20.2.3

The nurse is caring for a 24-year-old postpartum client in a mother-newborn care unit.

History and Physical	Nurses' Notes	Orders	Laboratory Results

1010: G3P2 client delivered a viable male at 38 weeks' gestation via repeat cesarean section for breech presentation. Apgar scores 6, 8, and 9 at 1, 5, and 10 minutes, respectively. Weight 6 lb, 4 ounces (2.8 kg). Cord blood sent for typing. Estimated blood loss 1200 mL.

1130: Transferred to mother-newborn care unit. Client alert and oriented × 4. VS: T 99.3°F (37.3°C), HR 89 beats/min and regular, BP 112/62 mm Hg, RR 14 breaths/min, SpO$_2$ 96% on RA. Partner at bedside and exhibiting appropriate bonding with newborn.

1600: Client alert and oriented × 4. Cradling newborn with skin-to-skin contact. Respirations equal and unlabored with no adventitious breath sounds. Skin warm and dry with 1+ pitting edema in bilateral lower extremities. Abdomen round with bowel sounds present in all quadrants. Positive flatus and tenderness noted with light palpation. Abdominal incision well-approximated with staples intact. Erythema, swelling, and moderate amount of serosanguineous drainage present. Fundus soft at umbilicus. Moderate amount of lochia rubra noted; no clots. Client uses toilet with standby assist due to reports of light-headedness. Voids 775 mL dark-yellow urine; no burning or difficulty urinating. VS: T 100.6°F (38.1°C), HR 112 beats/min and regular, RR 16 breaths/min, BP 94/69 mm Hg, SpO$_2$ 95% on RA.

The nurse reviews the collected client data with the registered nurse. Complete the following sentence by selecting from the lists of options below.

The nurse recognizes that the client is *most likely* experiencing postpartum **1 [Select]** resulting from **2 [Select]**.

OPTIONS FOR 1	OPTIONS FOR 2
Depression	Cesarean section
Hemorrhage	Uterine atony
Infection	Vaginal hematoma

Thinking Exercise 20.2.4

The nurse is caring for a 24-year-old postpartum client in a mother-newborn care unit.

History and Physical	Nurses' Notes	Orders	Laboratory Results

1010: G3P2 client delivered a viable male at 38 weeks' gestation via repeat cesarean section for breech presentation. Apgar scores 6, 8, and 9 at 1, 5, and 10 minutes, respectively. Weight 6 lb, 4 ounces (2.8 kg). Cord blood sent for typing. Estimated blood loss 1200 mL.

1130: Transferred to mother-newborn care unit. Client alert and oriented × 4. VS: T 99.3°F (37.3°C), HR 89 beats/min and regular, BP 112/62 mm Hg, RR 14 breaths/min, SpO$_2$ 96% on RA. Partner at bedside and exhibiting appropriate bonding with newborn.

1600: Client alert and oriented × 4. Cradling newborn with skin-to-skin contact. Respirations equal and unlabored with no adventitious breath sounds. Skin warm and dry with 1+ pitting edema in bilateral lower extremities. Abdomen round with bowel sounds present in all quadrants. Positive flatus and tenderness noted with light palpation. Abdominal incision well-approximated with staples intact. Erythema, swelling, and moderate amount of serosanguineous drainage present. Fundus soft at umbilicus. Moderate amount of lochia rubra noted; no clots. Client uses toilet with standby assist due to reports of light-headedness. Voids 775 mL dark-yellow urine; no burning or difficulty urinating. VS: T 100.6°F (38.1°C), HR 112 beats/min and regular, RR 16 breaths/min, BP 94/69 mm Hg, SpO$_2$ 95% on RA.

The nurse collaborates with the registered nurse to determine the client's priority for care. Complete the following sentence by selecting from the list of word choices below.

Based on the client's condition, the most appropriate potential nursing actions are [**Word Choice**] and [**Word Choice**].

WORD CHOICES
Applying a perineal ice pack
Emptying the bladder
Maintaining bedrest
Massaging the uterus
Promoting breast-feeding

Thinking Exercise 20.2.5

The nurse is caring for a 24-year-old postpartum client in a mother-newborn care unit.

History and Physical	Nurses' Notes	Orders	Laboratory Results

1010: G3P2 client delivered a viable male at 38 weeks' gestation via repeat cesarean section for breech presentation. Apgar scores 6, 8, and 9 at 1, 5, and 10 minutes, respectively. Weight 6 lb, 4 ounces (2.8 kg). Cord blood sent for typing. Estimated blood loss 1200 mL.

1130: Transferred to mother-newborn care unit. Client alert and oriented × 4. VS: T 99.3°F (37.3°C), HR 89 beats/min and regular, RR 14 breaths/min, BP 112/62 mm Hg, SpO$_2$ 96% on RA. Partner at bedside and exhibiting appropriate bonding with newborn.

1600: Client alert and oriented × 4. Cradling newborn with skin-to-skin contact. Respirations equal and unlabored with no adventitious breath sounds. Skin warm and dry with 1+ pitting edema in bilateral lower extremities. Abdomen round with bowel sounds present in all quadrants. Positive flatus and tenderness noted with light palpation. Abdominal incision well-approximated with staples intact. Erythema, swelling, and moderate amount of serosanguineous drainage present. Fundus soft at umbilicus. Moderate amount of lochia rubra noted; no clots. Client uses toilet with standby assist due to reports of light-headedness. Voids 775 mL dark-yellow urine; no burning or difficulty urinating. VS: T 100.6°F (38.1°C), HR 112 beats/min and regular, RR 16 breaths/min, BP 94/69 mm Hg, SpO$_2$ 95% on RA.

1620: Fundal massage performed until midline and firm. Client and newborn positioned for breast-feeding. Lactation consultant at bedside.

2030: Client alert and oriented × 4. Newborn sleeping in bassinet at bedside. Abdomen soft and nontender. Incision erythematous but well-approximated with staples intact. No drainage or swelling noted. Fundus midline and firm. Denies light-headedness. Ambulates to the toilet, and voids clear, yellow urine without difficulty. Light amount of lochia rubra with several small clots noted on perineal pad. Reviewed plan for discharge home in the morning.

The nurse assists the registered nurse with discharge planning and health teaching. Which of the following statements would the nurse include when reinforcing health teaching with the client? **Select all that apply.**

○ "Breast-feeding will delay the return of ovulation, which will provide reliable contraception for several months."

○ "Contact your provider if you notice a foul smell from your vaginal discharge or experience increasing pain."

○ "It is common to feel a huge range of emotions for several months after delivery including feelings of not enjoying your life."

○ "Postpartum bleeding will continue for several weeks and become increasingly lighter in color and flow."

○ "Shower daily, and continue perineal care until the flow of bleeding stops."

○ "Take it easy for the next few weeks. Start with low-impact activities, and progress slowly."

Thinking Exercise 20.2.6

The nurse is caring for a 24-year-old postpartum client at an ambulatory obstetric clinic. The nurse reviews the most recent nurses' notes with the registered nurse to evaluate client outcomes. Highlight the client findings that indicate the client is *effectively* transitioning to becoming a new parent.

History and Physical	Nurses' Notes	Orders	Laboratory Results

Mother-Newborn Unit

1010: G3P2 client delivered a viable male at 38 weeks' gestation via repeat cesarean section for breech presentation. Apgar scores 6, 8, and 9 at 1, 5, and 10 minutes, respectively. Weight 6 lb, 4 ounces (2.8 kg). Cord blood sent for typing. Estimated blood loss 1200 mL.

1130: Transferred to mother-newborn care unit. Client alert and oriented × 4. VS: T 99.3°F (37.3°C), HR 89 beats/min and regular, RR 14 breaths/min, BP 112/62 mm Hg, SpO$_2$ 96% on RA. Partner at bedside and exhibiting appropriate bonding with newborn.

1600: Client alert and oriented × 4. Cradling newborn with skin-to-skin contact. Respirations equal and unlabored with no adventitious breath sounds. Skin warm and dry with 1+ pitting edema in bilateral lower extremities. Abdomen round with bowel sounds present in all quadrants. Positive flatus and tenderness noted with light palpation. Abdominal incision well-approximated with staples intact. Erythema, swelling, and moderate amount of serosanguineous drainage present. Fundus soft at umbilicus. Moderate amount of lochia rubra noted; no clots. Client uses toilet with standby assist due to reports of light-headedness. Voids 775 mL dark-yellow urine; no burning or difficulty urinating. VS: T 100.6°F (38.1°C), HR 112 beats/min and regular, RR 16 breaths/min, BP 94/69 mm Hg, SpO$_2$ 95% on RA.

1620: Fundal massage performed until midline and firm. Client and newborn positioned for breast-feeding. Lactation consultant at bedside.

2030: Client alert and oriented × 4. Newborn sleeping in bassinet at bedside. Abdomen soft and nontender. Incision erythematous but well-approximated with staples intact. No drainage or swelling noted. Fundus midline and firm. Denies light-headedness. Ambulates to the toilet, and voids clear, yellow urine without difficulty. Light amount of lochia rubra with several small clots noted on perineal pad. Reviewed plan for discharge home in the morning.

Ambulatory Clinic—3 Days After Hospital Discharge

1210: Client arrives for postpartum follow-up appointment and staple removal for lower abdominal incision. Alert and oriented × 4. Reports breast-feeding every 2–3 hours including during the night and taking naps during the day when the newborn sleeps. Eats small snacks throughout the day, but has not felt hungry enough to eat a full meal. Abdomen soft, round, and nontender. Denies having a bowel movement since discharge. Lower abdominal incision well approximated. No redness or drainage noted. VS: T 98.6°F (37°C), HR 75 beats/min and regular, RR 14 breaths/min, BP 124/66 mm Hg, SpO$_2$ 97% on RA. Denies pain. Reports a scheduled appointment with the lactation clinic this afternoon and with the obstetrician in 10 days.

Stand-Alone Thinking Exercise 20.1

The nurse is caring for a client who presents at 26 weeks' gestation for follow-up prenatal visit.

History and Physical	Nurses' Notes	Orders	Laboratory Results
Glucose Tolerance Fasting glucose	Test #1 77 mg/dL	Test #2 82 mg/dL	Reference Range 70–110 mg/dL (3.9–6.1 mmol/L)
1 hour after glucose	198 mg/dL	206 mg/dL	<180 mg/dL (10 mmol/L)
2 hours after glucose	159 mg/dL	162 mg/dL	<155 mg/dL (8.6 mmol/L)
3 hours after glucose	147 mg/dL	150 mg/dL	<140 mg/dL (7.8 mmol/L)

History and Physical	Nurses' Notes	Orders	Laboratory Results

0900: Alert and oriented × 4. Obstetric history: G3P2. Skin warm and dry. Respirations equal and unlabored with no adventitious breath sounds noted. Abdomen round. Client reports frequent fetal movement. Fetal HR 144 beats/min. Client's spouse is present and expresses concern that the client is experiencing frequent episodes of dizziness, chills, and clamminess. VS: 98.2°F (36.8°C), HR 76 beats/min and regular, BP 112/68 mm Hg, RR 14 breaths/min, SpO$_2$ 98% on RA. Denies pain. FSBG 102 mg/dL (5.7 mmol/L). (Normal range 70–110 mg/dL [3.9–6.1 mmol/L].) Physician at bedside reviewing results from glucose tolerance tests.

The nurse reviews the client findings with the registered nurse. Which of the following orders would the nurse anticipate for this client? **Select all that apply.**

○ Consult with a registered dietitian nutritionist.
○ Provide a balanced diet divided into three meals and three to four snacks daily.
○ Administer glargine insulin 5 units subcutaneously twice a day.
○ Administer glucose tablets or another oral fast-acting sugar as needed.
○ Instruct the client on proper methods for obtaining and monitoring FSBG levels.
○ Administer regular insulin subcutaneously per sliding scale before meals.
○ Teach the client about signs and symptoms of hyperglycemia and hypoglycemia.

Stand-Alone Thinking Exercise 20.2—Pharmacology

The nurse is caring for a 21-year-old client in the emergency department (ED).

Progress Notes	Nurses' Notes	Orders	Diagnostic Results

0230: Client brought to ED by spouse due to persistent headache accompanied by nausea, vomiting, and dizziness. Client is alert and oriented × 4. Reports headache began early in the morning and continues to worsen despite acetaminophen administration. Client is pregnant at 25 weeks' gestation with first child and states current nausea and vomiting are different from morning sickness previously experienced. Spouse shares that the obstetrician expressed concern regarding the client's blood pressure during their prenatal visit last week. Respirations equal and unlabored with no adventitious breath sounds. Skin warm and dry. 2+ pitting edema present in bilateral lower extremities. Abdomen soft and round. Client reports frequent fetal movement. Fetal HR 138 beats/min. Fundal height 25 cm. Client ambulates with assistance to the toilet. Reports dizziness and "seeing stars." Voids 250 mL clear, yellow urine; sample collected for point-of-care testing. No vaginal discharge or bleeding present. Denies chest pain or shortness of breath. Reports headache pain rated 8/10.

0245: Point-of-care dipstick results demonstrate protein in urine.

Nursing Flow Sheet	Nurses' Notes	Orders	Laboratory Results	
Parameters	Results: 16 Weeks' Gestation	Results: 20 Weeks' Gestation	Results: 24 Weeks' Gestation	Results: 25 Weeks' Gestation (Current)
Temperature	98.8°F (37.1°C)	98.6°F (37°C)	98.4°F (36.8°C)	98°F (36.7°C)
Heart rate	76 beats/min	88 beats/min	85 beats/min	100 beats/min
Respiratory rate	13 breaths/min	14 breaths/min	14 breaths/min	22 breaths/min
Blood pressure	126/67 mm Hg	138/80 mm Hg	162/110 mm Hg	188/115 mm Hg
SpO$_2$	99% on RA	98% on RA	97% on RA	98% on RA
Weight	116 lb (52.6 kg)	120 lb (54.4 kg)	124 lb (56.2 kg)	129 lb (58.5 kg)

The nurse reviews the collected client data with the registered nurse. Complete the following sentence by selecting from the lists of options below.

The nurse recognizes that the client is *most likely* experiencing **1 [Select]** and would anticipate administration of **2 [Select]** and **3 [Select]**.

OPTIONS FOR 1	OPTIONS FOR 2	OPTIONS FOR 3
Hyperemesis gravidarum	Intravenous fluids	Hydralazine
Placenta previa	Magnesium sulfate	Morphine
Preeclampsia	Oxytocin	Vasopressin

Stand-Alone Thinking Exercise 20.3

The nurse is caring for a client at 39 weeks' gestation on a labor and delivery unit.

Progress Notes	Nurses' Notes	Orders	Diagnostic Results

2210: Client admitted after spontaneous rupture of membranes. Alert and oriented × 4 with partner at bedside. Respirations equal and unlabored with no adventitious lung sounds. Skin warm and dry. Abdomen round. Fetal HR 139 beats/min. 3-cm cervical dilation, 80% effacement, −1 fetal station. Denies contractions. VS: 98.9°F (37.1°C), HR 88 beats/min and regular, RR 18 breaths/min, BP 139/59 mm Hg, SpO$_2$ 99% on RA. Reports pain rated 3/10.

2350: Client reports contractions every 4–5 minutes, with each lasting 40–60 seconds and increasing in intensity. Variable decelerations noted on fetal monitor. 5-cm cervical dilation, 90% effacement, −3 fetal station. VS: HR 100 beats/min and regular, RR 23 breaths/min, BP 144/78 mm Hg, SpO$_2$ 99% on RA. Reports pain rated 6/10.

2355: Fetal monitor alarms with HR 85 beats/min.

The nurse reviews the collected client data with the registered nurse. Complete the diagram by selecting from the choices below to specify what potential condition the client is likely experiencing, **2** nursing actions that are appropriate to take, and **2** parameters the nurse would monitor to assess the client's progress.

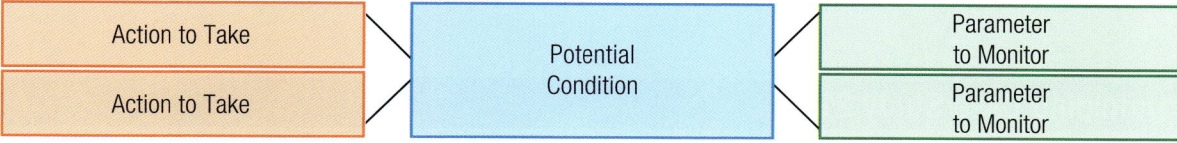

Actions to Take	Potential Conditions	Parameters to Monitor
Administer intravenous oxytocin	Hypertonic labor	Cervical dilation
Apply supplemental oxygen	Premature labor	Contraction strength
Assist the client to the knee-chest position	Prolapsed umbilical cord	Fetal heart rate
Carefully replace the cord back into the client's uterus	Uterine rupture	Fetal movement
Prepare for emergency cesarean delivery		Vaginal bleeding

Commonly Occurring Client Conditions Affecting Newborns

Unfolding Case Study 21.1

Thinking Exercise 21.1.1

The nurse is caring for a newborn client in a maternal-newborn unit.

History and Physical	Nurses' Notes	Orders	Laboratory Results

0215: Baby delivered vaginally at 32 weeks' gestation. Apgar scores of 5 at 1 minute and 6 at 5 minutes. Neuromuscular and physical maturity Ballard score is 20. Pale-pink, mottled thorax with cyanotic extremities. Vernix caseosa abundant, and lanugo present on forehead and shoulders. Abdomen distended. Nasal flaring, grunting, and intercostal and sternal retractions noted. VS: T 96.6°F (35.8°C), HR 98 beats/min, RR 72 breaths/min, SpO_2 88% on RA. Weight 5 lb, 14 ounces (2.6 kg).

The nurse reviews the collected client data with the registered nurse. Complete the following sentence by selecting from the list of word choices below.

The nurse recognizes that the client's **[Word Choice]** requires *immediate* follow-up by the health care team.

WORD CHOICES
Apgar scores
Ballard score
Heart rate
SpO_2 level
Temperature

Thinking Exercise 21.1.2

The nurse is caring for a newborn client in a maternal-newborn unit.

History and Physical	Nurses' Notes	Orders	Laboratory Results

0215: Baby delivered vaginally at 32 weeks' gestation. Apgar scores of 5 at 1 minute and 6 at 5 minutes. Neuromuscular and physical maturity Ballard score is 20. Pale-pink, mottled thorax with cyanotic extremities. Vernix caseosa abundant, and lanugo present on forehead and shoulders. Abdomen distended. Nasal flaring, grunting, and intercostal and sternal retractions noted. VS: T 96.6°F (35.8°C), HR 98 beats/min, RR 72 breaths/min, SpO_2 88% on RA. Weight 5 lb, 14 ounces (2.6 kg).

The nurse reviews the collected client data with the registered nurse. Select the **3** potential complications for which the client is at high risk.

○ Asphyxia
○ Cold stress
○ Fluid and electrolyte imbalances
○ Phenylketonuria
○ Polycythemia
○ Respiratory distress syndrome
○ Spina bifida

Thinking Exercise 21.1.3

The nurse is caring for a newborn client in a maternal-newborn unit.

History and Physical	Nurses' Notes	Orders	Laboratory Results

0215: Baby delivered vaginally at 32 weeks' gestation. Apgar scores of 5 at 1 minute and 6 at 5 minutes. Neuromuscular and physical maturity Ballard score is 20. Pale-pink, mottled thorax with cyanotic extremities. Vernix caseosa abundant, and lanugo present on forehead and shoulders. Abdomen distended. Nasal flaring, grunting, and intercostal and sternal retractions noted. VS: T 96.6°F (35.8°C), HR 98 beats/min, RR 72 breaths/min, SpO_2 88% on RA. Weight 5 lb, 14 ounces (2.6 kg).

The nurse reviews the client findings with the registered nurse. Complete the following sentence by selecting from the lists of options below.

The nurse determines the *priority* for care at this time is **1 [Select]** administered via **2 [Select]**.

OPTIONS FOR 1	OPTIONS FOR 2
Enteral nutrition	Gastric feeding tube
Humidified oxygen	Peripheral venous device
Intravenous fluids	Skin-to-skin contact
Kangaroo care	Warm incubator

Thinking Exercise 21.1.4

The nurse is caring for a newborn client in a maternal-newborn unit.

History and Physical	Nurses' Notes	Orders	Laboratory Results

0215: Baby delivered vaginally at 32 weeks' gestation. Apgar scores of 5 at 1 minute and 6 at 5 minutes. Neuromuscular and physical maturity Ballard score is 20. Pale-pink, mottled thorax with cyanotic extremities. Vernix caseosa abundant, and lanugo present on forehead and shoulders. Abdomen distended. Nasal flaring, grunting, and intercostal and sternal retractions noted. VS: T 96.6°F (35.8°C), HR 98 beats/min, RR 72 breaths/min, SpO_2 88% on RA. Weight 5 lb, 14 ounces (2.6 kg).

0230: Client sleeping in warmed incubator. Peripheral vascular access device inserted in right dorsal arch. 5% D/NS infusing at 6 mL/h. Arterial and venous blood drawn and sent to lab. VS: T 96.8°F (36°C), HR 102 beats/min, RR 65 breaths/min, SpO_2 94% on 40% humidified O_2.

The nurse reviews the most recent nurses' notes with the registered nurse and contributes to the client's plan of care. For each priority condition, select the potential nursing actions that would be appropriate for the client's plan of care.

CLIENT CONDITIONS	POTENTIAL NURSING ACTIONS
Fluid and electrolyte imbalance	O Assess the status of fontanelles and tissue turgor. O Document urine output by weighing the client's wet diapers. O Monitor serum calcium and glucose levels.
Poor control of body temperature	O Adjust the incubator to maintain optimal body temperature. O Monitor respirations for periods of apnea. O Place a skin probe on the client's abdomen below the diaper.
Respiratory distress	O Assess arterial blood gas results. O Initiate continuous pulse oximetry. O Maintain emergency respiratory equipment at the bedside.

Thinking Exercise 21.1.5

The nurse is caring for a newborn client in a maternal-newborn unit.

History and Physical	Nurses' Notes	Orders	Laboratory Results

0215: Baby delivered vaginally at 32 weeks' gestation. Apgar scores of 5 at 1 minute and 6 at 5 minutes. Neuromuscular and physical maturity Ballard score is 20. Pale-pink, mottled thorax with cyanotic extremities. Vernix caseosa abundant, and lanugo present on forehead and shoulders. Abdomen distended. Nasal flaring, grunting, and intercostal and sternal retractions noted. VS: T 96.6°F (35.8°C), HR 98 beats/min, RR 72 breaths/min, SpO$_2$ 88% on RA. Weight 5 lb, 14 ounces (2.6 kg).

0230: Client sleeping in warmed incubator. Peripheral vascular access device inserted in right dorsal arch. D5NS infusing at 6.5 mL/h. Arterial and venous blood drawn and sent to lab. VS: T 96.8°F (36°C), HR 102 beats/min, RR 65 breaths/min, SpO$_2$ 94% on 40% humidified O$_2$.

0500: Client's eyes open. Moves all extremities. Respirations equal and unlabored. VS: T 98.2°F (36.7°C), HR 144 beats/min, RR 54 breaths/min, SpO$_2$ 98% on 35% humidified O$_2$. Client removed from incubator and placed skin-to-skin with parent.

0505: Client continues to bond with parent, rooting for breast. VS: HR 148 beats/min, RR 52 breaths/min, SpO$_2$ 98% on low-flow humidified O$_2$. Client latches to breast with assistance. Sucking is inconsistent and weak, lasting only 2 to 3 minutes before client falls asleep.

The nurse reviews the collected client data with the registered nurse to implement the client's plan of care. Which actions would be appropriate for the nurse to implement at this time? **Select all that apply.**

O Assess bowel sounds and monitor for the passage of meconium.
O Consult a certified lactation consultant for suck-training exercises.
O Encourage manual expression of breast milk after feeding attempts.
O Evaluate the strength of the client's suck reflex.
O Initiate gavage feedings via nasogastric tube.
O Use a small, soft nipple with a large hole when bottle-feeding.
O Wake the client and promote breast-feeding every 2 to 3 hours.

Thinking Exercise 21.1.6

The nurse is caring for a newborn client in a maternal-newborn unit.

History and Physical	Nurses' Notes	Orders	Laboratory Results

0215: Baby delivered vaginally at 32 weeks' gestation. Apgar scores of 5 at 1 minute and 6 at 5 minutes. Neuromuscular and physical maturity Ballard score is 20. Pale-pink, mottled thorax with cyanotic extremities. Vernix caseosa abundant, and lanugo present on forehead and shoulders. Abdomen distended. Nasal flaring, grunting, and intercostal and sternal retractions noted. VS: T 96.6°F (35.8°C), HR 98 beats/min, RR 72 breaths/min, SpO$_2$ 88% on RA. Weight 5 lb, 14 ounces (2.6 kg).

0230: Client sleeping in warmed incubator. Peripheral vascular access device inserted in right dorsal arch. D5NS infusing at 6.5 mL/h. Arterial and venous blood drawn and sent to lab. VS: T 96.8°F (36°C), HR 102 beats/min, RR 65 breaths/min, SpO$_2$ 94% on 40% humidified O$_2$.

0500: Client's eyes open. Moves all extremities. Respirations equal and unlabored. VS: T 98.2°F (36.7°C), HR 144 beats/min, RR 54 breaths/min, SpO$_2$ 98% on 35% humidified O$_2$. Client removed from incubator and placed skin-to-skin with parent.

0505: Client continues to bond with parent, rooting for breast. VS: HR 148 beats/min, RR 52 breaths/min, SpO$_2$ 98% on low-flow humidified O$_2$. Client latches to breast with assistance. Sucking is inconsistent and weak, lasting only 2 to 3 minutes before client falls asleep.

2 Days Later
0600: Client alert in bedside warmer. Moves all extremities and responds to stimulation appropriately. Thorax and extremities warm with no mottling or cyanosis noted. Heart tones regular. Respirations equal and unlabored with no adventitious breath sounds. Abdomen soft and round with active bowel sounds in all quadrants. VS: T 98.2°F (36.7°C), HR 140 beats/min, RR 48 breaths/min, SpO$_2$ 97% on RA. 24-hour intake: 170 mL; 24-hour urine output: 140 mL. Yellow, seedy, loose stool this morning. Weight 5 lb, 6 ounces (2.4 kg).

0610: Client transferred to parent. Laches with minimal assistance.

0635: Fed for 5 to 7 minutes on each breast. Supplemental bottle-feeding of 2 ounces (60 mL) expressed breast milk provided after breast-feeding by parent. VS: T 97.1°F (36.1°C), HR 133 beats/min, RR 54 breaths/min, SpO$_2$ 96% on RA.

The nurse reviews the most recent nurses' notes and is assisting to evaluate the client's current status with findings from 2 days ago. For each data collection finding, select whether each finding indicates the client's status is improving or not improving.

DATA COLLECTION FINDINGS	IMPROVING	NOT IMPROVING
Breast-feeding		
Fluid balance		
Oxygenation		
Temperature		

Unfolding Case Study 21.2

Thinking Exercise 21.2.1

The nurse is caring for a newborn client born at 40 weeks' gestation with a unilateral cleft lip and palate in the maternal-newborn unit.

History and Physical	Nurses' Notes	Orders	Laboratory Results

0630: Two-day-old infant is lethargic, lying supine in the bedside bassinet. Moro reflex normal with movement of the bassinet. Eyes open with repetitive physical stimulation. Depressed anterior fontanelle present. Respirations audibly wet with frequent coughing. Small amount of pale-yellow drainage from right nostril. Rhonchi auscultated throughout lung fields. Heart tones regular. Abdomen soft and round. Parent confirms client fed for 40 minutes and ingested 3 ounces (88.7 mL) of expressed breast milk by bottle. Diaper is dry. Parent states, "My spouse changed the diaper before going home last night." VS: T 98.6°F (37°C), HR 154 beats/min and regular, RR 56 breaths/min, SpO$_2$ 95% on RA. Parent expresses frustration with feedings and states, "I wish I could breast-feed as I did with my previous children. The bottle is a mess. More milk comes out of my baby's nose and mouth than goes into the stomach."

The nurse reviews collected client data with the registered nurse. Select the **4** client findings that require **immediate** follow-up.

○ Auscultated breath sounds
○ Last diaper change
○ Length of feeding
○ Level of consciousness
○ Parent's expressed frustration
○ Quality of respirations
○ Vital signs

Thinking Exercise 21.2.2

The nurse is caring for a newborn client born at 40 weeks' gestation with a unilateral cleft lip and palate in the maternal-newborn unit.

History and Physical	Nurses' Notes	Orders	Laboratory Results

0630: Two-day-old infant is lethargic, lying supine in the bedside bassinet. Moro reflex normal with movement of the bassinet. Eyes open with repetitive physical stimulation. Depressed anterior fontanelle present. Respirations audibly wet with frequent coughing. Small amount of pale-yellow drainage from right nostril. Rhonchi auscultated throughout lung fields. Heart tones regular. Abdomen soft and round. Parent confirms client fed for 40 minutes and ingested 3 ounces (88.7 mL) of expressed breast milk by bottle. Diaper is dry. Parent states, "My spouse changed the diaper before going home last night." VS: T 98.6°F (37°C), HR 154 beats/min and regular, RR 56 breaths/min, SpO$_2$ 95% on RA. Parent expresses frustration with feedings and states, "I wish I could breast-feed as I did with my previous children. The bottle is a mess. More milk comes out of my baby's nose and mouth than goes into the stomach."

The nurse reviews collected client data with the registered nurse. Complete the following sentence by selecting from the list of word choices below.

The nurse recognizes that client findings are *most likely* caused by [**Word Choice**] and [**Word Choice**].

WORD CHOICES
Aspiration
Cephalohematoma
Dehydration
Maple syrup urine disease
Trisomy 21 syndrome

Thinking Exercise 21.2.3

The nurse is caring for a newborn client born at 40 weeks' gestation with a unilateral cleft lip and palate in the maternal-newborn unit.

History and Physical	Nurses' Notes	Orders	Laboratory Results

0630: Two-day-old infant is lethargic, lying supine in the bedside bassinet. Moro reflex normal with movement of the bassinet. Eyes open with repetitive physical stimulation. Depressed anterior fontanelle present. Respirations audibly wet with frequent coughing. Small amount of pale-yellow drainage from right nostril. Rhonchi auscultated throughout lung fields. Heart tones regular. Abdomen soft and round. Parent confirms client fed for 40 minutes and ingested 3 ounces (88.7 mL) of expressed breast milk by bottle. Diaper is dry. Parent states, "My spouse changed the diaper before going home last night." VS: T 98.6°F (37°C), HR 154 beats/min and regular, RR 56 breaths/min, SpO$_2$ 95% on RA. Parent expresses frustration with feedings and states, "I wish I could breast-feed as I did with my previous children. The bottle is a mess. More milk comes out of my baby's nose and mouth than goes into the stomach."

The nurse reviews the client findings with the registered nurse. Complete the following sentences by selecting from the lists of options below.

The nurse determines the *priority* for care at this time is to manage the client's __1 [Select]__. The nurse's *priority* action would be to __2 [Select]__.

OPTIONS FOR 1	OPTIONS FOR 2
Airway	Administer supplemental oxygen.
Congenital anomaly	Insert a peripheral venous device for fluid resuscitation.
Fluid status	Place the client in the high Fowler position.
Nutrition	Reinforce teaching related to feeding and orofacial clefts.

Thinking Exercise 21.2.4

The nurse is caring for a newborn client born at 40 weeks' gestation with a unilateral cleft lip and palate in the maternal-newborn unit.

History and Physical	Nurses' Notes	Orders	Laboratory Results

0630: Two-day-old infant is lethargic, lying supine in the bedside bassinet. Moro reflex normal with movement of the bassinet. Eyes open with repetitive physical stimulation. Depressed anterior fontanelle present. Respirations audibly wet with frequent coughing. Small amount of pale-yellow drainage from right nostril. Rhonchi auscultated throughout lung fields. Heart tones regular. Abdomen soft and round. Parent confirms client fed for 40 minutes and ingested 3 ounces (88.7 mL) of expressed breast milk by bottle. Diaper is dry. Parent states, "My spouse changed the diaper before going home last night." VS: T 98.6°F (37°C), HR 154 beats/min and regular, RR 56 breaths/min, SpO$_2$ 95% on RA. Parent expresses frustration with feedings and states, "I wish I could breast-feed as I did with my previous children. The bottle is a mess. More milk comes out of my baby's nose and mouth than goes into the stomach."

0700: Care transferred to RN. Shift-change report provided at bedside. Parent sitting upright in chair, and client sleeping skin-to-skin against parent's chest. RR 40 breaths/min, SpO$_2$ 98% on RA.

0900: Client is alert. Respirations equal and unlabored with no adventitious breath sounds. Parent expressed breast milk and is preparing to bottle-feed the client.

The nurse reviews the collected client data with the registered nurse and reinforces teaching with the parent. Which health teaching would the nurse reinforce with the parent to promote client safety? **Select all that apply.**

○ "Breast-feeding is the best way to meet your baby's nutritional needs."
○ "Feedings should be about 30 minutes or less to prevent exhaustion and calorie loss."
○ "Milk leaking from the client's nose and mouth during feedings is a sign of choking."
○ "Place your baby in an upright, sitting position to prevent the backflow of milk."
○ "Tilt the bottle so the nipple is always filled and pointed down away from the cleft."
○ "Use the specialized cleft palate bottle provided to you by the lactation consultant."
○ "You should burp your baby two to three times during feedings."

Thinking Exercise 21.2.5

The nurse is caring for a newborn client born at 40 weeks' gestation with a unilateral cleft lip and palate in the pediatric unit.

History and Physical	Nurses' Notes	Orders	Laboratory Results

Maternal-Newborn Unit

0630: Two-day-old infant is lethargic, lying supine in the bedside bassinet. Moro reflex normal with movement of the bassinet. Eyes open with repetitive physical stimulation. Depressed anterior fontanelle present. Respirations audibly wet with frequent coughing. Small amount of pale-yellow drainage from right nostril. Rhonchi auscultated throughout lung fields. Heart tones regular. Abdomen soft and round. Parent confirms client fed for 40 minutes and ingested 3 ounces (88.7 mL) of expressed breast milk by bottle. Diaper is dry. Parent states, "My spouse changed the diaper before going home last night." VS: T 98.6°F (37°C), HR 154 beats/min and regular, RR 56 breaths/min, SpO$_2$ 95% on RA. Parent expresses frustration with feedings and states, "I wish I could breast-feed as I did with my previous children. The bottle is a mess. More milk comes out of my baby's nose and mouth than goes into the stomach."

0700: Care transferred to RN. Shift-change report provided at bedside. Parent sitting upright in chair, and client sleeping skin-to-skin against parent's chest. RR 40 breaths/min, SpO$_2$ 98% on RA.

0900: Client is alert. Respirations equal and unlabored with no adventitious breath sounds. Parent expressed breast milk and is preparing to bottle-feed the client.

Ambulatory Pediatric Clinic

1320: 10-week-old client scheduled for cheiloplasty (lip restoration) presents to clinic with parents for presurgical screening. Client alert and moves all extremities. Parent states client has been eating 2 to 3 ounces (59.1–88.7 mL) of expressed breast milk every 3 hours and has a wet diaper after every feeding. Client has not had any episodes of choking or respiratory distress. Respirations equal and unlabored with no adventitious breath sounds. Heart tones regular. Abdomen soft and round with active bowel sounds in all quadrants. VS: T 98.8°F (37.1°C), HR 122 beats/min and regular, RR 24 breaths/min, SpO$_2$ 99% on RA. Weight 12.6 lb (5.7 kg). Parent bonding is appropriate. Client cleared for surgery.

Pediatric Unit

1800: Client admitted post-cheiloplasty from PACU. Alert and crying; parent attempts to console. Surgical incision well approximated. Scant serous drainage noted. VS: T 98.5°F (36.9°C), HR 130 beats/min and regular, RR 22 breaths/min, SpO$_2$ 99% on RA.

The nurse reviews the collected client data with the registered nurse to implement the plan of care. Select the **2 priority** actions the nurse would implement.

○ Assess pain using the Wong-Baker FACES® scale.
○ Carefully position the client on the abdomen to rest.
○ Encourage the client to use a pacifier.
○ Ensure that the client is adequately swaddled.
○ Gently cleanse the suture line with sterile water.
○ Provide tube feedings until the incision heals.

Thinking Exercise 21.2.6

The nurse is caring for a newborn client born at 40 weeks' gestation with a unilateral cleft lip and palate.

History and Physical	Nurses' Notes	Orders	Laboratory Results

Maternal-Newborn Unit

0630: Two-day-old client is lethargic, lying supine in the bedside bassinet. Moro reflex normal with movement of the bassinet. Eyes open with repetitive physical stimulation. Depressed anterior fontanelle present. Respirations audibly wet with frequent coughing. Small amount of pale-yellow drainage from right nostril. Rhonchi auscultated throughout lung fields. Heart tones regular. Abdomen soft and round. Parent confirms client fed for 40 minutes and ingested 3 ounces (88.7 mL) of expressed breast milk by bottle. Diaper is dry. Parent states, "My spouse changed the diaper before going home last night." VS: T 98.6°F (37°C), HR 154 beats/min and regular, RR 56 breaths/min, SpO$_2$ 95% on RA. Parent expresses frustration with feedings and states, "I wish I could breast-feed as I did with my previous children. The bottle is a mess. More milk comes out of my baby's nose and mouth than goes into the stomach."

0700: Care transferred to RN. Shift-change report provided at bedside. Parent sitting upright in chair, and client sleeping skin-to-skin against parent's chest. RR 40 breaths/min, SpO$_2$ 98% on RA.

0900: Client is alert. Respirations equal and unlabored with no adventitious breath sounds. Parent expressed breast milk and is preparing to bottle-feed the client.

Ambulatory Pediatric Clinic

1320: 10-week-old client scheduled for cheiloplasty (lip restoration) presents to clinic with parents for presurgical screening. Client alert and moves all extremities. Parent states client has been eating 2 to 3 ounces (59.1–88.7 mL) of expressed breast milk every 3 hours and has a wet diaper after every feeding. Client has not had any episodes of choking or respiratory distress. Respirations equal and unlabored with no adventitious breath sounds. Heart tones regular. Abdomen soft and round with active bowel sounds in all quadrants. VS: T 98.8°F (37.1°C), HR 122 beats/min and regular, RR 24 breaths/min, SpO$_2$ 99% on RA. Weight 12.6 lb (5.7 kg). Parent bonding is appropriate. Client cleared for surgery.

Pediatric Unit

1800: Client admitted post-cheiloplasty from PACU. Alert and crying; parent attempts to console. Surgical incision well approximated. Scant serous drainage noted. VS: T 98.5°F (36.9°C), HR 130 beats/min and regular, RR 22 breaths/min, SpO$_2$ 99% on RA.

0830: Client alert and cooing. Moves all extremities and interacts appropriately with parents. Surgical incision well approximated. No redness, swelling, or drainage noted. Respirations equal and unlabored with no adventitious breath sounds. Heart tones regular. Active bowel sounds in all quadrants. Client tolerates bottle-feeding every 2 to 3 hours, eating 2 to 3 ounces (59.1–88.7 mL) of expressed breast milk with each feeding. Wet diaper every 3 to 4 hours. Yellow, seedy, loose stool this morning. Discharge teaching reinforced.

The nurse collaborates with the registered nurse to determine if discharge teaching is effective. Select whether the following statements by the client's parent indicate understanding or no understanding of the discharge teaching provided.

CLIENT STATEMENTS	UNDERSTANDING	NO UNDERSTANDING
"Cuddling with my baby will provide emotional support for us both."		
"I will administer children's aspirin to manage my baby's pain."		
"It is important to prevent bumping or scratching of the lip and nose areas."		
"Now that the cleft lip is fixed, I can breast-feed instead of using the bottle."		
"I will use a cotton-tipped applicator to gently cleanse the sutures and apply topical ointment."		

Stand-Alone Thinking Exercise 21.1

The nurse is caring for a newborn who was delivered 30 hours ago at $36^{5}/_{7}$ weeks' gestation to a 36-year-old parent who has an obstetric history of G4P3.

Nursing Flow Sheet	Nurses' Notes	Orders	Laboratory Results

0900: Newborn client was delivered 30 hours ago at $36^{5}/_{7}$ weeks' gestation to a 36-year-old parent who has an obstetric history of G4P3. Client alert. Cephalohematoma and extensive facial bruising noted. Client put to breast for feeding. Difficulty latching noted. Parent expresses desire to exclusively breast-feed and requests that no supplementation be offered.

1210: Parent reports that client is too sleepy to eat and has had no wet diapers. Supplemental formula or expressed colostrum offered. Parent refuses. Reinforced breast-feeding instructions, and encouraged parent to put client to each breast for at least 10 minutes.

1500: Client lethargic. Parent reports that client has not been fed in 6 hours. Jaundice noted on palms, upper chest, face, and sclera. Physician notified. Laboratory results reviewed: Total bilirubin elevated. Orders received. Phototherapy initiated.

1820: Lactation consultant at bedside. Client is difficult to arouse but wakes with repeated stimulation. Adequately latches and feeds for 5 to 10 minutes on each breast.

2140: Client under phototherapy. Easily aroused. Jaundice noted on face and sclera. Client put to breast for first time since lactation consultation visit. Client latches and feeds for 5 to 10 minutes on each breast.

Nursing Flow Sheet	Nurses' Notes	Orders	Laboratory Results	
Parameters	**0900**	**1210**	**1500**	**2140**
Temperature	98.6°F (37°C)	98.9°F (37.1°C)	98.9°F (37.1°C)	97.3°F (36.3°C)
Heart rate	146 beats/min	134 beats/min	112 beats/min	130 beats/min
Respiratory rate	48 breaths/min	42 breaths/min	44 breaths/min	42 breaths/min
SpO$_2$	99% on RA	99% on RA	100% on RA	100% on RA
Urine output	Voids once: Yellow urine	None	Voids: Brick-red colored urine	Voids: Orange-yellow urine
Bowel output	Meconium	None	None	Yellowish-green, seedy stool
	Birth		**1500 (Day 1)**	
Weight	2.66 kg (5 lb 13 ounces)		2.44 kg (5 lb 6 ounces)	
Length	16 cm (40.6 inches)		16 cm (40.6 inches)	

The nurse collaborates with the registered nurse to determine if the treatment plan is effective for the client. For each data collection finding, select whether each finding indicates the client is improving or not improving.

DATA COLLECTION FINDINGS	IMPROVING	NOT IMPROVING
Breast-feeding		
Jaundice		
Level of consciousness		
Temperature		
Weight		

Stand-Alone Thinking Exercise 21.2

A nurse is caring for a newborn client in a maternal-newborn unit.

Health History	Nurses' Notes	Orders	Diagnostic Results

Perinatal Ambulatory Clinic Visit

41-year-old multiparous parent at 37 weeks' gestation in clinic for perinatal checkup. Alert and oriented × 4. Describes birthing plan and support systems in place to care for current children during hospitalization and for a few weeks after discharge. Fetal HR 136 beats/min. Fundal height 39 cm (15.4 inches). VS: T 98.6°F (37°C), HR 76 beats/min and regular, BP 134/74 mm Hg, RR 16 breaths/min, SpO_2 95% on RA. FSBG 220 mg/dL.

Obstetric History

- G3P2
- Blood type A+
- Rubella immune
- HIV negative
- Hepatitis B negative

Medical History

- Obesity (BMI 34.2)
- Hyperlipidemia
- Type 2 diabetes mellitus

Progress Notes	Nurses' Notes	Orders	Diagnostic Results

Maternal-Newborn Unit

2200: Client born by assisted vaginal delivery at 39 weeks' gestation. Birth weight 11 lb, 7.4 ounces (5.2 kg), length 19.4 inches (49.2 cm), head circumference 14.8 inches (37.6 cm). Apgar scores 6, 8, and 9 at 1, 5, and 10 minutes, respectively. Client placed on parent's chest and allowed to root to find breast. Client latches on to nipple with minimal assist. Umbilical cord clamped; 3-vessel cord noted.

2300: Client alert with eyes open. Crys lustily. Heart tones regular. Lung fields clear. Abdomen soft and round. VS: T 98.3°F (36.8°C), HR 148 beats/min, RR 54 breaths/min, SpO_2 97% on RA. Blood type O+.

0030: Client sleeping but easily aroused when put to breast. Successfully latches and feeds for 10 to 15 minutes on each breast. Parents demonstrate appropriate bonding behaviors.

0200: Client is irritable with weak, high-pitched cry. Skin warm and diaphoretic. Mild respiratory distress and nasal flaring noted. Tremors present in all extremities. VS: T 98.6°F (37°C), HR 154 beats/min, RR 76 breaths/min, SpO_2 95% on RA.

The nurse reviews the collected client data with the registered nurse. Complete the diagram by selecting from the choices below to specify what potential condition the client is likely experiencing, **2** nursing actions that are appropriate to take, and **2** parameters the nurse would monitor to assess the client's progress.

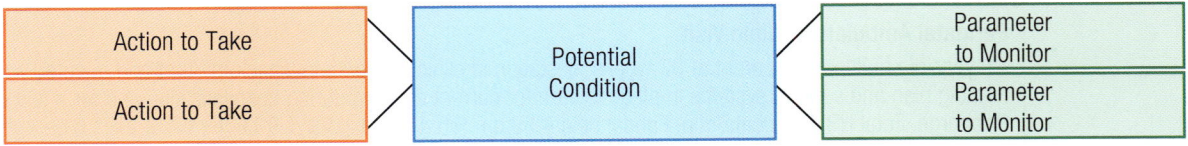

Actions to Take	Potential Conditions	Parameters to Monitor
Administer Rh₀(D) immune globulin (RhoGAM®)	Congenital kidney defect	Blood glucose level
Apply supplemental oxygen	Hypoglycemia	Creatinine level
Encourage breast-feeding every 1.5 to 2 hours	Isoimmunization	Heat loss
Obtain a fingerstick blood glucose (FSBG) level	Phenylketonuria	Level of consciousness
Swaddle the baby in a blanket		Urinary output

Commonly Occurring Client Conditions Affecting Children

Unfolding Case Study 22.1

Thinking Exercise 22.1.1

The nurse is caring for a 7-year-old postoperative client at a same-day surgical center. The nurse reviews collected client data with the registered nurse. Highlight the client findings that require **immediate** follow-up.

History and Physical	Nurses' Notes	Orders	Laboratory Results

1540: Child transferred to PACU following tonsillectomy and adenoidectomy for recurrent upper respiratory infections; parent at bedside. Child placed in side-lying position; ice collar in place. Child whimpering and stating throat hurts "a lot." No nausea or vomiting. Small amount of pinkish drainage from mouth on tissue. Eating a few ice chips. IV infusing in left forearm. VS: 99°F (37.2°C), HR 100 beats/min, RR 24 breaths/min, BP 98/50 mm Hg, SpO$_2$ 94% on RA. Acetaminophen administered per agency protocol.

1645: Child dozing intermittently; restless at times. Swallowing frequently while sleeping. VS: 98.6°F (37°C), HR 104 beats/min, RR 24 breaths/min, BP 94/50 mm Hg, SpO$_2$ 93% on RA.

Thinking Exercise 22.1.2

The nurse is caring for a 7-year-old postoperative client at a same-day surgical center.

History and Physical	Nurses' Notes	Orders	Laboratory Results

1540: Child transferred to PACU following tonsillectomy and adenoidectomy for recurrent upper respiratory infections; parent at bedside. Child placed in side-lying position; ice collar in place. Child whimpering and stating throat hurts "a lot." No nausea or vomiting. Small amount of pinkish drainage from mouth on tissue. Eating a few ice chips. IV infusing in left forearm. VS: 99°F (37.2°C), HR 100 beats/min, RR 24 breaths/min, BP 98/50 mm Hg, SpO$_2$ 94% on RA. Acetaminophen administered per agency protocol.

1645: Child dozing intermittently; restless at times. Swallowing frequently while sleeping. VS: 98.6°F (37°C), HR 104 beats/min, RR 24 breaths/min, BP 94/50 mm Hg, SpO$_2$ 93% on RA.

The nurse reviews the collected client data with the registered nurse. Complete the following sentence by selecting from the lists of options below.

The client is *most likely* experiencing **1 [Select]** as evidenced by **2 [Select]** and **3 [Select]**.

OPTIONS FOR 1	OPTIONS FOR 2	OPTIONS FOR 3
Infection	Fever	Hypoxemia
Sleep apnea	Restlessness	Severe pain
Hemorrhage	Hypotension	Frequent swallowing

Thinking Exercise 22.1.3

The nurse is caring for a 7-year-old postoperative client at a same-day surgical center.

History and Physical	Nurses' Notes	Orders	Laboratory Results

1540: Child transferred to PACU following tonsillectomy and adenoidectomy for recurrent upper respiratory infections; parent at bedside. Child placed in side-lying position; ice collar in place. Child whimpering and stating throat hurts "a lot." No nausea or vomiting. Small amount of pinkish drainage from mouth on tissue. Eating a few ice chips. IV infusing in left forearm. VS: 99°F (37.2°C); HR 100 beats/min, RR 24 breaths/min, BP 98/50 mm Hg, SpO$_2$ 94% on RA. Acetaminophen administered per agency protocol.

1645: Child dozing intermittently; restless at times. Swallowing frequently while sleeping. VS: 98.6°F (37°C), HR 104 beats/min, RR 24 breaths/min, BP 94/50 mm Hg, SpO$_2$ 93% on RA.

The nurse reviews the collected client data with the registered nurse. Complete the following sentence by selecting from the list of word choices below.

The *priority* for client care at this time is to prevent **[Word Choice]**.

WORD CHOICES
Pneumonia
Surgical site infection
Hypovolemic shock

Thinking Exercise 22.1.4

The nurse is caring for a 7-year-old postoperative client at a same-day surgical center.

History and Physical	Nurses' Notes	Orders	Laboratory Results

1540: Child transferred to PACU following tonsillectomy and adenoidectomy for recurrent upper respiratory infections; parent at bedside. Child placed in side-lying position; ice collar in place. Child whimpering and stating throat hurts "a lot." No nausea or vomiting. Small amount of pinkish drainage from mouth on tissue. Eating a few ice chips. IV infusing in left forearm. VS: 99°F (37.2°C), HR 100 beats/min, RR 24 breaths/min, BP 98/50 mm Hg, SpO$_2$ 94% on RA. Acetaminophen administered per agency protocol.

1645: Child dozing intermittently; restless at times. Swallowing frequently while sleeping. VS: 98.6°F (37°C), HR 104 beats/min, RR 24 breaths/min, BP 94/50 mm Hg, SpO$_2$ 93% on RA.

The nurse collaborates with the registered nurse and contributes to the client's plan of care. Select whether the following potential nursing actions are indicated or not indicated for the client at this time.

POTENTIAL NURSING ACTIONS	INDICATED	NOT INDICATED
Transfer care of the client to the registered nurse.		
Decrease the IV infusion rate.		
Observe the client carefully for bleeding.		
Monitor vital signs every 30 minutes.		
Report relevant client findings to the surgeon.		

Thinking Exercise 22.1.5

The nurse is caring for a 7-year-old postoperative client at a same-day surgical center.

History and Physical	Nurses' Notes	Orders	Laboratory Results

1540: Child transferred to PACU following tonsillectomy and adenoidectomy for recurrent upper respiratory infections; parent at bedside. Child placed in side-lying position; ice collar in place. Child whimpering and stating throat hurts "a lot." No nausea or vomiting. Small amount of pinkish drainage from mouth on tissue. Eating a few ice chips. IV infusing in left forearm. VS: 99°F (37.2°C), HR 100 beats/min, RR 24 breaths/min, BP 98/50 mm Hg, SpO_2 94% on RA. Acetaminophen administered per agency protocol.

1645: Child dozing intermittently; restless at times. Swallowing frequently while sleeping. VS: 98.6°F (37°C), HR 104 beats/min, RR 24 breaths/min, BP 94/50 mm Hg, SpO_2 93% on RA.

1715: Coughing up small amount of bright-red blood. Child reports worsening throat pain. IV infusion rate increased per agency protocol. Parent and child reassured that bleeding commonly occurs after this type of surgery and can be managed. VS: 98.4°F (36.9°C), HR 100 beats/min, RR 22 breaths/min, BP 96/52 mm Hg, SpO_2 92% on RA.

The nurse collaborates with the registered nurse and contributes to the client's plan of care. Which of the following potential nursing actions would be appropriate for the nurse to implement at this time? **Select all that apply.**

O Monitor the client for indications of fluid overload after increasing the IV infusion rate.
O Encourage the client to drink fluids to prevent dehydration.
O Keep the client in the sitting position with the head elevated.
O Administer the ordered opioid medication for pain management.
O Prepare the parent and client for a possible treatment procedure in the operating suite.

Thinking Exercise 22.1.6

The nurse is caring for a 7-year-old postoperative client at a same-day surgical center.

History and Physical	Nurses' Notes	Orders	Laboratory Results

1540: Child transferred to PACU following tonsillectomy and adenoidectomy for recurrent upper respiratory infections; parent at bedside. Child placed in side-lying position; ice collar in place. Child whimpering and stating throat hurts "a lot." No nausea or vomiting. Small amount of pinkish drainage from mouth on tissue. Eating a few ice chips. IV infusing in left forearm. VS: 99°F (37.2°C), HR 100 beats/min, RR 24 breaths/min, BP 98/50 mm Hg, SpO_2 94% on RA. Acetaminophen administered per agency protocol.

1645: Child dozing intermittently; restless at times. Swallowing frequently while sleeping. VS: 98.6°F (37°C); HR 104 beats/min; RR 24 breaths/min; BP 94/50 mm Hg, SpO_2 93% on RA.

1715: Coughing up small amount of bright-red blood. Child reports worsening throat pain. IV infusion rate increased per agency protocol. Parent and child reassured that bleeding commonly occurs after this type of surgery and can be managed. VS: 98.4°F (36.9°C), HR 100 beats/min, RR 22 breaths/min, BP 96/52 mm Hg, SpO_2 92% on RA.

1735: Surgeon in to examine client. Order to continue monitoring child and notify surgeon if additional bleeding occurs. Opioid analgesic administered per agency protocol.

1950: No additional bleeding noted since 1715. No excessive swallowing noted during sleeping. Pain rating decreased from 5/10 to 1/10 on the Wong-Baker FACES Pain Rating Scale. Preparing for discharge to home with instructions for home care. Parent very anxious that bleeding could occur after discharge. Discharge instructions provided about when to contact the surgeon or visit ED for bleeding or other complications.

The nurse reviews the most recent nurses' notes with the registered nurse. Complete the following sentence by selecting from the lists of options below.

The client's condition has **1 [Select]** as evidenced by **2 [Select]**.

OPTIONS FOR 1	OPTIONS FOR 2
Improved	Continued pain
Not changed	Severe anxiety
Worsened	No additional bleeding

Unfolding Case Study 22.2

Thinking Exercise 22.2.1

The nurse is caring for a 3-week-old infant in the pediatric emergency department (ED).

History and Physical	Nurses' Notes	Orders	Laboratory Results

1025: Infant brought to pediatric ED by parents, who report that infant has had projectile vomiting immediately after taking each bottle for the past few days. Parents have tried to burp infant more often and feed more slowly, but nothing has helped. Infant constantly hungry and will take bottle after vomiting. Parents report that infant weighed 8 lb (3.6 kg) at birth. Noticed infant has not needed as many diaper changes this week compared with last week. Infant has sunken frontal fontanelle, inelastic skin turgor, and dry mucous membranes. Diaper currently dry. Current weight 7 lb, 14 ounces (3.57 kg). VS: T 99.3°F (37.4°C) axillary, HR 200 beats/min, RR 66 breaths/min, BP 68/40 mm Hg, SpO_2 94% on RA.

The nurse reviews the collected client data with the registered nurse. Select the **5** client findings that require **immediate** follow-up.

O Temperature
O Heart rate
O Respiratory rate
O Blood pressure
O SpO_2
O Weight
O Skin turgor/mucous membranes
O Decreased urine output

Thinking Exercise 22.2.2

The nurse is caring for a 3-week-old infant in the pediatric emergency department.

History and Physical	Nurses' Notes	Orders	Laboratory Results

1025: Infant brought to pediatric ED by parents, who report that infant has had projectile vomiting immediately after taking each bottle for the past few days. Parents tried to burp infant more often and feed more slowly, but nothing has helped. Infant constantly hungry and will take bottle after vomiting. Parents report that infant weighed 8 lb (3.6 kg) at birth. Noticed infant has not needed as many diaper changes this week compared with last week. Infant has sunken frontal fontanelle, inelastic skin turgor, and dry mucous membranes. Diaper currently dry. Current weight 7 lb, 14 ounces (3.57 kg). VS: T 99.3°F (37.4°C) axillary, HR 200 beats/min, RR 66 breaths/min, BP 68/40 mm Hg, SpO_2 94% on RA.

The nurse reviews the collected client data with the registered nurse. For which of the following complications is the infant at high risk? **Select all that apply.**

O Urinary tract infection
O Electrolyte imbalance
O Intussusception
O Aspiration pneumonia
O Urinary calculi

Thinking Exercise 22.2.3

The nurse is caring for a 3-week-old infant in the pediatric emergency department.

History and Physical	Nurses' Notes	Orders	Laboratory Results

1025: Infant brought to pediatric ED by parents, who report that infant has had projectile vomiting immediately after taking each bottle for the past few days. Parents tried to burp infant more often and feed more slowly, but nothing has helped. Infant constantly hungry and will take bottle after vomiting. Parents report that infant weighed 8 lb (3.6 kg) at birth. Noticed infant has not needed as many diaper changes this week compared with last week. Infant has sunken frontal fontanelle, inelastic skin turgor, and dry mucous membranes. Diaper currently dry. Current weight 7 lb, 14 ounces (3.57 kg). VS: T 99.3°F (37.4°C) axillary, HR 200 beats/min, RR 66 breaths/min, BP 68/40 mm Hg, SpO_2 94% on RA.

The nurse collaborates with the registered nurse and contributes to the client's plan of care. Complete the following sentence by selecting from the list of word choices below.

The *priority* for the client's care at this time is to prevent [**Word Choice**].

WORD CHOICES
Malnutrition
Delayed development
Major organ dysfunction
Metabolic acidosis
Urinary tract infection

Thinking Exercise 22.2.4

The nurse is caring for a 3-week-old infant in the pediatric emergency department.

History and Physical	Nurses' Notes	Orders	Laboratory Results

1025: Infant brought to pediatric ED by parents, who report that infant has had projectile vomiting immediately after taking each bottle for the past few days. Parents tried to burp infant more often and feed more slowly, but nothing has helped. Infant constantly hungry and will take bottle after vomiting. Parents report that infant weighed 8 lb (3.6 kg) at birth. Noticed infant has not needed as many diaper changes this week compared with last week. Infant has sunken frontal fontanelle, inelastic skin turgor, and dry mucous membranes. Diaper currently dry. Current weight 7 lb, 14 ounces (3.57 kg). VS: T 99.3°F (37.4°C) axillary, HR 200 beats/min, RR 66 breaths/min, BP 68/40 mm Hg, SpO_2 94% on RA.

1110: Bedside abdominal ultrasound examination performed. Infantile pyloric stenosis confirmed.

The nurse collaborates with the registered nurse and contributes to the client's plan of care. Select whether the following potential nursing actions are indicated or not indicated for the client at this time.

POTENTIAL NURSING ACTIONS	INDICATED	NOT INDICATED
Establish peripheral IV access for fluids.		
Continue to feed the infant as usual.		
Draw labs per orders.		
Prepare for emergency surgery.		
Document the diaper count per agency protocol.		

Thinking Exercise 22.2.5

The nurse is caring for a 3-week-old infant in the acute pediatric unit.

History and Physical	Nurses' Notes	Orders	Laboratory Results

Emergency Department

1025: Infant brought to pediatric ED by parents, who report that infant has had projectile vomiting immediately after taking each bottle for the past few days. Parents tried to burp infant more often and feed more slowly, but nothing has helped. Infant constantly hungry and will take bottle after vomiting. Parents report that infant weighed 8 lb (3.6 kg) at birth. Noticed infant has not needed as many diaper changes this week compared with last week. Infant has sunken frontal fontanelle, inelastic skin turgor, and dry mucous membranes. Diaper currently dry. Current weight 7 lb, 14 ounces (3.57 kg). VS: T 99.3°F (37.4°C) axillary, HR 200 beats/min, RR 66 breaths/min, BP 68/40 mm Hg, SpO$_2$ 94% on RA.

1110: Bedside abdominal ultrasound examination performed. Infantile pyloric stenosis confirmed.

Day of Surgery

1305: Infant returned from PACU following pyloromyotomy. IV infusing in right foot. Alert and crying; calmer with pacifier. Moving all extremities. Surgical dressing dry and intact. Parent at bedside. Current VS: T 98.6°F (37°C) axillary, HR 152 beats/min, RR 48 breaths/min, BP 78/44 mm Hg, SpO$_2$ 94% on RA.

The nurse collaborates with the registered nurse and contributes to the client's postoperative plan of care. Which of the following nursing actions would be appropriate for the nurse to implement at this time?

O Monitor vital signs every 1 to 2 hours.
O Connect the nasogastric tube to low continuous suction.
O Place the infant in the prone position.
O Assess the infant for pain, and manage accordingly.
O Advise the parents that the infant can be fed as usual later today.
O Insert an indwelling urinary catheter to assess output.
O Take daily weights each morning before feeding.

Thinking Exercise 22.2.6

The nurse is caring for a 3-week-old infant in the acute pediatric unit.

History and Physical	Nurses' Notes	Orders	Laboratory Results

Emergency Department

1025: Infant brought to pediatric ED by parents, who report that infant has had projectile vomiting immediately after taking each bottle for the past few days. Parents tried to burp infant more often and feed more slowly, but nothing has helped. Infant constantly hungry and will take bottle after vomiting. Parents report that infant weighed 8 lb (3.6 kg) at birth. Noticed infant has not needed as many diaper changes this week compared with last week. Infant has sunken frontal fontanelle, inelastic skin turgor, and dry mucous membranes. Diaper currently dry. Current weight 7 lb, 14 ounces (3.57 kg). VS: T 99.3°F (37.4°C) axillary, HR 200 beats/min, RR 66 breaths/min, BP 68/40 mm Hg, SpO$_2$ 94% on RA.

1110: Bedside abdominal ultrasound examination performed. Infantile pyloric stenosis confirmed.

Day of Surgery

1305: Infant returned from PACU following pyloromyotomy. IV infusing in right foot. Alert and crying; calmer with pacifier. Moving all extremities. Surgical dressing dry and intact. Parent at bedside. Current VS: T 98.6°F (37°C) axillary, HR 152 beats/min, RR 48 breaths/min, BP 78/44 mm Hg, SpO$_2$ 94% on RA.

Postoperative Day 2

1655: Infant taking 3 to 4 ounces (90–120 mL) for each feeding. No vomiting. Parents taught to burp infant frequently and place the infant in the sitting position after feeding. Surgical incision dry and intact. Morning weight 8 lb, 5 ounces (3.8 kg). Parents provided with discharge instructions earlier today.

1800: VS: T 101°F (38.3°C) axillary, HR 198 beats/min, RR 52 breaths/min, BP 74/42 mm Hg, SpO$_2$ 93% on RA.

The nurse reviews the most recent nurses' notes and is assisting to determine if the client's treatment plan was effective. For each data collection finding, select whether the finding indicates that the client's status has improved or not improved.

CLIENT FINDINGS	IMPROVED	NOT IMPROVED
Feeding		
Heart rate		
Weight		
Temperature		

Unfolding Case Study 22.3

Thinking Exercise 22.3.1

The nurse is caring for a 12-year-old client at a pediatric ambulatory care clinic.

History and Physical	Nurses' Notes	Orders	Laboratory Results

1740: Child brought to clinic by grandparent, who is the child's legal guardian. Grandparent reports that child has had joint pain that moves from one joint to another and a rash on the chest and abdomen for several days. Child reports lack of appetite, fatigue, and occasional dyspnea on exertion. Grandparent reports that the child had a very sore throat with a "little fever" about 3 weeks ago but does not have a sore throat now. Did not take child for medical attention 3 weeks ago due to lack of health insurance. Borrowed money from a family member to pay for today's clinic visit. Child currently presents with swollen knee joints bilaterally and left wrist redness and swelling, but can move all extremities. Reddened circular rash on anterior thorax and abdomen noted. No adventitious breath sounds throughout lung fields. No respiratory distress; denies chest pain. VS: T 102.6°F (39.2°C), HR 90 beats/min and regular, RR 20 breaths/min, BP 100/62 mm Hg, SpO_2 95% on RA.

The nurse reviews the collected client data with the registered nurse. For each body system, select the client findings that require **immediate** follow-up.

BODY SYSTEMS	CLIENT FINDINGS
Respiratory	O Occasional dyspnea O Decreased SpO_2
Skin/musculoskeletal	O Thoracic and abdominal rash O Joint pain and swelling
Metabolic	O Fever O Fatigue

Thinking Exercise 22.3.2

The nurse is caring for a 12-year-old client at a pediatric ambulatory care clinic.

History and Physical	Nurses' Notes	Orders	Laboratory Results

1740: Child brought to clinic by grandparent, who is the child's legal guardian. Grandparent reports that child has had joint pain that moves from one joint to another and a rash on the chest and abdomen for several days. Child reports lack of appetite, fatigue, and occasional dyspnea on exertion. Grandparent reports that the child had a very sore throat with a "little fever" about 3 weeks ago but does not have a sore throat now. Did not take child for medical attention 3 weeks ago due to lack of health insurance. Borrowed money from a family member to pay for today's clinic visit. Child currently presents with swollen knee joints bilaterally and left wrist redness and swelling, but can move all extremities. Reddened circular rash on anterior thorax and abdomen noted. No adventitious breath sounds throughout lung fields. No respiratory distress; denies chest pain. VS: T 102.6°F (39.2°C); HR 90 beats/min and regular, RR 20 breaths/min, BP 100/62 mm Hg, SpO_2 95% on RA.

The nurse reviews the collected client data with the registered nurse. For each client finding, select whether the finding is consistent with the health conditions of rubella (German measles), systemic juvenile idiopathic arthritis, or rheumatic fever. Some findings may be consistent with more than one condition.

CLIENT FINDINGS	RUBELLA (GERMAN MEASLES)	SYSTEMIC JUVENILE IDIOPATHIC ARTHRITIS	RHEUMATIC FEVER
Fever			
Rash			
Fatigue			
Pain that moves from joint to joint			

Thinking Exercise 22.3.3

The nurse is caring for a 12-year-old client at a pediatric ambulatory care clinic.

History and Physical	Nurses' Notes	Orders	Laboratory Results

1740: Child brought to clinic by grandparent, who is the child's legal guardian. Grandparent reports that child has had joint pain that moves from one joint to another and a rash on the chest and abdomen for several days. Child reports lack of appetite, fatigue, and occasional dyspnea on exertion. Grandparent reports that the child had a very sore throat with a "little fever" about 3 weeks ago but does not have a sore throat now. Did not take child for medical attention 3 weeks ago due to lack of health insurance. Borrowed money from a family member to pay for today's clinic visit. Child currently presents with swollen knee joints bilaterally and left wrist redness and swelling, but can move all extremities. Reddened circular rash on anterior thorax and abdomen noted. No adventitious breath sounds throughout lung fields. No respiratory distress; denies chest pain. VS: T 102.6°F (39.2°C), HR 90 beats/min and regular, RR 20 breaths/min, BP 100/62 mm Hg, SpO$_2$ 95% on RA.

The nurse collaborates with the registered nurse and contributes to the child's plan of care. Complete the following sentence by selecting from the lists of options below.

The ***priority*** for the client's care is to monitor for findings associated with **1 [Select]** because the client's condition can cause **2 [Select]**.

OPTIONS FOR 1	OPTIONS FOR 2
Pyelonephritis	Carditis
Heart failure	Acute kidney injury
Respiratory failure	Pneumonia

Thinking Exercise 22.3.4

The nurse is caring for a 12-year-old client at a pediatric ambulatory care clinic.

History and Physical	Nurses' Notes	Orders	Laboratory Results

1740: Child brought to clinic by grandparent, who is the child's legal guardian. Grandparent reports that child has had joint pain that moves from one joint to another and a rash on the chest and abdomen for several days. Child reports lack of appetite, fatigue, and occasional dyspnea on exertion. Grandparent reports that the child had a very sore throat with a "little fever" about 3 weeks ago but does not have a sore throat now. Did not take child for medical attention 3 weeks ago due to lack of health insurance. Borrowed money from a family member to pay for today's clinic visit. Child currently presents with swollen knee joints bilaterally and left wrist redness and swelling, but can move all extremities. Reddened circular rash on anterior thorax and abdomen noted. No adventitious breath sounds throughout lung fields. No respiratory distress; denies chest pain. VS: T 102.6°F (39.2°C), HR 90 beats/min and regular, RR 20 breaths/min, BP 100/62 mm Hg, SpO$_2$ 95% on RA.

The nurse collaborates with the registered nurse and contributes to the client's plan of care. Which of the following nursing actions would be appropriate for the nurse to implement at this time? **Select all that apply.**

○ Draw blood for anti-streptolysin O (ASO) titer.
○ Perform an electrocardiogram.
○ Draw blood for erythrocyte sedimentation rate.
○ Prepare to transfer the client to an acute care pediatric unit.
○ Anticipate an order for one of the penicillin drugs.

Thinking Exercise 22.3.5—Pharmacology

The nurse is caring for a 12-year-old client at a pediatric ambulatory care clinic.

History and Physical	Nurses' Notes	Orders	Laboratory Results

1740: Child brought to clinic by grandparent, who is the child's legal guardian. Grandparent reports that child has had joint pain that moves from one joint to another and a rash on the chest and abdomen for several days. Child reports lack of appetite, fatigue, and occasional dyspnea on exertion. Grandparent reports that the child had a very sore throat with a "little fever" about 3 weeks ago but does not have a sore throat now. Did not take child for medical attention 3 weeks ago due to lack of health insurance. Borrowed money from a family member to pay for today's clinic visit. Child currently presents with swollen knee joints bilaterally and left wrist redness and swelling, but can move all extremities. Reddened circular rash on anterior thorax and abdomen noted. No adventitious breath sounds throughout lung fields. No respiratory distress; denies chest pain. VS: T 102.6°F (39.2°C), HR 90 beats/min and regular, RR 20 breaths/min, BP 100/62 mm Hg, SpO$_2$ 95% on RA.

1815: Blood drawn for BMP, ASO titer, and ESR. ECG performed: Normal sinus rhythm. No abnormalities noted.

1850: Health teaching for child discharge to home with grandparent. Advised grandparent to allow child to rest and play quietly. Prescription for penicillin V potassium and naproxen; given discount coupons for drugs.

The nurse reviews the collected client data with the registered nurse and reinforces teaching with the client and grandparent. Select the **5** statements that would be appropriate for the nurse to include in the discharge teaching.

○ "Take medications with food because they can cause gastrointestinal distress, especially diarrhea."
○ "Make arrangements to have the penicillin injection given every 28 days."
○ "Even if the client is feeling better, be sure to give all of the prescribed doses."
○ "Penicillin V potassium will help relieve the client's joint pain and fever."
○ "Inform the health care provider if the client has any allergies to penicillin or other antibiotics."
○ "Call the clinic if the client experiences any episodes of bleeding or excessive bruising."
○ "The client will need to take a prophylactic antibiotic prior to any medical or dental procedure."

Thinking Exercise 22.3.6

The nurse is caring for a 12-year-old client at a pediatric ambulatory care clinic and reviews the most recent nurses' notes with the registered nurse. Highlight the client findings in the follow-up visit notes that indicate the client's condition may be **worsening**.

History and Physical	Nurses' Notes	Orders	Laboratory Results

Pediatric Clinic Initial Visit

1740: Child brought to clinic by grandparent, who is the child's legal guardian. Grandparent reports that child has had joint pain that moves from one joint to another and a rash on the chest and abdomen for several days. Child reports lack of appetite, fatigue, and occasional dyspnea on exertion. Grandparent reports that the child had a very sore throat with a "little fever" about 3 weeks ago but does not have a sore throat now. Did not take child for medical attention 3 weeks ago due to lack of health insurance. Borrowed money from a family member to pay for today's clinic visit. Child currently presents with swollen knee joints bilaterally and left wrist redness and swelling, but can move all extremities. Reddened circular rash on anterior thorax and abdomen noted. No adventitious breath sounds throughout lung fields. No respiratory distress; denies chest pain. VS: T 102.6°F (39.2°C), HR 90 beats/min and regular, RR 20 breaths/min, BP 100/62 mm Hg, SpO$_2$ 95% on RA.

1815: Blood drawn for BMP, ASO titer, and ESR. ECG performed: Normal sinus rhythm. No abnormalities noted.

1850: Health teaching for child discharge to home with grandparent. Advised grandparent to allow child to rest and play quietly. Prescription for penicillin V potassium and naproxen; given discount coupons for drugs.

Pediatric Clinic Follow-up Visit—2 Weeks Later

0830: Follow-up visit for rheumatic fever diagnosed 2 weeks ago and treated at home with drug therapy and rest. Grandparent reports that child wanted to visit with friends and go to school, so did not rest as much during drug therapy as intended. Took all of the antibiotic doses as prescribed. Joint pain and swelling decreased; rash barely visible. Yesterday, child had several episodes of shortness of breath and chest discomfort. Appetite remains poor. Has intermittent fevers, mostly in the evenings. VS: 99.4°F (37.4°C), HR 88 beats/min and irregular, RR 26 breaths/min, BP 104/56 mm Hg, SpO$_2$ 91% on RA.

Stand-Alone Thinking Exercise 22.1

The nurse is caring for a 9-year-old client at an acute pediatric unit.

History and Physical	Nurses' Notes	Orders	Laboratory Results

1510: Child admitted with anemia and thrombocytopenia caused by 6-month history of acute lymphoblastic leukemia (ALL). Started packed RBCs via infusion pump. Parent at bedside. VS: T 98.6°F (37°C), HR 106 beats/min, RR 26 breaths/min, BP 96/50 mm Hg, SpO$_2$ 96% on 2 L/min O$_2$ via NC.

1625: Parent at nurses' station yelling, "Something is wrong with my little girl." Child's lips cyanotic; dyspneic with report of dry cough. Alert and oriented × 4; crackles in both lower lung bases. VS: T 98.6°F (37°C), HR 112 beats/min, RR 30 breaths/min, BP 104/58 mm Hg, SpO$_2$ 92% on 2 L/min O$_2$ via NC.

The nurse reviews the collected client data with the registered nurse. Complete the diagram by selecting from the choices below to specify what potential condition the client is likely experiencing, **2** nursing actions that are appropriate to take, and **2** parameters the nurse would monitor to assess the client's progress.

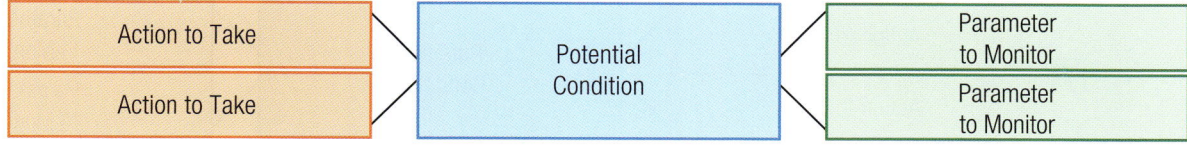

Actions to Take	Potential Conditions	Parameters to Monitor
Decrease the rate of the blood transfusion	Allergic reaction	SpO$_2$
Administer diphenhydramine immediately	Hypovolemic shock	Vital signs
Place the child in the supine position	Fluid overload	Urine output
Stop the blood transfusion	Acute exacerbation of acute lymphoblastic leukemia	Presence of bleeding
Increase the oxygen rate		Hemoglobin and hematocrit

Stand-Alone Thinking Exercise 22.2

The nurse is caring for a 6-month-old infant at a community clinic that provides free health care for migrants.

History and Physical	Nurses' Notes	Orders	Laboratory Results

1705: Brought to clinic by parent, who reports that infant has been having difficulty breathing due to heavy congestion with mucus for the past 2 days. Infant congested; clear drainage from nose noted. Chest retractions and nasal flaring present. Coughing periodically. Expiratory wheezing auscultated throughout lung fields. Parent reports that grandparent has been caring for child for a couple of days while family looked for shelter and possible work. VS: T 102.2°F (39°C) axillary, HR 164 beats/min, RR 72 breaths/min, BP 100/58 mm Hg, SpO$_2$ 89% on RA.

1725: Nasal swab obtained for rapid antigen test.

The nurse reviews the collected client data with the registered nurse. Complete the diagram by selecting from the choices below to specify what potential condition the client is likely experiencing, **2** nursing actions that are appropriate to take, and **2** parameters the nurse would monitor to assess the client's progress.

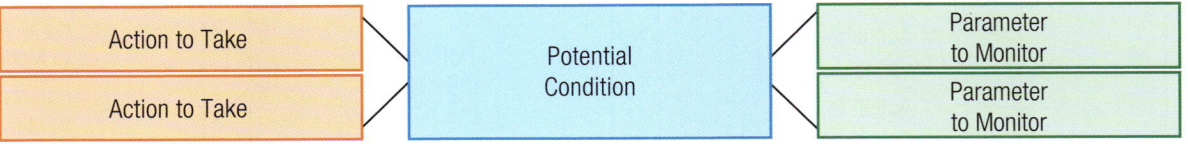

Actions to Take	Potential Conditions	Parameters to Monitor
Initiate oxygen therapy	Croup	SpO$_2$
Administer a steroid via inhaler	Asthma	Presence of wheezing
Transfer the infant to the acute care unit	Epiglottitis	Color and quantity of nasal drainage
Place the infant on a mechanical ventilator	Respiratory syncytial virus (RSV)	Respiratory status
Teach the parent about how to give amoxicillin		Arterial blood gases

CHAPTER 23

Commonly Occurring Client Conditions Affecting Adolescents

Unfolding Case Study 23.1

Thinking Exercise 23.1.1

The nurse is caring for a 15-year-old client in the emergency department (ED).

History and Physical	Nurses' Notes	Orders	Laboratory Results

2025: Client brought to ED by family with report of abdominal pain that started last evening. According to the client, the pain began "in the middle of my belly, but is now lower and more on the right. It hurts to touch my abdomen." Rates pain as 8/10. Has not eaten much today due to lack of appetite and occasional nausea. Lung sounds clear; heart tones present. Abdomen distended with right lower quadrant pain on palpation. Able to move all extremities, but moving right leg aggravates right lower quadrant pain. VS: 100°F (37.8°C), HR 92 beats/min, RR 20 breaths/min, BP 112/66 mm Hg, SpO_2 97% on RA. Abdominal x-ray, urinalysis, and labs ordered. Peripheral IV access established in left forearm for fluid administration.

The nurse reviews the collected client data with the registered nurse. Select the **2** client findings that require **immediate** follow-up.

- ○ Body temperature
- ○ Heart rate
- ○ Distended abdomen
- ○ Blood pressure
- ○ Lack of appetite
- ○ Right lower quadrant abdominal pain

Thinking Exercise 23.1.2

The nurse is caring for a 15-year-old client in the emergency department.

History and Physical	Nurses' Notes	Orders	Laboratory Results

2025: Client brought to ED by family with report of abdominal pain that started last evening. According to the client, the pain began "in the middle of my belly, but is now lower and more on the right. It hurts to touch my abdomen." Rates pain as 8/10. Has not eaten much today due to lack of appetite and occasional nausea. Lung sounds clear; heart tones present. Abdomen distended with right lower quadrant pain on palpation. Able to move all extremities, but moving right leg aggravates right lower quadrant pain. VS: 100°F (37.8°C), HR 92 beats/min, RR 20 breaths/min, BP 112/66 mm Hg, SpO_2 97% on RA. Abdominal x-ray, urinalysis, and labs ordered. Peripheral IV access established in left forearm for fluid administration.

The nurse reviews the collected client data with the registered nurse. Complete the following sentence by selecting from the list of word choices below.

The complication for which the client is **most** at risk is [**Word Choice**].

WORD CHOICE
Dehydration
Hyponatremia
Perforated appendix
Small bowel obstruction

Thinking Exercise 23.1.3

The nurse is caring for a 15-year-old client in the emergency department.

History and Physical	Nurses' Notes	Orders	Laboratory Results

2025: Client brought to ED by family with report of abdominal pain that started last evening. According to the client, the pain began "in the middle of my belly, but is now lower and more on the right. It hurts to touch my abdomen." Rates pain as 8/10. Has not eaten much today due to lack of appetite and occasional nausea. Lung sounds clear; heart tones present. Abdomen distended with right lower quadrant pain on palpation. Able to move all extremities, but moving right leg aggravates right lower quadrant pain. VS: 100°F (37.8°C), HR 92 beats/min, RR 20 breaths/min, BP 112/66 mm Hg, SpO$_2$ 97% on RA. Abdominal x-ray, urinalysis, and labs ordered. Peripheral IV access established in left forearm for fluid administration.

2135: Client reports that pain has lessened to 3/10, although no analgesia administered. Becoming irritated; wants to go home and spend time with friends online to play computer game.

The nurse collaborates with the registered nurse and contributes to the client's plan of care. Complete the following sentence by selecting from the list of options below.

The *priority* for client care at this time is to **1 [Select]**.

OPTIONS
Manage the client's nutritional status.
Monitor for changes in SpO$_2$.
Manage the client's pain.
Observe for signs of peritonitis.

Thinking Exercise 23.1.4

The nurse is caring for a 15-year-old client in the emergency department.

History and Physical	Nurses' Notes	Orders	Laboratory Results

2025: Client brought to ED by family with report of abdominal pain that started last evening. According to the client, the pain began "in the middle of my belly, but is now lower and more on the right. It hurts to touch my abdomen." Rates pain as 8/10. Has not eaten much today due to lack of appetite and occasional nausea. Lung sounds clear; heart tones present. Abdomen distended with right lower quadrant pain on palpation. Able to move all extremities, but moving right leg aggravates right lower quadrant pain. VS: 100°F (37.8°C), HR 92 beats/min, RR 20 breaths/min, BP 112/66 mm Hg, SpO$_2$ 97% on RA. Abdominal x-ray, urinalysis, and labs ordered. Peripheral IV access established in left forearm for fluid administration.

2135: Client reports that pain has lessened to 3/10, although no analgesia administered. Becoming irritated; wants to go home and spend time with friends online to play computer game.

2145: VS: 101.8°F (38.8°C), HR 106 beats/min, RR 22 breaths/min, BP 110/58 mm Hg, SpO$_2$ 97% on RA. Client shaking and requesting additional covers. Reports pain rated 3/10.

The nurse collaborates with the registered nurse and contributes to the client's plan of care. Complete the following sentence by selecting from the lists of options below.

The nurse anticipates that the client will have **1 [Select]** because the client could develop **2 [Select]**.

OPTIONS FOR 1	OPTIONS FOR 2
A nasogastric tube inserted	Peritonitis
Emergency surgery	Constipation
An enema	Hyperactive bowel sounds

Thinking Exercise 23.1.5

The nurse is caring for a 15-year-old client in the emergency department.

History and Physical	Nurses' Notes	Orders	Laboratory Results

2025: Client brought to ED by family with report of abdominal pain that started last evening. According to the client, the pain began "in the middle of my belly, but is now lower and more on the right. It hurts to touch my abdomen." Rates pain as 8/10. Has not eaten much today due to lack of appetite and occasional nausea. Lung sounds clear; heart tones present. Abdomen distended with right lower quadrant pain on palpation. Able to move all extremities, but moving right leg aggravates right lower quadrant pain. VS: 100°F (37.8°C), HR 92 beats/min, RR 20 breaths/min, BP 112/66 mm Hg, SpO$_2$ 97% on RA. Abdominal x-ray, urinalysis, and labs ordered. Peripheral IV access established in left forearm for fluid administration.

2135: Client reports that pain has lessened to 3/10, although no analgesia administered. Becoming irritated; wants to go home and spend time with friends online to play computer game.

2145: VS: 101.8°F (38.8°C), HR 106 beats/min, RR 22 breaths/min, BP 110/58 mm Hg, SpO$_2$ 97% on RA. Client shaking and requesting additional covers. Reports pain rated 3/10.

2220: Surgeon in to discuss emergency surgery with client and family. Explained the need to perform laparoscopic surgery later today to remove perforated appendix and irrigate abdominal area.

The nurse assists with implementation of nursing actions in preparation for the client's surgery. Which of the following nursing actions would the nurse plan to implement at this time? **Select all that apply.**

O Keep the client NPO with an intravenous fluid infusion.
O Obtain informed consent for abdominal surgery.
O Place the client in the sitting or semireclining position.
O Administer an opioid analgesic for abdominal pain.
O Observe the abdomen for rigidity and increased distention.
O Monitor vital signs every 30 to 60 minutes.
O Check for body jewelry, and cover or remove it.

Thinking Exercise 23.1.6

The nurse is caring for a 15-year-old client in the emergency department.

History and Physical	Nurses' Notes	Orders	Laboratory Results

Emergency Department

2025: Client brought to ED by family with report of abdominal pain that started last evening. According to the client, the pain began "in the middle of my belly, but is now lower and more on the right. It hurts to touch my abdomen." Rates pain as 8/10. Has not eaten much today due to lack of appetite and occasional nausea. Lung sounds clear; heart tones present. Abdomen distended with right lower quadrant pain on palpation. Able to move all extremities, but moving right leg aggravates right lower quadrant pain. VS: 100°F (37.8°C), HR 92 beats/min, RR 20 breaths/min, BP 112/66 mm Hg, SpO$_2$ 97% on RA. Abdominal x-ray, urinalysis, and labs ordered. Peripheral IV access established in left forearm for fluid administration.

2135: Client reports that pain has lessened to 3/10, although no analgesia administered. Becoming irritated; wants to go home and spend time with friends online to play computer game.

2145: VS: 101.8°F (38.8°C), HR 106 beats/min, RR 22 breaths/min, BP 110/58 mm Hg, SpO$_2$ 97% on RA. Client shaking and requesting additional covers. Reports pain level rated 3/10.

2220: Surgeon in to discuss emergency surgery with client and family. Explained the need to perform laparoscopic surgery later today to remove perforated appendix and irrigate abdominal area.

Postoperative Day 1

0950: Preparing for discharge to home with family this afternoon. Alert and oriented × 4. Reports surgical pain rated 1/10. Incisions dry and intact. Lung sounds clear throughout. Abdomen soft and round. Bowel sounds present × 4. Able to walk to bathroom without assistance. VS: 98.8°F (37.1°C), HR 74 beats/min, RR 16 breaths/min, BP 116/70 mm Hg, SpO$_2$ 98% on RA.

The nurse reviews the most recent nurses' notes and is assisting to determine the clients' readiness for discharge. Complete the following sentence by selecting from the list of word choices below.

Based on current client findings, the nurse determines that the client's condition has **[Word Choice]**.

WORD CHOICES
Improved
Not improved
Worsened

Unfolding Case Study 23.2

Thinking Exercise 23.2.1

The nurse is caring for a 13-year-old client in the pediatric emergency department (PED).

History and Physical	Nurses' Notes	Orders	Laboratory Results

1400: Child brought to PED by family after school nurse notified them of child's new-onset drowsiness, abdominal pain, cough, nasal congestion, and increased thirst. Child has had type 1 diabetes mellitus for 8 years, which has been controlled by glargine and lispro insulin for the past year. Planning to obtain a continuous glucose monitoring system to use with an insulin pump next year. No other medical history or medications. Family reports that child attended a large birthday party this past weekend where "several kids had colds or some sort of respiratory illness." Child reports feeling very tired and wanting to sleep. Drowsy but oriented × 4. Face flushed; lips reddened and dry. Breath smells fruity. Occasional expiratory wheezing; deep, rapid respirations. Abdomen soft and round with bowel sounds present × 4. All pulses 2+; cap refill <3 sec. Skin turgor poor; skin and mucous membranes dry. VS: 102.6°F (39.2°C), HR 112 beats/min, RR 30 breaths/min, BP 88/48 mm Hg, SpO$_2$ 95% on RA. Denies dyspnea; has been voiding frequently today. FSBG 285 mg/dL (15.8 mmol/L).

1420: Labs drawn, and peripheral IV access established in right forearm.

The nurse reviews the collected client data with the registered nurse. For each body system, select the findings that require **immediate** follow-up.

BODY SYSTEM	CLIENT FINDINGS
Respiratory	O Occasional expiratory wheezing O Deep, rapid respirations O Cough and chest congestion
Integumentary/metabolic	O Temperature O Finger stick blood glucose (FSBG) O Fruity breath
Cardiovascular	O Fatigue O Heart rate O Blood pressure

Thinking Exercise 23.2.2

The nurse is caring for a 13-year-old client in the pediatric emergency department.

History and Physical	Nurses' Notes	Orders	Laboratory Results

1400: Child brought to PED by family after school nurse notified them of child's new-onset drowsiness, abdominal pain, cough, nasal congestion, and increased thirst. Child has had type 1 diabetes mellitus for 8 years, which has been controlled by glargine and lispro insulin for the past year. Planning to obtain a continuous glucose monitoring system to use with an insulin pump next year. No other medical history or medications. Family reports that child attended a large birthday party this past weekend where "several kids had colds or some sort of respiratory illness." Child reports feeling very tired and wanting to sleep. Drowsy but oriented × 4. Face flushed; lips reddened and dry. Breath smells fruity. Occasional expiratory wheezing; deep, rapid respirations. Abdomen soft and round with bowel sounds present × 4. All pulses 2+; cap refill <3 sec. Skin turgor poor; skin and mucous membranes dry. VS: 102.6°F (39.2°C), HR 112 beats/min, RR 30 breaths/min, BP 88/48 mm Hg, SpO_2 95% on RA. Denies dyspnea; has been voiding frequently today. FSBG 285 mg/dL (15.8 mmol/L).

1420: Labs drawn, and peripheral IV access established in right forearm.

1515: PED physician notified of lab results.

History and Physical	Nurses' Notes	Orders	Laboratory Results
Laboratory Test and Reference Range (Serum)			**1500 Results**
Blood urea nitrogen (BUN) (5–18 mg/dL [1.79–6.43 mmol/L])			47 mg/dL (16.78 mmol/L)
Creatinine (0.5–1.0 mg/dL [44.2–88.4 μmol/L])			0.9 mg/dL (79.6 μmol/L)
Sodium (136–145 mEq/L [136–145 mmol/L])			137 mEq/L (137 mmol/L)
Potassium (3.5–5.0 mEq/L [3.5–5.0 mmol/L])			5.7 mEq/L (5.7 mmol/L)
Glucose (nonfasting) (<200 mg/dL [<11.1 mmol/L])			297 mg/dL (16.5 mmol/L)
pH (7.35–7.45)			7.29
Bicarbonate (21–28 mEq/L [21–28 mmol/L])			17 mEq/L (17 mmol/L)
Laboratory Test and Reference Range (Urine)			**1500 Results**
Ketones (negative)			Positive

The nurse reviews the collected client data with the registered nurse. Which of the following conditions is the client likely experiencing? **Select all that apply.**

O Hyperglycemia
O Ketoacidosis
O Hyponatremia
O Dehydration
O Hyperkalemia

Thinking Exercise 23.2.3

The nurse is caring for a 13-year-old client in the pediatric emergency department.

History and Physical	Nurses' Notes	Orders	Laboratory Results

1400: Child brought to PED by family after school nurse notified them of child's new-onset drowsiness, abdominal pain, cough, nasal congestion, and increased thirst. Child has had type 1 diabetes mellitus for 8 years, which has been controlled by glargine and lispro insulin for the past year. Planning to obtain a continuous glucose monitoring system to use with an insulin pump next year. No other medical history or medications. Family reports that child attended a large birthday party this past weekend where "several kids had colds or some sort of respiratory illness." Child reports feeling very tired and wanting to sleep. Drowsy but oriented × 4. Face flushed; lips reddened and dry. Breath smells fruity. Occasional expiratory wheezing; deep, rapid respirations. Abdomen soft and round with bowel sounds present × 4. All pulses 2+; cap refill <3 sec. Skin turgor poor; skin and mucous membranes dry. VS: 102.6°F (39.2°C), HR 112 beats/min, RR 30 breaths/min, BP 88/48 mm Hg, SpO$_2$ 95% on RA. Denies dyspnea; has been voiding frequently today. FSBG 285 mg/dL (15.8 mmol/L).

1420: Labs drawn, and peripheral IV access established in right forearm.

1515: PED physician notified of lab results.

History and Physical	Nurses' Notes	Orders	Laboratory Results
Laboratory Test and Reference Range (Serum)			**1500 Results**
Blood urea nitrogen (BUN) (5–18 mg/dL [1.79–6.43 mmol/L])			47 mg/dL (16.78 mmol/L)
Creatinine (0.5–1.0 mg/dL [44.2–88.4 μmol/L])			0.9 mg/dL (79.6 μmol/L)
Sodium (136–145 mEq/L [136–145 mmol/L])			137 mEq/L (137 mmol/L)
Potassium (3.5–5.0 mEq/L [3.5–5.0 mmol/L])			5.7 mEq/L (5.7 mmol/L)
Glucose (nonfasting) (<200 mg/dL [<11.1 mmol/L])			297 mg/dL (16.5 mmol/L)
pH (7.35–7.45)			7.29
Bicarbonate (21–28 mEq/L [21–28 mmol/L])			17 mEq/L (17 mmol/L)
Laboratory Test and Reference Range (Urine)			**1500 Results**
Ketones (negative)			Positive

The nurse collaborates with the registered nurse and contributes to the client's plan of care. Complete the following sentence by selecting from the list of word choices below.

The **priority** for the client's care at this time is to manage the client's [**Word Choice**].

WORD CHOICES
Hyponatremia
Hyperkalemia
Respiratory condition
Chronic kidney disease
Diabetic ketoacidosis

Thinking Exercise 23.2.4

The nurse is caring for a 13-year-old client in the pediatric emergency department.

History and Physical	Nurses' Notes	Orders	Laboratory Results

1400: Child brought to PED by family after school nurse notified them of child's new-onset drowsiness, abdominal pain, cough, nasal congestion, and increased thirst. Child has had type 1 diabetes mellitus for 8 years, which has been controlled by glargine and lispro insulin for the past year. Planning to obtain a continuous glucose monitoring system to use with an insulin pump next year. No other medical history or medications. Family reports that child attended a large birthday party this past weekend where "several kids had colds or some sort of respiratory illness." Child reports feeling very tired and wanting to sleep. Drowsy but oriented × 4. Face flushed; lips reddened and dry. Breath smells fruity. Occasional expiratory wheezing; deep, rapid respirations. Abdomen soft and round with bowel sounds present × 4. All pulses 2+; cap refill <3 sec. Skin turgor poor; skin and mucous membranes dry. VS: 102.6°F (39.2°C), HR 112 beats/min, RR 30 breaths/min, BP 88/48 mm Hg, SpO$_2$ 95% on RA. Denies dyspnea; has been voiding frequently today. FSBG 285 mg/dL (15.8 mmol/L).

1420: Labs drawn, and peripheral IV access established in right forearm.

1515: PED physician notified of lab results.

History and Physical	Nurses' Notes	Orders	Laboratory Results
Laboratory Test and Reference Range (Serum)			**1500 Results**
Blood urea nitrogen (BUN) (5–18 mg/dL [1.79–6.43 mmol/L])			47 mg/dL (16.78 mmol/L)
Creatinine (0.5–1.0 mg/dL [44.2–88.4 μmol/L])			0.9 mg/dL (79.6 μmol/L)
Sodium (136–145 mEq/L [136–145 mmol/L])			137 mEq/L (137 mmol/L)
Potassium (3.5–5.0 mEq/L [3.5–5.0 mmol/L])			5.7 mEq/L (5.7 mmol/L)
Glucose (nonfasting) (<200 mg/dL [<11.1 mmol/L])			297 mg/dL (16.5 mmol/L)
pH (7.35–7.45)			7.29
Bicarbonate (21–28 mEq/L [21–28 mmol/L])			17 mEq/L (17 mmol/L)
Laboratory Test and Reference Range (Urine)			**1500 Results**
Ketones (negative)			Positive

The nurse collaborates with the registered nurse and contributes to the client's plan of care. Select whether the following potential nursing actions are indicated or not indicated for the client at this time.

POTENTIAL NURSING ACTIONS	INDICATED	NOT INDICATED
Monitor a continuous regular insulin infusion.		
Administer antibiotic therapy per agency protocol.		
Encourage oral fluids including water.		
Administer a 5%D/0.45% NS intravenous infusion.		
Perform rapid testing for respiratory infections.		

Thinking Exercise 23.2.5

The nurse is caring for a 13-year-old client in the pediatric emergency department.

History and Physical	Nurses' Notes	Orders	Laboratory Results

1400: Child brought to PED by family after school nurse notified them of child's new-onset drowsiness, abdominal pain, cough, nasal congestion, and increased thirst. Child has had type 1 diabetes mellitus for 8 years, which has been controlled by glargine and lispro insulin for the past year. Planning to obtain a continuous glucose monitoring system to use with an insulin pump next year. No other medical history or medications. Family reports that child attended a large birthday party this past weekend where "several kids had colds or some sort of respiratory illness." Child reports feeling very tired and wanting to sleep. Drowsy but oriented × 4. Face flushed; lips reddened and dry. Breath smells fruity. Occasional expiratory wheezing; deep, rapid respirations. Abdomen soft and round with bowel sounds present × 4. All pulses 2+; cap refill <3 sec. Skin turgor poor; skin and mucous membranes dry. VS: 102.6°F (39.2°C), HR 112 beats/min, RR 30 breaths/min, BP 88/48 mm Hg, SpO_2 95% on RA. Denies dyspnea; has been voiding frequently today. FSBG 285 mg/dL (15.8 mmol/L).

1420: Labs drawn, and peripheral IV access established in right forearm.

1515: PED physician notified of lab results.

1520: Orders received. Rapid bedside testing negative for COVID, RSV, and influenza.

History and Physical	Nurses' Notes	Orders	Laboratory Results
Laboratory Test and Reference Range (Serum)			**1500 Results**
Blood urea nitrogen (BUN) (5–18 mg/dL [1.79–6.43 mmol/L])			47 mg/dL (16.78 mmol/L)
Creatinine (0.5–1.0 mg/dL [44.2–88.4 μmol/L])			0.9 mg/dL (79.6 μmol/L)
Sodium (136–145 mEq/L [136–145 mmol/L])			137 mEq/L (137 mmol/L)
Potassium (3.5–5.0 mEq/L [3.5–5.0 mmol/L])			5.7 mEq/L (5.7 mmol/L)
Glucose (nonfasting) (<200 mg/dL [<11.1 mmol/L])			297 mg/dL (16.5 mmol/L)
pH (7.35–7.45)			7.29
Bicarbonate (21–28 mEq/L [21–28 mmol/L])			17 mEq/L (17 mmol/L)
Laboratory Test and Reference Range (Urine)			**1500 Results**
Ketones (negative)			Positive

The nurse collaborates with the registered nurse and contributes to the client's plan of care. Select the **3** nursing actions that would be essential for the nurse to implement at this time.

O Begin antiviral therapy per PED protocol.
O Redraw labs to monitor for changes.
O Monitor finger stick blood glucose (FSBG) levels every 30 to 60 minutes.
O Begin continuous cardiac monitoring.
O Initiate supplemental oxygen therapy.

Thinking Exercise 23.2.6

The nurse is caring for a 13-year-old client in the pediatric emergency department. The nurse collaborates with the registered nurse to determine the effectiveness of the plan of care. Highlight the client findings in the 1645 nurses' note that indicate the client's condition is **improving**.

History and Physical	Nurses' Notes	Orders	Laboratory Results

1400: Child brought to PED by family after school nurse notified them of child's new-onset drowsiness, abdominal pain, cough, nasal congestion, and increased thirst. Child has had type 1 diabetes mellitus for 8 years, which has been controlled by glargine and lispro insulin for the past year. Planning to obtain a continuous glucose monitoring system to use with an insulin pump next year. No other medical history or medications. Family reports that child attended a large birthday party this past weekend where "several kids had colds or some sort of respiratory illness." Child reports feeling very tired and wanting to sleep. Drowsy but oriented × 4. Face flushed; lips reddened and dry. Breath smells fruity. Occasional expiratory wheezing; deep, rapid respirations. Abdomen soft and round with bowel sounds present × 4. All pulses 2+; cap refill <3 sec. Skin turgor poor; skin and mucous membranes dry. VS: 102.6°F (39.2°C), HR 112 beats/min, RR 30 breaths/min, BP 88/48 mm Hg, SpO$_2$ 95% on RA. Denies dyspnea; has been voiding frequently today. FSBG 285 mg/dL (15.8 mmol/L).

1420: Labs drawn, and peripheral IV access established in right forearm.

1515: PED physician notified of lab results.

1520: Orders received. Rapid bedside testing negative for COVID, RSV, and influenza.

1645: Continuous regular insulin infusing per protocol. Child less drowsy; oriented × 4. Face remains flushed; lips dry. Breath continues to smell fruity. No report of abdominal pain. Continues with occasional coughing and nasal congestion. VS: 100.6°F (38.1°C), HR 102 beats/min, RR 26 breaths/min, BP 100/52 mm Hg, SpO$_2$ 95% on RA, FSBG 188 mg/dL (10.4 mmol/L). Repeat labs drawn.

History and Physical	Nurses' Notes	Orders	Laboratory Results
Laboratory Test and Reference Range (Serum)			**1500 Results**
Blood urea nitrogen (BUN) (5–18 mg/dL [1.79–6.43 mmol/L])			47 mg/dL (16.78 mmol/L)
Creatinine (0.5–1.0 mg/dL [44.2–88.4 μmol/L])			0.9 mg/dL (79.6 μmol/L)
Sodium (136–145 mEq/L [136–145 mmol/L])			137 mEq/L (137 mmol/L)
Potassium (3.5–5.0 mEq/L [3.5–5.0 mmol/L])			5.7 mEq/L (5.7 mmol/L)
Glucose (nonfasting) (<200 mg/dL [<11.1 mmol/L])			297 mg/dL (16.5 mmol/L)
pH (7.35–7.45)			7.29
Bicarbonate (21–28 mEq/L [21–28 mmol/L])			17 mEq/L (17 mmol/L)
Laboratory Test and Reference Range (Urine)			**1500 Results**
Ketones (negative)			Positive

Unfolding Case Study 23.3

Thinking Exercise 23.3.1

The nurse is caring for a 17-year-old client in the emergency department (ED).

History and Physical	Nurses' Notes	Orders	Laboratory Results

1400: Client brought to ED by family after client developed a fever, headache, vomiting, and occasional confusion yesterday. Client lives in college dormitory; was screened this morning by campus health clinic practitioner, who recommended ED visit. Has had several sinus infections during the past few months but most recently developed a sore throat and "runny" nose. Client reports headache currently rated 9/10, and neck feels a little stiff. Feels nauseated, but better than this morning. History of Duchenne muscular dystrophy since client was 4 years of age. Uses motorized wheelchair or scooter most of the time to move around campus but is ADL independent. Drowsy but oriented × 4; PERRLA. Skin warm and dry with few petechiae noted on chest. Lung sounds clear throughout all lobes. No adventitious breath sounds. Abdomen soft and round with bowel sounds present × 4. Bilateral enlarged calf muscles. All pulses 2+; cap refill <3 sec. VS: 103°F (39.4°C), HR 110 beats/min, RR 22 breaths/min, BP 96/52 mm Hg, SpO_2 94% on RA. Denies dyspnea or chest pain.

The nurse reviews the collected client data with the registered nurse. Which of the following client findings require **immediate** follow-up? **Select all that apply.**

O Fever
O Tachycardia
O Tachypnea
O SpO_2
O Headache
O Nausea and vomiting
O Neck stiffness
O Enlarged calf muscles
O Duchenne muscular dystrophy

Thinking Exercise 23.3.2

The nurse is caring for a 17-year-old client in the emergency department.

History and Physical	Nurses' Notes	Orders	Laboratory Results

1400: Client brought to ED by family after client developed a fever, headache, vomiting, and occasional confusion yesterday. Client lives in college dormitory; was screened this morning by campus health clinic practitioner, who recommended ED visit. Has had several sinus infections during the past few months but most recently developed a sore throat and "runny" nose. Client reports headache currently rated 9/10, and neck feels a little stiff. Feels nauseated, but better than this morning. History of Duchenne muscular dystrophy since client was 4 years of age. Uses motorized wheelchair or scooter most of the time to move around campus but is ADL independent. Drowsy but oriented × 4; PERRLA. Skin warm and dry with few petechiae noted on chest. Lung sounds clear throughout all lobes. No adventitious breath sounds. Abdomen soft and round with bowel sounds present × 4. Bilateral enlarged calf muscles. All pulses 2+; cap refill <3 sec. VS: 103°F (39.4°C), HR 110 beats/min, RR 22 breaths/min, BP 96/52 mm Hg, SpO_2 94% on RA. Denies dyspnea or chest pain.

The nurse reviews the collected client data with the registered nurse. Complete the following sentence by selecting from the lists of options below.

The client *most likely* has **1 [Select]** as evidenced by **2 [Select]** and **3 [Select]**.

OPTIONS FOR 1	OPTIONS FOR 2	OPTIONS FOR 3
Meningitis	Tachypnea	SpO$_2$
Brain tumor	Hypotension	Fever
Traumatic brain injury	Neck stiffness	Tachycardia

Thinking Exercise 23.3.3

The nurse is caring for a 17-year-old client in the emergency department.

History and Physical	Nurses' Notes	Orders	Laboratory Results

1400: Client brought to ED by family after client developed a fever, headache, vomiting, and occasional confusion yesterday. Client lives in college dormitory; was screened this morning by campus health clinic practitioner, who recommended ED visit. Has had several sinus infections during the past few months but most recently developed a sore throat and "runny" nose. Client reports headache currently rated 9/10, and neck feels a little stiff. Feels nauseated, but better than this morning. History of Duchenne muscular dystrophy since client was 4 years of age. Uses motorized wheelchair or scooter most of the time to move around campus but is ADL independent. Drowsy but oriented × 4; PERRLA. Skin warm and dry with few petechiae noted on chest. Lung sounds clear throughout all lobes. No adventitious breath sounds. Abdomen soft and round with bowel sounds present × 4. Bilateral enlarged calf muscles. All pulses 2+; cap refill <3 sec. VS: 103°F (39.4°C), HR 110 beats/min, RR 22 breaths/min, BP 96/52 mm Hg, SpO$_2$ 94% on RA. Denies dyspnea or chest pain.

The nurse collaborates with the registered nurse and contributes to the client's plan of care. Complete the following sentence by selecting from the list of word choices below.

The *priority* for client care at this time would be to **[Word Choice]**.

WORD CHOICES
Manage the headache pain.
Control the nausea and vomiting.
Manage the central nervous system infection.
Prevent decreasing level of consciousness.

Thinking Exercise 23.3.4

The nurse is caring for a 17-year-old client in the emergency department.

History and Physical	Nurses' Notes	Orders	Laboratory Results

1400: Client brought to ED by family after client developed a fever, headache, vomiting, and occasional confusion yesterday. Client lives in college dormitory; was screened this morning by campus health clinic practitioner, who recommended ED visit. Has had several sinus infections during the past few months but most recently developed a sore throat and "runny" nose. Client reports headache currently rated 9/10, and neck feels a little stiff. Feels nauseated, but better than this morning. History of Duchenne muscular dystrophy since client was 4 years of age. Uses motorized wheelchair or scooter most of the time to move around campus but is ADL independent. Drowsy but oriented × 4; PERRLA. Skin warm and dry with few petechiae noted on chest. Lung sounds clear throughout all lobes. No adventitious breath sounds. Abdomen soft and round with bowel sounds present × 4. Bilateral enlarged calf muscles. All pulses 2+; cap refill <3 sec. VS: 103°F (39.4°C), HR 110 beats/min, RR 22 breaths/min, BP 96/52 mm Hg, SpO$_2$ 94% on RA. Denies dyspnea or chest pain.

The nurse collaborates with the registered nurse and contributes to the client's plan of care. Select whether the following potential nursing actions are indicated or not indicated for the client at this time.

POTENTIAL NURSING ACTIONS	INDICATED	NOT INDICATED
Prepare for probable lumbar puncture.		
Obtain peripheral venous access.		
Start high-flow oxygen via facemask.		
Monitor for seizure activity.		
Place the client on Droplet Precautions.		

Thinking Exercise 23.3.5

The nurse is caring for a 17-year-old client in the emergency department.

History and Physical	Nurses' Notes	Orders	Laboratory Results

1400: Client brought to ED by family after client developed a fever, headache, vomiting, and occasional confusion yesterday. Client lives in college dormitory; was screened this morning by campus health clinic practitioner, who recommended ED visit. Has had several sinus infections during the past few months but most recently developed a sore throat and "runny" nose. Client reports headache currently rated 9/10, and neck feels a little stiff. Feels nauseated, but better than this morning. History of Duchenne muscular dystrophy since client was 4 years of age. Uses motorized wheelchair or scooter most of the time to move around campus but is ADL independent. Drowsy but oriented × 4; PERRLA. Skin warm and dry with few petechiae noted on chest. Lung sounds clear throughout all lobes. No adventitious breath sounds. Abdomen soft and round with bowel sounds present × 4. Bilateral enlarged calf muscles. All pulses 2+; cap refill <3 sec. VS: 103°F (39.4°C), HR 110 beats/min, RR 22 breaths/min, BP 96/52 mm Hg, SpO$_2$ 94% on RA. Denies dyspnea or chest pain.

1445: Peripheral venous access obtained in left forearm. NS infusing at 125 mL/h.

1540: Continues to be drowsy but oriented × 4. PERRLA. Lumbar puncture performed. CSF opening pressure 29 cm H$_2$O (normal value is ≤25 cm H$_2$O). CSF sample slightly cloudy and sent to lab for stat analysis. VS: 102.4°F (39.1°C), HR 106 beats/min, RR 20 breaths/min, BP 100/56 mm Hg, SpO$_2$ 95% on RA.

1655: CSF analysis positive for meningococcal meningitis.

1735: Admit to private room in acute care unit for treatment.

The nurse reviews the collected client data with the registered nurse. Select the **3** nursing actions that would be appropriate for the nurse to implement when admitting the client to the acute care unit.

○ Administer antibiotic therapy per protocol.
○ Place the client on protective (reverse) isolation.
○ Administer antiseizure drug therapy.
○ Monitor vital signs every 8 to 12 hours.
○ Monitor neurologic status frequently.
○ Keep the room as brightly lit as possible.

Thinking Exercise 23.3.6

The nurse is caring for a 17-year-old client in the emergency department.

History and Physical	Nurses' Notes	Orders	Laboratory Results

Emergency Department

1400: Client brought to ED by family after client developed a fever, headache, vomiting, and occasional confusion yesterday. Client lives in college dormitory; was screened this morning by campus health clinic practitioner, who recommended ED visit. Has had several sinus infections during the past few months but most recently developed a sore throat and "runny" nose. Client reports headache currently rated 9/10, and neck feels a little stiff. Feels nauseated, but better than this morning. History of Duchenne muscular dystrophy since client was 4 years of age. Uses motorized wheelchair or scooter most of the time to move around campus but is ADL independent. Drowsy but oriented × 4; PERRLA. Skin warm and dry with few petechiae noted on chest. Lung sounds clear throughout all lobes. No adventitious breath sounds. Abdomen soft and round with bowel sounds present × 4. Bilateral enlarged calf muscles. All pulses 2+; cap refill <3 sec. VS: T 103°F (39.4°C), HR 110 beats/min, RR 22 breaths/min, BP 96/52 mm Hg, SpO$_2$ 94% on RA. Denies dyspnea or chest pain.

1445: Peripheral venous access obtained in left forearm. NS infusing at 125 mL/h.

1540: Continues to be drowsy but oriented × 4. PERRLA. Lumbar puncture performed. CSF opening pressure 29 cm H$_2$O (normal value is ≤25 cm H$_2$O). CSF sample slightly cloudy and sent to lab for stat analysis. VS: T 102.4°F (39.1°C), HR 106 beats/min, RR 20 breaths/min, BP 100/56 mm Hg, SpO$_2$ 95% on RA.

1655: CSF analysis positive for meningococcal meningitis.

1735: Admit to private room in acute care unit for treatment.

Acute Care Unit—3 Days Later

0810: Alert and oriented × 4, PERRLA. No seizure activity for past 24 hours. Reports headache rated 2/10. No nausea or vomiting. VS: T 99.4°F (37.4°C), HR 88 beats/min, RR 16 breaths/min, BP 146/92 mm Hg, SpO$_2$ 95% on RA.

The nurse collaborates with the registered nurse to evaluate the effectiveness of the client's plan of care. For each data collection finding, select whether the finding indicates that the client's status has improved or not improved.

CLIENT FINDINGS	IMPROVED	NOT IMPROVED
Headache pain rated 2/10		
Alert and oriented × 4		
Temperature 99.4°F (37.4°C)		
Heart rate 88 beats/min		
Blood pressure 146/92 mm Hg		

Stand-Alone Thinking Exercise 23.1

The nurse is caring for an 18-year-old client at the campus health care center.

History and Physical	Nurses' Notes	Orders	Laboratory Results

0850: Client brought to campus health care center by friends 2 weeks after returning from a college spring break trip to a Caribbean island. Client developed a fever 3 days ago with headache (7/10 pain), anorexia, abdominal pain, and fatigue. Yesterday a friend at college noticed the client's skin and corner of the sclerae had a yellowish appearance. Client has asthma triggered by seasonal allergies but reports no other significant medical history. Has noticed voiding darker than usual urine for the past few days. Alert and oriented × 4. Skin warm, dry, and jaundiced. Lung sounds clear throughout all lobes. No adventitious breath sounds. Abdomen soft, round, and tender with bowel sounds present × 4. All pulses 2+; cap refill <3 sec. VS: 102.4°F (39.1°C), HR 104 beats/min, RR 16 breaths/min, BP 118/74 mm Hg, SpO$_2$ 97% on RA.

The nurse reviews the collected client data with the registered nurse. Complete the diagram by selecting from the choices below to specify what potential condition the client is likely experiencing, **2** nursing actions that are appropriate to take, and **2** parameters the nurse would monitor to assess the client's progress.

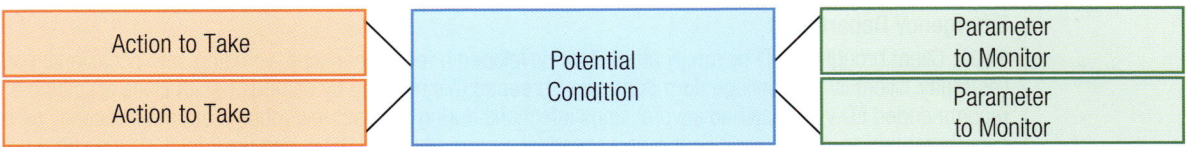

Actions to Take	Potential Conditions	Parameters to Monitor
Initiate oxygen therapy	Appendicitis	Body temperature
Use Standard Precautions when providing care	Influenza	Appetite
Administer an appropriate vaccine immediately	Hepatitis A	SpO_2
Provide supportive therapy including intravenous fluids and rest	Acute kidney injury	Skin and sclerae
Prepare the client for hemodialysis		Serum creatinine

Stand-Alone Thinking Exercise 23.2

The nurse is caring for a 14-year-old client at the urgent care center.

History and Physical	Nurses' Notes	Orders	Laboratory Results

0635: Client brought to urgent care center by family after client developed finger swelling, severe joint pain, abdominal pain, and muscle spasms in the lower legs for the past 24 hours. Client also reports fatigue and anorexia. Client's medical history includes gastroesophageal reflux disorder (GERD), iron deficiency anemia, and recent COVID-19 infection. Alert and oriented × 4. PERRLA. Skin warm and dry. Lung sounds clear throughout all lobes. No adventitious breath sounds. Abdomen distended and very tender when touched; bowel sounds present × 4. All pulses 2+; cap refill <3 sec. VS: 100.8°F (38.2°C), HR 98 beats/min, RR 14 breaths/min, BP 106/68 mm Hg, SpO_2 96% on RA.

0745: Peripheral venous access established. Stat labs drawn.

History and Physical	Nurses' Notes	Orders	Laboratory Results
Serum Laboratory Test and Reference Range		**0810 Today**	**3 Months Ago**
Red blood cells 4.3 × 10⁶/μL (4.3 × 10¹²/L)		2.1 × 10⁶/μL (2.1 × 10¹²/L)	4.3 × 10⁶/μL (4.3 × 10¹²/L)
Hemoglobin (10–15 g/dL [6.21 mmol/L])		5.9 g/dL (3.66 mmol/L)	10.1 g/dL (5.65 mmol/L)
Hematocrit (32%–44% [0.32–0.44 volume fraction])		17% (0.17 volume fraction)	32% (0.32 volume fraction)
White blood cells (5000–10,000/mm³ [5–10 × 10⁹/L])		10,500/mm³ (10.5 × 10⁹/L)	10,000/mm³ (10 × 10⁹/L)
Platelets (150,000–400,000/mm³ [150–400 × 10⁹/L])		398,000/mm³ (398 × 10⁹/L)	365,000/mm³ (365 × 10⁹/L)

The nurse reviews the collected client data with the registered nurse and contributes to the client's plan of care. Complete the following sentence by selecting from the list of options below.

The *priority* need for client care at this time is to **1 [Select]** because the client most likely has **2 [Select]**.

OPTIONS FOR 1	OPTIONS FOR 2
Manage pain	Hemophilia
Reduce fever	Leukemia
Ensure adequate nutrition	Sickle cell anemia
Ensure adequate tissue perfusion	Thalassemia

CHAPTER 3 Client Conditions Affecting Perfusion

Answers With Rationales for Thinking Exercises

Unfolding Case Study 3.1

Thinking Exercise 3.1.1

Answer

History and Physical	Nurses' Notes	Orders	Laboratory Results

1150: Client arrives for routine colostomy and cancer screening. Health history includes hypertension, dyslipidemia, and iron deficiency anemia. Client reports nonadherence to antihypertensive drugs due to fear that they will cause sexual dysfunction. Alert and oriented × 4, but appears restless; reports, "my vision seems foggy around the edges." Heart tones regular. Respirations are equal with lung fields clear throughout upon auscultation. Abdomen soft, round, and nontender. Bowel sounds present in all quadrants. Client confirms completing procedural preparations, stating "I haven't had anything to eat or drink besides the laxative preparation, which I finished early this morning. Currently, I feel nauseous, and I may vomit." VS: T 98.4°F (36.9°C), HR 104 beats/min, BP 194/138 mm Hg, RR 14 breaths/min, SpO$_2$ 95% on RA. Client reports headache at the back of the head, rated 6/10.

Rationale

The nurse must recognize the client's restless behavior as immediately concerning. Restlessness and fidgety behaviors are associated with many serious conditions that the nurse would want to follow up on immediately. Pain must always be addressed as a priority. Headaches can have a variety of causes including some life-threatening conditions. A headache with an accompanying report of nausea and vision changes is especially concerning, and the nurse must urgently follow up on these symptoms. The client's heart rate and blood pressure are not within normal limits. Although the client has a history of hypertension, the current blood pressure is significantly elevated. It is essential for the nurse to follow up on the blood pressure to determine if it is related to the client's tachycardia, headache, visual changes, and restlessness. Other client findings are expected or do not require immediate follow-up.
CJ Cognitive Skill: Recognize Cues
References: Linton & Matteson, 2023, pp. 673

Thinking Exercise 3.1.2

Answer

CLIENT FINDINGS	ANEMIA	HYPERTENSIVE CRISIS	HYPOGLYCEMIA
Blurred vision		X	X
Restless	X	X	X
Headache	X	X	X
Nausea		X	X
Tachycardia	X	X	X

Rationale

Anemia is a condition of too few red blood cells (RBCs). The body compensates for anemia by increasing heart and respiratory rates to circulate oxygen-carrying RBCs more quickly, shifting blood from the extremities to the brain and the heart and increasing production of erythropoietin to stimulate production of more RBCs. This client has a history of iron deficiency anemia and presents with current symptoms of anemia including tachycardia, restlessness, and headache. Other manifestations of anemia are tachypnea, cool hands and feet, pallor, fatigue, weakness, and decreased exercise tolerance. A hypertensive crisis is a sudden, severe increase in BP that is usually associated with an elevated diastolic BP of 130 mm Hg or higher. Client symptoms that correlate with a hypertensive crisis are tachycardia, headache, blurred vision, nausea, and restlessness. Clients experiencing a hypertensive crisis may also have tachypnea, confusion, chest pain, and shortness of breath. Hypoglycemia exists when the blood glucose level drops below normal. Symptoms occur based on how low the blood glucose level is and the client's ability to tolerate that level. This client exhibits signs of hypoglycemia including tachycardia, irritability, blurred vision, headache, and nausea. Additional symptoms of hypoglycemia include weakness, hunger, diaphoresis, tremors, irritability, and pallor.

CJ Cognitive Skill: Analyze Cues
References: Linton & Matteson, 2023, pp. 567–568, 673, 1023

Thinking Exercise 3.1.3

Answer

The client is *most likely* experiencing a **hypertensive crisis**. Without immediate treatment, the client is at *high risk* for **cardiac failure**, **acute kidney injury**, and **stroke**.

Rationale

The client's fingerstick blood glucose (FSBG) level is within normal limits. The client is not experiencing hypotension, diaphoresis, cool extremities, or pallor, which are commonly associated with hypoglycemia and anemia. Additionally, the client confirms not taking prescribed antihypertensive drugs for the past 5 to 6 days. These findings assist the nurse to determine that the client's condition is most consistent with hypertensive crisis, a life-threatening medical emergency. Hypertensive crisis usually occurs because a client has stopped taking antihypertensives drugs (especially beta-adrenergic antagonists, which can have a significant rebound effect) or the client has existing malignant hypertension, hypertensive encephalopathy, eclampsia, or pheochromocytoma. During a hypertensive crisis, the client's blood pressure will be high enough to cause organ damage, therefore the nurse must take immediate action. If appropriate treatment is not provided, death may follow because of cardiac failure, acute kidney injury, and stroke.

CJ Cognitive Skill: Prioritize Hypotheses
References: Linton & Matteson, 2023, pp. 567–568, 673-674, 1023; Willihnganz et al., 2022, pp. 181–187

Thinking Exercise 3.1.4

Answer

POTENTIAL NURSING ACTIONS	INDICATED	NOT INDICATED
Frequently assess for changes in level of consciousness	✗	
Establish peripheral venous access	✗	
Keep the head of the bed at less than 30 degrees		✗
Insert an indwelling urinary catheter		✗
Place oral airway and suction equipment at the bedside	✗	

Rationale

The nurse needs to establish peripheral venous access in anticipation of IV diuretics and potent vasodilators, which will most likely be administered to lower the client's blood pressure. The nurse must monitor for signs of decreased perfusion including decreased level of consciousness, seizures, chest pain, shortness of breath, decreased SpO_2, and decreased urinary output. Assessing the client's neurologic status and vital signs frequently and monitoring cardiac and renal function will assist the nurse to identify changes in the client's status. Although the nurse will be monitoring intake and output carefully, inserting an indwelling urinary catheter increases the client's risk for a health care–associated infection and is not appropriate at this time. The nurse would elevate the head of the bed to facilitate breathing and decrease intracranial pressure and place an oral airway and suction equipment at the bedside in case the client experiences cardiac or respiratory failure.

CJ Cognitive Skill: Generate Solutions
References: Linton & Matteson, 2023, pp. 673–674

Thinking Exercise 3.1.5

Answer

- ○ Administer the prescribed furosemide dose
- ○ Assist the medical technician to obtain an ECG
- ✗ Collaborate with the RN to administer IV labetalol
- ○ Consult with the cardiologist
- ○ Delegate 15-minute vital signs to assistive personnel
- ✗ Implement continuous pulse oximetry
- ○ Initiate O_2 therapy at 2 L/min via NC
- ✗ Obtain vital signs before and after each dose of labetalol

Rationale

The priority goal when treating a client experiencing a hypertensive crisis is to lower the BP as quickly as possible to prevent further organ damage. Therefore the nurse should prioritize administration of labetalol and obtain vital signs before and after each dose. Collaboration with the RN is essential as this client's condition is unstable and without predictable outcomes. Direct support from the RN is needed for the administration of IV labetalol. Continuous pulse oximetry will assist the nurse to monitor for hypoxia, a complication of inadequate perfusion. Therefore the nurse would prioritize the implementation of continuous pulse oximetry and administer supplemental oxygen if the client's SpO_2 decreases. Vital signs must be monitored every 15 minutes and should be delegated to assistive personnel after the client's condition has stabilized. The furosemide dose should be administered after the labetalol because it is an oral dose and will not lower the client's blood pressure as quickly. The ECG and cardiologist consultation would occur after initial treatment of the client's BP.

CJ Cognitive Skill: Take Actions
References: Linton & Matteson, 2023, pp. 673–674; Willihnganz et al., 2022, pp. 183–187, 365, 454–457

Thinking Exercise 3.1.6

Answer

- ✗ Accessory muscle use when breathing
- ✗ Coarse crackles auscultated in bilateral lungs
- ○ HR 82 beats/min
- ○ Headache rated 4/10

○ Resting with eyes closed
✗ RR 19 breaths/min
○ SpO$_2$ 98% on 2 L/min O$_2$ via NC
✗ Voided 140 mL of dark amber urine

Rationale

A decrease in the client's HR, BP, and pain level are signs of improvement, but other client findings should alert the nurse to the potential of organ damage and a worsening condition. Coarse crackles indicate excessive fluid on the lungs or pulmonary edema which may be caused by cardiac failure. The client's use of accessory muscles and tachypnea demonstrate a need to work harder to breath adequately and are signs the client has not improved. An oral dose of furosemide usually produces a positive effect within one hour and therefore, the nurse would expect to observe initial signs of diuresis. The client's urinary output does not reflect this expected outcome and may be a sign the client is not improving. The nurse must monitor urinary output closely and report limited effects of the diuretic to the RN and provider as this could be a sign of renal damage from hypertension.
CJ Cognitive Skill: Evaluate Outcomes
References: Linton & Matteson, 2023, pp. 673–674; Willihnganz et al., 2022, pp. 183–187

Unfolding Case Study 3.2

Thinking Exercise 3.2.1

Answer

○ Blood pressure
○ Chest diameter ratio
✗ Dyspnea
○ Emesis
✗ Pain
✗ Pale and diaphoretic
✗ SpO$_2$ level

Rationale

The nurse must recognize signs of inadequate perfusion and gas exchange and follow up on these symptoms immediately, as they are usually associated with life-threatening conditions. Pain is always a priority, especially chest pain, because it may be a sign of inadequate blood flow to the cardiac muscle. Dyspnea and hypoxemia are signs of a gas exchange problem and inadequate oxygen levels in the body. If not addressed immediately, these conditions may lead to tissue and organ death. The nurse should also recognize pallor and diaphoresis as the sympathetic nervous system response to inadequate arterial blood flow and prioritize these findings for follow-up. The client's anteroposterior-to-transverse chest diameter ratio is not within normal limits, but this is a chronic condition and does not need immediate attention. The client's elevated blood pressure and emesis are not priority concerns as these are most likely secondary responses to the client's acute condition. Prioritizing actions to address the client's pain, dyspnea, and hypoxia will subsequently resolve the client's elevated BP and nausea.
CJ Cognitive Skill: Recognize Cues
References: Linton & Matteson, 2023, pp. 461–465, 511, 617–628

Thinking Exercise 3.2.2

Answer

✗ Acute coronary syndrome
○ Alcohol withdrawal

✗ Emphysema
✗ Gastroesophageal reflux disease
○ Hyperosmolar hyperglycemia nonketotic syndrome
✗ Pulmonary embolism

Rationale

Acute coronary syndrome (ACS) is a term used to describe a range of cardiac conditions including myocardial infarction and unstable angina. Hypertension, obesity, tobacco use, and poor dietary practices are all risk factors for ACS. Chest pain, the primary sign of ACS, is usually described as burning or squeezing, and it may radiate to the arm, shoulder, neck, jaw, or epigastrium. Other client symptoms that relate to ACS are diaphoresis, dyspnea, nausea, and vomiting. The client's health history includes gastroesophageal reflux disease (GERD), therefore the nurse must evaluate if the current symptoms are potentially an exacerbation of this chronic condition. GERD symptoms may appear suddenly, commonly occur after a meal, and include severe pain that may radiate to the back, neck, or jaw. The client's symptoms began suddenly after breakfast with pain, rated 8/10, radiating to the left shoulder. The client's tobacco use via cigarettes should alert the nurse to potential lung damage resulting in chronic emphysema and chronic bronchitis. Manifestations of emphysema exhibited by the client are dyspnea (especially with exertion or when lying flat), decreased SpO_2, heaviness in the chest, use of accessory muscles for breathing, and increased anteroposterior diameter of the chest (barrel chest). The client's obesity (BMI 31) is a risk factor for the development of an emboli, and current symptoms are consistent with classic signs of a pulmonary embolism including dyspnea, chest pain, and diaphoresis. Although the client drinks alcohol daily, there is no indication that the client recently stopped or decreased alcohol use, and current symptoms do not align with those of alcohol withdrawal. Hyperosmolar hyperglycemia nonketotic syndrome (HHNS) is a life-threatening complication of uncontrolled diabetes mellitus. This client has many risk factors for diabetes mellitus, including hypertension, obesity, and poor dietary practices, but is not currently experiencing symptoms of hyperglycemia or HHNS.

CJ Cognitive Skill: Analyze Cues

References: Linton & Matteson, 2023, pp. 518, 531–533, 677–682, 759–760, 999–1006; Willihnganz et al., 2022, pp. 363–367, 371–373, 521–523

Thinking Exercise 3.2.3

Answer

The nurse recognizes that the client is **_most likely_** experiencing <u>**acute coronary syndrome**</u> as evidenced by <u>**ECG rhythm changes**</u> and <u>**chest pain not relieved with nitroglycerin**</u>.

Rationale

Although the client is experiencing symptoms associated with several conditions, additional client findings assist the nurse to focus on acute coronary syndrome as the most likely condition. ST-segment and T-wave changes on a 12-lead ECG accompanied by angina (chest pain) are signs of an ischemic myocardium and appear with stable angina or ACS. Stable angina usually occurs during physical activity or stress and resolves with rest and nitrates. Chest pain associated with ACS (unstable angina or myocardial infarction) may occur at rest or with minimal exertion and is not relieved by changing positions. Nitrates increase blood flow to the myocardium but may not eliminate chest pain when a client is experiencing unstable angina or a myocardial infarction. Additional client findings also help the nurse eliminate other conditions. Symptoms associated with GERD are commonly reduced by oral antacids and changing positions, specifically raising the head of the bed. Clients experiencing emphysema exacerbation commonly exhibit wheezing or other adventitious breath sounds, and breathing effort becomes easier when sitting in the high-Fowler or tripod position.

CJ Cognitive Skill: Prioritize Hypotheses

References: Linton & Matteson, 2023, pp. 518–519, 531–534, 677–682, 759–760; Willihnganz et al., 2022, pp. 397–403

Thinking Exercise 3.2.4

Answer

POTENTIAL NURSING ACTIONS	INDICATED	NOT INDICATED
Administer second dose of nitroglycerin sublingual	✗	
Ask spouse to remain in the waiting room		✗
Establish peripheral venous access	✗	
Initiate continuous cardiac monitoring	✗	
Request order for IV pain medication	✗	

Rationale

The nurse understands that the client's acute pain is related to inadequate myocardial tissue perfusion and would plan to implement nursing interventions to relieve pain and enhance oxygen to the myocardium. Nitroglycerin is administered to dilate coronary arteries and increase blood flow to cardiac tissue. Sublingual nitroglycerin may be administered every 5 minutes × 3 doses in an attempt to relieve chest pain. Dysrhythmias including premature ventricular contractions (PVCs), ventricular tachycardia, and ventricular fibrillation may result from myocardial tissue damage. The nurse would therefore initiate continuous cardiac monitoring to promptly identify ECG changes. Peripheral venous access must also be established to administer emergency drugs quickly and directly as needed. Finally, the nurse would request IV pain medications if not already ordered. Morphine is usually administered to relieve pain, decrease anxiety, and relax bronchial smooth muscles. The nurse would not ask the spouse to leave the bedside. Instead, the nurse would establish a calm environment for the client and spouse by providing simple explanations of procedures and equipment as well as reinforcing information given by the physician about the diagnosis and treatment.

CJ Cognitive Skill: Generate Solutions

References: Linton & Matteson, 2023, pp. 681–686; Willihnganz et al., 2022, pp. 310–315, 397–403

Thinking Exercise 3.2.5

Answer

The nurse would *prioritize* **laboratory tests** and **informed consent** so the client may be urgently transported to the **cardiac catheterization lab**.

Rationale

Emergency percutaneous coronary intervention (PCI) is the first-line treatment for myocardial infarction with the goal of reopening the occluded artery within 90 minutes of onset of chest pain. Several PCI procedures can be performed in the cardiac catheterization laboratory. Baseline laboratory tests and informed consent must be completed prior to any procedure, therefore the nurse would prioritize these activities in preparation for emergent transport off the unit. The nurse would also administer interventions for pain but would not expect the client to be pain free prior to the PCI procedure. The client would be kept NPO for the procedure and may be transferred to the intensive care unit after PCI. Cardiac rehabilitation services would be initiated after the client is stable.

CJ Cognitive Skill: Take Actions

References: Linton & Matteson, 2023, pp. 681–686

Thinking Exercise 3.2.6—Pharmacology

Answer

CLIENT STATEMENTS	UNDERSTANDING	NO UNDERSTANDING
"Chest pain may occur with activity, so I will always carry nitroglycerin tablets and contact EMS if the pain is not relieved after 3 doses."		✗
"I don't like fish, but I plan to eat more walnuts and food items that contain soybeans."	✗	
"I will begin exercising every day by walking around my city block 3 times."		✗
"My heart wouldn't need to work so hard if I lost some weight and stopped smoking."	✗	
"Spices, garlic, and onions can add flavor to my food without adding more sodium."	✗	
"Wearing a telemetry monitor when I exercise will help me become more active in a safe manner."	✗	

Rationale

The client should begin exercising by walking the same distance at home as in the hospital 3 times a day, usually around 400 feet. The client would be taught to gradually increase walking distance every other week as tolerated and directed by the health care provider. Wearing a telemetry monitor during exercise increases client safety by allowing the health care provider to monitor cardiac function, identify complications, and adjust the individualized rehabilitation plan. The client may experience angina with activity and therefore should be taught to always carry nitroglycerin tablets or spray. The nurse would also teach the client to cease activity, sit down, and place 1 nitroglycerin tablet or spray under the tongue at the first indication of chest discomfort. Within 5 minutes, if no relief results, the client would be taught to call emergency medical services (EMS) and then repeat the nitroglycerin dose while waiting for services to arrive. The client should not take 3 doses of nitroglycerin before calling for medical assistance. A major treatment component for clients with heart disease is nutrition to maintain normal weight or lose weight if obese. The client would be taught strategies to decrease sodium, decrease saturated fats, and eliminate unsaturated fats in the diet. Foods containing omega-3 fatty acids, such as certain fish, walnuts, and soybeans, may help lower serum triglycerides and decrease mortality from heart disease. Smoking stimulates the heart rate and causes blood vessels to constrict, which makes the heart work harder. Smoking cessation is essential.

CJ Cognitive Skill: Evaluation Outcomes
References: Linton & Matteson, 2023, pp. 681–686; Willihnganz et al., 2022, pp. 397–403

Stand-Alone Thinking Exercise 3.1

Answer

Initiate IV fluids			Intake and output
Administer pain medication		Sickle cell crisis	Vital signs

Rationale

The client is most likely experiencing a sickle cell crisis. A sickle cell crisis occurs when sickled cells become stuck in larger blood vessels of the body, obstructing blood flow and causing severe pain. Symptoms vary depending on where the circulation is blocked, but circulation to the chest, abdomen, and extremities is commonly compromised during a sickle cell crisis. There is no test to confirm sickle cell crisis, but clients with known sickle cell disease who complain of severe pain are believed to be in crisis. This client has a history of sickle cell anemia and presents with severe pain in the bilateral upper extremities as well as discomfort in the chest and abdomen. Additionally, client findings correlate with some of the stressors that can trigger a sickle cell crisis, including infection, cold weather changes, and dehydration. For this client, infection may be suspected based on the client's elevated temperature, elevated white blood cell count, and right lower leg assessment (hyperpigmentation, edema, and multiple venous ulcers). The client appears to also have been caught unprepared for cold weather. Finally, the client's heart rate and blood pressure as well as BUN and creatine levels indicate potential dehydration. The nurse would administer IV fluids to correct any dehydration and help the kidneys clear metabolic wastes from ruptured RBCs. Pain medication would also be administered to manage severe pain that occurs during these episodes. The nurse would monitor intake and output to evaluate the client's hydration status and measure vital signs frequently for further signs of infection (sepsis) and dehydration. Supplemental O_2 can be administered but has little benefit in reversing the crisis, and the client's SpO_2 is currently 96%. Hydroxyurea is prescribed as a preventive treatment for clients who experience frequent crises. Once a client is in crisis, hydroxyurea does not work quickly enough to reduce either the severity or duration of the crisis. The client's leg wounds would be addressed after prioritizing treatments for symptoms of sickle cell crisis. The nurse would recognize that client findings of the right lower extremity are most likely due to peripheral venous insufficiency, not an arterial embolism, which usually presents with pain, pallor, pulselessness, paresthesia, and paralysis. The client has a history of type 2 diabetes mellitus and an elevated blood glucose level. The nurse would provide oral antidiabetic medication or SQ insulin to lower the glucose level. DKA is associated with insulin-dependent or type 1 diabetes mellitus, not type 2. The jaundice noted in the client's sclera and conjunctiva is most likely related to chronic sickle cell disease. Sickle cells do not live as long as normal RBCs and die faster than the liver can filter them out. Bilirubin, from broken down cells, builds up and causes jaundice.

CJ Cognitive Skill: Recognize Cues, Analyze Cues, Prioritize Hypotheses, Generate Solutions, Take Actions, Evaluate Outcomes

References: Linton & Matteson, 2023, pp. 569–571, 702–708, 1005; Pagana et al., 2023, pp. 150, 296, 449, 749, 946

Stand-Alone Thinking Exercise 3.2

Answer

Based on assessment findings and medical history, the client is ***most likely*** experiencing **symptomatic bradycardia.** The nurse would **insert a peripheral venous device** in anticipation of **atropine administration** and prepare for **transcutaneous pacing** if the client's condition does not improve.

Rationale

The client is experiencing bradycardia (HR <60 beats/min). Bradycardia can occur after a myocardial infarction or cardiac surgery as a result of damage to heart tissue. Clients with bradycardia may be asymptomatic except for the decreased pulse rate, or they may be symptomatic, indicating that the decreased pulse rate is failing to adequately perfuse the body. Client findings consistent with symptomatic bradycardia are hypotension, chest pain, shortness of breath, and light-headedness. The administration of intravenous atropine sulfate is prioritized to increase the client's HR and cardiac output. Other interventions for symptomatic bradycardia,, including administration of supplemental oxygen (to increase SpO_2) and intravenous fluids (to increase BP), focus on treating underlying causes and managing symptoms. If the HR does not increase sufficiently, transcutaneous pacing would be used to produce a faster pulse rate. Classic signs of pulmonary embolism are dyspnea, chest pain, hemoptysis, cough, orthopnea, tachycardia, and wheezing or crackles heard upon auscultation. The client is experiencing dyspnea and chest pain, but other client findings assist the nurse to eliminate pulmonary embolism as the most likely option. Cardiopulmonary resuscitation is the restoration of heart and lung function after cardiac arrest. This client has a pulse and is breathing, therefore the client is not experiencing cardiac arrest. Defibrillation is the delivery of an electrical shock to the heart to restore normal cardiac conduction and contraction in a client experiencing ventricular fibrillation or pulseless ventricular tachycardia. Defibrillation is not used if the client has a pulse.

CJ Cognitive Skill: Recognize Cues, Analyze Cues, Prioritize Hypotheses, Generate Solutions, Take Actions

References: Linton & Matteson, 2023, pp. 518, 635–636, 647, 652

Stand-Alone Thinking Exercise 3.3

Answer

| Administer drugs to correct the cardiac rhythm and control the pulse rate | → | Atrial fibrillation | → | Level of orientation |
| Teach the client about anticoagulation | | | | Urine output |

Rationale

The nurse must recognize that the client findings are caused by the client's heart rhythm, which is fast (tachycardia) and irregular. The current rhythm is interfering with the heart's ability to properly pump, resulting in decreased cardiac output and inadequate perfusion of the body. Although there are many cardiac rhythms that negatively affect cardiac output, the client's history of hyperthyroidism and current symptoms most closely align with atrial fibrillation (Afib). Afib is characterized as a very irregular rhythm with an arterial rate above 400 beats/min and a ventricular rate from 100 to 150 beats/min. Symptoms of Afib are heart palpitations and signs of decreased cardiac output including dizziness or light-headedness, dyspnea, and angina. Treatment goals for Afib focus on correcting the rhythm and controlling the rate of the rhythm to increase cardiac output and prevent embolus formation due to pooling blood in the atria. Therefore the nurse anticipates administration of drugs, such as calcium channel blockers or beta-adrenergic blockers, to slow conduction and decrease the ventricular rate; antidysrhythmic drugs, such amiodarone or ibutilide, to restore a normal rhythm; and anticoagulant drugs, such as warfarin or dabigatran, to prevent embolus formation. Client education should be provided for all medications administered; specific teachings related to anticoagulation therapy are signs of bleeding and safety measures to prevent injury. The nurse would closely monitor for further signs of decreased cardiac output including neurologic changes, decreased urine output, abdominal pain, cold and clammy extremities, tachycardia, and hypotension. The nurse would also monitor for signs of bleeding, a complication of anticoagulant therapy. Clinical manifestations of internal bleeding are similar to those of decreased cardiac output and include confusion; vision changes; abdominal pain; dark, tarry stools; dyspnea; tachycardia; and hypotension. Although the client has a history of hyperthyroidism, symptoms of a thyroid storm are high fever, delirium, loss of consciousness, and congestive heart failure, which the client is not currently experiencing. The client's swollen and bulging eyes are most likely a symptom of hyperthyroidism (exophthalmos) and not caused by an allergic reaction. Cardiomyopathy may cause an abnormally fast heart rate and rhythm, but the client is not experiencing abdominal bloating, peripheral edema, or hypertension, which are common signs of cardiomyopathy.

CJ Cognitive Skill: Recognize Cues, Analyze Cues, Prioritize Hypotheses, Generate Solutions, Take Actions, Evaluate Outcomes

References: Linton & Matteson, 2023, pp. 636; Willihnganz et al., 2022, pp. 382–396, 424–433

Answers With Rationales for Thinking Exercises

Thinking Exercise 4.1.1

Answer

History and Physical	Nurses' Notes	Orders	Laboratory Results

1115: Client assessed in the emergency department. Alert and oriented × 4, but unable to speak full sentences due to shortness of breath. Client's spouse is a bedside and states, "Feelings of breathless with moderate activity started several days ago. It has progressively worsened to difficulty breathing at rest and an inability to sleep at night." Heart tones regular and pulses palpable throughout. Client denies chest pain. Bilateral lower extremity 2+ pitting edema present. Barrel chest; wheezing and bilateral rhonchi auscultated in lung fields. Productive cough present with a large amount of yellow-green sputum. Abdomen soft and obese with normal bowel sounds. VS: T 97.3°F (36.2°C), HR 84 beats/min, RR 24 breaths/min, BP 109/56 mm Hg, SpO_2 90% on 2 L/min O_2 via NC.

Rationale

The client's dyspnea, occurring at rest and interfering with speech and sleep, requires immediate follow-up by the nurse and health care team. Tachypnea and decreased oxygen saturation level are signs of potential hypoxemia and must be addressed immediately to prevent organ and tissue damage. Adventitious breath sounds may be causing or resulting from various life-threatening conditions, therefore the nurse should further assess these findings. A large amount of yellow-green sputum is concerning, but the client is currently able to expectorate with a productive cough, therefore sputum amount and color are not life-threatening. The client's barrel chest, obesity, and lower extremity edema are abnormal but not priorities at this time. Other client findings are within normal parameters.
CJ Cognitive Skill: Recognize Cues
References: Linton & Matteson, 2023, pp. 531–532

Thinking Exercise 4.1.2

Answer

✗ Acute COPD exacerbation
○ Acute severe asthma
✗ Heart failure
○ Gastroesophageal reflux disease
○ Liver cirrhosis
✗ Pneumonia

Rationale

The client's health history, including chronic hypertension, hyperlipidemia, morbid obesity, and tobacco smoking, increased the client's risk for heart failure (HF). Symptoms of HF exhibited by the client are dyspnea with activity and progressing to dyspnea at rest, orthopnea, pitting edema, and pulmonary congestion (rhonchi). The client also has a history of chronic obstructive pulmonary disease (COPD), which increases the client's risk for pneumonia and the probability of an acute COPD exacerbation (flare-up). Client symptoms correlating with pneumonia are dyspnea and cough with yellow-green sputum. Increased dyspnea, increased sputum production, wheezing, peripheral edema, and difficulty sleeping are client findings that correlate with an exacerbation of COPD. Barrel chest is a sign of chronic pulmonary disease. Obesity is a risk factor for liver cirrhosis and gastroesophageal reflux disease, but the client is not presenting with any findings that correlate with these disorders. The client does not have a history of asthma, and client findings progressed slowly over several days, which is inconsistent with acute severe asthma (status asthmaticus).

CJ Cognitive Skill: Analyze Cues

References: Linton & Matteson, 2023, pp. 509–510, 524–527, 531–532, 687–688, 759–760, 799–801

Thinking Exercise 4.1.3

Answer

The nurse recognizes that the client is most likely experiencing **acute COPD exacerbation**.
The nurse would prioritize **breathing techniques** and **airway clearance** to improve gas exchange.

Rationale

Based on client findings and health history, the nurse would determine that the client is most likely experiencing an acute exacerbation of COPD, a chronic inflammatory lung disease that causes obstructed gas exchange within the lungs. COPD is characterized by bronchoconstriction, bronchial inflammation, and damaged alveoli. Interventions to improve gas exchange focus on improving ventilation and maintaining airway clearance. Breathing techniques such as tripod breathing, effective coughing, and positioning promote gas exchange. Fluid restrictions are not helpful for acute COPD exacerbation. There is no indication that the client has a bacterial infection, so antibiotic therapy is not appropriate at this time. Airway clearance may be facilitated by drug therapy such as bronchodilators and nebulizer treatments. Cardiac rehabilitation is appropriate after a cardiac event like a myocardial infarction. The client is already receiving supplemental oxygen therapy. Increasing the oxygen flow may not be safe for this client depending on the amount of carbon dioxide that is being retained.

CJ Cognitive Skill: Prioritize Hypothesis

References: Linton & Matteson, 2023, pp. 531–535

Thinking Exercise 4.1.4

Answer

POTENTIAL NURSING INTERVENTIONS	INDICATED	NOT INDICATED
Place the client in an upright position with the head of the bed elevated	✗	
Use supplemental oxygen to keep oxygen saturation levels at 88% to 92%	✗	
Perform nasotracheal suction to clear the client's airway		✗
Assist the care team to obtain an arterial blood sample to assess ABGs	✗	
Encourage the client to remain out of bed for 3 hours twice a day		✗

Rationale

Client findings indicate acute respiratory distress as a result of COPD exacerbation. Therefore the client would remain in bed but be placed in an upright position with the head of the bed elevated. This position will help alleviate the client's dyspnea by promoting increased chest expansion and keeping the diaphragm in the proper position to contract. When the client can tolerate sitting in a chair, the nurse would encourage the client to get out of bed for 1-hour periods two to three times a day. Arterial blood gas (ABG) values provide essential information related to the client's gas exchange, oxygenation, ventilation, and acid-base status. The nurse would assist the health care team to obtain baseline ABG values, which will be used to guide the plan of care and evaluate the client's response to treatments. All hypoxic clients, including those with COPD, should receive oxygen therapy at rates appropriate to reduce hypoxia. Supplemental oxygen would be titrated to keep the client's PaO_2 level greater than 60 mm Hg and SpO_2 level between 88% and 92%, depending on the amount of arterial carbon dioxide. This client's SpO_2 is currently within range at 90% on 2 L/min O_2 via NC; the nurse would continue to monitor saturation levels carefully. Nasotracheal suction is not appropriate for this client; it is only used for clients with a weak cough, weak pulmonary muscles, and an inability to expectorate effectively.

CJ Cognitive Skill: Generate Solutions

References: Linton & Matteson, 2023, pp. 531–539; Pagana et al., 2023, pp. 100–107

Thinking Exercise 4.1.5—Pharmacology

Answer

PRESCRIBED MEDICATIONS	NURSING ACTIONS
Albuterol 2.5 mg/ipratropium bromide 0.5 mg by nebulizer every 6 hours	✗ Assess the client's HR and rhythm prior to and during nebulizer treatments. ✗ Report an increase in HR of 20 beats/min or more to the provider. ✗ Encourage the client to suck on ice chips or hard candy.
Budesonide 2 inhalations 2 times per day	✗ Assess the client for signs and symptoms of pneumonia. ✗ Assist the client to gargle and rinse the mouth with a nonalcoholic mouthwash after each dose. ○ Position the client with the head of the bed elevated at 30 degrees during administration of inhalants.
Guaifenesin 200 mg orally every 4 hours	○ Administer 1 hour before or 2 hours after meals. ✗ Promote fluid intake of 8 to 12 8-ounce glasses of water daily. ✗ Use a humidifier when providing supplemental oxygen.

Rationale

The client should be placed in the high-Fowler position for nebulizer and inhalant medications to increase airway patency and medication perfusion throughout the respiratory tract. The client's nebulizer treatment is a combination of albuterol (a beta-adrenergic bronchodilation agent) and ipratropium bromide (an anticholinergic bronchodilation agent). Both drugs can cause tachycardia and palpitations. Therefore the nurse would assess the client's heart rate and rhythm at regular intervals throughout treatment and report a 20 beats/min or more increase in heart rate to the provider. Anticholinergic effects may cause dry mouth. The nurse would encourage the client to alleviate dryness by sucking on ice chips or hard candy. Budesonide is an inhaled corticosteroid used to decrease respiratory inflammation. Corticosteroids increase the client's risk for the development of oral thrush. Therefore the nurse would instruct the client to perform good oral hygiene techniques and gargle and rinse the mouth with a nonalcoholic mouthwash after each treatment. An increased risk of pneumonia is associated with the use of inhaled corticosteroids in clients with COPD, therefore the nurse would monitor for symptoms of pneumonia. Guaifenesin is an expectorant that acts by enhancing the output of respiratory tract fluid. The increased flow of secretions decreases mucus viscosity and promotes ciliary action. A combination of ciliary action and coughing then expels the phlegm from the pulmonary system. The nurse would encourage the client to drink 8 to 12 8-ounce glasses of water daily and humidify supplemental oxygen to assist with thinning of bronchial secretions for expectoration of mucus. Guaifenesin may be administered without regard to food.

CJ Cognitive Skill: Take Actions

References: Willihnganz et al., 2022, pp. 481–504

Thinking Exercise 4.1.6

Answer

CLIENT STATEMENTS	UNDERSTANDING	NO UNDERSTANDING
"I will perform controlled coughing exercises in the morning and at night before bed to help clear my lungs."	✗	
"When I feel breathless, sitting forward in my chair and leaning against a table may help me catch my breath."	✗	
"Taking my ipratropium inhaler routinely will help prevent symptoms of dyspnea."	✗	
"When my breathing rate increases, I should hold a paper bag over my mouth and nose and try to take normal breaths."		✗
"Losing some weight may decrease my symptoms and help me tolerate more activity."	✗	

Rationale

Effective coughing can improve gas exchange by increasing airflow and removing secretions in the airways. The client should perform controlled coughing upon rising in the morning to eliminate mucus that collected during the night and in the evening before bed to help clear lungs for a less interrupted night's sleep. Sitting forward and leaning on a table will assist the client to relax and resume normal breathing after periods of breathlessness. This position increases chest expansion, improves diaphragm contractions, and conserves energy by supporting the client's arms and upper body. Breathing into a paper bag is contraindicated as this would increase the concentration of inspired CO_2 in a client who already likely has issues exhaling CO_2 and is consequently retaining a high level of this gas in the body. The client should sit in a chair, lean forward, and use diaphragmatic or pursed lip breathing when experiencing episodes of hyperventilation (tripod or orthopneic position). Excess weight increases the work of breathing and contributes to symptoms of breathlessness, dyspnea, and fatigue. Clients with COPD frequently experience weight loss and become underweight. This client's health history indicates morbid obesity, therefore weight loss would be beneficial and may decrease symptoms and improve activity tolerance.

CJ Cognitive Skill: Evaluate Outcomes
References: Linton & Matteson, 2023, pp. 531–539

Unfolding Case Study 4.2

Thinking Exercise 4.2.1

Answer

○ Anorexia
✗ Chest pain
○ Fatigue
✗ Dyspnea
○ Body temperature
○ Pedal pulses
✗ SpO_2

Rationale

The nurse should recognize a change in the client's status including new-onset chest pain and dyspnea, which could be caused by a life-threatening condition. These findings need immediate follow-up by the nurse. Several of the client's vital signs are outside of normal parameters. The client's peripheral oxygen saturation level (SpO_2) is low (<95%), presenting a high risk for serious damage to vital organs, and needs to be addressed immediately. The client's heart rate is most likely a response to hypoxemia and should be followed up. The client's temperature is not life-threatening. The client's pulses are weak but palpable throughout. Anorexia and fatigue are common responses to cancer and chemotherapy; these are not emergent issues.

CJ Cognitive Skill: Recognize Cues
References: Linton & Matteson, 2023, pp. 518–519

Thinking Exercise 4.2.2

Answer

The nurse recognizes that the client is most likely experiencing **pulmonary embolism** as evidenced by **sudden onset of dyspnea** and **stabbing chest pain**.

Rationale

This client is most likely experiencing pulmonary embolism (PE), which typically presents with sudden onset of dyspnea and stabbing chest pain. Vital signs associated with PE include tachycardia, tachypnea, low-grade fever, and low SpO_2, indicating hypoxemia. Apprehension and diaphoresis may also occur with PE, but these are vague symptoms and do not assist the nurse to differentiate the potential conditions. PE most often occurs when a blood clot breaks loose from a deep vein thrombosis (DVT), travels through the right side of the heart, and lodges within the pulmonary artery or one or more of its branches. Clients with cancer and those receiving chemotherapy treatment are at high risk for venous thromboembolism (VTE) (either DVT, PE, or both). This client's right leg assessment is consistent with a DVT. The client is also at risk for pneumonia and metastatic cancer, but these conditions do not present with sudden onset of symptoms.

CJ Cognitive Skill: Analyze Cues
References: Linton & Matteson, 2023, pp. 509–510, 518–519, 546–547

Thinking Exercise 4.2.3

Answer

The nurse determines that the *priority* for care at this time is to manage the client's **hypoxemia**.

Rationale

The client's priority, life-threatening problem is hypoxemia or low blood oxygen saturation levels (SpO_2). Pulmonary embolism creates a mismatch of ventilation (air breathed in) and perfusion (blood flow), which causes hypoxemia. If not treated emergently, the client risks hypoxia (low levels of oxygen in body tissues) and tissue and organ death. Anxiety, chest pain, and tachycardia are most likely symptoms from a lack of oxygen and may be relieved by addressing the client's hypoxemia.

CJ Cognitive Skill: Prioritize Hypotheses
References: Linton & Matteson, 2023, pp. 518–519

Thinking Exercise 4.2.4

Answer

POTENTIAL NURSING ACTIONS	INDICATED	NOT INDICATED
Transfer the client to a bed, and position with the head of the bed elevated 30 degrees.		X
Apply a continuous pulse oximetry device to assess oxygenation.	X	
Perform chest percussion to assist the client with expectoration.		X
Monitor respiratory status including rate, effort, and lung sounds.	X	
Contact the provider and arrange an ambulance for transport to the hospital.	X	

Rationale

The nurse would place the client in the high-Fowler position (rather than the semi-Fowler position at 30 degrees) to improve ventilation and would assess the client's oxygenation continuously with pulse oximetry to determine if a higher flow of oxygen is needed to achieve an SpO_2 >94%. The client needs further medical care than can be provided at an outpatient infusion center. Therefore the nurse would contact the provider and arrange transportation for the client to be taken to a hospital. Additionally, the nurse would monitor the client's respiratory rate, effort and breath sounds, pulse rate, blood pressure, and skin color frequently for improvement or possible decline in status. The client may experience a cough and hemoptysis; chest percussion will not improve expectoration of this sputum and may negatively affect the client by increasing anxiety or pain.

CJ Cognitive Skill: Generate Solutions
References: Linton & Matteson, 2023, pp. 518–519

Thinking Exercise 4.2.5

Answer

- ✗ Apply a 5-lead telemetry monitor
- ○ Initiate a heparin infusion
- ○ Contact dietary for a lunch tray
- ○ Increase the supplemental oxygen rate
- ✗ Assess vital signs
- ○ Obtain a wheelchair for a radiology test
- ✗ Collaborate with the laboratory for serum blood tests

Rationale

The nurse would prioritize the application of the telemetry monitor and vital signs. Baseline assessment is necessary to determine client needs, generate appropriate interventions, and take actions in a timely manner. The client's oxygen saturation is greater than 94% on 4 L/min O_2 via NC; increasing the supplemental oxygen rate is not needed. Initiating anticoagulation therapy is important, but serum blood test results must be assessed prior to starting the infusion. Therefore the nurse will prioritize collaboration with the laboratory to complete serum blood tests and obtain results. The provider ordered a portable chest x-ray, meaning the client will not need to be transported off the unit for the radiology test. Dietary needs will be addressed after the client is stabilized and no procedures requiring NPO status are anticipated.

CJ Cognitive Skill: Take Actions
References: Linton & Matteson, 2023, pp. 518–519

Thinking Exercise 4.2.6

Answer

DATA COLLECTION FINDING	IMPROVED	NOT IMPROVED
Heart rate	✗	
Lung sounds		✗
Oxygen saturation	✗	
Pain	✗	
Respiratory rate		✗

Rationale

The client's plan of care to manage hypoxemia was effective as evidenced by increased oxygen saturation and decreased heart rate. The client also denies dyspnea and chest pain, which are significant signs of improvement. The client continues to experience tachypnea and crackles within lung fields. A pulmonary embolism may take weeks or months to totally dissolve. The client's symptoms should continue to improve as the clot gets smaller. The client reports generalized discomfort, rated 4/10, which is most likely related to cancer and associated therapy and was previously identified as an acceptable pain level by the client.

CJ Cognitive Skill: Evaluate Outcomes
References: Linton & Matteson, 2023, pp. 518–519

Stand-Alone Thinking Exercise 4.1

Answer

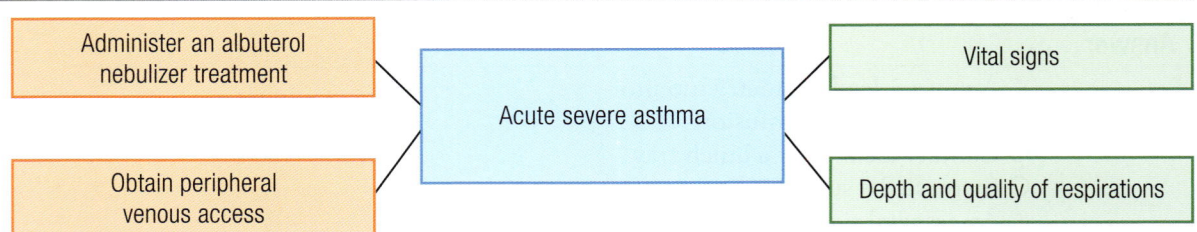

Rationale

Client findings are most consistent with an acute exacerbation of asthma, which correlates with the client's medical history. Acute severe asthma (status asthmaticus) is a severe, life-threatening acute episode of airway obstruction that intensifies once it begins and often does not respond to usual therapy. Symptoms of acute severe asthma are labored breathing, wheezing, use of accessory muscles for breathing, distention of neck veins, tachypnea, tachycardia, and diaphoresis. The client's condition must be addressed immediately to prevent cardiac or respiratory arrest. The nurse would administer an albuterol nebulizer treatment and start a peripheral venous device for IV fluids, systemic bronchodilators, steroids, and potentially epinephrine if the client does not respond to other therapies. Although the client's SpO_2 is currently within normal limits, the nurse would monitor the client's vital signs and oxygen saturation level to identify client decline and need for additional oxygen or ventilation support. The nurse will also monitor the depth and quality of the client's respirations to evaluate therapeutic outcomes and identify signs of respiratory failure. Airway obstruction and hypoxemia are most likely causing the client's tachypnea. Although the client does not verbalize feelings of anxiety, fear, or uneasiness, these symptoms may be present because of the client's breathlessness and chest tightness. Acute bronchitis is usually caused by a viral infection and presents with a productive cough, fever, chills, chest discomfort, and mild shortness of breath. The client denies having a recent infection, and client findings do not include cough or fever. Allergic rhinitis is inflammation of the nasal passages caused by an allergen. This client does not have symptoms of allergic rhinitis, which include nasal congestion, clear rhinorrhea, sneezing, and nasal pruritus.

CJ Cognitive Skills: Recognize Cues, Analyze Cues, Priority Hypotheses, Generate Solutions, Take Actions, Evaluate Outcomes
Reference: Linton & Matteson, 2023, pp. 524–530

Stand-Alone Thinking Exercise 4.2

Answer

POTENTIAL NURSING ACTIONS	INDICATED	NOT INDICATED
Assist the client to change position at least every 2 hours.	✗	
Teach the client to hold a pillow firmly over the abdominal incision prior to performing coughing and deep breathing exercises.	✗	
Encourage the client to perform coughing and deep breathing exercises every hour.	✗	
Instruct the client to take a deep breath and then blow out the air through the incentive spirometer mouthpiece.		✗
Promote early ambulation by assisting the client to walk in the hallway several times daily.	✗	
Collaborate with the client to properly manage pain with pharmacologic and nonpharmacologic therapies.	✗	

Rationale

The client is at risk for postoperative pulmonary complications due to a history of chronic respiratory disease and cigarette smoking. With chronic respiratory disease, increased chest rigidity and loss of lung elasticity reduce anesthetic excretion, and cigarette smoking damages cilia, which leads to retention of secretions. Both physiologic processes reduce gas exchange and increase the risk for pneumonia and atelectasis (alveolar collapse). Postoperative atelectasis usually occurs within 24 hours of anesthesia, while the onset for hospital-acquired pneumonia is 48 to 72 hours. Therefore the client is most likely experiencing atelectasis as evidence by dyspnea, rapid and shallow respirations, pulmonary crackles, and diminished breath sounds. A cough and low-grade fever are also common with atelectasis. Additionally, the client has had limited mobility since surgery and is reluctant to take medication for pain, which is most likely limiting the client's ability to take deep breaths or cough. Nursing actions would focus on deep breathing and coughing, mobility, and pain management. The nurse would teach proper techniques for splinting the incision site and encourage the client to perform splinting, coughing, and deep breathing exercises every 1 to 2 hours. An incentive spirometer may be used to improve inspiratory muscle action and reverse atelectasis. The nurse would teach the client to use the incentive spirometer (i.e., performing 5 to 10 breaths per session every hour by taking a long, slow, deep breath through the mouthpiece, raising the piston as high as possible, and then holding the breath for 2 to 4 seconds before slowly exhaling). Immobility limits lung expansion and allows fluids to pool in the lungs, therefore the nurse would assist the client to change position at least every 2 hours and plan for the client to be out of bed, unless contraindicated, on the first postoperative day. The nurse would also help the client ambulate several times daily, beginning on the second postoperative day. Adequate pain management is essential for the client to take deep breaths, cough, and ambulate in the hallway. Therefore, the nurse would further assess the client's reluctance to pain medication and collaborate with the client and provider to properly manage the client's pain with both pharmacologic and nonpharmacologic therapies.

CJ Cognitive Skills: Recognize Cues, Analyze Cues, Priority Hypotheses, Generate Solutions, Take Actions

Reference: Linton & Matteson, 2023, pp. 291–302

Answers With Rationales for Thinking Exercises

Unfolding Case Study 5.1

Thinking Exercise 5.1.1

Answer

- ○ Pain
- ○ Temperature
- ✗ Heart rate
- ✗ Respiratory rate
- ○ Blood pressure
- ○ SpO$_2$
- ○ Blood glucose
- ✗ Blood on surgical dressing
- ○ Client's concern about driving

Rationale

The client's heart rate and respiratory rate are increased above normal limits for an adult and would require immediate follow-up. These vital signs often increase in response to loss of fluid in the body. The client's blood pressure, temperature, FSBG, and peripheral oxygen saturation (SpO$_2$) are within expected normal limits, although the blood pressure has decreased slightly. The client's pain level is expected given that the client had surgery yesterday and was not using the PCA as needed. The bright-red blood on the surgical dressing requires immediate follow-up because the client had surgery yesterday. If bleeding worsens, the client could become hypovolemic, which would be potentially life threatening. The client's concern about not being able to drive would not require immediate follow-up, although it should be addressed at a later time when the client's immediate condition is managed.

CJ Cognitive Skill: Recognize Cues
Reference: Linton & Matteson, 2023, pp. 935–938

Thinking Exercise 5.1.2

Answer

The nurse should recognize that the client is likely experiencing **hemorrhage** and **phantom limb pain**.

Rationale

Based on the client findings of blood on the surgical dressing, increased respiratory rate, and increased heart rate, the client is probably experiencing hemorrhage as a postoperative complication. The client is also reporting pain in the amputated foot, which indicates phantom limb pain. There is no evidence of infection or acute compartment syndrome (ACS). ACS usually occurs in the calf of the leg due to decreased arterial perfusion. This client's lower leg has been amputated. There are also no client findings that are consistent with hypoxia because the SpO$_2$ is within the normal expected range.

CJ Cognitive Skill: Analyze Cues
Reference: Linton & Matteson, 2023, pp. 935–938

Thinking Exercise 5.1.3

Answer

The nurse determines that the *priority* for care at this time is to manage the client's **hemorrhage** as evidenced by **elevated heart rate** and **blood on dressing**.

Rationale

The client is experiencing hemorrhage and phantom limb pain. Hemorrhage is potentially life threatening, making this condition the priority for client care. Phantom limb pain is not potentially life threatening. The client likely does not have an infection because the surgery was only the day before, and the client has no signs or symptoms of an infection. When bleeding occurs, the client loses blood volume (hypovolemia). To compensate for this loss, the heart rate increases to circulate less blood more often to oxygenate vital organ tissues; respirations also typically increase to provide more oxygen for vital organ functioning. The client is experiencing hemorrhage because bright-red blood is present on the surgical dressing.

CJ Cognitive Skill: Prioritize Hypotheses
Reference: Linton & Matteson, 2023, pp. 935–938

Thinking Exercise 5.1.4

Answer

POTENTIAL NURSING ACTIONS	INDICATED	NOT INDICATED
Apply a pressure dressing over surgical dressing	X	
Keep the right residual limb flat on the bed		X
Monitor vital signs every 8 hours		X
Maintain bedrest for the rest of the day	X	

Rationale

When postoperative hemorrhage occurs following a leg amputation, pressure needs to be applied over the site to slow the bleeding. Therefore applying a pressure dressing is indicated. The residual limb should be elevated to slow the bleeding rather than remaining flat, and the client needs to stay in bed to prevent excessive movement that could cause increased bleeding. Vital signs should be taken more frequently than every 8 hours to monitor subtle or early changes. Therefore this action is not indicated or appropriate in this client situation.

CJ Cognitive Skill: Generate Solutions
Reference: Linton & Matteson, 2023, pp. 935–938

Thinking Exercise 5.1.5

Answer

X Elevate the right residual limb on 1 to 2 pillows.
X Check under the residual limb for bleeding.
O Apply a heat compress to the right residual limb.
X Apply a pressure dressing over the surgical dressing.
O Mark and label the area where blood is located on the dressing.
X Monitor vital signs every 1 to 2 hours.
X Start peripheral IV fluids.
X Maintain bedrest today.

Rationale

Applying pressure to the surgical site and elevating the residual limb should slow the postoperative bleeding. At times, bleeding is not obvious on the visible (anterior) side of the residual limb. However, the blood could ooze and pool under the affected limb. Therefore the nurse would place the hands under the surgical (residual) limb to feel for dampness or pooling of blood. Bedrest is important to prevent excessive movement that could worsen the bleeding. The nurse would start peripheral IV fluids to replace lost fluid volume and prevent or manage hypovolemia and possible shock. The client's vital signs need to be taken and recorded frequently to monitor the client during this situation. Heat would dilate the blood vessels and worsen bleeding. Therefore heat compresses are not appropriate for this client. Although marking and labeling any new drainage on a surgical dressing was the standard of care in the past, this action is not reliable and is no longer recommended or necessary.

CJ Cognitive Skill: Take Actions
Reference: Linton & Matteson, 2023, pp. 935–938

Thinking Exercise 5.1.6

Answer

DATA COLLECTION FINDING	IMPROVED	WORSENED
Heart rate	X	
Pain intensity		X
Respiratory rate	X	
Blood pressure	X	
Bleeding from surgical site	X	

Rationale

The postoperative bleeding slowed or stopped because the client now has normal vital signs. In addition, there is no new blood on the dressing. Starting IV fluids has increased the blood volume, which helped improve the client's heart rate and blood pressure; the client's respiratory rate decreased in response to these improvements. The phantom limb pain, however, has increased, showing worsening of the client's overall pain level.

CJ Cognitive Skill: Evaluate Outcomes
Reference: Linton & Matteson, 2023, pp. 935–938

Unfolding Case Study 5.2

Thinking Exercise 5.2.1

Answer

O Pain level
X Absent pedal pulse
O Heart rate
O Respiratory rate
O Blood pressure
X Capillary refill
X Cool, pale left foot

Rationale

The client experienced multiple fractures and soft tissue trauma of the left leg and pelvis as a result of being hit by a truck. These injuries cause inflammation, which includes swelling that can decrease distal perfusion. Therefore the nurse would recognize that the most relevant client findings requiring follow-up are the result of impaired arterial perfusion to the lower leg and foot, including an absent pedal pulse, increased capillary refill time, and a cool and pale left foot. These findings can become limb threatening or life threatening. The client's pain would need to be addressed at some point, but it is not a life-threatening finding. The severe pain, though, is likely causing an elevated blood pressure and an increased heart rate. However, these vital signs are not life threatening at this time. The client's respiratory rate is within normal limits for an adult.

CJ Cognitive Skill: Recognize Cues
Reference: Linton & Matteson, 2023, pp. 915, 917–918

Thinking Exercise 5.2.2

Answer

The nurse should recognize that the client is likely experiencing **compartment syndrome**.

Rationale

The lower leg has compartments, or areas enclosed in fascia (fibrous tissue), in which muscle, blood vessels, and nerves are located. The most recent assessment data indicate that the client's injury is causing decreased arterial blood flow and motor/sensory impairment in the affected foot. This neurovascular compromise suggests that the client is likely experiencing an uncommon but emergent complication of musculoskeletal trauma known as *acute compartment syndrome.* Deep vein thrombosis usually presents in the lower or upper leg with swelling, redness/hyperpigmentation, warmth, and pain. Peripheral vascular disease is a chronic problem that can occur in clients who have diabetes. However, it does not suddenly affect circulation over a few hours. There is no evidence that the client was using any substances. Withdrawal from substance use presents as behavioral and physiologic changes and is not confined to one extremity.

CJ Cognitive Skill: Analyze Cues
Reference: Linton & Matteson, 2023, pp. 915, 917–918

Thinking Exercise 5.2.3

Answer

The nurse determines that the ***priority*** for care at this time is to manage the client's **left leg pressure** as evidenced by a **pale, cool left foot** and **absent left pedal pulse**.

Rationale

Compartment syndrome causes increased pressure within small areas in the lower leg enclosed by fascia (compartments), which then decreases blood flow. This complication can be caused by internal pressure (swelling within compartments) or external pressure (by casts, dressings, or splints). The nurse loosened the splint and cut the lower part of the dressing near the foot to ensure that external pressure was not causing the client's problem. However, the client continued to have relevant findings consistent with compartment syndrome. The client's pale, cool foot and absent pedal pulse are the result of this complication. Therefore the priority is to relieve compartmental pressure to restore blood flow and adequate nerve function. The client's pain will likely decrease when the internal pressure is relieved. The client does not have findings consistent with thrombosis.

CJ Cognitive Skill: Prioritize Hypotheses
Reference: Linton & Matteson, 2023, pp. 915, 917–918

Thinking Exercise 5.2.4

Answer

○ Elevate the affected leg on 2 pillows.
○ Increase the rate of peripheral IV fluids.
○ Start oxygen therapy via nasal cannula.
✗ Notify the surgeon about the most recent client findings.
○ Apply heat to the affected lower leg to promote circulation.
✗ Request an order for additional analgesia to manage the client's pain.
✗ Prepare the client for a potential fasciotomy to relieve leg pressure.

Rationale

Although the surgeon was notified about changes in the client's condition according to the 0810 note, the client clinically deteriorated several hours later. The nurse would need to notify the surgeon about these more recent client findings. The client's pain intensity is markedly increased and needs to be addressed to promote comfort. However, the increased internal pressure in the lower leg that is causing severe neurovascular compromise can only be relieved by a surgical procedure known as *fasciotomy*. In this procedure, the surgeon would cut into affected compartments to relieve the pressure and would likely keep the surgical wound open for several days. Later, the surgical wound could be closed using a skin graft or other surgical procedure. The affected leg should not be elevated because that would decrease arterial perfusion to the distal leg and foot. There is no indication for increasing IV fluids or using oxygen at this time. Heat would not be used because it would dilate the arteries and increase compartment pressure.

CJ Cognitive Skill: Generate Solutions
Reference: Linton & Matteson, 2023, pp. 915, 917–918

Thinking Exercise 5.2.5

Answer

BODY SYSTEM	NURSING ACTION
Cardiovascular	✗ Take and record vital signs every 2–4 hours per protocol ✗ Perform a circulation check on the left foot every 2–4 hours per surgeon protocol ✗ Empty and record JP drainage every 8–12 hours per agency protocol
Respiratory	✗ Monitor SpO_2 and titrate supplemental oxygen per surgeon protocol ✗ Encourage deep breathing every hour while awake ○ Encourage use of an incentive spirometer every 8 hours
Neurologic	✗ Assess pain level with other vital signs ✗ Document the location and quality of pain for each assessment ○ Monitor for substance withdrawal behaviors

Rationale

Any client having surgery needs to have vital sign and pain level monitoring, including documenting the location and quality of the pain. The nurse would continue to carefully and frequently monitor circulation to the affected foot to assess the effectiveness of the surgery. The JP drain needs to be emptied and the amount of drainage recorded as part of intake and output measurement. The client has impaired mobility and therefore is at risk for complications of immobility, such as hypostatic pneumonia and atelectasis. Therefore the nurse would encourage the client to cough, deep breathe, and use the incentive spirometer every 1 to 2 hours while awake (not every 8 hours). The client's oxygen would be adjusted as needed and could be discontinued as soon as the SpO_2 remains within normal limits. There is no indication that the client has been using any substance.

CJ Cognitive Skill: Take Actions
Reference: Linton & Matteson, 2023, pp. 294–304, 915, 917–918

Thinking Exercise 5.2.6

Answer

DATA COLLECTION FINDING	IMPROVED	WORSENED
Pain reported at 3/10	✗	
Left pedal pulse 1+	✗	
Foot and toe movement	✗	
Vital signs	✗	
Skin integrity of injured foot		✗

Rationale

The most recent client findings indicate that the client's condition has improved, including a palpable pedal pulse, foot and toe movement, and decreased pain. The client's vital signs also returned to baseline as the client's pain level improved. However, the splint apparently caused excessive pressure on the client's left heel, which resulted in a necrotic pressure injury. This complication adds to the client's pain and healing process.

CJ Cognitive Skill: Evaluate Outcomes
Reference: Linton & Matteson, 2023, pp. 294–304, 915, 917–918

Unfolding Case Study 5.3

Thinking Exercise 5.3.1

Answer

History and Physical	Nurses' Notes	Orders	Laboratory Results

1550: Client admitted yesterday for acute rehabilitation program following cervical (C7–C 8) spinal cord injury resulting from diving into a shallow pool. Evaluated yesterday by PT and OT. Alert and oriented × 4; reports pain rated 2/10 after pain meds administered. Anterior neck surgical incision intact and healing. Halo fixator in place; no redness or drainage around screws. Breath sounds clear throughout lung fields; no dyspnea. Skin dry with usual pigmentation. Bowel sounds present in all quadrants. Abdomen soft, round, and nondistended. Urinary catheter draining medium-yellow urine with sediment. High-top shoes and antiembolism stockings in place. VS: T 98.6°F (37°C), HR 82 beats/min and regular, RR 18 breaths/min, BP 118/56 mm Hg, SpO$_2$ 95% on RA. Scheduled for first PT session to begin mobility training at 1600.

1815: Reports developing severe "pounding" frontal headache about 10 minutes ago. Face and neck flushed and diaphoretic. States vision is blurred and nose suddenly began feeling "stuffy." VS: T 99°F (37.2°C), HR 58 beats/min and regular, RR 22 breaths/min, BP 194/116 mm Hg, SpO$_2$ 94% on RA.

Rationale

The client was stabilized in the acute care setting after having an open reduction internal fixation of the fractured cervical vertebra. The client now has a sudden onset of severe headache with blurred vision, facial and neck flushing, and diaphoresis (excessive sweating). These findings may be caused by the client's highly elevated blood pressure, which can cause a stroke if it continues or increases further. These findings are potentially life-threatening clinical findings. As a compensatory response to severe hypertension with vagal stimulation, the client's heart rate decreased below the normal range for an adult and is therefore significant at this time. The peripheral oxygen saturation (SpO$_2$) of 94% is slightly lower than the ideal of 95%, but the client is not demonstrating respiratory distress. The respiratory rate is only slightly increased, which may be due to anxiety caused by the client's condition.

CJ Cognitive Skill: Recognize Cues
Reference: Linton & Matteson, 2023, pp. 444–445

Thinking Exercise 5.3.2

Answer

The nurse should recognize that the client is likely experiencing **autonomic dysreflexia**.

Rationale

Most clients who have a cervical spinal injury have muscle spasticity because the upper motor neurons are affected. However, there is no documentation about the client's spasticity as part of the new clinical findings. Spinal shock occurs immediately after the injury and results in flaccid paralysis, loss of reflexes, and absent bowel and bladder control. This client's injury was managed by surgical intervention before the client was transferred for acute rehabilitation. Neurogenic shock is an autonomic nervous system response that causes hypotension rather than the high blood pressure that this client is manifesting. The client's clinical findings are most consistent with autonomic dysreflexia (AD), an emergent situation. AD is an exaggerated sympathetic nervous system reaction to a noxious stimulus and can occur in clients whose spinal injury is above T6. The client with AD typically presents with increased blood pressure, bradycardia (as a result of vagal nerve stimulation), flushing and profuse sweating above the injury, nausea, severe pounding headache, and nasal congestion. These findings are all present in this client situation.
CJ Cognitive Skill: Analyze Cues
Reference: Linton & Matteson, 2023, pp. 444–445

Thinking Exercise 5.3.3

Answer

The nurse determines that the *priority* for care at this time is to manage the client's **blood pressure** because the client could develop a(n) **stroke**.

Rationale

Managing the client's severely elevated blood pressure is the priority for care because it can cause a hemorrhagic stroke, which is potentially life threatening. The client's heart rate is just below the usual range for adults and is likely not life threatening in a young adult. Pain as a clinical finding is not life threatening. Aneurysms are usually congenital or the result of long-term hypertension for many years. PE usually results from deep vein thrombosis, when a piece of the clot breaks off and lodges in one or more pulmonary blood vessels.
CJ Cognitive Skill: Prioritize Hypotheses
Reference: Linton & Matteson, 2023, pp. 444–445

Thinking Exercise 5.3.4

Answer

○ Lower the head of the client's bed to a flat position.
✗ Check the indwelling urinary catheter tubing for kinks.
○ Administer an analgesic medication.
✗ Ask the client about bowel habits, especially constipation.
✗ Notify the health care provider immediately.

Rationale

The nurse would notify the health care provider immediately because autonomic dysreflexia (AD) is an emergent clinical situation. The nurse would try to determine the source of the noxious stimulus causing the AD; a blocked or kinked indwelling urinary catheter or stool impaction are common causes. Therefore checking the urinary catheter and asking the client about bowel habits are indicated at this time. The nurse could check for impaction by rectal exam, but the exam could be another stimulus that could worsen the client's situation. Treating the client's headache pain with an analgesic is not the priority at this time. The client's headache should subside when the hypertension is managed. Lowering the head of the bed can increase blood return to the heart and therefore increase blood pressure. Conversely, elevating the head of the bed decreases the amount of blood going to the heart due to gravity. This decreased blood return to the heart can help decrease blood pressure.

CJ Cognitive Skill: Generate Solutions

Reference: Linton & Matteson, 2023, pp. 444–445

Thinking Exercise 5.3.5

Answer

○ Check BP every 5 minutes.
○ Perform a bladder scan.
○ Test urine for the presence of bacteria.
✗ Administer immediate-release nifedipine.
○ Monitor the client for seizure activity.
○ Notify the ICU of a possible transfer.

Rationale

Managing the client's elevated blood pressure (BP) is the priority for nursing care. Although seeking and removing/treating the source of noxious stimuli that could be causing hypertension is important, it does not typically lead to an immediate decrease in BP. Instead, giving the fast-acting antihypertensive drug nifedipine is the order that needs to be implemented first so it can begin to rapidly decrease the client's blood pressure within a few minutes. This drug is not used to manage chronic hypertension but it used in situations in which the blood pressure increases quickly. All of the other orders need to be implemented *after* medication administration. The client's BP needs frequent monitoring for the effectiveness of nifedipine. If the systolic blood pressure does not decrease to less than 150 mm Hg, the client would likely be transferred to a critical care unit. The bladder scan can determine if the client is retaining urine; the urine needs to be screened to check for infection that can sometimes cause AD in clients with a spinal cord injury. Acute hypertension can cause seizures for which the nurse would monitor.

CJ Cognitive Skill: Take Actions

Reference: Linton & Matteson, 2023, pp. 444–445, Willihnganz et al., 2022, pp. 374

Thinking Exercise 5.3.6

Answer

DATA COLLECTION FINDING	IMPROVED	NOT IMPROVED
Vision	✗	
Flushing	✗	
Nausea		✗
Heart rate	✗	
Blood pressure	✗	

Rationale

As documented in the last few nurses' notes, the client's blood pressure has markedly decreased, and the heart rate has increased to being within the normal range for an adult (60 to 100 beats/min). The client no longer has blurred vision or facial and neck flushing, indicating an improvement in the client's condition. However, the client continues to report the presence of nausea, which has apparently not improved.

CJ Cognitive Skill: Evaluate Outcomes

Reference: Linton & Matteson, 2023, pp. 444–445

Stand-Alone Thinking Exercise 5.1

Answer

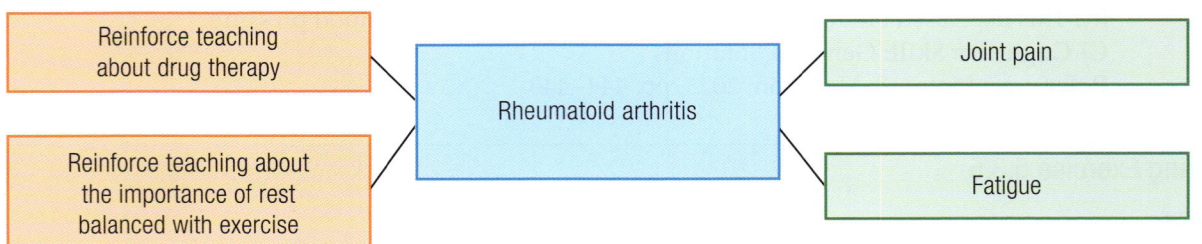

Rationale

The client has typical clinical findings that are consistent with early rheumatoid arthritis (RA). RA is a systemic inflammatory autoimmune disease that commonly affects small synovial (movable) joints of the body in a bilateral, symmetric pattern. Many of this client's hand joints are red, swollen, warm, and painful. If this disease continues to progress, the client can develop joint deformities and experience impaired mobility and functional ability. Osteoarthritis is not a primary inflammatory disease and is confined to one or more joints. Acute gout causes sudden and severe joint inflammation as a result of uric acid buildup in the body. It is usually extremely painful and usually resolves over several days. Systemic findings like anorexia, fever, and fatigue are not commonly seen in clients who have either acute gout or osteoarthritis. Clients typically do not know they have osteoporosis unless they experience a fracture or have a screening bone density scan. The primary health care provider would prescribe the client one or more drugs to decrease joint inflammation and decrease the progression of the disease. These drugs are referred to as *disease-modifying antirheumatic drugs* (DMARDs). The nurse would reinforce teaching regarding safe drug administration and the need to monitor for side effects and adverse effects. The nurse would also reinforce teaching about joint protection and the need to balance rest with exercise. It is not appropriate for the nurse to suggest that the client change jobs. Bisphosphonates are used to treat osteoporosis, and a low-purine diet is appropriate for clients who have acute gout. The nurse would monitor and teach the client to monitor for the level of fatigue and joint pain, which will hopefully improve as a result of the plan of care. Uric acid is monitored in clients who have gout.

CJ Cognitive Skills: Recognize Cues, Analyze Cues, Prioritize Hypotheses, Generate Solutions, Take Actions, Evaluate Outcomes
Reference: Linton & Matteson, 2023, pp. 897–901

Stand-Alone Thinking Exercise 5.2

Answer

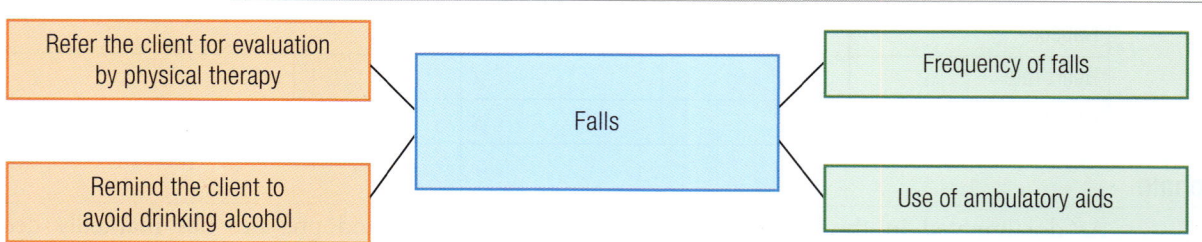

Rationale

The client has muscle weakness and spasticity and has recently experienced several falls. As a result, the client is using a cane when ambulating. When a client has a history of falling combined with impaired mobility, the client is most at risk for additional falls. Maintaining safety is the priority client outcome for a client who has mobility issues. The client is also at risk for decreased ADL ability, but this finding is not the priority condition or the condition for which the client is most at risk. Because the client has muscle spasticity, the client is also at risk for joint contractures. However, this is also not the condition for which the client is most at risk. The client is already receiving oxybutynin, which helps manage urinary incontinence. Because the client is most at risk for additional falls, the nurse would refer the client to physical therapy for evaluation. As a result of this evaluation, the client may need muscle-strengthening exercises or perhaps need to use a walker rather than a cane for ambulation to prevent falls. Falls often occur due to dizziness or light-headedness from drinking alcohol. Therefore the nurse would remind the client to avoid alcohol to help prevent falls. Although the client is at risk for infection due to taking glatiramer acetate for MS, reminding the client how to help prevent infection would not be an appropriate action to help prevent falls. Range-of-motion exercises may help prevent joint contractures but would not necessarily help prevent falls. Wearing contact lenses does not help to decrease diplopia. Wearing an eye patch helps some clients with this symptom, which would improve vision and could help prevent falls. The nurse would tell the client and family to monitor for any additional falls and the type of ambulatory aid the client was using and to report this information to the nurse to help monitor the client's progress. Although reporting the client's ADL ability, infections, and urinary function is important for the client who has MS, these parameters are not related to the client's risk for additional falls.

CJ Cognitive Skills: Recognize Cues, Analyze Cues, Prioritize Hypotheses, Generate Solutions, Take Actions, Evaluate Outcomes

Reference: Linton & Matteson, 2023, pp. 398–404

Answers With Rationales for Thinking Exercises

Unfolding Case Study 6.1

Thinking Exercise 6.1.1

Answer

✗ Nausea and vomiting
✗ Blood glucose level
○ Fatigue
○ Body temperature
○ SpO$_2$
○ Respiratory rate

Rationale

The client is currently experiencing nausea and vomiting, which can cause fluid and electrolyte imbalances; these imbalances could become life threatening. Therefore this finding needs immediate follow-up by the nurse and health care team. The client's blood glucose is elevated to the level that the client's breath is fruity. This finding indicates a possible diabetic emergency and needs to be addressed as soon as possible. The client's temperature and respiratory rate are not at a potentially life-threatening level; fatigue is also not life threatening. The client's peripheral oxygen saturation level as measured by pulse oximetry (SpO$_2$) is within the normal expected range of 95% or higher on room air (RA).

CJ Cognitive Skill: Recognize Cues
Reference: Linton & Matteson, 2023, pp. 1005–1006.

Thinking Exercise 6.1.2

Answer

The nurse recognizes that the client is likely experiencing early **diabetic ketoacidosis**.

Rationale

Diabetic ketoacidosis (DKA) occurs in clients who have type 1 diabetes mellitus (DM). The client has several findings that are consistent with DKA, including rapid breathing, fruity breath (due to ketones), headache, fatigue, dry skin, nausea and vomiting, and hyperglycemia (elevated blood glucose often above 600 mg/dL [33.3 mmol/L]). Hyperosmolar hyperglycemic nonketotic syndrome (HHNS) occurs in clients who have type 2 DM. The client is alert and oriented, and there is no evidence that the client has alcohol poisoning. The client's temperature is elevated, but there are no other data that support the presence of an infection. However, the client likely would be evaluated for an infection because infection can cause an increased blood glucose level.

CJ Cognitive Skill: Analyze Cues
Reference: Linton & Matteson, 2023, pp. 1005–1006.

Thinking Exercise 6.1.3

Answer

The nurse determines the priority for care at this time is to manage the client's **<u>dehydration</u>** as evidenced by **<u>tachycardia</u>** and **<u>hypotension</u>**.

Rationale

The client's blood glucose is elevated (hyperglycemia), but the level is not life threatening at this time. Clients who have DKA typically experience dehydration, which is potentially life threatening. This client's findings are consistent with dehydration, including dry skin, elevated body temperature, tachycardia, and low blood pressure. If dehydration is not treated as the priority, the client could experience shock. The client is not hypoxic as evidenced by a normal SpO_2. After treating the client's dehydration, the focus would be to decrease the client's glucose level. Once the glucose decreases to closer to a normal level, the client's vital signs, headache, abdominal discomfort, and nausea and vomiting would likely improve. Diuresis occurs because the client's kidneys are trying to rid the body of excess glucose; deep, rapid respirations occur because the body is trying to rid itself of ketone bodies that are causing metabolic acidosis. This finding should also improve as the client's hyperglycemia improves.
CJ Cognitive Skill: Prioritize Hypotheses
Reference: Linton & Matteson, 2023, pp. 1005–1006.

Thinking Exercise 6.1.4

Answer

POTENTIAL NURSING ACTIONS	INDICATED	NOT INDICATED
Monitor IV fluid infusion of 5% dextrose/normal saline.		X
Monitor the client's heart rate and rhythm.	X	
Monitor serum electrolyte levels.	X	
Begin supplemental oxygen via nasal cannula.		X
Monitor FSBG levels during IV regular insulin administration.	X	

Rationale

The client would receive an IV fluid bolus followed by a high continuous rate of IV fluids to manage the client's priority condition of dehydration. However, the client would likely receive normal saline rather than an IV solution containing dextrose, which breaks down in the body into glucose. If 5%D/NS were administered, the client's glucose level would continue to increase. When a client who has type 1 DM experiences hyperglycemia, the client typically has hyperkalemia (increased serum potassium). Hyperkalemia can cause cardiac dysrhythmias. Therefore the nurse would monitor serum electrolyte levels as well as the client's heart rate and rhythm. After actions to manage dehydration are implemented, the client would receive fast-acting insulin, usually intravenously. Some clients may receive subcutaneous ultrarapid-acting insulin such as insulin lispro or aspart instead. Regardless of how insulin is administered, the nurse would closely monitor the client's finger stick blood glucose (FSBG) levels with the expectation that they would eventually decrease to a normal range.
CJ Cognitive Skill: Generate Solutions
Reference: Linton & Matteson, 2023, pp. 1005–1006.

Thinking Exercise 6.1.5

Answer

✗ Continue to monitor and record blood glucose levels frequently per agency protocol.
✗ Encourage water and other appropriate fluids as tolerated.
✗ Record fluid intake and urine output per agency protocol.
○ Increase supplemental oxygen from 3 L/min to 4 L/min via NC.
✗ Maintain continuous cardiac monitoring.
○ Insert an indwelling urinary catheter for hourly monitoring.
✗ Collaborate with the registered nurse regarding potassium administration.

Rationale

The nurse would implement interventions that assist in managing the client's dehydration, including encouraging oral fluids if the client can tolerate them. To help determine the effectiveness of those interventions, the nurse would monitor and record fluid intake and urine output. An indwelling urinary catheter is not needed at this time because the client is continent and does not require 1- to 2-hour urine measurements. An indwelling urinary catheter can cause a catheter-associated urinary tract infection (CAUTI), especially in clients who are susceptible to infections such as those who have DM. Although the client's serum potassium is currently elevated, insulin administration to treat hyperglycemia moves potassium from the bloodstream into the cells, which then lowers the serum potassium level. As a result, clients who are treated for DKA usually require potassium supplementation. Supplemental oxygen is not needed because the client's SpO_2 is within the normal range.
CJ Cognitive Skill: Take Actions
References: Linton & Matteson, 2023, pp. 1005–1006; Pagana et al., 2023, pp. 150, 296, 451, 707, 803

Thinking Exercise 6.1.6

Answer

DATA COLLECTION FINDING	IMPROVED	UNCHANGED
Blood glucose	✗	
Cardiac rhythm		✗
Temperature	✗	
Blood pressure	✗	

Rationale

The client's plan of care to manage dehydration was effective as evidenced by decreased body temperature, decreased heart rate, and increased blood pressure since admission to the ED. These findings demonstrate improvement in the client's condition. The client's current blood glucose of 275 mg/dL (15.26 mmol/L) shows a significant improvement (decreased) since the client was admitted to the ED. However, the client's heart rhythm is unchanged and continues to be irregular, most likely due to hyperkalemia.
CJ Cognitive Skill: Evaluate Outcomes
Reference: Linton & Matteson, 2023, pp. 1005–1006.

Unfolding Case Study 6.2

Thinking Exercise 6.2.1

Answer

History and Physical	Nurses' Notes	Orders	Laboratory Results

1435: Friend brought client to center due to new-onset signs and symptoms including shakiness, irritability, light-headedness, and diaphoresis. Medical history includes anorexia nervosa, anemia, and recent diagnosis of type 1 diabetes mellitus (DM). Alert and oriented × 3 (person, place, and event). Breath sounds clear throughout lung fields. Client states has not eaten today except for a protein bar at around 0730. Abdomen soft, round, and nontender. Skin cool and very moist. Bowel sounds present in all quadrants. Able to move all extremities; cap refill <3 sec. VS: T 98.6°F (37°C), HR 58 beats/min and irregular, RR 18 breaths/min, BP 92/56 mm Hg, SpO$_2$ 96% on RA. FSBG 50 mg/dL (2.77 mmol/L). (Normal range 70–110 mg/dL [3.89–6.11 mmol/L].) Reported height 5 ft 10 inches (178 cm), reported weight 110 lb (49.9 kg).

Rationale

The client's new-onset findings require immediate follow-up and include shakiness, irritability, light-headedness, diaphoresis, and disorientation (not oriented to time). The client's FSBG is below the normal range of 70 to 110 mg/dL (3.89–6.11 mmol/L) and needs to be followed up immediately because a low glucose level can become life threatening. Neurons in the brain require glucose and oxygen to adequately function. If glucose continues to decrease, the client can lose consciousness and experience seizures or even death. The client's recent diagnosis of DM is very important and helps explain the client's findings. The client's history of anorexia nervosa does not require follow-up at this time but helps explain why the client has irregular bradycardia and hypotension. Neither vital sign value is life threatening at this time. The client's cool and moist skin is caused by excessive sweating (diaphoresis).
CJ Cognitive Skill: Recognize Cues
References: Linton & Matteson, 2023, pp. 1004–1005; Pagana et al., 2023, p. 451

Thinking Exercise 6.2.2

Answer

The nurse recognizes that the client is experiencing **acute hypoglycemia** as evidenced by the client's **FSBG** and **diaphoresis**.

Rationale

The client's FSBG is well below the normal range and is considered to be moderate acute hypoglycemia. When a client's glucose level falls below the normal range, the body experiences an adrenergic nervous system response typically manifested by shakiness, nervousness, irritability, diaphoresis, hunger, anxiety, and/or tingling or numbness of the lips. Most clients also develop tachycardia, but this client has a history of anorexia nervosa, which often causes bradycardia and hypotension. Clients who have diabetic ketoacidosis have hyperglycemia in which the blood glucose is *above* the normal range. There is no evidence that a stroke occurred because the client did not lose mobility, speech, and/or language ability.
CJ Cognitive Skill: Analyze Cues
References: Linton & Matteson, 2023, pp. 1004–1005; Pagana et al., 2023, p. 451

Thinking Exercise 6.2.3

Answer

The nurse determines the *priority* for care is to manage the client's **hypoglycemia**.

Rationale

The client's immediate acute condition is hypoglycemia, which is potentially life threatening if not treated promptly. Body cells require glucose to adequately function. There are no client findings that support dehydration because the client's skin is moist rather than dry, and the client has bradycardia rather than tachycardia. Although the client is underweight, the anorexia causing the client's weight is likely not life threatening at this time. The client's neurologic findings, such as shakiness and mild disorientation, are caused by hypoglycemia. Therefore managing the hypoglycemia would also treat these neurologic changes.

CJ Cognitive Skill: Prioritize Hypotheses
References: Linton & Matteson, 2023, pp. 1004–1005; Pagana et al., 2023, p. 451

Thinking Exercise 6.2.4

Answer

POTENTIAL NURSING ACTIONS	INDICATED	NOT INDICATED
Administer subcutaneous glucagon per agency protocol.		✗
Give 15 g of fast-acting carbohydrates such as 4 oz (120 mL) of apple juice.	✗	
Start 50 mL of 50% dextrose IV per agency protocol.		✗
Retest FSBG following the initial intervention to treat hypoglycemia.	✗	

Rationale

The client is conscious and able to consume food and fluids by mouth. Therefore the best way to treat hypoglycemia in a conscious client is to give the client 15 g of oral fast-acting carbohydrates, wait 15 minutes, and then perform another FSBG. This procedure should be continued every 15 to 30 minutes until the blood glucose is above 80 mg/dL (4.44 mmol/L). Parenteral glucagon or IV dextrose is only administered for hypoglycemia being experienced by an unconscious client. Therefore these actions are not indicated.

CJ Cognitive Skill: Generate Solutions
References: Linton & Matteson, 2023, pp. 1004–1005; Pagana et al., 2023, p. 451

Thinking Exercise 6.2.5

Answer

○ Establish peripheral intravenous access.
○ Administer subcutaneous glucagon per agency protocol.
✗ Give 15 g of fast-acting carbohydrates such as 4 oz (120 mL) of apple juice.
○ Provide discharge teaching about diabetes to improve glucose control.
✗ Retest FSBG following the initial intervention to treat hypoglycemia.

Rationale

The client is conscious and able to consume food and fluids. Therefore the best way to treat hypoglycemia in a conscious client is to give the client 15 g of fast-acting carbohydrates, wait 15 minutes, and then perform another FSBG. This procedure should be continued every 15 to 30 minutes until the blood glucose is above 80 mg/dL (4.44 mmol/L). As long as the client can consume oral fluids, IV access is likely not needed. Subcutaneous glucagon is given to clients who are unconscious. Discharge teaching is important but is not appropriate at this time until the diabetic emergency of acute hypoglycemia is resolved.

CJ Cognitive Skill: Take Actions
References: Linton & Matteson, 2023, pp. 1004–1005; Pagana et al., 2023, p. 451

Thinking Exercise 6.2.6—Pharmacology

Answer

CLIENT STATEMENTS	UNDERSTANDING	NO UNDERSTANDING
"I need to more carefully follow the prescribed diet to control this disorder."	✗	
"I should follow up with my primary care provider to monitor my hemoglobin A1c."	✗	
"I should carry some hard candies with me in case my sugar drops too low."	✗	
"I plan to get an insulin pump, which will control my diabetes."		✗
"I should keep injectable glucagon on hand just in case."	✗	

Rationale

All of the client's statements except one show understanding of the health teaching. The client likely became hypoglycemic due to nonadherence to the prescribed diet. Clients on insulin therapy need to balance this drug with food. Therefore the client needs to adhere to the diet and follow up with the provider to determine if the glucose is under control. Carrying hard candies or having access to any fast-acting carbohydrates is highly recommended for all clients who have DM. Clients should also have glucagon on hand for family or friends to administer if the client becomes unconscious from severely low blood glucose. The client does not understand how an insulin pump works because this device requires the client to self-monitor blood glucose and administer insulin boluses as needed. The pump would not independently control the client's diabetes.

CJ Cognitive Skill: Evaluate Outcomes

References: Linton & Matteson, 2023, pp. 1004–1005, 1012; Pagana et al., 2023, p. 451

Unfolding Case Study 6.3

Thinking Exercise 6.3.1

Answer

- O Fatigue
- O Varicose veins
- O Eczema on legs
- ✗ Blood pressure
- O Heart rate
- ✗ Blood glucose
- O BMI

Rationale

The client has an elevated blood pressure and blood glucose that need to be managed immediately because if these findings progress, they could rapidly become life threatening. Blood pressure and blood glucose can worsen quickly. None of the other findings are likely to worsen quickly or become imminently life threatening. The client's heart rate is within normal limits and is not relevant in this clinical situation. Therefore the findings that need immediate follow-up are blood pressure and glucose. The client's BMI, eczema, and varicose veins need to be addressed after the immediate issues. The client's fatigue would likely resolve when hyperglycemia and hypertension improve.

CJ Cognitive Skill: Recognize Cues

References: Linton & Matteson, 2023, pp. 661–674, 1015–1021; Pagana et al., 2023, p. 462

Thinking Exercise 6.3.2

Answer

The nurse recognizes that the client is most at risk for developing **stroke** and **hyperosmolar hyperglycemic nonketotic syndrome**.

Rationale

The client's blood pressure is very high and could cause a hemorrhagic stroke. The client's elevated blood glucose could worsen and develop into a diabetic emergency. A hyperglycemic emergency in clients with type 2 DM is called *hyperosmolar hyperglycemic nonketotic syndrome* (HHNS). Diabetic ketoacidosis only occurs in clients who have type 1 DM. There is no evidence that the client has an infection or sepsis at this time. However, any client who has DM is at risk for infection. The client is already obese as evidenced by a BMI over 30.
CJ Cognitive Skill: Analyze Cues
References: Linton & Matteson, 2023, pp. 418, 661–674, 1006–1007, 1015–1021; Pagana et al., 2023, p. 462

Thinking Exercise 6.3.3

Answer

○ Treating the eczema
○ Providing health teaching about diet
✗ Managing the hypertension
○ Treating the fatigue
✗ Decreasing the blood glucose level

Rationale

Managing the elevated blood pressure is a major priority because the client is at risk for stroke or hypertensive crisis, which are life-threatening conditions. A random elevated blood glucose and hemoglobin A1c over 9 demonstrate poor diabetic control. Therefore the client is at risk for diabetic emergencies, especially HHNS, a potentially life-threatening condition. The client's eczema, fatigue, and apparent nonadherence to the prescribed diet are not life threatening and therefore are not priorities for nursing care at this time.
CJ Cognitive Skill: Prioritize Hypotheses
References: Linton & Matteson, 2023, pp. 418, 661–674, 1006–1007, 1015–1021; Pagana et al., 2023, p. 462

Thinking Exercise 6.3.4

Answer

BODY SYSTEM/PROCESS	POTENTIAL NURSING ACTIONS
Endocrine	✗ Reinforce teaching about new diabetic medication to replace metformin. ○ Give the client a fast-acting insulin bolus in the office. ✗ Teach the client about the need to wear an emergency ID card, bracelet, or necklace.
Cardiovascular	○ Schedule a cardiac catheterization procedure. ✗ Explain the need to increase the daily antihypertensive drug dosage. ✗ Schedule vascular studies of the lower extremities.
Nutrition	○ Refer the client to a registered dietitian nutritionist. ✗ Explain the relationship of BMI to glucose control. ✗ Reinforce teaching about the need for regular exercise.

Rationale

The nurse would provide health teaching to help ensure that the client is familiar with the new prescribed diabetic medication and the need to increase the amlodipine. Insulin administration is not necessary because the client's glucose level is not yet life threatening. The client has findings that are consistent with poor circulation (absent pulse and varicosities) and therefore would need vascular studies. This diagnostic test is particularly important for clients who have diabetes because they frequently have peripheral vascular disease and ulcers. There are no findings that indicate a need for a cardiac catheterization. The client is able to verbalize what is needed on the prescribed diet for diabetes and hypertension, therefore referral to a registered dietitian nutritionist is not needed.

CJ Cognitive Skill: Generate Solutions

References: Linton & Matteson, 2023, pp. 661–674, 1006–1007, 1015–1021; Pagana et al., 2023, p. 462

Thinking Exercise 6.3.5—Pharmacology

Answer

✗ "This drug works to eliminate excess glucose through your urine."
○ "You may gain weight while taking this drug."
✗ "Report any symptoms of urinary tract infection such as burning and frequency."
✗ "You will need follow-up laboratory testing to check your electrolyte levels."
✗ "This drug will help decrease your hemoglobin A1c level to 7% or lower.
✗ "This drug will help reduce your risk of long-term complications of diabetes."

Rationale

All of these statements would be included when reinforcing health teaching about this drug, except that the client usually loses weight rather than gaining it. Empagliflozin is a sodium-glucose cotransporter-2 (SGLT2) inhibitor drug given to clients who have type 2 DM. The drug works in the kidneys to eliminate excess glucose into the urine, which increases the urine glucose concentration. As a result, the client is at slight risk for urinary tract infections, especially yeast infections. The drug can also decrease serum potassium levels, which need to be monitored. However, the drug's benefits outweigh these side effects, including the ability to reduce hemoglobin A1c and the long-term complications associated with diabetes such as kidney disease.

CJ Cognitive Skill: Take Actions

References: Linton & Matteson, 2023, pp. 1014; Willihnganz et al., 2023, pp. 586–588

Thinking Exercise 6.3.6

Answer

DATA COLLECTION FINDING	IMPROVED	UNCHANGED
Hemoglobin A1c	✗	
Blood pressure	✗	
FSBG	✗	
Heart rate		✗
Body weight	✗	

Rationale

The new plan of care for the client has been very effective in improving the client's blood pressure, glucose, and hemoglobin A1c levels. The newly prescribed diabetic drug and perhaps the client's adherence to diet and exercise resulted in significant weight loss in a 1-month period. This improvement can help the client avoid complications of both hypertension and DM. The client's heart rate has basically stayed the same and is therefore unchanged and within normal limits for an adult.

CJ Cognitive Skill: Evaluate Outcomes

References: Linton & Matteson, 2023, pp. 661–674, 1006–1007, 1015–1021; Pagana et al., 2023, p. 462

Stand-Alone Thinking Exercise 6.1

Answer

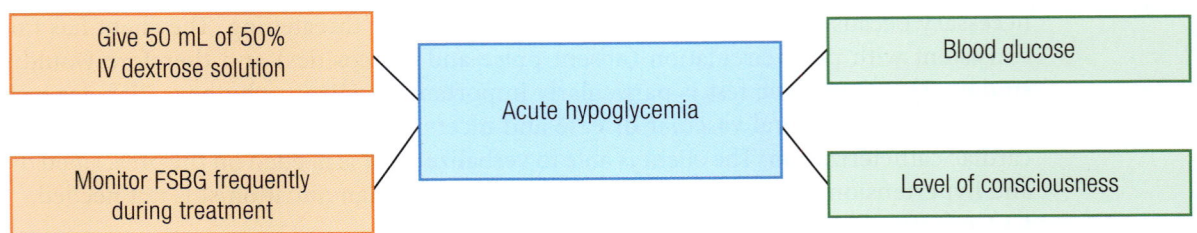

Rationale

The client has hypoglycemia, which is defined as a blood glucose level below 70 mg/dL (3.89 mmol/L). It is not known whether the client has a history of DM, but the client "smells strongly of alcohol," indicating a recent moderate to large alcohol consumption. When a moderate to large amount of alcohol is consumed by a chronically malnourished client, hypoglycemia can result within 6 to 36 hours after alcohol consumption. There are no client findings that support the presence of stroke or traumatic brain injury except for a decreased level of consciousness (LOC). If treatment for hypoglycemia is not effective in improving the client's LOC, the client would have a head CT to rule out these neurologic conditions. Because the client is unconscious, the nurse would administer 50 mL of IV 50% dextrose solution. The nurse would monitor the client's FSBG after dextrose administration per agency protocol. If the client was conscious, the nurse would give 15 g of fast-acting carbohydrates instead. Glucagon is not effective for clients who have hypoglycemia without DM. There is no indication at this time that the client needs supplemental oxygen. Total parenteral nutrition (TPN) is not a treatment for hypoglycemia. Additionally, the client would need to be referred to a registered dietitian nutritionist to assess the client's nutritional status before interventions were implemented. During and after treatment for hypoglycemia, the client's neurologic status, especially LOC, needs to be monitored to ensure that the client gains alertness and orientation. During and after the client's blood glucose level returns to its usual range, the client's FSBG should be monitored to ensure that it remains stable. When hypoglycemia resolves, the client's vital signs would likely return to the client's usual range. Intake and output documentation is not needed at this point in the client's care.

CJ Cognitive Skills: Recognize Cues, Analyze Cues, Priority Hypotheses, Generate Solutions, Take Actions, Evaluate Outcomes

Reference: Linton & Matteson, 2023, pp. 1023–1025

Stand-Alone Thinking Exercise 6.2

Answer

The nurse recognizes that the client is at high risk for **hyperosmolar hyperglycemic nonketotic syndrome**.

Rationale

HHNS is a diabetic emergency that occurs in clients who have type 2 DM due to lack of adequate or effective insulin in the body. The blood glucose of clients who have HHNS is typically very high (600 mg/dL [33.3 mmol/L] or higher), which causes osmotic diuresis with fluid and electrolyte imbalances. This client has type 2 DM with an increasing blood glucose. The laboratory results include an elevated BUN indicating either kidney disease, dehydration, high protein intake, or increased metabolism. Because the client's creatinine is within normal range, it is unlikely that the client has chronic kidney disease. Diabetic ketoacidosis only occurs in clients who have type 1 DM. The dehydration associated with HHNS can cause electrolyte imbalances (such as hypernatremia) and metabolic acidosis, not alkalosis.

CJ Cognitive Skill: Analyze Cues

References: Linton & Matteson, 2023, pp. 1006–1007; Pagana et al., 2023, pp. 150, 187, 220, 296, 451, 707, 805

Answers With Rationales for Thinking Exercises

Unfolding Case Study 7.1

Thinking Exercise 7.1.1

Answer

- ✗ Blood pressure
- ✗ Cardiac rhythm
- ○ Flatulence
- ✗ Light-headedness
- ✗ Pain
- ○ Respirations
- ○ Temperature
- ✗ Vomiting

Rationale

Several of the client's vital signs are abnormal. The client's body temperature, heart rate, and respiratory rate are all slightly elevated, but these findings are not life threatening. The client's low blood pressure and irregular cardiac rhythm are very concerning and most likely contributed to the client's light-headedness when getting out of bed. The nurse must follow up on these findings immediately to prevent potentially life-threatening perfusion issues. The client's projectile vomiting and abdominal pain are also priority findings that must be followed up on by the nurse and health care team. Not only are these symptoms uncomfortable for the client, but they are most likely signs of a serious gastrointestinal condition and could cause dehydration or another life-threatening condition. Flatulence is generally a positive sign of gastrointestinal motility and does not require immediate follow-up by the nurse.

CJ Cognitive Skill: Recognize Cues

References: Linton & Matteson, 2023, pp. 90–99, 778–779

Thinking Exercise 7.1.2

Answer

DATA COLLECTION FINDINGS	ACUTE APPENDICITIS	ACUTE PANCREATITIS	SMALL BOWEL OBSTRUCTION
Abdominal pain	✗	✗	✗
Hyperactive, high-pitched bowel sounds			✗
Nausea and vomiting	✗	✗	✗
Fever	✗	✗	
Flatulence	✗		✗

Rationale

Acute appendicitis is a condition in which the appendix becomes inflamed and filled with pus resulting in acute abdominal pain (usually peri-umbilical or right lower quadrant pain) that may worsen with coughing or movement. Clients may also experience nausea and vomiting, bloating and flatulence, and fever and chills. Acute pancreatitis is inflammation of the pancreas resulting in severe abdominal pain in the upper quadrants and frequently radiating to the client's back or left shoulder. Eating or drinking may worsen the pain. Clients with pancreatitis also experience nausea and vomiting, tachycardia, and fever. Small bowel obstruction is a blockage of the bowel that prevents the normal passage of food, air, and fluid. Classic signs of small bowel obstruction are nausea and vomiting (possibly projectile vomiting) as well as abdominal distention, tenderness, and guarding. Early signs may also include bloating and flatulence along with hyperactive, high-pitched bowel sounds as the bowel attempts to overcome the obstruction.
CJ Cognitive Skill: Analyze Cues
References: Linton & Matteson, 2023, pp. 777–780, 812–816

Thinking Exercise 7.1.3

Answer

The nurse recognizes that the client is *most likely* experiencing **small bowel obstruction**. The client is at the highest risk for **dehydration** and **electrolyte imbalance**.

Rationale

The client findings and health history correlate most closely with a diagnosis of small bowel obstruction. Intestinal obstruction can be caused by many factors including a strangulated hernia, a tumor, paralytic ileus, strictures, volvulus, intussusception, and postoperative adhesions. Scar tissue from previous abdominal trauma and surgery increases this client's risk for bowel obstruction. The client has no known risk factors for pancreatitis including diabetes, obesity, or excessive alcohol consumption. The client's lipase is also within normal limits and would be elevated if the pancreas were inflamed. Although acute appendicitis frequently occurs in clients between 10 and 30 years of age, the client denies recent infections or constipation, which can cause appendicitis. The client's white blood cell (WBC) count and C-reactive protein (CRP) are also within normal limits, which indicates that no inflammation or infectious processes are present. Vomiting large amounts of emesis leads to losses of fluid and electrolytes, which increases the client's risk for dehydration and electrolyte imbalances. Client findings including elevated heart rate, low blood pressure, and dizziness upon rising are all signs of potential dehydration. The client's irregular heart rhythm may be caused by an electrolyte imbalance. The client's red blood cell (RBC) count does not indicate a risk of anemia. Ascites can occur when pancreatic secretions collect in the peritoneum; the client is not at risk for this condition.
CJ Cognitive Skill: Prioritize Hypothesis
References: Linton & Matteson, 2023, pp. 777–780, 812–816; Pagana et al., 2023, pp. 292, 554, 688, 749, 946

Thinking Exercise 7.1.4

Answer

POTENTIAL NURSING ACTIONS	INDICATED	NOT INDICATED
Insert a nasogastric tube and connect to suction.	X	
Infuse isotonic fluids via peripheral venous access.	X	
Request a breakfast tray with bland foods.		X
Monitor intake and output.	X	
Prepare for an abdominal computed tomography (CT) scan.	X	

Rationale

An intestinal obstruction may be suspected based on the client's history, physical examination, and laboratory studies, but a radiology test, usually a CT scan, is required to confirm the diagnosis. The nurse would anticipate this test and prepare the client for the CT scan. Initial treatment of an intestinal obstruction is often gastrointestinal decompression unless emergency surgery is indicated first. The nurse would insert a nasogastric tube, connect it to suction, monitor output, and ensure that it is consistently draining. Intravenous fluids would also be prescribed to promote fluid balance, therefore the nurse would establish peripheral venous access and anticipate administration of isotonic fluids such as 0.9% normal saline. The client would remain NPO to rest the bowels. The nurse would closely monitor fluid balance via intake and output and frequent weights.

CJ Cognitive Skill: Generate Solutions

References: Linton & Matteson, 2023, pp. 777–778

Thinking Exercise 7.1.5

Answer

The nurse would *prioritize* the administration of **potassium chloride IV** and monitoring for **cardiac dysrhythmias**.

Rationale

The client's serum potassium level is significantly low. Hypokalemia can cause life-threatening dysrhythmias, therefore the nurse must first address this condition. The nurse would prioritize the administration of supplemental potassium chloride via the IV route because the client is currently NPO and initiate continuous ECG monitoring for early identification of dysrhythmias. Although the nurse would administer prescribed morphine sulfate and monitor the client's response, pain is not a life-threatening condition, therefore pain management would occur after initiating potassium replacement protocols and continuous ECG monitoring. The client's SpO_2 level is within normal limits, and there are no signs of respiratory distress or hypoxemia present. Supplemental oxygen is not a priority action. Dehydration can cause elevated BUN and sodium levels with normal serum creatinine levels. Intravenous fluids currently infusing will help replace lost fluids.

CJ Cognitive Skill: Take Actions

References: Linton & Matteson, 2023, pp. 90–99, 777–778; Pagana et al., 2023, pp. 150, 292, 296, 451, 554, 688, 707, 749, 803, 946

Thinking Exercise 7.1.6

Answer

DATA COLLECTION FINDINGS	IMPROVED	NOT IMPROVED
Abdominal pain		X
Blood pressure	X	
Cardiac rhythm	X	
Fever		X
Urine output	X	

Rationale

The client's fluid and electrolyte imbalances are correcting as evidenced by the client's improved blood pressure, normal sinus cardiac rhythm, and urine output. The client's pain was previously relieved per the 1200 nurses' notes but has returned and is greater than it was earlier. Sudden sharp pain accompanied by abdominal rigidity and fever are signs of a bowel perforation, a serious complication of intestinal obstruction. These findings must be reported to the health care provider immediately. If untreated, bowel perforation can cause peritonitis and sepsis.

CJ Cognitive Skill: Evaluate Outcomes
References: Linton & Matteson, 2023, pp. 90–95, 777–779

Unfolding Case Study 7.2

Thinking Exercise 7.2.1

Answer

The client's **pulmonary congestion** and **urinary output** are *most concerning* and must be followed up by the nurse immediately.

Rationale

The nurse is most concerned with the client's pulmonary congestion. An increasing respiratory rate, decreasing SpO_2 level, labored respirations, crackles auscultated throughout lung fields, and pale, frothy secretions are all signs of respiratory distress, which can be life threatening. The nurse must follow up on these findings immediately to prevent hypoxemia and respiratory failure. Additionally, the nurse would be concerned with the client's low amount of urine output. Since arriving on the unit, the client's intake is 2300 mL and output is only 350 mL. Normal urine output is at least 30 mL/h, and this client's output is significantly less. Oliguria, abnormally small amounts of urine, may be caused by many conditions that can lead to organ failure if not treated immediately. Incisional redness and swelling around the umbilical area, pitting edema in the lower extremities, and bounding radial pulses are abnormal findings, but they are not life threatening and therefore not the nurse's priority concerns. The client's pain level is an expected finding and does not need immediate follow-up because it is not life threatening.

CJ Cognitive Skill: Recognize Cues
References: Linton & Matteson, 2023, pp. 294–304, 858–861

Thinking Exercise 7.2.2

Answer

The nurse recognizes that the client is *most likely* experiencing **acute kidney injury** as manifested by **oliguria** and **BUN and creatinine levels**.

Rationale

Client findings most closely align with acute kidney injury (AKI). The most current definition of AKI is an increase in serum creatinine by 0.3 mg/dL (26.2 µmol/L) within 48 hours (or 1.5 to 1.9 × baseline) and a urine volume less than 0.5 mL/kg/h for 6 hours. Current oliguria and increased creatinine levels match this definition and indicate that the kidneys are not functioning at the client's baseline level. The client's health history, including diabetes, hypertension, and obesity, increases the risk for both acute and chronic kidney dysfunction. Preoperative BUN and creatinine results demonstrate that the client already had possible kidney dysfunction, most likely a complication of poorly controlled blood glucose levels (elevated HbA1c), which increases the risk of AKI, especially after major surgery and an episode of hypotension (PACU vital signs). During the oliguria phase of AKI, urine output may decrease to less than 400 mL/day, causing hypervolemia (fluid overload) and resulting in increased creatinine levels. Although the client's blood glucose level is elevated, it is not high enough to be consistent with a hyperglycemic hyperosmolar state (HHS). Additionally, clients with HHS usually experience polyuria and dehydration. Hypoactive bowel sounds after a major abdominal surgery are normal. The client is currently passing flatulence, which is a positive sign of bowel function, and normal bowel sounds should resume within 1 or 2 days after surgery.

CJ Cognitive Skill: Analyze Cues

References: Linton & Matteson, 2023, pp. 294–304, 858–861; Pagana et al., 2023, pp. 150, 296, 451, 462, 688, 707, 749, 803, 946

Thinking Exercise 7.2.3

Answer

- ◯ Anemia
- ◯ Bone fractures
- ✗ Fluid volume excess
- ✗ Hyperglycemia
- ✗ Inadequate nutrition
- ◯ Peripheral neuropathy
- ◯ Uremic halitosis

Rationale

Anemia, bone fractures, peripheral neuropathy, and uremic halitosis are complications of chronic kidney disease and not consistent with acute kidney injury (AKI). The client is experiencing fluid volume excess secondary to oliguria. Pulmonary complications of excess fluid volume are life threatening, therefore the nurse would identify fluid overload as a priority condition. Although the client has a history of diabetes mellitus, current hyperglycemia may be a result of the stress of illness and increases in blood levels of catecholamines, cortisol, and glucagon. The nurse would prioritize the management of blood glucose levels to prevent complications, including neurologic changes and risk of infection. Finally, the nurse would identify the client's increased nutritional needs for postoperative healing and due to the AKI diagnosis. Clients who have AKI often have a high rate of catabolism (protein breakdown) and may be too ill or their appetite too poor to meet caloric needs. The client has unique nutritional needs that must be addressed by the nurse and health care team.

CJ Cognitive Skill: Prioritize Hypotheses

References: Linton & Matteson, 2023, pp. 294–304, 858–861

Thinking Exercise 7.2.4

Answer

PRIORITY CONDITIONS	POTENTIAL NURSING ACTIONS
Fluid volume excess	◯ Administer a diuretic, such as spironolactone ✗ Restrict fluid intake ✗ Continuously assess and document fluid status
Hyperglycemia	◯ Administer oral antihyperglycemic medications ✗ Frequently monitor blood glucose levels ◯ Monitor for urinary ketones
Inadequate nutrition	✗ Assess food intake during every shift ✗ Collaborate with a registered dietitian nutritionist (RDN) ✗ Provide supplemental nutrition if needed

Rationale

To address the client's fluid volume excess, the nurse would closely monitor intake and output and assess for complications of fluid overload, especially pulmonary complications. The nurse would expect fluids to be restricted and intravenous fluids to be discontinued. The nurse would also plan to administer prescribed diuretics. An intravenous loop diuretic, such as furosemide, would most likely be prescribed. Spironolactone is a potassium-sparing diuretic and would be contraindicated due to the client's risk of hyperkalemia. The nurse would address the client's hyperglycemia by frequently monitoring blood glucose levels and administering insulin as prescribed. Oral hypoglycemia medications would not be used during the client's state of acute illness, and urinary ketones are monitored in clients with type 1 diabetes mellitus. To address the client's nutritional needs, the nurse would collaborate with a registered dietitian nutritionist to ensure that the client's protein and caloric needs are met. The nurse would also assess food intake during every shift, encourage the client to eat, and provide supplemental nutrition if needed to ensure that caloric intake is adequate. Weight would also be monitored to assess fluid and nutritional status.

CJ Cognitive Skill: Generate Solutions
References: Linton & Matteson, 2023, pp. 858–861

Thinking Exercise 7.2.5

Answer

- ✗ Assist the client to identify desired fluids to drink throughout the day.
- ✗ Collaborate with the client to develop a plan for fluid intake.
- ○ Encourage the client to suck on ice chips as desired to prevent dry mouth.
- ✗ Explain the purpose of fluid restriction and the goals of the current treatment plan.
- ✗ Offer oral care with swish-and-spit mouthwash to moisten oral mucosa.
- ○ Only allow fluids with meals to ensure that restrictions are not exceeded.
- ○ Provide a glass of iced water with directions to sip it slowly throughout the day.
- ○ Suggest eating foods higher in sodium to retain ingested fluids.

Rationale

It is essential for the client to understand the purpose of fluid restriction and the goals of treatment. The nurse would reinforce teaching to help minimize client anxiety related to fluid restriction. The nurse would also help the client cope with fluid limitations by assisting the client to choose desired fluids and collaborating with the client to develop a plan for fluid intake throughout waking hours. Small amounts of fluids should be provided throughout the day, not only with meals, and a full glass should not be left at the bedside. Ice chips may be offered to address dry mouth, but they must be counted toward fluid intake and therefore cannot be ingested as desired. The nurse may offer oral care with swish-and-spit mouthwash to moisten the oral mucosa but must ensure that the client does not drink additional fluids during oral care. A high-sodium diet would be contraindicated for this client and would not address the client's concerns related to dry mouth.

CJ Cognitive Skill: Take Actions
References: Linton & Matteson, 2023, pp. 294–304, 858–861

Thinking Exercise 7.2.6

Answer

History and Physical	Nurses' Notes	Laboratory Results	Nursing Flow Sheet

Surgical Day

1430: Client arrived from postanesthesia care unit. Health history includes type 2 diabetes mellitus, hypertension, and obesity. Alert and oriented × 4. Follows commands and moves extremities appropriately. Respirations equal and unlabored. Bilateral upper lobes clear, and lower lobes diminished on auscultation. Heart tones regular, pulses palpable throughout. Peripheral venous devices present in each arm; 0.9% NS infusing at 100 mL/h with no signs of infiltration present. Abdomen large and soft. Bowel sounds hypoactive in all quadrants. Midline abdominal incision covered with dry dressing, no drainage present. Indwelling urinary catheter draining clear-yellow urine to gravity. Reinforced deep breathing and coughing exercises. Client accurately demonstrates use of incentive spirometer and abdominal splinting. Patient-controlled anesthesia (PCA) device set as prescribed. Client denies pain.

Postoperative Day 1

0730: Client drowsy, easily aroused, and oriented × 4. Skin warm and dry. 1+ pitting edema present in bilateral lower extremities. Heart tones regular, bilateral radial pulses bounding, and pedal pulses palpable throughout. Respirations labored. Crackles noted throughout lung fields on auscultation. Client splints abdomen and performs deep breathing and coughing exercises. Expectorates pale, frothy secretions. Abdomen large, round, and soft. Hypoactive bowel sounds in all quadrants. Client reports passing small amounts of flatulence. No bowel movement. Midline abdominal incision well approximated, redness and swelling present around umbilicus, normal temperature, no drainage noted on dressing. Client reports incisional pain rated 3/10. Client demonstrates appropriate use of PCA. Indwelling urinary catheter drains dark-amber urine to gravity. Discuss daily plan including out of bed for breakfast. Client states being too tired to get out of bed and does not feel like eating breakfast.

0820: Physician at bedside. Orders received. Intravenous fluids discontinued. Furosemide 20 mg IV administered. Registered dietitian nutritionist consult initiated. Client oriented × 4. Remains in bed for breakfast, eating less than 50% of meal. Fluids restricted to 1500 mL daily.

1130: Client requests a glass of iced water, stating "My mouth is so dry. I can't believe I am only allowed a liter and a half of fluid today. That won't be enough."

1400: Client alert and oriented × 4. Skin warm and dry. Nonpitting edema is present in bilateral lower extremities. Heart tones regular and pulses palpable throughout. Respirations equal and unlabored. Crackles noted in bilateral lower lobes of lungs on auscultation. Abdomen large, round, and soft. Bowel sounds present in all quadrants. Client reports passing flatulence. No bowel movement. Midline abdominal incision well approximated, redness and swelling present around umbilicus, normal temperature, no drainage noted on dressing. Client splints abdomen, uses incentive spirometer, and performs deep breathing and coughing exercises. Dry cough: No sputum expectorated. Client reports incisional pain rated 2/10 with breathing exercises; demonstrates appropriate use of PCA. Indwelling urinary catheter draining clear-yellow urine to gravity.

History and Physical	Nurses' Notes	Laboratory Results	Nursing Flow Sheet

		Medical-Surgical Unit			
	Postanesthesia Care Unit	Surgical Day 1430	Surgical Day 2000	Postoperative Day 1 0730	Postoperative Day 1 1400
Vital Signs					
T	98.1°F (36.7°C)	98.5°F (36.9°C)	98.7°F (37°C)	98.9°F (37.1°C)	98.7°F (37°C)
HR	72 beats/min	80 beats/min	86 beats/min	92 beats/min	86 beats/min
BP	88/45 mm Hg	110/49 mm Hg	118/50 mm Hg	143/72 mm Hg	114/69 mm Hg
RR	12 breaths/min	14 breaths/min	12 breaths/min	18 breaths/min	14 breaths/min
SpO_2	96%	98%	98%	94%	98%
O_2	40% facemask	4 L/min via NC	2 L/min via NC	2 L/min via NC	2 L/min via NC
Intake					
IV	2500 mL	–	550 mL	1150 mL	100 mL
Oral	–	–	240 mL	360 mL	450 mL
Output					
Urinary	–	300 mL	150 mL	200 mL	720 mL
Approximate blood loss	1750 mL	–	–	–	–

Rationale

The client presents several signs of improved respiratory function. Respirations are currently unlabored, the respiratory rate has decreased, and the SpO_2 level is within normal limits on 2 L/min O_2 via nasal cannula. The client continues to perform deep breathing and coughing exercises as expected but is no longer expectorating pale, frothy secretions. The client's blood pressure and urinary output are also within normal limits, indicating improved kidney function. Urinary output is averaging 110 mL/h and is clear and yellow. Incisional pain has decreased from 3/10 to 2/10 when doing breathing exercises. Finally, bowel sounds are active in all quadrants. This is a positive postoperative sign of returning to normal bowel function.

CJ Cognitive Skill: Evaluate Outcomes
References: Linton & Matteson, 2023, pp. 294–304, 858–861

Stand-Alone Thinking Exercise 7.1

Answer

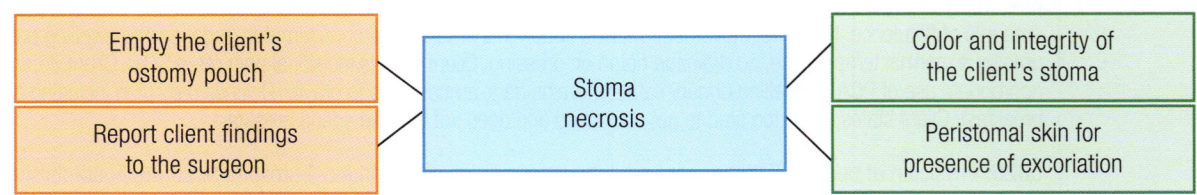

Rationale

The nurse would recognize dark-purple discoloration of the stoma as a sign of stoma necrosis, an early postoperative complication resulting from inadequate stomal blood supply or ischemia. Stoma necrosis is often related to tension on the mesentery, ligation of the primary blood vessel, or excessive mesenteric dissection, and it most frequently develops in obese patients and those undergoing emergency stoma creation. Signs of ischemia, arising in the superficial mucosa, typically present with partial discoloration of the stoma and tenderness at the stoma site. Ongoing ischemia may result in full-thickness stoma necrosis, which is usually not evident until several postoperative days. Superficial necrosis may resolve without surgical intervention, but severe necrosis is an emergency requiring timely revision of the stoma. Therefore the nurse would report data collection findings to the surgeon and frequently monitor the client's stoma for changes in color and integrity, carefully assessing for additional signs of ischemia. The nurse would also decrease pressure around the stoma site to promote blood flow by expelling excessive flatulence from the bag, emptying stool when the ostomy pouch is one-third full, and ensuring that the appliance template fits well and is not too tight around the stoma. Keeping the stoma warm and increasing client activity also helps increase blood flow. It is normal to have liquid stool and flatulence in the first few days after abdominal surgery and colostomy placement. With time, the stool becomes firm, and the sigmoid colostomy should produce stools similar to those previously passed through the anus. Because the stool is currently in liquid form, the nurse would monitor the client's peristomal skin for the presence of excoriation. The nurse would also reinforce nutritional teaching focused on foods that can cause increased flatulence including vegetables and other high-fiber foods. There are no signs of opioid-induced respiratory depression or fluid imbalance. The client's respiratory rate and oxygen saturation are within normal limits, and the client is alert and oriented. Additionally, the client is voiding clear-yellow urine, and the client's weight has not increased or decreased significantly during admission.

CJ Cognitive Skills: Recognize Cues, Analyze Cues, Prioritize Hypotheses, Generate Solutions, Take Actions, Evaluate Outcomes
Reference: Linton & Matteson, 2023, pp. 309–326

Stand-Alone Thinking Exercise 7.2

Answer

POTENTIAL ORDERS	INDICATED	NOT INDICATED
Acetaminophen for pain and fever management	✗	
Blood culture and sensitivity	✗	
Broad-spectrum antibiotic	✗	
Fetal ultrasound		✗
Fluid restriction		✗
Serum HbA1c level		✗
Urine culture and sensitivity	✗	

Rationale

The client is most likely experiencing acute pyelonephritis. Hormonal changes as well as obstruction caused by the fetus during pregnancy make acute pyelonephritis more common during the second trimester and beginning of the third trimester. Data collection findings consistent with acute pyelonephritis are fever, tachycardia, flank or back pain, abdominal discomfort, nausea, general malaise, nocturia, and burning, urgency, or frequency of urination. The client's urinalysis also shows positive leukocyte esterase and nitrites and the presence of white blood cells (WBCs). The nurse would anticipate obtaining a urine sample for culture and sensitivity testing and blood cultures to determine the source and spread of the infectious organism. While awaiting results from urine and blood cultures, the nurse would expect a broad-spectrum antibiotic to be prescribed. The nurse would also reinforce patient teaching focused on recommended fluid intake of 2 to 3 L/day to promote urine output and on pain and fever management with acetaminophen, which does not interfere with kidney blood flow and is safe during pregnancy. The client does not have a history of diabetes mellitus, and blood glucose levels have been stable. Therefore the nurse would not expect the client's HbA1c to be assessed. Additionally, the client reports an active fetus, and the fetal heart rate is normal for 26 weeks' gestation. The provider may order an ultrasound examination of the kidneys, but a fetal ultrasound examination is not required at this time.

CJ Cognitive Skills: Recognize Cues, Analyze Cues, Prioritize Hypotheses, Generate Solutions
Reference: Linton & Matteson, 2023, pp. 844–845; Pagana et al., 2023, pp. 150, 296, 451, 462, 688, 707, 749, 803, 905, 946

Answers With Rationales for Thinking Exercises

Unfolding Case Study 8.1

Thinking Exercise 8.1.1

Answer

The nurse recognizes that the client's **dysuria** and **pelvic pain** require follow-up by the nurse and health care team.

Rationale

The client has a history of dysmenorrhea or pain associated with menstruation. This is a chronic problem, but the nurse must recognize that the client's pelvic pain (abdominal and back pain) has worsened and is now occurring between menstrual cycles. Therefore the nurse would prioritize this finding and communicate it to the health care team for follow-up. Additionally, the nurse would recognize dysuria or pain when urinating as an abnormal finding requiring immediate follow-up. Dysuria is a symptom of many conditions including various infections that can cause tissue or organ failure. The client's alcohol intake is greater than recommended but not an immediate concern. Fatigue is also an abnormal finding associated with many conditions and may be a secondary symptom from chronic pain. The nurse would plan to address the client's fatigue after following up on the pelvic and urinary pain. The client's urine is within normal limits.
Cognitive Skill: Recognize Cues
Reference: Linton & Matteson, 2023, pp. 1052–1056

Thinking Exercise 8.1.2

Answer

CLIENT FINDINGS	ENDOMETRIOSIS	INTERSTITIAL CYSTITIS	PELVIC INFLAMMATORY DISEASE
Pelvic pain not related to menstruation	✗	✗	✗
Dysmenorrhea	✗		✗
Painful sexual intercourse (dyspareunia)	✗	✗	✗
Dysuria	✗	✗	✗

Rationale

Endometriosis is a condition in which cells similar to the lining of the uterus, or endometrium, grow outside the uterus. Pelvic inflammatory disease (PID) is an infection within the female reproductive system that is often caused by bacteria from a sexually transmitted infection such as chlamydia. Endometriosis and PID share similar symptoms of pelvic pain, dysmenorrhea, dyspareunia, and dysuria. Clients with endometriosis may also experience pain during defecation and blood in the urine (hematuria) or stool. Unusual vaginal discharge, especially yellow, green, or odorous discharge, occurs with PID but not with endometriosis. Interstitial cystitis is a non-infectious condition of bladder inflammation. Like endometriosis and PID, female clients with interstitial cystitis may also experience dysuria, pelvic pain, and dyspareunia. Dysmenorrhea is not a sign of interstitial cystitis, but urinary frequency and urgency are.
Cognitive Skill: Analyze Cues
Reference: Linton & Matteson, 2023, pp. 1052–1056

Thinking Exercise 8.1.3

Answer

The client is *most likely* experiencing **endometriosis**. The nurse determines that the *priority* for care at this time is **pain management**.

Rationale

Although the client's symptoms are common to all three conditions, hematuria and the presence of pelvic masses are signs of endometriosis, not interstitial cystitis or PID. Treatment of endometriosis varies with severity of the condition and may include pain medication, oral contraceptives, laparoscopy for diagnosis and removal of endometrial implants, and total abdominal hysterectomy with bilateral salpingo-oophorectomy. Although not life-threatening, the nurse would prioritize pain management, validating that the pain is real and providing information about pain relief measures. Endometriosis is not caused by an infection, therefore antibiotic therapy is not needed. The client and partner may benefit from counseling, but physical pain needs to be managed first.
Cognitive Skill: Prioritize Hypotheses
Reference: Linton & Matteson, 2023, pp. 1052–1056

Thinking Exercise 8.1.4

Answer

POTENTIAL NURSING ACTIONS	INDICATED	NOT INDICATED
Encourage expression of anxiety and concerns related to sexuality and reproduction.	✗	
Discuss postoperative care including incentive spirometry, early ambulation, and pain management.	✗	
Assess the client's understanding of the procedure, and answer questions as appropriate.	✗	
Suggest the use of creams and lubricants to manage loss of libido or vaginal changes.	✗	
Reinforce preoperative teaching focused on laboratory tests and preparations the night before surgery.	✗	

Rationale

All of the nursing actions would be included in the client's presurgical care. A total abdominal hysterectomy with bilateral salpingo-oophorectomy involves removal of the entire uterus and cervix along with the fallopian tubes and ovaries from both sides of the body. The nurse must complete psychosocial assessments and explore the significance of the surgery for the client and partner related to sexuality and reproduction. Many females relate their uterus to self-image, femininity, and/or sexuality. Therefore the nurse would facilitate a safe and therapeutic discussion with the client and partner, correct any misperceptions such as surgically induced masculinization and weight gain, and educate the client about vaginal estrogen creams, lubricants, and gentle dilation that can help if loss of libido or vaginal changes occur. The nurse would also evaluate the client's understanding of the procedure to obtain informed consent and reinforce preoperative teaching focused on surgical preparation, laboratory tests, and NPO status. The nurse would also discuss postoperative care including incentive spirometry, early ambulation, and pain management.
Cognitive Skill: Generate Solutions
Reference: Linton & Matteson, 2023, pp. 1052–1056

Thinking Exercise 8.1.5

Answer

POTENTIAL POSTOPERATIVE COMPLICATIONS	POTENTIAL NURSING ACTION
Postoperative bleeding	✗ Assess the client's abdominal dressing and perineal pad every hour. ○ Monitor vital signs every 12 hours and then once a shift until discharge. ✗ Report vaginal bleeding that saturates more than one perineal pad per hour to the surgeon.
Urinary retention	✗ Assist the client to the bathroom, and provide privacy and assistive measures to promote spontaneous voiding. ✗ Record urinary output and the color, clarity, and odor of urine. ✗ Teach the client to perform perineal hygiene after voiding and at least every 8 hours.
Pain	✗ Administer analgesics as ordered. ✗ Assess pain location, character, and severity. ✗ Assist the client to brace the abdomen when performing breathing exercises.

Rationale

The nurse must monitor the client carefully to identify postoperative complications that may occur during the first 12 to 24 hours after a total hysterectomy. The nurse would assess the client's abdominal dressing and perineal pad at least every hour for the first 12 hours and report any incisional drainage or excessive vaginal bleeding (saturating more than one perineal pad per hour). Vital signs would also be monitored frequently, usually every 4 hours, to evaluate adequacy of fluid volume and peripheral circulation. Urinary retention is a common complication due to surgical manipulation, local tissue edema, and temporary sensory or motor impairment. The nurse would assess and record urinary output and the color, clarity, and odor of the urine. The nurse would also assist the client to the bathroom and provide assistive measures (running water in the sink or pouring warm water over the perineum) as needed to promote spontaneous voiding. If the client is unable to void spontaneously, intermittent catheterization may be required. Additionally, the nurse would teach and assist the client to perform perineal hygiene after every voiding and at least every 8 hours. Perineal hygiene includes washing the vulva with warm, soapy water and then rinsing with warm water from an irrigating apparatus. Frequent pain assessments would also be completed and include location, character, and severity of pain. The nurse would administer analgesics as ordered and implement comfort measures such as frequent repositioning and bracing techniques when performing breathing exercises.

Cognitive Skill: Take Actions
Reference: Linton & Matteson, 2023, pp. 1052–1056

Thinking Exercise 8.1.6

Answer

✗ "I will report any increased redness or drainage from my incision to the surgeon."

○ "Resting in bed for at least 1 week will minimize surgical complications and promote wound healing."

✗ "I will avoid lifting anything more than 10 lb (4.5 kg) for the next 6 weeks."

○ "My menstrual periods may be irregular for the first few months after surgery."

✗ "I will monitor my temperature and contact the surgeon if I have a fever at or above 100°F (37.8°C)."

✗ "I may experience hot flashes, night sweats, and vaginal dryness due to the surgical procedure."

✗ "If I experience any acute leg pain, swelling, or redness, I should contact the surgeon."

Rationale

The client and partner should be taught to provide personal home care after surgery and report potential complications and/or changes to the surgeon. The client correctly understands to contact the surgeon with signs of an incisional infection (wound redness and drainage, fever) or deep vein thrombosis (leg pain, swelling, and redness). The client also understands activity restrictions. The client should not remain in bed as this may increase complications of thrombosis or respiratory infections. The client should avoid strenuous activity including lifting anything heavier than 5 to 10 lb. The client's uterus and ovaries were removed, therefore the client will no longer menstruate. The client may have some vaginal discharge for a few days after going home and may experience menopause symptoms such as hot flashes, night sweats, and vaginal dryness.

Cognitive Skill: Evaluate Outcomes

Reference: Linton & Matteson, 2023, pp. 1052–1056

Unfolding Case Study 8.2

Thinking Exercise 8.2.1

Answer

History and Physical	Nurses' Notes	Orders	Laboratory Results

1220: Male client presents with dysuria and hematuria. Client reports difficulty starting urination, unable to maintain a constant stream, and burning during urination. States, "I thought I should come to the emergency room when I noticed blood in my urine." Alert and oriented × 4. Reports recent fatigue and some expected weight loss. Heart tones regular, skin warm and dry, pulses palpable throughout. Bilateral lower extremity nonpitting edema present. Respirations equal and unlabored. Lung fields clear upon auscultation. Abdomen soft and flat with active bowel sounds in all quadrants. Last bowel movement this morning; soft, light-brown stool. Client reports recent rectal pressure and painful defecation. Denies penile discharge or blisters/sores on genitals or anus. VS: T 98.8°F (37.1°C), HR 72 beats/min, RR 14 breaths/min, BP 136/49 mm Hg, SpO₂ 98% on RA. Denies pain. The client is a tax accountant, lives alone, and is divorced with no children.

Rationale

The nurse must recognize abnormal genitourinary symptoms such as urinary hesitancy (difficulty initiating or maintaining a urine stream), dysuria (pain or burning sensation during urination), and hematuria (blood in urine). These symptoms may be caused by an infection or urinary obstruction and require immediate follow-up to prevent postrenal acute kidney injury, a potentially life-threatening condition. The nurse would also plan to follow up on the client's report of rectal pressure and painful defecation as these may be signs of a serious urinary or bowel condition. The other client findings are within normal limits or are not life threatening.

CJ Cognitive Skill: Recognize Cues

Reference: Linton & Matteson, 2023, pp. 1094–1095, 1099–1100, 1112–1125

Thinking Exercise 8.2.2

Answer

✗ Benign prostatic hyperplasia
○ Constipation
✗ Cystitis
○ Hemorrhoids
✗ Prostate cancer
✗ Sexually transmitted infection
✗ Renal calculi

Rationale

Dysuria, urinary hesitancy, and hematuria correlate with several conditions including benign prostatic hyperplasia (BPH), cystitis, prostate cancer, sexually transmitted infections (STIs), and renal calculi. STIs commonly present with perineal itchiness, blisters or sores on the genitals or the anus, and abnormal discharge from the penis. This client is not experiencing these symptoms, but many STIs are asymptomatic, therefore they should not be ruled out at this time. Rectal pressure and painful defecation may occur with constipation and hemorrhoids as well as with an enlarged prostate due to BPH or prostate cancer. The client's last bowel movement was this morning, and no anal blisters or sores are present; therefore the constipation and hemorrhoids are not potential health problems.

CJ Cognitive Skill: Analyze Cues
Reference: Linton & Matteson, 2023, pp. 842–843, 848, 1094–1095, 1099–1100, 1112–1125

Thinking Exercise 8.2.3

Answer

The nurse determines the ***priority*** for care at this time is to establish a **therapeutic environment** for **expressing concerns and asking questions**.

Rationale

The client is in the emergency department alone and received diagnostic results that may be confusing and scary. The nurse must establish a therapeutic environment with trust and mutual respect for the client to discuss concerns, ask questions, and fully understand the situation and scheduled exam. Although a clear pathway to the bathroom is important, it is not the highest priority at this time. The client is alert and oriented × 4, has no known fall risks, and is not receiving the Fleet enema in the emergency department. The outpatient procedure will require the client to administer the enema at home 2 hours prior to the procedure. The client's postvoid residual (PVR) volume is 125 mL. A PVR volume greater than 200 mL is considered abnormal; therefore intermittent urinary catheterization is not currently needed.

CJ Cognitive Skill: Prioritize Hypotheses
Reference: Linton & Matteson, 2023, pp. 1099–1100

Thinking Exercise 8.2.4

Answer

✗ Case manager consult for discharge home in the morning
○ Discontinue urinary catheter once ambulating
✗ Docusate sodium 50 mg orally each day PRN
✗ Monitor intake and output every shift
✗ Oxybutynin 5 mg orally every 8 hours PRN
✗ Patient-controlled anesthesia (PCA)
○ Sequential compression devices when in bed

Rationale

The nurse would anticipate postoperative orders typical for any client undergoing a surgical procedure including frequent vital signs, fluids to maintain hydration, pain management, wound care, and interventions to prevent pulmonary complications and blood clots including sequential compression devices when the client is in bed. Patient-controlled analgesia (PCA) is a common method of opioid delivery during the first 24 hours after surgery. The client would have an indwelling urinary catheter, and the nurse will be expected to monitor intake and output at least every shift. The nurse would not anticipate an order to remove the urinary catheter immediately after surgery. The nurse would expect a stool softener, such as docusate sodium, to prevent possible constipation and an antispasmodic drug, such as oxybutynin, to decrease bladder spasm induced by the indwelling urinary catheter. Clients who have minimally invasive procedures are discharged 1 to 2 days after surgery and can resume usual activities in about 1 or 2 weeks.

CJ Cognitive Skill: Generate Solutions
Reference: Linton & Matteson, 2023, pp. 1095–1100

Thinking Exercise 8.2.5

Answer

POTENTIAL NURSING ACTION	INDICATED	NOT INDICATED
Teach the client how to empty the indwelling urinary catheter collection bag.	✗	
Demonstrate how to inspect the incisional sites for signs of infection.	✗	
Obtain a blood sample for a postsurgical PSA blood test.		✗
Remove the wound closure tape, and cleanse each laparoscopic wound with sterile saline.		✗
Teach the client proper urinary meatus cleansing.	✗	

Rationale

The client would most likely be discharged with an indwelling urinary catheter. Therefore the nurse would reinforce teaching related to catheter care including cleansing the urinary meatus, maintaining straight drainage to promote urinary elimination, and emptying the collection bag. Clients who had a laparoscopic procedure can usually shower 1 to 2 days after surgery. The 2 × 2 bandages may be removed, but the wound closure tape must be left in place and allowed to fall off naturally in about 1 week to 10 days. Clients should be shown how to inspect the incision or puncture site(s) daily for signs of infection. PSA blood tests are usually performed 6 weeks after surgery and then every 4 to 6 months to monitor progress. A PSA test is not indicated at this time.

CJ Cognitive Skill: Take Actions
Reference: Linton & Matteson, 2023, pp. 1095–1100

Thinking Exercise 8.2.6

Answer

The nurse recognizes that the client is likely experiencing **erectile dysfunction** and **urinary incontinence**, which indicates that the client is not progressing as expected.

Rationale

Urge incontinence and erectile dysfunction (ED) are potential long-term complications of prostatectomy and indicate that the client is not progressing as expected. Urinary incontinence occurs because the internal and external sphincters of the bladder lie close to the prostate gland and can potentially be damaged during surgery. The nurse must recognize that the client is experiencing this complication and reinforce teaching related to Kegel perineal exercises. The nurse can teach the client a variety of ways to stimulate the perineal muscles. The nurse would also further explore the client's concern related to achieving an erection to determine the extent of ED present. Drugs such as sildenafil may be effective in treating ED, so the nurse would communicate this condition to the surgeon. The client's activity level and wound assessment are within normal limits for 6 weeks after surgery. Although the nurse would follow up on the client's daily use of a stool softener to ensure that it is not being misused, there are no signs indicating that the client is experiencing constipation or painful defecation.

CJ Cognitive Skill: Evaluate Outcomes

Reference: Linton & Matteson, 2023, pp. 1095–1100

Unfolding Case Study 8.3

Thinking Exercise 8.3.1

Answer

History and Physical	Nurses' Notes	Orders	Laboratory Results

0620: Client presents with dysuria and testicular pain. Reports symptoms started yesterday afternoon and noticed a creamy, green-colored discharge from his penis this morning. Alert and oriented × 4. Heart tones regular, skin warm and dry, pulses palpable throughout. Respirations equal and unlabored. Lung fields clear upon auscultation. Abdomen soft and flat with active bowel sounds in all quadrants. Last bowel movement yesterday morning. Client reports urinary frequency and urgency throughout the night. Testicles are swollen and tender to touch. No swelling, discoloration, or wounds present on penis or meatus. VS: T 99.9°F (37.7°C), HR 68 beats/min, RR 14 breaths/min, BP 127/42 mm Hg, SpO_2 97% on RA. The client is single, works as a waiter, and is sexually active with more than one partner.

Rationale

The nurse must recognize abnormal reproductive and genitourinary findings including dysuria, creamy, green penile discharge, and urinary frequency and urgency. These symptoms are most likely caused by an infection and require immediate follow-up to prevent potential life-threatening complications. The nurse would also plan to follow up on the client's swollen and tender testicles as these may be signs of trauma, infection, or other testicular disorders. Finally, the nurse would ask follow-up questions to better understand the client's sexual history and recent experiences. All other client findings are within normal limits.

CJ Cognitive Skill: Recognize Cues

Reference: Linton & Matteson, 2023, pp. 1112–1125

Thinking Exercise 8.3.2

Answer

The nurse recognizes that the client is likely experiencing **sexually transmitted infection.**

Rationale

Client findings are most consistent with sexually transmitted infections (STIs) including painful or burning urination (dysuria), discharge from the penis, and swollen and tender testicles. Other conditions may manifest with similar signs and symptoms but are not consistent with all of the client's findings. For example, prostatitis (inflammation of the prostate gland) manifests with dysuria, hematuria, and a weak urinary stream, and inguinal hernia presents with a bulge in the scrotum and feelings of pain, heaviness, or burning in the groin. Neither condition includes discharge from the penis or is associated with a history of multiple sexual partners.

CJ Cognitive Skill: Analyze Cues

Reference: Linton & Matteson, 2023, pp. 842–843, 1083–1085, 1093, 1112–1118

Thinking Exercise 8.3.3

Answer

The nurse determines the *priority* for care at this time is to obtain **specimen for culture** prior to **administering anti-infective agents**.

Rationale

Discharge from the client's penis must be collected and studied to determine the exact infecting organism and proper treatments. The specimen for a culture or other laboratory test must be collected before giving the first dose of an anti-infective agent. Therefore the nurse would obtain the specimen first and then administer medications, provide patient education, and report to the local health department. Confirmed cases of many STIs must be reported to the local health department. Client consent is not needed as this action is considered mandatory reporting. A health department investigator would most likely follow up with the client to obtain the names of sexual partners. This is not the responsibility of the nurse.

CJ Cognitive Skill: Prioritize Hypotheses
Reference: Linton & Matteson, 2023, pp. 1112–1114

Thinking Exercise 8.3.4

Answer

POTENTIAL NURSING ACTIONS	INDICATED	NOT INDICATED
Assess the client's psychological response to being diagnosed with the sexually transmitted infections.	X	
Explain the risk for multiple sexually transmitted infections and other medical complications.	X	
Prepare the client for prostate and rectal examinations.		X
Suggest wearing supportive underwear and applying an ice pack to the groin area to reduce testicular pain.	X	
Transfer the client to an inpatient acute care unit.		X

Rationale

A diagnosis of STI can be very distressing. Clients may exhibit anxiety about treatment and potential complications, fear of rejection by others, anger at the person who transmitted the infection, concern about infecting others, or other emotions. This client responded by stating the need to go to work. The nurse must conduct an assessment to understand the client's response and intervene appropriately to address any concerns. Diagnosis with more than one STI is common in clients who have multiple sexual partners. Gonorrhea and chlamydia often occur together. STIs can cause sterility and damage other body organs including heart tissue and joints. The nurse must explain these conditions and complications to the client. The client may already be experiencing epididymitis, a complication of gonorrhea. The nurse can suggest supportive underwear and ice compresses to decrease inflammation and pain. STIs are usually treated in outpatient settings. There is no indication that the client needs to be transferred to an inpatient unit or that the client needs a prostate or rectal exam.

CJ Cognitive Skill: Generate Solutions
Reference: Linton & Matteson, 2023, pp. 1112–1125

Thinking Exercise 8.3.5

Answer

✗ Assess for allergies before administering antimicrobials.
○ Teach the client proper techniques for administering IM medication.
✗ Advise the client to be retested for sexually transmitted infections in 3 to 4 months.
○ Schedule a follow-up appointment with the client's primary health care provider.
○ Teach the client to take the antibiotics until symptoms are eliminated.

Rationale

Treatment for gonorrhea usually consists of a single dose of ceftriaxone IM, which in most cases cures the client quickly and safely. The nurse would administer the IM dose within the emergency department prior to discharging the client. The nurse always assesses for allergies prior to administering any antimicrobial. Treatment for chlamydia usually involves a 7-day anti-infective course. The nurse would teach the client to take the full course of the antibiotic even if symptoms are no longer present. The nurse would advise the client to schedule a follow-up appointment with the primary health care provider and be retested 3 to 4 months after treatment to confirm successful results of treatment. The nurse is not responsible for scheduling follow-up appointments for the client.

CJ Cognitive Skill: Take Actions
Reference: Linton & Matteson, 2023, pp. 1112–1125

Thinking Exercise 8.3.6

Answer

CLIENT STATEMENTS	UNDERSTANDING	NO UNDERSTANDING
"I will use a latex condom when engaging in sexual activities that involve genital contact."	✗	
"I should engage in oral sex because my sexually transmitted infections cannot be spread by oral-genital contact."		✗
"Decreasing the number of sexual partners will decrease my risk for future sexually transmitted infections."	✗	
"Treatment will eliminate symptoms, but I will always have these sexually transmitted infections."		✗

Rationale

Sexually transmitted infections are most commonly transmitted by contact with mucous membranes in the mouth, eyes, urethra, vagina, and rectum. Therefore the client can spread and contract STIs during oral-genital contact. A condom or latex barrier over the genitals should be used for genital, anal, and oral sexual contact. Decreasing the number of sexual partners, practicing abstinence, practicing mutual monogamy, and wearing a condom are all safe sexual practices and reduce the risk of STIs. Bacterial infections, such as chlamydia and gonorrhea, can be cured by the treatments prescribed, but the client will need to be retested to ensure that the treatments worked.

CJ Cognitive Skill: Evaluate Outcomes
Reference: Linton & Matteson, 2023, pp. 1112–1125

Stand-Alone Thinking Exercise 8.1

Answer

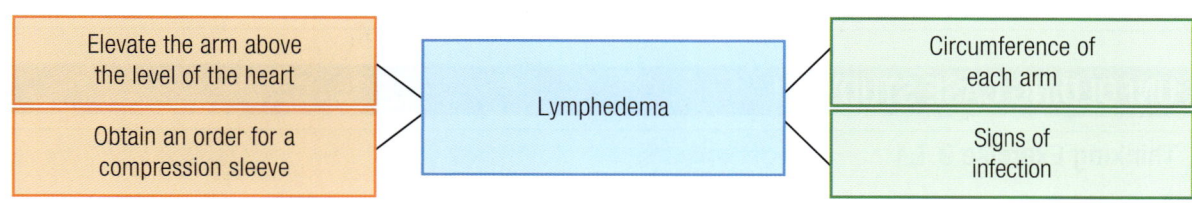

Rationale

This client is most likely experiencing lymphedema. A modified radical mastectomy includes removal of lymph nodes in the axilla. Because lymph nodes normally help return tissue fluid to the bloodstream, their removal can result in lymphedema or the accumulation of fluid in the affected area. Early signs of lymphedema are limb heaviness, aching or soreness, numbness, tingling, and stiffness. Clients may also experience limb weakness and impaired mobility of the shoulder, arm, elbow, wrist, and fingers. As the fluid increases, the limb may become visibly swollen with an observable increase in limb size. Lymphedema may be managed with a compression garment, self-massage, and gravity lymphatic drainage. Therefore the nurse would elevate the client's arm above the level of the heart and obtain an order for a compression sleeve to promote fluid removal from the arm. Monitoring and recording limb size or girth with a flexible nonstretch tape measure provides data for evaluating treatments and determining whether the client's condition is improving or not improving. The nurse would teach the client to measure both affected and nonaffected limbs at multiple points along each arm from the wrist up to the axilla. The most common complication of lymphedema is infection. Therefore the nurse would assess and teach the client to monitor for signs of infection, especially cellulitis. Angina pain is usually described as a sudden onset of squeezing, pressure, heaviness, tightness, or pain in the chest. Although females may not experience classic signs of angina, this client's symptoms did not start abruptly, and chest pain, dyspnea, and/or gastrointestinal symptoms are not present. Carpal tunnel syndrome manifests with arm numbness, tingling, weakness, and pain, but the client has no risk factors for carpal tunnel syndrome such as an occupation or hobby involving repetitive movements. The client fell recently and could have sprained a wrist using it to stop the fall. Signs of a sprained wrist are swelling, bruising, and pain that increases with touch or movement. This client did not report or show signs of pain when the extremity was assessed.

CJ Cognitive Skills: Recognize Cues, Analyze Cues, Prioritize Hypotheses, Generate Solutions, Take Actions, Evaluate Outcomes

Reference: Linton & Matteson, 2023, pp. 1064–1068

Answers With Rationales for Thinking Exercises

Thinking Exercise 9.1.1

Answer

History and Physical	Nurses' Notes	Orders	Laboratory Results

1145: Client brought to clinic by friend after concern that client was becoming isolated at home. Friend states that client recently "lost his wife, who was his best friend," and now is being evicted from a small apartment due to financial issues. Wife's health care bills were "overwhelming." Client's two adult children live out of state and seldom visit. Client states "There's no need to worry about me; nothing really matters." Reports recent anorexia, insomnia, and bad moods, especially in the mornings. Reports losing 30 lb (13.6 kg) in the past month. Other medical history includes substance use disorder (alcohol), hypertension, type 2 diabetes mellitus, H/O myocardial infarction, and early COPD. Alert and oriented × 4. VS: T 98.6°F (37°C), HR 78 beats/min and regular, RR 20 breaths/min, BP 126/82 mm Hg.

Rationale

Being a middle-aged adult experiencing stressful events (loss of wife and finances) and having a history of substance use, this client is susceptible to concerning emotional and behavioral findings. This client was becoming isolated with report of anorexia, insomnia, and irritable moods. These findings require immediate follow-up because they are consistent with possible life-threatening conditions as indicated by the client's reported apathy and worthlessness. Losing 30 lb (13.6 kg) also requires immediate follow-up due to anorexia. The other history shows the presence of chronic conditions that are not currently life threatening. The client's vital signs are within normal limits.
Cognitive Skill: Recognize Cues
Reference: Halter & Fratena, 2023, pp. 104–118

Thinking Exercise 9.1.2

Answer

The nurse recognizes that the client is likely experiencing **major depressive disorder**.

Rationale

The client's findings are most consistent with major depressive disorder. Common findings include agitated, sad, or irritable moods; anorexia or overeating; trouble sleeping; diminished interest or pleasure in participating in any activity; feelings of worthlessness and apathy; and lack of concentration and memory. There is no evidence that the client has findings that indicate any of the other choices. Additionally, clients on the schizophrenia spectrum are usually psychotic with delusions and/or hallucinations. The hallmark behavior associated with generalized anxiety disorder is excessive worry, which the client has not expressed. Bipolar disorder can include mania, hypomania, depression, or a combination.
Cognitive Skill: Analyze Cues
Reference: Halter & Fratena, 2023, pp. 104–118

Thinking Exercise 9.1.3

Answer

The nurse determines the ***priority*** for care at this time is to ensure the client's __safety__ because the client __feels worthless__ and __is becoming isolated__.

Rationale

The client likely has major depressive disorder, which places the client at risk for suicide or suicidal ideation, a life-threatening situation. Feelings of worthlessness, isolation, and apathy suggest that the client may feel there is nothing to live for. Therefore safety is the priority for the client's care. The client's nutritional and financial status need to be addressed, but there is no evidence that these issues are life threatening.
Cognitive Skill: Prioritize Hypotheses
Reference: Halter & Fratena, 2023, pp. 104–118

Thinking Exercise 9.1.4

Answer

POTENTIAL NURSING ACTIONS	INDICATED	NOT INDICATED
Transfer the client to an inpatient acute psychiatric facility.		✗
Reinforce health teaching about antidepressant drug therapy.	✗	
Consult with a social worker to ensure a safe home environment.	✗	
Assist the client in developing a safety plan.	✗	
Assess the client's support systems.	✗	

Rationale

At this time, there is no indication that the client needs to be admitted to an acute psychiatric facility. However, the client needs to begin antidepressant therapy, and the nurse needs to reinforce health teaching about the medication. The client also needs support and a plan to ensure safety. Assessing for support systems and ensuring a safe home environment can help the client remain in the community instead of being hospitalized.
Cognitive Skill: Generate Solutions
Reference: Halter & Fratena, 2023, pp. 104–118

Thinking Exercise 9.1.5

Answer

✗ "Do you feel like hurting yourself at this time?"
✗ "Do you feel like hurting someone else at this time?"
○ "Do you have a plan for paying your wife's medical bills?"
○ "Do you have a plan for where to live after your eviction?"
✗ "Do you have a plan to hurt yourself now or in the future?"

Rationale

Although the client is concerned about financial and living arrangements, the most important questions regarding safety include whether the client has a desire to hurt self or others. Assessing if the client has a plan for suicide is even more important because suicide occurs most often when a plan has been carefully thought out.
Cognitive Skill: Take Actions
Reference: Halter & Fratena, 2023, pp. 104–118

Thinking Exercise 9.1.6

Answer

DATA COLLECTION FINDING	IMPROVED	NOT IMPROVED
Client safety	✗	
Nutrition status	✗	
Feelings of worthlessness	✗	
Sleep		✗

Rationale

The client has been taking medication to treat depression and has improved as a result as demonstrated by no suicidal ideation, small weight gain indicating consuming more food, and being happy about being a new grandfather. Having this new role to look forward to helps improve self-worth and provide energy and excitement. However, the client continues to have difficulty sleeping, which has not improved.

Cognitive Skill: Evaluate Outcomes
Reference: Halter & Fratena, 2023, pp. 104–118

UNFOLDING CASE STUDY 9.2

Thinking Exercise 9.2.1

Answer

○ Skin dirty and odorous
○ Wearing only underwear
○ History of schizophrenia
✗ Threatening to kill people
○ History of substance use disorder
✗ Having auditory hallucinations

Rationale

The client's threat to kill others is obviously life-threatening and would require immediate follow-up to ensure safety. The client is hearing voices that may be calling the client worthless or instructing the client to kill self or others. Therefore the presence of auditory hallucinations requires immediate follow-up. Wearing few clothes and being dirty are not life-threatening findings. A history of substance use disorder and schizophrenia is also not imminently life threatening.

CJ Cognitive Skill: Recognize Cues
Reference: Halter & Fratena, 2023, pp. 75–88

Thinking Exercise 9.2.2

Answer

The nurse recognizes that the client is likely experiencing **psychosis**.

Rationale

The client believes that the voices being heard are real and that the client was selected to decide "who goes to heaven." This delusion combined with auditory hallucinations represents loss of contact with reality, or psychosis. Dementia is chronic confusion that is insidious in onset. Although psychotic behaviors can occur in clients who have dementia, this client has a history of schizophrenia and substance

use disorder. Anxiety causes fear, uncertainty, and apprehension. This client does not display findings associated with anxiety. Depression refers to mood and includes sadness, apathy, and changes in appetite and sleep, which this client does not have.
CJ Cognitive Skill: Analyze Cues
Reference: Halter & Fratena, 2023, pp. 75–88

Thinking Exercise 9.2.3

Answer

The nurse determines the *priority* for care at this time is to ensure **safety for self and others** because the client is **threatening to kill people**.

Rationale

Client safety is always the most important priority for nursing care. This client is threatening to kill people, which demonstrates that safety could be jeopardized. There is no evidence that the client is at risk for infection, and lack of housing is not more important that violence toward self or others.
CJ Cognitive Skill: Prioritize Hypotheses
Reference: Halter & Fratena, 2023, pp. 75–88

Thinking Exercise 9.2.4

Answer

POTENTIAL NURSING ACTIONS	INDICATED	NOT INDICATED
Contact the hospital administrator.		✗
Initiate a response code for agitation/potential violence.	✗	
Speak in a low voice when communicating with the client.	✗	
Restrain the client to prevent harm to self or others.		✗
Ask if the voices are telling the client to harm others.	✗	

Rationale

At this time, other methods to de-escalate the client should be used rather than using restraints because the client is verbally rather than physically threatening using a weapon or other device. The nurse would ask the client about what the voices are saying while speaking in a low voice. The nurse would initiate a response code for potential violence so security and other key personnel will be available to help if needed. The client is not using a weapon at this time, so the nurse would not need to contact the administrator. However, if the situation escalates, the nurse would notify the administrator.
CJ Cognitive Skill: Generate Solutions
Reference: Halter & Fratena, 2023, pp. 75–88

Thinking Exercise 9.2.5

Answer

✗ Provide time for the client to verbalize the outburst.
✗ Actively listen to what the client is saying before responding.
✗ Remove any equipment or items that could be a source of injury.
✗ Ask any unnecessary staff to leave the immediate area.
✗ Try to redirect the client's attention away from the internal voices.
✗ Maintain a distance of 2 to 3 feet from the client.

Rationale

All of the choices are correct and appropriate actions to ensure client and staff safety. The staff needs to be patient and allow the client to verbalize feelings while actively listening. Few staff should be in the area to decrease the number of individuals who could be injured. Keeping a distance of 2 to 3 feet prevents being hit by the client. Equipment or items that could be used as weapons also should be removed.

CJ Cognitive Skill: Take Actions
Reference: Halter & Fratena, 2023, pp. 75–88

Thinking Exercise 9.2.6

Answer

DATA COLLECTION FINDING	IMPROVED	NOT IMPROVED
Attention to internal voices	✗	
Dress and hygiene	✗	
Communication with others	✗	
Aggressive behaviors	✗	

Rationale

The client has been very adherent to planned interventions including participating in group therapy sessions. This demonstrates improved communication with others. The client continues to hear voices but pays less attention to them. Aggressive behaviors like threatening staff have subsided, and the client is now well-groomed. All of these findings show improvement in the client's condition.

CJ Cognitive Skill: Evaluate Outcomes
Reference: Halter & Fratena, 2023, pp. 75–88

UNFOLDING CASE STUDY 9.3

Thinking Exercise 9.3.1

Answer

- ○ Family history of major depressive disorder
- ✗ Alert and oriented × 2
- ✗ Isolated from family
- ✗ Has not eaten or slept for 8 days
- ✗ Irritable and using excessive profanity
- ✗ Mood changes from euphoria to anger
- ○ Conversation difficult to follow
- ○ History of generalized anxiety disorder

Rationale

The client is only 22 years of age but is only oriented to person and place, which is very concerning and should be immediately followed up. The client has been awake, has not eaten for 8 days, and remained isolated from the family. Along with the client's mood changes, including anger and irritability, these behaviors are very concerning to the nurse because the client could be at risk for injury to self or others. A history of anxiety and family history of depression are not as important at this time. Being unable to follow the client's conversation is also not a factor for possible self-harm or harm to others.

CJ Cognitive Skill: Recognize Cues
Reference: Halter & Fratena, 2023, pp. 89–102

Thinking Exercise 9.3.2

Answer

The nurse recognizes that the client is likely experiencing **acute mania**.

Rationale

The client findings that are most concerning to the nurse indicate that the client is experiencing acute mania. Clients who have acute mania stay awake and do not eat for at least 1 week.
CJ Cognitive Skill: Analyze Cues
Reference: Halter & Fratena, 2023, pp. 89–102

Thinking Exercise 9.3.3

Answer

The nurse determines the *priority* for care at this time is to prevent **injury** because the client **is irritable, impulsive, and angry**.

Rationale

The client findings suggest that the client is at risk for injury to self or others. The client demonstrates negative behaviors (irritability, impulsivity, and anger) that suggest the possibility of harm or violence. The nurse is always focused on maintaining safety as the priority for any client's care. It is not known if the client is dehydrated because the family reported the client had no food for 8 days. The client could have inadequate nutrition, but this possible condition is not more important than client safety.
CJ Cognitive Skill: Prioritize Hypotheses
Reference: Halter & Fratena, 2023, pp. 89–102

Thinking Exercise 9.3.4

Answer

POTENTIAL NURSING ACTIONS	INDICATED	NOT INDICATED
Assess whether the client is a danger to self or others.	X	
Assess the family's understanding of the client's situation.	X	
Use a firm and calm approach to the client.	X	
Provide thorough explanations to the client.		X
Monitor food intake and sleep pattern.	X	

Rationale

The nurse would continue assessing the client for safety, including determining if the client is at risk to self or others. Food intake and sleep pattern would also be continually assessed. Being calm but firm would likely elicit a positive client response, but presenting long, thorough explanations is not appropriate. The nurse would present short, concise information because the client likely has a short attention span or inattentiveness. The nurse would also ensure that the client's family is well informed about the client's situation.
CJ Cognitive Skill: Generate Solutions
Reference: Halter & Fratena, 2023, pp. 89–102

Thinking Exercise 9.3.5

Answer

✗ Provide frequent rest periods.
✗ Provide high-calorie fluids and finger foods.
○ Encourage the client to participate in structured group activities.
✗ Decrease environmental stimuli when possible.
✗ Provide one-on-one client observation on admission to ensure safety.

Rationale

Clients experiencing acute mania do not sleep and can become overly fatigued. Therefore providing frequent rest periods is very important. To maintain client safety as the priority for care, providing one-on-one observation is preferred at least for the first 24 hours after admission. Because the client does not take time to eat, the client should be offered high-calorie fluids like protein-rich smoothies or milkshakes and finger foods that can be accessed easily and eaten intermittently. When possible, stimuli in the environment should be removed or decreased to prevent adding to the client's irritability and restlessness. Having the client participate in group activities could present additional stimulation, therefore it would be best to have the client participate in individual structured activities.
CJ Cognitive Skill: Take Actions
Reference: Halter & Fratena, 2023, pp. 89–102

Thinking Exercise 9.3.6—Pharmacology

Answer

CLIENT STATEMENTS	UNDERSTANDING	NO UNDERSTANDING
"My blood lithium levels will be monitored while I am taking this drug."	✗	
"I will restrict my intake of fluids while taking this drug."		✗
"I know that I might gain weight while taking this drug."	✗	
"I should take this drug with meals to help decrease stomach irritation."	✗	

Rationale

Lithium is often the mood stabilizer of choice for clients who have bipolar disorder with mania. Drug blood levels must be monitored until the desired therapeutic level is reached and then every 3 to 6 months after that. Because lithium is a salt, fluid and sodium balance should be maintained on a consistent basis and not restricted. Weight gain can occur due to fluid retention, particularly in females. Taking the drug with meals can help decrease stomach irritation.
CJ Cognitive Skill: Evaluate Outcomes
Reference: Halter & Fratena, 2023, pp. 89–102, 357–358

Stand-Alone Thinking Exercise 9.1

Answer

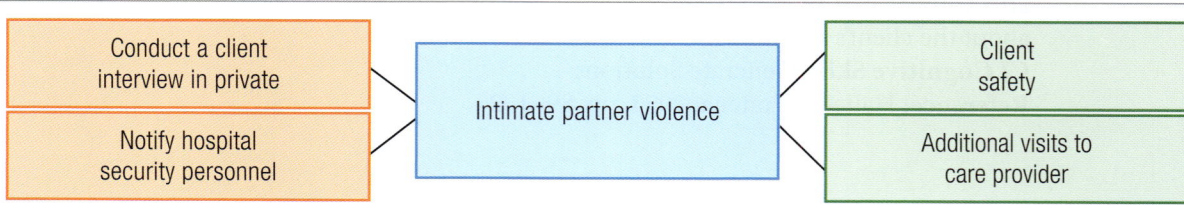

Rationale

The collected data are commonly seen in clients who experience intimate partner violence, including fear, unexplained bruising and other injuries, and frequent visits to the ED. There are no data that support substance use disorder, suicidal ideation, or major depressive disorder. The client's crying could be fear or concern about the client's children. To gain more information about the client's potential condition, the nurse would interview the client privately. Because the client's partner arrived at the ED and was demanding, angry, and intimidating, the nurse would want to notify hospital security immediately to stand by in case they are needed. The client's children are apparently safe, and the nurse would not need to contact CPS at this point. Counseling may have already been explored, so the nurse would ask if counseling has been sought in the past as part of the interview. As a result of nursing actions, the nurse and other health care professionals would want to ensure that the client is safe and that the client does not need to seek additional health care for future injuries. There is no evidence that the client needs neurologic assessment or vital signs monitoring and no indication that the client plans to commit suicide.

CJ Cognitive Skills: Recognize Cues, Analyze Cues, Prioritize Hypotheses, Generate Solutions, Take Actions, Evaluate Outcomes

Reference: Halter & Fratena, 2023, pp. 292–300

Stand-Alone Thinking Exercise 9.2

Answer

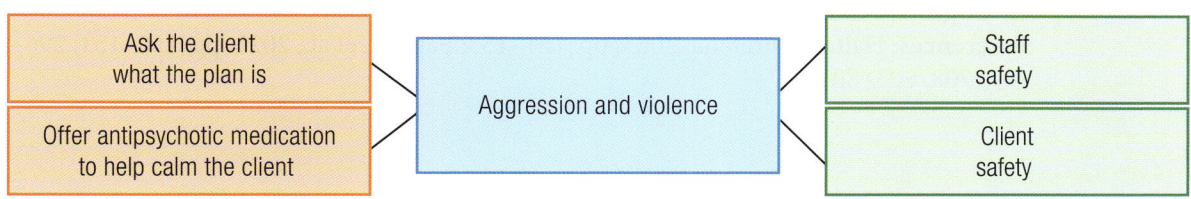

Rationale

The client is demonstrating anger, aggression, and violence. Although anger is a normal emotion, aggression is the behavioral manifestation of anger. Violence is an extreme type of aggression in which intentional physical or other type of injury or death is directed toward others. This client's findings support this condition rather than the other choices such as major depressive disorder or anxiety. Antisocial personality is typically manifested by lack of empathy, callousness, lack of concern for others, and impulsivity. The best action to take at this time is to offer antipsychotic medication that can help calm the client rather than restraints. Restraints may increase the client's anger and aggression. Contacting the social worker may be needed at some point, but not immediately. It is more important to determine what the client's plan is regarding potentially harming others. The safety of both the client and staff is most important for monitoring. At this time, knowing the client's blood alcohol level is not the most important parameter to monitor. There is no indication that the client has a plan for suicide; vital signs monitoring is not relevant in this client situation.

CJ Cognitive Skills: Recognize Cues, Analyze Cues, Prioritize Hypotheses, Generate Solutions, Take Actions, Evaluate Outcomes

Reference: Halter & Fratena, 2023, pp. 278–284

Stand-Alone Thinking Exercise 9.3

Answer

The nurse determines that the client is most at risk for **cardiac dysrhythmias** at this time.

Rationale

The client has a history of anorexia nervosa, which is characterized by an intense fear of gaining weight. Added to the history of major depressive disorder, clients with anorexia nervosa do not eat, or they eat and then purge their food. As a result, vital nutrients and electrolytes are not adequate to meet the body's needs. The laboratory test results indicate that the client's sodium, potassium, and glucose are below normal ranges. The client's sodium is low, but not at a critical value. Mild hyponatremia can cause weakness but would be unlikely to cause acute confusion or seizures. The client's glucose is low (hypoglycemia) but is not at a life-threatening level. The client's body has likely adjusted to this glucose level. Diabetic ketoacidosis is a hyperglycemia emergency. Potassium is needed for muscle function, including the myocardium. The client's potassium level is very low and approaching the critical value of 2.4 mEq/L. Severe hypokalemia can cause cardiac dysfunction that could manifest as a life-threatening cardiac dysrhythmia. The client's BUN and creatinine are slightly elevated indicating possible dehydration, increased catabolism (protein breakdown), and/or early kidney dysfunction. The most current definition of *acute kidney injury* is an increase in serum creatinine by 0.3 mg/dL (26.2 μmol/L) within 48 hours or 1.5 to 1.9 times baseline. The nurse would monitor the client's kidney function, but this is not the condition for which the client is most at risk.

CJ Cognitive Skills: Recognize Cues, Analyze Cues

References: Halter & Fratena, 2023, pp. 151–153; Pagana, et al., 2023, pp. 150–151, 296–297, 451–453, 707–708, 803–804

Answers With Rationales for Thinking Exercises

Unfolding Case Study 10.1

Thinking Exercise 10.1.1

Answer

- ○ History of generalized anxiety disorder
- ○ Inability to concentrate and problem-solve
- ✗ Difficulty sleeping
- ✗ Irritability and lack of patience
- ○ Palpitations and nausea when anxious
- ✗ Drinks excessive alcohol every night
- ✗ Tachycardia
- ✗ Elevated blood pressure

Rationale

The client's heart rate and blood pressure are elevated, which could be due to anxiety or a physiologic cause. Although these abnormalities are not currently life threatening, they could worsen. The client has insomnia for which the client is using excessive alcohol. Lack of sleep and excessive alcohol potentially could be life threatening and are immediately concerning. The client's irritability and lack of patience with family members could lead to abuse and require immediate follow-up by the health care team. Palpitations and nausea due to anxiety and the inability to concentrate or problem solve are not usually harmful or potentially harmful. Knowing that the client has a history of anxiety is helpful to understand the client's current situation, but it does not require immediate follow-up.
CJ Cognitive Skill: Recognize Cues
Reference: Halter & Fratena, 2023, pp. 264–277

Thinking Exercise 10.1.2

Answer

The nurse recognizes that the client is likely experiencing a **situational crisis**.

Rationale

Crises can be categorized into three types: (1) maturational (developmental) crises, (2) situational crises, and (3) adventitious crises. Situational crises are caused by an unanticipated life event such as job loss or the death of a family member. Coping with this type of crisis is often ineffective for clients who have a history of mental or behavioral disorders. The client is not out of touch with reality and therefore is not psychotic. Multiple types of personality disorders have been identified. Clients who have these disorders generally manifest odd or eccentric behaviors, erratic or dramatic behaviors, or fearful behaviors. This client does not demonstrate any of these findings. However, the client has a history of panic attacks. Panic is the most extreme manifestation of anxiety. Clients who have panic anxiety, sometimes called a *panic attack,* may try to withdraw from a situation by pacing, running, or screaming. Physical findings include sweating, chills, hot flashes, shortness of breath, palpitations,

chest pain, abdominal cramping, and headache. This client experienced an unexpected job loss, which increased the symptoms associated with anxiety. However, the client does not present with multiple findings associated with panic.
CJ Cognitive Skill: Analyze Cues
Reference: Halter & Fratena, 2023, pp. 264–277

Thinking Exercise 10.1.3

Answer

The nurse determines the ***priority*** for care at this time is to ensure the client's __safety__ because the client __is irritable and impatient__ and __is drinking alcohol every night__.

Rationale

The priority for care of any client is always keeping the client and others safe. This client is displaying behaviors, such as irritability and impatience, that could jeopardize the client's own safety or the safety of others. Additionally, regular consumption of alcohol could have short- and long-term effects such as increased risk of violent behaviors, hypertension, cancer, and other life-threatening conditions. The client's current tachycardia and high blood pressure could be temporary due to anxiety or long-term due to a cardiovascular condition. However, cardiovascular health is not more important than overall client safety. Financial security is also desired for the client, but it is not more important than the need for client safety.
CJ Cognitive Skill: Prioritize Hypotheses
Reference: Halter & Fratena, 2023, pp. 264–277

Thinking Exercise 10.1.4

Answer

✗ "Are you considering killing or hurting yourself?"
✗ "If you are thinking about suicide, do you have a plan?"
○ "Do you have a gun in your house or car?"
✗ "Have you ever attempted suicide before?"
✗ "Are you considering hurting any of your family members?"
○ "What do you have to live for now that you lost your job?"

Rationale

A safety assessment is needed for this client because the client indicates that family could be financially secure if they had access to the client's life insurance benefits. Access to these funds could only occur upon the client's death. To determine if the client is considering hurting self or others, the nurse would ask if the client has any thoughts of suicide and, if so, if the client has a plan. Having a suicide plan signals the need for immediate intervention, such as hospitalization. If the client has a plan, it is appropriate to obtain more details about the plan. However, it is not appropriate to ask specifically about owning a gun because of possible legal and ethical issues related to firearm ownership. It is also not appropriate to ask the client what there is to live for because this validates the devastation of losing a job.
CJ Cognitive Skill: Generate Solutions
Reference: Halter & Fratena, 2023, pp. 252–263

Thinking Exercise 10.1.5

Answer

MENTAL HEALTH NEEDS	POTENTIAL NURSING ACTIONS
Coping	✗ Identify the client's usual coping styles. ✗ Teach the client about newly prescribed antianxiety drug therapy. ○ Teach the client about new ways to cope with crises.
Safety	○ Instruct the client to remove any weapons in the house or car, including guns. ✗ Remind the client to report any thoughts of harm to self or others. ✗ Identify any cultural or religious beliefs that may help the client experiencing crisis.
Support	✗ Refer the client to community resources for substance use disorder. ○ Refer the client to a community vocational rehabilitation program. ✗ Remind the client to regularly participate in outpatient group therapy for crisis stabilization and rehabilitation.

Rationale

The nurse would help the client identify usual coping styles or skills that could be used in this situational crisis. However, the nurse would not use personal knowledge to teach new coping skills to the client. Individuals need to determine their own coping skills and develop new ones as each situation requires. The nurse would conduct health teaching about the newly prescribed antianxiety drug therapy. To help promote safety, the nurse would remind the client to immediately report thoughts of suicide or violence and identify cultural or religious beliefs that may influence the client's coping ability. The nurse would not ask the client to remove potential weapons due to possible legal and ethical issues. Referrals that are appropriate for this client include group therapy and substance use disorder resources. Vocational rehabilitation is designed for clients who are disabled and need new job skills. This client does not meet this criterion and should not be referred to this community resource for support.

CJ Cognitive Skill: Take Actions
Reference: Halter & Fratena, 2023, pp. 264–277

Thinking Exercise 10.1.6

Answer

DATA COLLECTION FINDING	IMPROVED	NOT IMPROVED
Heart rate	✗	
Palpitations	✗	
Sleep	✗	
Substance use		✗

Rationale

The client's heart rate has returned to normal range for an adult (60 to 100 beats/min), which shows improvement when compared with previous tachycardia. The client also shared that sleep and palpitations improved in the past 2 weeks. Additionally, the client is more patient and less irritable. However, the client continues to drink alcohol on a regular basis, which shows lack of improvement in this area.

CJ Cognitive Skill: Evaluate Outcomes
Reference: Halter & Fratena, 2023, pp. 264–277

Unfolding Case Study 10.2

Thinking Exercise 10.2.1

Answer

      ✗ Level of consciousness (LOC)
      ○ Body temperature
      ✗ Respiratory rate
      ✗ Heart rate
      ✗ Blood pressure
      ✗ Oxygen saturation

Rationale

The client is not alert and oriented, which indicates a decreased LOC that could worsen. This neurologic finding is potentially life threatening and requires immediate follow-up in case the LOC continues to decline. All of the client's vital signs are below normal limits, but the temperature is not low enough to be concerning at this time. The client's respiratory and heart rates, blood pressure, and oxygen saturation are all very low and potentially life threatening, particularly if they worsen, because major organs may not be adequately perfused.
CJ Cognitive Skill: Recognize Cues
Reference: Halter & Fratena, 2023, pp. 192–194

Thinking Exercise 10.2.2

Answer

The nurse recognizes that the client is *most likely* experiencing **alcohol intoxication**.

Rationale

The client's findings are consistent with rapid alcohol intoxication, sometimes called *alcohol poisoning.* A client who has a blood alcohol content (BAC) greater than 0.08 g/dL is identified in most geographic locations as having alcohol intoxication; this client's BAC is 0.27 g/dL. The client apparently drank a large amount of alcohol in a short period. At this high level of blood alcohol, the client would be expected to experience nausea and vomiting, memory blackouts, and decreased vital sign values.
CJ Cognitive Skill: Analyze Cues
Reference: Halter & Fratena, 2023, pp. 192–194; Pagana et al., 2022, pp. 240, 388, 440, 917

Thinking Exercise 10.2.3

Answer

The *priority* for care at this time is to manage the client's **airway and breathing** because alcohol is a **depressant**.

Rationale

The client has a decreased LOC, diminished gag reflex, bradypnea (low respiratory rate), and low peripheral oxygen saturation. All of these findings are likely the result of large amounts of alcohol and its effects on the brain. Alcohol is a central nervous system depressant that can affect the vital sign center (medulla and pons); the cerebellum, causing balance and gait changes; and the cerebral cortex, causing decreased LOC and cognitive changes. Using the ABCs for priority setting, airway and breathing are the priority focus for care at this time.
CJ Cognitive Skill: Prioritize Hypotheses
Reference: Halter & Fratena, 2023, pp. 192–194; Pagana et al., 2022, pp. 240, 388, 440, 917

Thinking Exercise 10.2.4

Answer

POTENTIAL NURSING ACTIONS	INDICATED	NOT INDICATED
Maintain the client in an upright sitting position.	✗	
Administer naloxone per agency protocol.		✗
Establish peripheral access for IV fluid and electrolyte replacement.	✗	
Assess vital signs, including LOC, every 15 to 30 minutes.	✗	
Administer supplemental oxygen.	✗	

Rationale

The nurse would place and maintain the client in an upright sitting position to facilitate breathing by expanding the thorax. IV fluids are needed to dilute serum alcohol levels and flush this toxic substance from the body via the kidneys. Alcohol also contributes to dehydration, which requires IV fluid replacement. The nurse would not offer oral fluids at this time because the client's gag reflex is diminished. Electrolytes, especially sodium and potassium, also need to be replaced to prevent complications such as increasing confusion and dysrhythmias. Supplemental oxygen is needed because the client has a low respiratory rate and peripheral oxygen saturation level. Vital signs, including assessing the client's neurologic status, should be taken frequently to determine any change that could indicate clinical deterioration or improvement in the client's condition. Naloxone would not be given because it is used to treat opioid overdose rather than alcohol intoxication or poisoning.

CJ Cognitive Skill: Generate Solutions

Reference: Halter & Fratena, 2023, pp. 192–194; Pagana et al., 2022, pp. 240, 388, 440, 917

Thinking Exercise 10.2.5

Answer

✗ Reorient the client frequently, including explaining what led up to the ED visit.
O Schedule the client for a cranial CT scan.
✗ Observe the client carefully for psychotic behaviors such as hallucinations.
✗ Initiate continuous cardiac monitoring.
O Plan to discharge the client to home with a friend.
✗ Continue to monitor vital signs and neurologic status every 15 to 30 minutes.

Rationale

The client has impaired neurologic functioning as evidenced by decreased LOC, disorientation, respiratory depression, and hypotension caused by excessive alcohol. Therefore the nurse would continue to monitor vital signs and neurologic status every 15 to 30 minutes until the client becomes stable. Excessive alcohol can cause psychosis, which needs to be monitored, especially observing for hallucinations. The nurse would reorient the client frequently to help the client recall the current time, place, and situation. The client's low and irregular heart rate requires more specific assessment of possible dysrhythmia, which would be evidenced by continuous cardiac monitoring. There is no need at this time for cranial imaging because the client did not experience a head injury. The client would not be discharged at this time because of neurologic and possible cardiac impairment.

CJ Cognitive Skill: Take Actions

Reference: Halter & Fratena, 2023, pp. 192–194; Pagana et al., 2022, pp. 240, 388, 440, 917

Thinking Exercise 10.2.6

Answer

CURRENT CLIENT FINDING	IMPROVED	NOT IMPROVED
LOC	✗	
Seizure activity		✗
Blood pressure	✗	
SpO_2	✗	

Rationale

The client was drowsy, oriented to self only, and unable to follow a conversation on admission to the ED. The client is currently alert, which is an improvement in condition, but is still only oriented to self. The client's blood pressure also has improved from 88/50 to 106/66. Although the SpO_2 decreased while on oxygen therapy, the value remains above 90%. On admission, the SpO_2 was 88%, so it has improved. However, the client has new seizure activity that was not present on admission. This finding demonstrates that the client's condition has not improved.

CJ Cognitive Skill: Evaluate Outcomes
Reference: Halter & Fratena, 2023, pp. 192–198

Unfolding Case Study 10.3

Thinking Exercise 10.3.1

Answer

- ○ History of clinical depression
- ○ History of frequent STIs
- ✗ Nonadherence with prescribed drug therapy
- ✗ Recent deep wounds from cuts
- ✗ Nutritional status
- ○ Feeling more stressed than usual
- ✗ Frequent insomnia
- ○ Heart rate

Rationale

Cutting is a form of self-injury and needs immediate follow-up because clients may consider more serious self-harm such as suicide. The client is also having other potentially life-threatening findings including insomnia and inadequate nutrition as evidenced by a low BMI and a statement about eating pattern. Having a history of depression is not immediately concerning, but nonadherence in taking prescribed drug therapy for depression requires immediate follow-up. A history of STIs and being more stressed than usual are notable but not potentially life threatening at this time. Therefore these findings do not need immediate follow-up.

CJ Cognitive Skill: Recognize Cues
Reference: Halter & Fratena, 2023, pp. 319–326

Thinking Exercise 10.3.2

Answer

DATA COLLECTION FINDINGS	MAJOR DEPRESSIVE DISORDER	DYSFUNCTIONAL GRIEF
Sadness due to grandfather's death 18 months ago	✗	✗
Anorexia and insomnia	✗	✗
Self-injury (cutting)		✗
Frequent nightmares		✗

Rationale

Clients who have major depressive disorder experience a severely sad mood and distress that interferes with social, occupational, or other aspects of a client's life, such as causing changes in sleep and nutritional patterns. Findings associated with grief may mimic those of depression, but with grief, the client has feelings of emptiness and loss. Clients with major depressive disorder have lost any feelings of joy, which are often replaced with guilt and self-loathing. Dysfunctional grief occurs when the usual grieving process takes more than 1 year to resolve. Clients who experience dysfunctional grief often have maladaptive behaviors such as aggression, impulsive spending, and indiscriminate sexual behaviors. Emotional surges can lead the client to self-injury or suicidal ideation. Changes in eating and sleeping behaviors are also common.

CJ Cognitive Skill: Analyze Cues
Reference: Halter & Fratena, 2023, pp. 104–106, 319–326

Thinking Exercise 10.3.3

Answer

The nurse determines the *priority* for care at this time is to ensure the client's **safety** because the client **continues cutting** and **continues to feel very sad**.

Rationale

Any client who has depression and/or dysfunctional grief is at risk for harm to self or others. The client is already cutting as a way to deal with the emotional pain of losing a loved one. Continued sadness could result in suicidal thoughts or ideation and supports the priority need of client safety. Although the client has impaired skin integrity and inadequate nutrition, neither of these conditions is potentially life threatening at this time. Being nonadherent with drug therapy is important but is not a major reason why the client's safety may be at risk.

CJ Cognitive Skill: Prioritize Hypotheses
Reference: Halter & Fratena, 2023, pp. 319–326

Thinking Exercise 10.3.4

Answer

- ✗ Encourage the client to express feelings about the loss.
- ○ Provide a reminder that the client will get over the loss with time.
- ✗ Refer the client to comprehensive grief and bereavement services.
- ✗ Assess the client for suicidal thoughts or ideation.
- ✗ If the client does not wish to talk about the loss, suggest journaling or drawing.
- ✗ Encourage the client to recall positive memories of the grandfather.

Rationale

The client needs to continue to process the loss to help resolve the grief. First, the nurse would assess the client for suicidal thoughts or ideation to ensure the priority need of safety. One of the most important ways to process grief is to encourage clients to express their feelings either verbally or in other ways such as journaling and drawing. Recalling positive memories is also reassuring and comforting. The nurse would refer the client to services for grieving and bereavement, including counseling. Nurses should never minimize the clients' feelings by falsely assuring them that they will get over the loss with time.

CJ Cognitive Skill: Generate Solutions
Reference: Halter & Fratena, 2023, pp. 319–326

Thinking Exercise 10.3.5

Answer

- ✗ "It is very important that you take your antidepressant as prescribed to help you cope with this loss."
- ✗ "Take care of yourself by eating regularly, exercising as often as possible, and getting at least 7 hours of sleep each night."
- ○ "Avoid any printed material about death and grieving to prevent you from getting more upset."
- ✗ "Seek support from friends, family, or others, and discuss your feelings about the loss with them."
- ✗ "Let's talk about other ways you might be able to cope with your emotional pain instead of cutting."
- ○ "You might want to consider changing to being a part-time college student to help lessen your stress level."

Rationale

Teaching clients to take care of themselves during the grieving process is essential in coping with a major loss. Healthy behaviors such as eating regularly, exercising, and getting adequate amounts of sleep are important for self-care. Alternatives for managing emotional pain are important because the client might cut too deeply causing excessive bleeding and possible infection. Friends, family, spiritual leaders, and others should be identified to help the client through this crisis. The nurse would also remind the client about the need to adhere to prescribed antidepressant drug therapy to help alleviate sadness and improve other activities such as sleeping and eating. The client may benefit from reading books or other printed materials related to coping with grief and bereavement. Therefore the nurse would not encourage the client to avoid these helpful resources. The nurse would also not suggest life changes for the client such as changing from a full-time to part-time student. The client is 20 years of age and may only have a short time to graduation, when a paying career may begin or the client can seek employment.

CJ Cognitive Skill: Take Actions
Reference: Halter & Fratena, 2023, pp. 319–326

Thinking Exercise 10.3.6

Answer

The nurse determines that the client has not improved regarding **nightmares**.

Rationale

The client findings show improvement in all areas, except the client continues to have nightmares. The client is adherent with drug therapy, has not been cutting recently, and is sleeping and eating better. These behaviors indicate that the client is coping with the situational crisis better than 4 weeks ago.

CJ Cognitive Skill: Evaluate Outcomes
Reference: Halter & Fratena, 2023, pp. 319–326

Stand-Alone Thinking Exercise 10.1

Answer

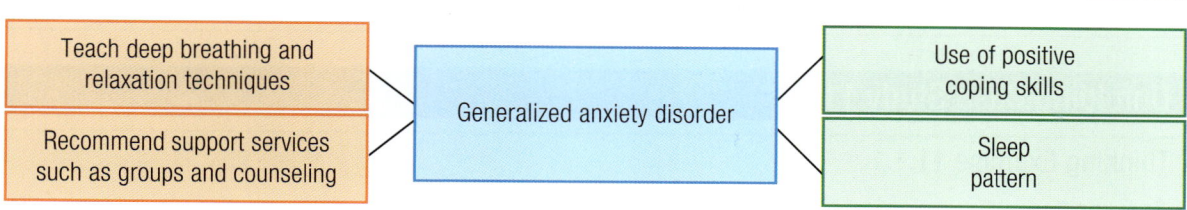

Rationale

The hallmark finding in clients who have generalized anxiety disorder is excessive worry that typically causes sleep pattern disturbance and subsequent fatigue. This client demonstrates these behaviors. Although the client has a glass of wine each night, this amount of alcohol does not support having substance use disorder. However, many clients are not truthful in reporting the amount of alcohol consumed. Besides the reported insomnia, the client does not appear sad or have other findings associated with major depressive disorder. The client's excessive worry apparently began after a recent hospital discharge. However, the client does not report nightmares, flashbacks, or other findings associated with posttraumatic stress disorder. Clients who have mild to moderate anxiety often benefit from practicing deep breathing and other relaxation techniques. For severe anxiety, drug therapy is usually prescribed. Support services, including self-help, groups, and counseling, can be very helpful in managing anxiety at any level. There is no indication at this time to assess blood alcohol level or suicidal ideation. There is also no indication that the client is abusing or neglecting the client's children, therefore there is no need to notify child protective services. After implementation of the appropriate actions, the nurse would monitor for the use of positive coping skills and an improvement in the client's sleep pattern. There is no evidence that the client is having panic attacks. The client's financial status does not definitively correlate with the client's anxiety level. Hopefully the client will visit the provider if needed; visiting the provider does not indicate the effectiveness of the plan of care.

CJ Cognitive Skills: Recognize Cues, Analyze Cues, Prioritize Hypotheses, Generate Solutions, Take Actions, Evaluate Outcomes

Reference: Halter & Fratena, 2023, pp. 124–136

Answers With Rationales for Thinking Exercises

Unfolding Case Study 11.1

Thinking Exercise 11.1.1

Answer

History and Physical	Nurses' Notes	Orders	Laboratory Results

0740: Client alert and oriented × 4. Ingested 100% of breakfast with 600 mL fluids. Health history includes atrial fibrillation, coronary artery disease, heart failure, and dyslipidemia. Morning medications administered: aspirin, atorvastatin, digoxin, and warfarin. Client transported off unit for PT as part of inpatient cardiac rehabilitation after recent hospitalization for myocardial infarction.

0910: Client returns to nursing unit after PT session. Alert and oriented × 4. Follows commands, and moves all extremities with equal strength. Client positioned in bedside chair in preparation for lunch. Respirations labored with use of accessory muscles. Chest rises and falls symmetrically. Crackles auscultated in lung fields. Skin warm and intact except for type 2 skin tear on right forearm with foam dressing. No bleeding or drainage noted; hyperpigmentation present around wound site. Dependent nonpitting edema present in bilateral lower extremities. VS: T 100.3°F (37.9°C), HR 122 beats/min and irregular, RR 28 breaths/min, BP 140/68 mmHg, SpO$_2$ 88% on RA. Denies pain but reports dyspnea. Client states "I can't seem to catch my breath, even after resting for a few minutes."

Rationale

The nurse must be aware of the client's cardiac health history and recognize signs of inadequate perfusion and gas exchange related to chronic and acute complications of heart disease. Low SpO$_2$ and reports of dyspnea while at rest are very concerning and signal inadequate perfusion and oxygen levels in the body. These symptoms must be addressed immediately to prevent tissue and organ death. Auscultated crackles in lung fields may be caused by a respiratory or cardiac condition and are most likely causing the client's dyspnea. Labored breathing, use of accessory muscles, and tachypnea are signs that the client is working hard to breath. The nurse must follow up on these client findings to prevent respiratory fatigue and failure. The client's irregular heart rate is potentially life-threatening and requires immediate follow-up. The client's temperature and blood pressure are elevated but not of immediate concern as these vital sign changes are most likely a response to the client's dyspnea and decreased SpO$_2$. Skin wounds in older adults are always troubling, but this is not a priority at this time.
CJ Cognitive Skill: Recognize Cues
References: Linton & Matteson, 2023, pp. 518, 636, 681–682, 687–688

Thinking Exercise 11.1.2

Answer

✗ Atrial fibrillation with rapid ventricular response
✗ Heart failure exacerbation
○ Lung cancer
✗ Myocardial infarction
○ Pneumothorax

Rationale

The client's history of coronary artery disease and a previous myocardial infarction would alert the nurse to another potential heart attack. Chest pain is the primary sign of a myocardial infarction, but some client's experience atypical symptoms and may not exhibit traditional burning or squeezing chest pain. Client symptoms that relate to myocardial infarction are dyspnea at rest, tachycardia, tachypnea, and decreased SpO_2. The client also has a history of atrial fibrillation (Afib) and is experiencing tachycardia or rapid ventricular rate. Afib is a cardiac dysrhythmia in which multiple rapid impulses depolarize the atria in a totally disorganized manner causing an arterial rate of 350 to 600 beats/min, a loss of atrial kick, and an irregular ventricular response. If the ventricles also beat with a rapid rate, ventricular filling is significantly decreased, and cardiac output is reduced. Afib with rapid ventricular rate is a serious condition and manifests with fatigue, dyspnea, anxiety, chest discomfort, hypotension, tachypnea, and decreased SpO_2. A history of coronary artery disease, Afib, and myocardial infarction increases the client's risk of heart failure, which the client experienced. When the heart was unable to effectively pump blood to meet the demands of the body, the client experienced insufficient perfusion of body tissues. Symptoms of heart failure depend on the affected side of the heart. The client is experiencing signs of heart failure including dyspnea at rest, labored breathing, pulmonary congestions (auscultated crackles), tachycardia, tachypnea, and decreased SpO_2. Dyspnea is also a symptom of lung cancer and pneumothorax, but the client's health history and other clinical findings do not align with these conditions.

CJ Cognitive Skill: Analyze Cues
References: Linton & Matteson, 2023, pp. 514–515, 518, 636, 681–682, 687–688

Thinking Exercise 11.1.3

Answer

The nurse recognizes that the client is *most likely* experiencing **inadequate cardiac output** and **pulmonary edema** from **left-sided heart failure**.

Rationale

The client's B-type natriuretic peptide (BNP) is greater than 400 mcg/L (400 pg/mL), which indicates that dyspnea is most likely related to a cardiac condition rather than a respiratory condition. BNP levels correlate with left ventricular pressures and therefore are a significant marker for left-sided heart failure (formally known as *congestive heart failure*), especially when the client has historical and physical findings associated with heart failure. Left-sided heart failure results in decreased cardiac output, which causes impaired tissue perfusion, and increased pulmonary venous pressure, which leads to pulmonary congestion (edema). Signs of inadequate cardiac output are anxiety, tachycardia, ashen or pale appearance, cool extremities, weak peripheral pulses, and oliguria. Clinical manifestations of pulmonary edema are dyspnea, tachypnea, auscultated crackles, and hacking cough. Chest radiology presenting an enlarged heart (cardiomegaly) and hazy lung fields (plural effusions) is also associated with a diagnosis of left-sided heart failure. Cardiac ischemia usually causes ST-segment and T-wave changes on an ECG. The client's ECG does not reveal these rhythm changes. Additionally, the client is not experiencing chest pain, nausea, diaphoresis, or other manifestations of an ischemic myocardium. The nurse would expect the client's prothrombin time and international normalized ratio (INR) to be elevated because the client is taking warfarin, a drug that inhibits an enzyme that produces vitamin K needed for clotting. The therapeutic range for a client on warfarin is generally an INR between 2.0 and 3.0. Warfarin increases the client's risk of hemorrhage, but there are no clinical findings that indicate bleeding, insufficient clotting, or anemia. The client's hemoglobin and hematocrit are within normal limits and most likely appear to have decreased due to dilution from increased fluid in the body.

CJ Cognitive Skill: Prioritize Hypotheses
References: Linton & Matteson, 2023, pp. 682–683, 687–688; Pagana et al., 2023, pp. 260, 265, 347, 412.

Thinking Exercise 11.1.4

Answer

POTENTIAL NURSING ACTIONS	INDICATED	NOT INDICATED
Collaborate with a registered dietitian nutritionist to provide a low-sodium diet.	X	
Promote rest by eliminating unnecessary activities including visitors.		X
Schedule essential activities with frequent periods of rest.	X	
Teach the client to utilize pursed-lip breathing techniques.		X
Weigh the client each morning at the same time on the same scale.	X	

Rationale

Nursing care for a client with heart failure focuses on improving cardiac output, reducing cardiac workload, improving pulmonary oxygenation, and normalizing fluid volume. The nurse would plan to give medications as ordered and monitor for therapeutic and adverse effects. Common medications administered to improve cardiac output are angiotensin-converting enzyme (ACE) inhibitors, diuretics, beta-adrenergic blockers, inotropic agents, cardiac glycosides, and nitrates. Bedrest and interventions to minimize stress and anxiety help decrease cardiac workload. Therefore the nurse would eliminate unnecessary activity and schedule essential activities with frequent periods of rest. The nurse would not prevent the client from having visitors but would instead advise them to visit quietly for short periods. To improve pulmonary oxygenation, the nurse would administer supplemental oxygen, assist the client into a comfortable semi-Fowler or high-Fowler (sitting) position, and teach the client to cough and deep breathe every 2 hours. Pursed-lip breathing is a technique used to control dyspnea related to asthma, COPD, and pulmonary fibrosis. It is not beneficial for a client with pulmonary edema. Fluid retention is a response to heart failure and unfortunately increases workload on the heart. The nurse would closely monitor intake and output, assess for signs of fluid retention, and collaborate with a registered dietitian nutritionist to provide a sodium-restricted diet. Obtaining and monitoring daily weights is the best indicator of fluid overload or loss.
CJ Cognitive Skill: Generate Solutions
References: Linton & Matteson, 2023, pp. 687–691

Thinking Exercise 11.1.5—Pharmacology

Answer

O Advise the client to eat foods low in potassium such as apples, carrots, and berries.
O Assist the client with frequent oral hygiene to prevent dry mouth.
X Assess the client for signs of acute confusion and dizziness.
O Check the client's finger stick blood glucose level before meals and at bedtime.
X Collaborate with unlicensed assistive personnel to routinely toilet the client.
X Evaluate laboratory results for potential electrolyte imbalances.
X Monitor the client's apical pulse rate and heart rhythm.

Rationale

Diuretics, such as furosemide, are administered to reduce preload and are the first-line drugs of choice in older adults with heart failure and fluid overload. Loop diuretics like furosemide promote fluid excretion and continue to work even after excess fluid is removed. Therefore the nurse must be alert for signs of dehydration in the older adult including acute confusion, decreased urinary output, and dizziness. Scheduled routine toileting promotes client safety and comfort after administration of furosemide. The nurse would also monitor the client for electrolyte imbalances, which is a common side effect of loop diuretics. Hypokalemia is especially concerning because a decrease in potassium can increase digoxin sensitivity and toxicity. Although the client's digoxin dose did not change, the nurse must recognize the client's increased risk and take actions to identify signs and symptoms of digoxin toxicity, which are often vague and nonspecific. The nurse would assess for nausea, anorexia, fatigue, blurred vision, and changes in mental status, especially in older adults. The nurse would also monitor the client's apical pulse rate and heart rhythm. Valsartan, an angiotensin II receptor blocker (ARB), is a potent vasodilator used to treat hypertension and heart failure. The nurse should be alert for orthostatic hypotension and implement fall precautions to ensure the client's safety. Dry mouth is a side effect of $alpha_2$ antagonist drugs, which this client is not prescribed.

CJ Cognitive Skill: Take Actions
References: Linton & Matteson, 2023, pp. 687–691; Willihnganz et al., 2022, pp. 438–461

Thinking Exercise 11.1.6

Answer

CLIENT FINDINGS	IMPROVED	NOT IMPROVED
Auscultated crackles in lung fields		✗
Cardiac rhythm: Afib with frequent PVCs		✗
Experiences breathlessness with activity		✗
Extremities warm with 2+ peripheral pulses throughout	✗	
Productive cough with scant white, frothy sputum		✗
Sleeping when undisturbed	✗	

Rationale

Client data that demonstrate improvement are sleeping when undisturbed and warm extremities with 2+ peripheral pulses throughout. These data illustrate that the client is comfortable, not anxious, not experiencing dyspnea at rest, and adequately perfusing all extremities with oxygenated blood. Auscultated crackles in lung fields remain present and not improved. Additionally, the client continues to experience dyspnea or breathlessness with activity. Client findings that indicate a worsened condition are frequent PVCs and a productive cough with scant white, frothy sputum. PVCs are commonly an early sign of hypokalemia, for which the client is at high risk. The nurse must identify this as a potential complication of therapy and take actions to prevent a life-threatening dysrhythmia. The client previously experienced an unproductive cough and is now coughing up white, frothy sputum. This is a sign that the client's pulmonary congestion has not improved.

CJ Cognitive Skill: Evaluation Outcomes
References: Linton & Matteson, 2023, pp. 687–691

Unfolding Case Study 11.2

Thinking Exercise 11.2.1

Answer

✗ Blood pressure
✗ Dysarthria
○ Heart rate
✗ Level of consciousness
✗ Orientation status
○ SpO_2 level

Rationale

The client's neurologic status has significantly changed from shift report 30 minutes earlier. The nurse must recognize lethargy, disorientation, left facial weakness, and slurred speech (dysarthria) as abnormal findings that could be caused by a life-threatening condition. The client's vital signs are within normal limits except for the client's blood pressure. The client has a history of hypertension, but the current blood pressure is significantly elevated and must be evaluated further to determine if is causing the client's condition or is a result of the condition.

CJ Cognitive Skill: Recognize Cues
References: Linton & Matteson, 2023, pp. 415–420, 1004

Thinking Exercise 11.2.2

Answer

CLIENT FINDING	BELL'S PALSY	HYPOGLYCEMIA	STROKE
Acute confusion		✗	✗
Drooling	✗		
Drowsiness		✗	✗
Facial weakness	✗		✗
Slurred speech		✗	✗

Rationale

The client has a history of diabetes mellitus and currently exhibits symptoms of hypoglycemia including disorientation, drowsiness, and slurred speech. Additional signs of hypoglycemia are tachycardia, diaphoresis, tremors, anxiety, and hunger. The client has several risk factors for a stroke including advanced age, recent surgery, diabetes mellitus, and hypertension. Current client findings consistent with a stroke are disorientation, drowsiness, facial weakness, inability to manage oral secretions (drooling), and slurred speech. Clients experiencing an acute stroke may also present with headache, visual problems, dysphagia, sensory impairment, and language problems. Bell's palsy is an acute disorder of the seventh cranial nerve that causes paralysis of muscles on the affected side of the face. The cause of Bell's palsy is not known, but the client currently exhibits findings consistent with Bell's palsy including facial palsy and drooling. Other common symptoms of Bell's palsy are headache, loss of taste sensation, hypersensitivity to sound, and inability to close the eye on the affected side.

CJ Cognitive Skill: Analyze Cues
References: Linton & Matteson, 2023, pp. 409, 415–420, 1004

Thinking Exercise 11.2.3

Answer

The client is *most likely* experiencing **stroke** and is **at *high risk*** for developing **aspiration pneumonia**.

Rationale

Additional client data assist the nurse to identify the most likely condition and eliminate other conditions. The client is experiencing left-sided hemiplegia and dysarthria, which are not associated with Bell's palsy. Additionally, the finger stick blood glucose (FSBG) level is within normal limits, and the client is not experiencing hypotension or pallor associated with hypoglycemia and anemia. Therefore the client is most likely experiencing a stroke. Complications of an acute stroke are related to impaired neuromuscular function and include dehydration, constipation, contractures, urinary tract infections, thrombophlebitis, pressure injuries, and pneumonia. The nurse must recognize the client's inability to manage secretions as a priority concern and take actions to prevent aspiration pneumonia.

CJ Cognitive Skill: Prioritize Hypotheses
References: Linton & Matteson, 2023, pp. 409, 415–421, 1004

Thinking Exercise 11.2.4

Answer

POTENTIAL NURSING ACTIONS	INDICATED	NOT INDICATED
Administer scheduled antihypertensive medications.		✗
Assist in completing the facility's approved stroke scale.	✗	
Position the client to comfort with the head of the bed flat.		✗
Provide a variety of tools to help the client communicate.	✗	
Report and document the time the symptoms began.	✗	
Use a gait belt to ambulate the client to the bathroom.		✗

Rationale

The client's significant change in health status requires care to be transferred to a registered nurse. When providing transition of care, the nurse must report the time symptoms began. The nurse assists the registered nurse to complete the facility's approved stroke scale. Establishing a baseline assessment with a valid and reliable tool assists in the diagnosis and determination of treatment options. The National Institutes of Health Stroke Scale (NIHSS) assessment is the most frequently used tool that assesses for level of consciousness, orientation, communication deficiencies, visual deficits, sensory impairment, and motor function. The nurse would provide several tools and resources to help the client communicate effectively. The client should choose the communication method that works best; the nurse should not decide. The client should remain NPO until a swallowing evaluation is complete. The client would be on bedrest in a comfortable position. Positioning the client in a flat position increases the risk of aspiration and is therefore not indicated. Intravenous antihypertensive medications maybe ordered to treat the client's elevated blood pressure.

CJ Cognitive Skill: Generate Solutions

References: Linton & Matteson, 2023, pp. 415–431

Thinking Exercise 11.2.5

Answer

The nurse determines the *priority* action at this time is to assess the client for **contrast media allergy** in preparation for **head computerized tomography (CT) scan**.

Rationale

A stroke is a medical emergency and requires prompt treatment to reduce or prevent permanent disability. Rapid response and stroke teams consist of experts in acute stroke assessment and management and must be notified immediately. Once the stroke team is at the bedside, the nurse can assist the team by preparing the client for diagnostic exams, most likely a computerized tomography perfusion (CTP) scan and/or computerized tomography angiography (CTA). Imaging scans are used to definitively diagnose a stroke and must be completed prior to administration of intravenous thrombolytic therapy. The nurse would assess for known allergies to contrast and remove all personal and medical equipment that would not be transported with the client to radiology. The nurse would position the client to decrease secretions from pooling in the back of the mouth, perform oral suctioning to remove secretions, and continuously monitor the client's oxygen saturation level. Nasotracheal suction would not be appropriate at this time.

CJ Cognitive Skill: Take Actions

References: Linton & Matteson, 2023, pp. 415–431

Thinking Exercise 11.2.6

Answer

BODY SYSTEMS	CLIENT FINDINGS
Respiratory	✗ Productive cough present ✗ RR 14 breaths/min ○ Rhonchi auscultated in lung fields
Cardiovascular	✗ BP 136/52 mm Hg ○ 2+ edema in left lower extremity ✗ Skin warm, dry, and normal coloration
Neurologic	✗ Symmetrical facial features and expressions ✗ Left upper extremity moves against gravity ○ Requires a picture board to communicate effectively

Rationale

Client findings including normal blood pressure, respiratory rate, and skin assessment indicate that the client is improving. The client's productive cough is a sign of improvement and demonstrates the ability to clear secretions from the airway. However, rhonchi auscultated in lung fields suggest that secretions are not being cleared completely and the client may be experiencing an acute pulmonary condition. A chopped and nectar-thickened diet implies that the client's ability to swallow is impaired, which increases the client's risk for aspiration and may be the cause of the adventitious breath sounds. The client's symmetrical facial features and expressions and the ability to move the left extremities are signs of improvement. Although strength on the left side is not normal, the ability to move the extremities at all and especially the left upper extremity against gravity is a positive sign. It is encouraging that the client can communicate and actively participate in care, but the client's speech remains undiscernible. Therefore requiring the use of a picture board to communicate effectively is not a sign of improvement. Finally, pitting edema in the left lower extremity is not normal and not a sign of improvement.

CJ Cognitive Skill: Evaluate Outcomes
References: Linton & Matteson, 2023, pp. 415–436

Stand-Alone Thinking Exercise 11.1

Answer

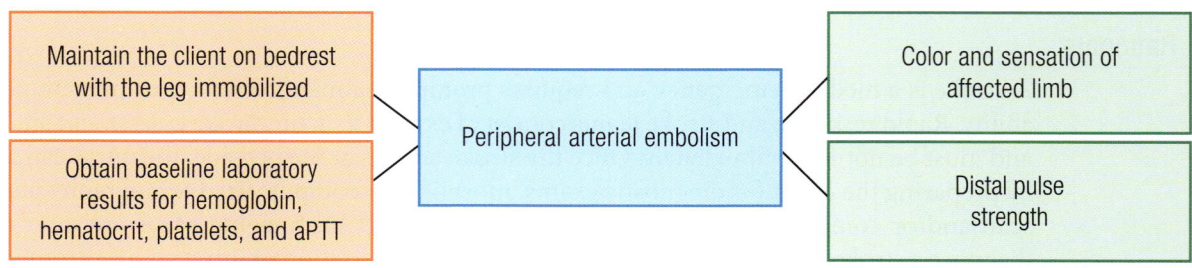

Rationale

The client is experiencing inadequate peripheral perfusion in the right lower extremity. Evidence of impaired arterial circulation is pain, coolness, pallor (or ashen in dark-brown or black skin), weak or absent pulses, and sluggish pulses. Inadequate peripheral perfusion is caused by an arterial embolism or occlusion, such as an arterial clot, which blocks blood from moving to the distal portion of the affected extremity. Deep vein thrombosis is a venous condition that blocks blood from effectively moving out of the affected extremity and back to the heart. An arterial embolism may be caused by prosthetic heart valves, mitral valve disease, infective endocarditis, atrial fibrillation, and cardiomyopathy. Arterial embolism is managed by intravenous heparin. The nurse would obtain baseline laboratory data including hemoglobin, hematocrit, platelets, and aPTT prior to initiation of heparin. Signs of bleeding would be monitored while the heparin is infusing. Until the clot is removed or dissolved, the client would remain on bedrest, and the affected limb may be immobilized. The client would also be kept NPO in preparation for potential intra-arterial thrombolysis or surgical embolectomy. The nurse would continue to monitor for the presence of distal pulses and signs of tissue death in the affected limb including irregular discoloration, coolness to touch, and decreased sensation. Muscle cramps and spasms (tetany) are manifestations of hypocalcemia, not hypercalcemia. Additionally, hypercalcemia causes a decrease in gastrointestinal function leading to hypoactive bowel sounds, nausea, and constipation. Dehydration can cause leg cramps, but the collected client data do not correlate with dehydration.

CJ Cognitive Skill: Recognize Cues, Analyze Cues, Prioritize Hypotheses, Generate Solutions, Take Actions, Evaluate Outcomes

References: Linton & Matteson, 2023, pp. 94–95, 99, 705–706; Clayton et al., 2022, pp. 427–431

Stand-Alone Thinking Exercise 11.2

Answer

Based on the assessment findings, the nurse would *prioritize* <u>supplemental oxygen</u> and anticipate administration of <u>IV fluids</u>.

Rationale

The nurse would recognize the client findings—increased heart rate and respiratory rate—as compensatory mechanisms to retain normal hemodynamics. The heart rate and respiratory rate continue to increase in an attempt to maintain normal blood pressure, SpO_2 levels, and blood flow to vital organs. Over time, these compensatory mechanisms begin to fail, and the client is unable to deliver a heart rate and respiratory rate required to provide adequate cardiac output and perfusion to vital organs. Early signs of inadequate tissue perfusion are changes in neurologic status such as restlessness, agitation, and confusion; decreased urinary output due to decreased blood flow to the kidneys; and increased blood glucose levels caused by increased glycogenolysis triggered the body's compensatory sympathetic response. Lactic acid blood levels are used to document the presence of tissue hypoxia and determine the degree of hypoxia. Lactic acid levels increase when conditions such as heart failure, sepsis, or shock lower the flow of blood and oxygen to the body. The nurse does not need to know the underlying cause of the client's condition to understand that intervention is essential to prevent progressive deterioration. Maintaining perfusion and oxygenation of vital organs is the priority. The nurse would administer supplemental oxygen and monitor the client's respiratory rate, pattern, and quality as well as SpO_2 to determine how much oxygen is required and if ventilatory support is needed. The nurse would also administer IV fluids to restore intravascular volume, cardiac output, and adequate tissue perfusion. A fluid challenge is usually administered (250 mL of crystalloid solution) followed by continuous IV fluid replacement until a mean arterial pressure of 60 mm Hg or greater is attained and evidence of adequate tissue perfusion is noted.

CJ Cognitive Skill: Recognize Cues, Analyze Cues, Prioritize Hypotheses, Generate Solutions

References: Linton & Matteson, 2023, pp. 158–169; Pagana et al., 2023, pp. 451, 545, 749, 946

Answers With Rationales for Thinking Exercises

Thinking Exercise 12.1.1

Answer

- ○ BMI 19
- ✗ Lateral chest pain
- ○ Cool, dry skin
- ○ Course crackles
- ✗ Oriented to self and family
- ○ Dependent edema
- ✗ SpO$_2$ 86% on RA

Rationale

The client lives independently and has no history of dementia, and the family expresses concern related to the client's orientation. The nurse must recognize acute confusion and only oriented to self and family as a change in status. In older adults, acute confusion is a common change indicating an acute health problem and requires immediate follow-up by the nurse. Chest pain is concerning for all clients and must be evaluated emergently to determine if the cause is a life-threatening cardiac or pulmonary condition. Clients with chronic lung disease frequently have a lower-than-normal SpO$_2$ level, usually between 92% and 88%. The client's current SpO$_2$ of 86% is too low, and this requires immediate follow-up by the nurse, especially since the client is showing signs of potential hypoxemia including tachycardia, tachypnea, and confusion. Course crackles are a common lung sound auscultated in clients with COPD. Although the nurse cannot confirm if the adventitious lung sound is related to the client's chronic disease or an acute condition, the finding is not life threatening and therefore would not be a priority for immediate follow-up. The client's cool, dry skin and dependent lower extremity edema do not indicate a life-threatening condition and may be chronic findings for the older adult client. The client's BMI indicates undernourishment because it is lower than the optimal value of 20 to 25, but this is not a priority and would be addressed after the client is stable.

CJ Cognitive Skill: Recognize Cues
Reference: Linton & Matteson, 2023, pp. 250, 509–510, 531–532

Thinking Exercise 12.1.2

Answer

CLIENT FINDING	COPD EXACERBATION	LUNG CANCER	PNEUMONIA
Productive cough	✗	✗	✗
Chest pain		✗	✗
Acute confusion			✗
Wheezing	✗		
Fatigue	✗	✗	✗

Rationale

The client has a history of chronic obstructive pulmonary disease (COPD), therefore the nurse would first analyze symptoms to determine whether an exacerbation has occurred. Client findings that correspond with symptoms of COPD exacerbation are productive cough, wheezing, course crackles, and use of accessory muscles to breathe. Clients may also experience dyspnea and fatigue during acute COPD exacerbation. The client has several risk factors for pneumonia including smoking history, chronic illness, and low weight (BMI = 19). Relevant clinical findings for pneumonia are chest pain, productive cough, hemoptysis (dark-red sputum), and fever. Acute onset of confusion and fatigue are also common symptoms exhibited in older adults with pneumonia. As a previous smoker, the client is also at risk for lung cancer. Lung cancer generally does not cause symptoms until advanced stages. Client findings that correlate with lung cancer are chronic productive cough, hemoptysis (dark-red sputum), chest pain, and fatigue. COPD and lung cancer are chronic conditions and do not usually present with acute confusion and fever. Wheezing is rare in both pneumonia and lung cancer.
CJ Cognitive Skill: Analyze Cues
Reference: Linton & Matteson, 2023, pp. 509–510, 531–532, 546

Thinking Exercise 12.1.3
Answer

The nurse determines the *priority* for care at this time is to manage the client's **hypoxemia**. The nurse's *first* action would be to **administer oxygen to keep the SpO$_2$ between 88% and 92%**.

Rationale

The client's oxygenation status including vital signs and mental status changes are most concerning and indicate the client is experiencing hypoxemia or low blood oxygen saturation levels, which can cause permanent damage to organs and is life threatening. The nurse would prioritize the client's hypoxemia and administer oxygen as needed to keep SpO$_2$ levels between 88% and 92%. Although SpO$_2$ levels greater than 94% are the normal goal, the client has COPD, and a lower goal would more accurately reflect the client's normal oxygen saturation level. Other respiratory interventions including administering a nebulizer treatment and placing the client in the high-Fowler position may help the client breathe better, but they will not increase blood oxygen levels and therefore would be secondary to the application of supplemental oxygen. Confusion and tachycardia are most likely symptoms of hypoxemia and will resolve with administration of supplemental oxygen. The client's acute pain is a concern, but it is not currently life threatening.
CJ Cognitive Skill: Prioritize Hypotheses
Reference: Linton & Matteson, 2023, pp. 509–511

Thinking Exercise 12.1.4
Answer

POTENTIAL NURSING ACTIONS	INDICATED	NOT INDICATED
Assist the client to perform deep-breathing and coughing exercises.	X	
Encourage the client to ambulate in the hallway at least twice each day.		X
Insert an indwelling urinary catheter to gravity drainage.		X
Organize patient care activities to allow periods of uninterrupted rest.	X	
Arrange for food options that are high in protein and preferred by the client.	X	
Place the client in a negative-airflow room, and provide surgical masks for all visitors and health care providers.		X

Rationale

Pneumonia causes an accumulation of secretions in the lungs that impairs gas exchange and may result in alveolar collapse. The nurse would implement interventions to promote the expectoration of secretions including assisting the client to change positions and perform deep-breathing and coughing exercises at least every 2 hours. Activity is commonly restricted for the client with pneumonia and would not include ambulating in the hallway twice daily during the acute phase. The nurse would organize patient care activities to prevent overtiring and allow periods of uninterrupted rest. Although strict intake and output monitoring is expected, the nurse would not insert an indwelling urinary catheter due to increased risk of catheter-associated urinary tract infection (CAUTI). Instead, the nurse would collaborate with the registered nurse and assistive personnel to facilitate use of a bedside commode or bedpan for urinary collection. Good nutrition is essential to healing. The nurse would anticipate a high-protein, soft diet and arrange for food options that are attractive and preferred by the client. The CDC infection control guideline for community-acquired pneumonia is Standard Precautions. Droplet Precautions are also recommended for specific types of pneumonia. There is no need to place the client in a negative-airflow room or provide masks for all visitors and health care providers.

CJ Cognitive Skill: Generate Solutions
Reference: Linton & Matteson, 2023, pp. 509–512

Thinking Exercise 12.1.5

Answer

- ✗ Blood cultures × 2
- O Chest physiotherapy
- O Ciprofloxacin 400 mg IV every 12 hours
- O Nutritional consultation
- O Oxycodone hydrochloride 2.5 mg/acetaminophen 325 mg, 1 tablet every 6 hours PRN for pain
- ✗ Sputum culture
- O Strict monitoring of intake and output
- O Titrate supplemental oxygen to keep SpO_2 between 88% and 92%

Rationale

Supplemental oxygen has already been administered, and the client's SpO_2 is within that expected range. The nurse does not need to further titrate oxygen at this time. Instead, the nurse would prioritize blood and sputum cultures. Clients with an infection are generally prescribed a broad-spectrum antibiotic until cultures reveal the actual microorganism causing the infection. Blood and sputum cultures must be completed prior to initiating antibiotic therapy to ensure that the organism is properly identified. After cultures are sent to the laboratory, the nurse would administer the prescribed antibiotic and reassess the client's pain to ensure that it remains at an acceptable level. Then the nurse would collaborate with the registered dietitian nutritionist for the nutritional consultation and with the respiratory therapist for chest physiotherapy.

CJ Cognitive Skill: Take Actions
Reference: Linton & Matteson, 2023, pp. 509–512

Thinking Exercise 12.1.6

Answer

CLIENT FINDING	IMPROVED	NOT IMPROVED
Alert and oriented × 4	✗	
SpO_2 93% on 4 L/min O_2 via NC	✗	
Dyspnea with activity and at rest		✗
Diminished right lobe breath sounds		✗
Drinks 1 protein shake between each meal	✗	

Rationale

The client's vital signs and mental status have improved and demonstrate signs of progression toward resolving the priority problem of hypoxemia. The client is alert and oriented × 4. An SpO_2 level of 93% on 4 L/min O_2 via NC exceeds the goal of 88% to 92%. The client may tolerate a decrease in the amount of supplemental oxygen currently being used. The client's cough has transitioned into a dry, unproductive cough, a common chronic finding experienced by clients with COPD and a sign of improvement. The client tolerates a significant portion of each meal and drinks three protein shakes daily, which is another positive sign. Clients with COPD frequently experience dyspnea with activity but not at rest. The client's shortness of breath at rest and diminished right lobe breath sounds are new findings. A pleural effusion, or accumulation of fluid between the pleura that surrounds the lungs and the pleura that lines the thoracic cavity, would result in diminished breath sounds and shortness of breath. Pleural effusions are a complication of pneumonia and an indication that the client's status has not improved.

CJ Cognitive Skill: Evaluate Outcomes

Reference: Linton & Matteson, 2023, pp. 509–512

Unfolding Case Study 12.2

Thinking Exercise 12.2.1

Answer

History and Physical	Nurses' Notes	Orders	Progress Notes

1320: Client admitted from surgical suite after an uncomplicated right total hip arthroplasty. Health history includes atrial fibrillation and osteoarthritis. Client is drowsy but easily aroused to voice and oriented × 4. Speech is clear, and simple commands followed appropriately. Skin cool and dry with palpable pulses throughout. Right hip dressing dry, wound drain intact, and 50 mL sanguineous drainage emptied. Respirations equal, unlabored, and without adventitious lung sounds. Abdomen soft with hypoactive bowel sounds. Denies nausea. Indwelling urinary catheter in place draining clear yellow urine to gravity. Urinary drainage bag emptied, 1500 mL output. Left forearm peripheral IV infusing 0.9% NS at 100 mL/h and morphine PCA with basal rate of 1 mg/h and demand rate of 0.5 mg every 8 minutes. VS: T 97.2°F (36.2°C), HR 102 beats/min and irregular, RR 13 beats/min, BP 120/58 mm Hg, SpO_2 98% on 4 L/min O_2 via NC. Surgical site pain rated 7/10. PCA teaching reinforced, and client demonstrates appropriate use of demand feature. Client's adult child at bedside; all questions answered.

1430: Client sleeping. Unable to awaken with verbal stimuli, but arouses with moderate stimuli and then drifts back to sleep quickly. VS: HR 105 beats/min and irregular, RR 11 breaths/min, BP 109/52 mm Hg, SpO_2 90% on 4 L/min O_2 via NC. Incisional dressing dry, and 20 mL sanguineous drainage in wound drain. Urinary drainage bag with 75 mL yellow urine. PCA reports 5 mg morphine infused. Adult child at bedside holding client's hand.

Rationale

The nurse must recognize that the client's level of consciousness has declined from the previous assessment. The client is now lethargic, arousing only to moderate stimuli and drifting back to sleep quickly. The respiratory rate, blood pressure, and SpO_2 have all decreased and are now lower than normal range. Changes in respiratory rate, blood pressure, SpO_2, and level of consciousness correlate with potential hypoxemia and require immediate follow-up to prevent organ failure. The client is experiencing tachycardia and an irregular heart rhythm, but these findings are not an acute change from the previous hour and are most likely related to the client's chronic condition of atrial fibrillation. The client's urinary output and other physical findings are within normal limits for a postoperative client. The client's PCA pump reports 5 mg morphine were infused, which is the maximum amount for the period presented. Although this dose is within the PCA programmed range, it is concerning due to the client's current lethargy and requires further analysis.

CJ Cognitive Skill: Recognize Cues

Reference: Linton & Matteson, 2023, pp. 149–155

Thinking Exercise 12.2.2

Answer

The nurse recognizes that the client is **_most likely_** experiencing **opioid overdose**.

Rationale

The client is showing hallmark signs of opioid overdose including hypoventilation and lethargy. The client is at risk for complete respiratory depression and possible anoxic brain injury if the team does not intervene in a timely manner. Opioid overdose depresses the central nervous system creating hypotension. The client's palpable pulses and adequate urinary output over the past hour indicate an adequate fluid status, not hypovolemic shock. There are no signs of airway obstruction, chest pain, shortness of breath, or other signs of an anaphylactic reaction or pulmonary embolism.
CJ Cognitive Skill: Analyze Cues
Reference: Linton & Matteson, 2023, pp. 81, 149–155, 158–161, 518–520

Thinking Exercise 12.2.3

Answer

The nurse determines the **_priority_** for care at this time is **ventilation support** because the client is experiencing **respiratory depression** and **hypoxemia**.

Rationale

The client is experiencing impaired gas exchange related to respiratory depression and hypoxemia (decreased oxygen saturation) secondary to an opioid overdose. The nurse must prioritize interventions that will improve the client's ventilation or breathing to prevent respiratory failure and death. The client's cardiac arrhythmia (atrial fibrillation) is a chronic condition and would not need continuous monitoring at this time. Signs of dehydration include a decrease in blood pressure and an increase in heart rate, but these symptoms could also be caused by hypoxemia. The client's urine output demonstrates adequate fluid volume, therefore fluid replacement would not be a priority at this time.
CJ Cognitive Skill: Prioritize Hypotheses
Reference: Linton & Matteson, 2023, pp. 81, 149–155, 158–161, 518–520

Thinking Exercise 12.2.4

Answer

- ✗ Ensure that bag-valve-mask ventilation equipment is at the bedside.
- ✗ Notify the health care provider.
- ✗ Position the client to maintain airway patency.
- ✗ Recommend discontinuing the PCA.
- ✗ Request an order for naloxone.
- ✗ Titrate supplemental oxygen until the SpO_2 is greater than 94%.

Rationale

Respiratory depression and hypoxemia require immediate intervention to prevent respiratory failure and death. Emergency care of the client requires positioning the client to keep the airway open and titrating supplemental oxygen to keep the SpO_2 greater than 94%. Both interventions will promote ventilation and oxygenation. Emergency equipment including an artificial airway and bag-valve-mask ventilation equipment must be at the bedside in case the client declines further, and manual ventilation is needed. Additionally, the provider and/or surgeon would be notified for orders to reverse analgesic effects with naloxone and prevent further occurrences of opioid-induced respiratory depression by discontinuing or reducing the PCA.
CJ Cognitive Skill: Generate Solutions
Reference: Linton & Matteson, 2023, pp. 149–155

Thinking Exercise 12.2.5

Answer

✗ Administer an additional dose of naloxone.
✗ Alert the Rapid Response Team.
○ Increase the intravenous infusion rate to 150 mL/h.
○ Initiate bag-valve-mask manual breathing.
○ Place the client in the high-Fowler position.

Rationale

Naloxone's onset of action is about 2 to 5 minutes with a duration of action lasting about 30 minutes. The client responded to the first dose of naloxone, but respiratory depression has recurred, therefore the nurse would administer an additional dose of naloxone. The Rapid Response Team would also be notified for additional support and to determine if the client requires mechanical ventilation for persistent respiratory depression. Bag-valve-mask manual breathing may be required if the client's respiratory rate decreases further, and increased IV fluids may be required if the client's blood pressure does not increase with opioid reversal. The nurse would reassess the client's respiratory rate and blood pressure after administering the second dose of naloxone. Due to the client's current neurologic state, the nurse would place the client in the semi-Fowler or Sims position, not the high-Fowler position.
CJ Cognitive Skill: Take Actions
Reference: Linton & Matteson, 2023, pp. 149–155

Thinking Exercise 12.2.6

Answer

The nurse determines the client's status has **_improved_** based on the client's **orientation status** and **oxygen saturation**.

Rationale

The client's neurologic status has improved. The client may sleep when undisturbed but is easily aroused and oriented × 4. The client's SpO_2 has also improved and is within normal limits on 4 L/min O_2 via NC. Active bowel sounds, adequate urine output, and serosanguinous drainage are all signs that indicate the client is recovering appropriately from surgery. These findings do not assist the nurse to evaluate the client's response to interventions focused on opioid overdose, hypoventilation, and hypoxemia.
CJ Cognitive Skill: Evaluate Outcomes
Reference: Linton & Matteson, 2023, pp. 149–155

Stand-Alone Thinking Exercise 12.1

Answer

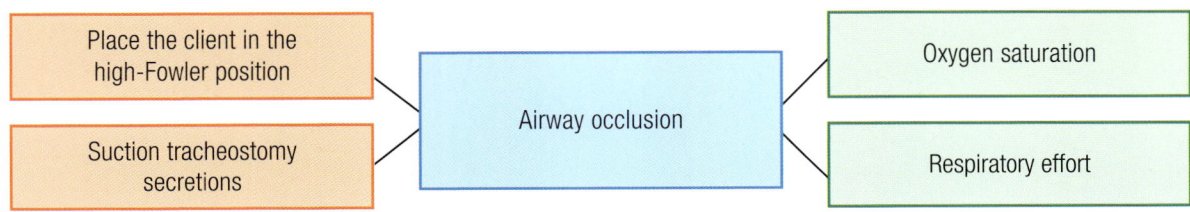

Rationale

Increased mucous production and a chronic cough are common symptoms of COPD, but the client may not be unable to effectively expectorate mucous secretions due to a weak cough and the viscosity (thickness) of the tracheal secretions. The nurse would recognize that pulmonary mucus is most likely causing an airway obstruction or occlusion of the tracheal cannula. The nurse would perform tracheal suctioning to remove secretions and place the client in the high-Fowler position to engage abdominal muscles and promote spontaneous breathing and coughing. The nurse would then monitor the client's SpO_2 and respiratory effort to determine if additional supplemental oxygen or a return to mechanical ventilation is required. Autonomic dysreflexia generally occurs in clients with spinal cord injuries and is caused by an overreaction of the autonomic nervous system to a noxious stimulus. The primary symptom of autonomic dysreflexia is a sudden and severe increase in blood pressure. This client's blood pressure did not increase drastically. The client has a history of substance use disorder but has maintained sobriety or abstinence from substance use for the past 10 years. The client would not have withdrawal symptoms at this time. The client is at risk for aspiration from tube feedings. Low residuals and active bowel sounds decrease the risk. Additionally, tube-feed aspiration leads to pneumonia, which would not take priority over an airway obstruction.

CJ Cognitive Skills: Recognize Cues, Analyze Cues, Prioritize Hypotheses, Generate Solutions, Take Actions, Evaluate Outcomes

Reference: Linton & Matteson, 2023, pp. 483, 499–502, 536

Stand-Alone Thinking Exercise 12.2

Answer

The nurse determines that *priority* actions for the client at this time are **encouraging deep-breathing and coughing exercises** and **monitoring oxygenation saturation**.

Rationale

The nurse would recognize that the client most likely aspirated on the carbonated beverage. The client is prescribed nectar thick fluids due to swallowing difficulties resulting from a recent left-hemisphere stroke. Carbonated beverages, such as soda, are not nectar thick and therefore put the client at high risk for fluid aspiration. The nurse would prioritize deep-breathing and coughing exercises to help the client expectorate fluid that entered the trachea and lungs. The nurse would also monitor the client's oxygen saturation carefully. The client's SpO_2 decreased to 94%. If it decreases further, the nurse may need to apply supplemental oxygen. The nurse must prioritize the client's airway and breathing before reinforcing teaching with the family or transferring the client back to the bed. The client's neurologic status has not changed, therefore there is no need to complete a stroke scale assessment at this time.

CJ Cognitive Skills: Recognize Cues, Analyze Cues, Priority Hypotheses, Generate Solutions, Take Actions

Reference: Linton & Matteson, 2023, pp. 420–429, 513

Answers With Rationales for Thinking Exercises

Unfolding Case Study 13.1

Thinking Exercise 13.1.1

Answer

History and Physical	Nurses' Notes	Orders	Laboratory Results

0410: Client found slumped forward, moaning, and wedged between toilet and wall. Apparently fell while using the bathroom. Alert, but orientation difficult to assess due to apparent pain. Usually ambulates with a rollator or cane, but no ambulatory device noted in bathroom. Crying out and grabbing right hip. Right leg shorter than left leg and externally rotated. Pedal pulses equal, and cap refill < 3 sec. Client has long history of osteoporosis managed with risedronate. Skin intact except for large skin tear on right forearm oozing serosanguinous fluid. Bruising beginning to develop near skin tear. VS: T 98.6°F (37°C), HR 110 beats/min and regular, BP 154/88 mm Hg, RR 24 breaths/min, SpO$_2$ 93% on RA.

Rationale

The client fell and experienced a right hip injury as a result. The nurse would immediately follow up on the injury because the right leg is externally rotated and shorter than the left leg. The hip injury could potentially be life threatening if blood vessels are damaged and bleeding occurs. When older adults experience a fall, they often become disoriented and acutely confused. Therefore this finding is expected and does not require immediate follow-up. The client also has a skin tear, but this finding is not life threatening or potentially life threatening at this time. The client's heart rate, respiratory rate, and blood pressure are higher than normal, but these vital signs often increase in the presence of acute pain and resulting anxiety. The heart rate, respiratory rate, and blood pressure are not at life-threatening levels. The client's SpO$_2$ is less than 95%, but 93% is acceptable for an older adult unless the client is experiencing respiratory distress.
CJ Cognitive Skill: Recognize Cues
Reference: Linton & Matteson, 2023, pp. 923–928

Thinking Exercise 13.1.2

Answer

The client *most likely* has a **fractured hip** as evidenced by **hip pain** and **shortened leg**.

Rationale

The client has all of the typical and expected findings of a fractured hip following the fall in the bathroom, including severe hip pain and an externally rotated and shortened affected leg when compared with the other leg. Some clients also have bruising or other tissue damage in the hip area. There is no evidence that the client has a fractured pelvis, which would cause pain in the pelvic area. Although the client has a skin tear on the right forearm, there is no other evidence of a fractured radius. However, an x-ray of the injured arm may be performed in the emergency department to ensure that there is no fracture.
CJ Cognitive Skill: Analyze Cues
Reference: Linton & Matteson, 2023, pp. 927–928

Thinking Exercise 13.1.3

Answer

The nurse determines that the *priority* for client care is to surgically repair the fracture to prevent **impaired blood flow to the hip** and **complications of immobility**.

Rationale

If the fracture is not surgically repaired, the client could experience impaired peripheral blood flow to the affected leg caused by soft tissue damage, fracture fragments, and/or edema. Inadequate circulation could lead to necrosis (cell death). The client would also experience complications of impaired mobility if the hip fracture is not repaired. Common complications include pressure injury, atelectasis, pneumonia, constipation, and venous thromboembolism (VTE), including deep vein thrombosis (DVT) and pulmonary embolism (PE). Repairing the fracture will not prevent worsening osteoporosis. Hip fracture repair would help to decrease pain and prevent hip contracture, but these conditions are not the priority reason for the surgery.
CJ Cognitive Skill: Prioritize Hypotheses
Reference: Linton & Matteson, 2023, pp. 197–208, 923–928

Thinking Exercise 13.1.4

Answer

O Reposition the client at least once every 8 hours.
✗ Apply sequential compression devices to both legs.
✗ Encourage the client to use the incentive spirometer.
O Administer an IV antibiotic per surgeon protocol.
✗ Administer an anticoagulant per surgeon protocol.
✗ Initiate physical and occupational therapy consults.

Rationale

To prevent possible venous thromboembolism (DVT or PE), the nurse would place sequential compression devices (SCDs) on both legs while the client is in bed. DVT commonly occurs when clients remain in bed, and venous blood flow slows and forms a thrombus (clot) in the calf of the leg. If a piece of the thrombus breaks off and travels to the lungs, this potentially life-threatening condition is a PE. SCDs apply intermittent pressure on the calf of each leg to promote venous blood return to help prevent a DVT. The nurse would also administer an anticoagulant in small doses to help prevent VTE and would ambulate the client as early as possible. Therefore physical therapy and occupational therapy consults are essential. Although the client was initially acutely confused and disoriented, the client should improve with reorientation and time. Therefore teaching and encouraging the client to use the incentive spirometer is important to prevent atelectasis and pneumonia. An antibiotic is usually not given after surgery to help prevent infection. However, many clients receive one dose immediately before or initially during surgery. To prevent pressure injury, the nurse would reposition the client every 1 to 2 hours, not every 8 hours.
CJ Cognitive Skill: Generate Solutions
Reference: Linton & Matteson, 2023, pp. 197–208, 923–928

Thinking Exercise 13.1.5

Answer

○ Notify the Rapid Response Team (RRT) immediately.
✗ Anticipate an order for an oral anticoagulant such as dabigatran.
✗ Elevate the client's left leg on a pillow.
○ Draw blood to test the client's platelet count.
✗ Monitor the client for shortness of breath, chest pain, and acute confusion.

Rationale

Although the nurse would contact the surgeon about the findings related to the client's calf, there is no need to notify the Rapid Response Team because this condition is not immediately life threatening. When contacting the surgeon, the nurse would expect an order for an oral anticoagulant used to treat DVT. An oral anticoagulant would be preferred because the client will continue on this drug after hospital discharge. It will be easier for the client to take an oral drug rather than one that requires an injection. Drugs such as dabigatran do not require lab test monitoring. The affected leg would be elevated because DVT usually causes edema, and elevation helps promote venous blood return to the heart. The client is at risk for PE, therefore the nurse would monitor for signs and symptoms of this complication such as shortness of breath, chest pain, and acute confusion.

CJ Cognitive Skill: Take Actions
Reference: Linton & Matteson, 2023, pp. 708–710, 923–928

Thinking Exercise 13.1.6 Pharmacology

Answer

CLIENT STATEMENT	UNDERSTANDING	NO UNDERSTANDING
"When the redness and soreness in my calf goes away, I still need to take this drug."	✗	
"I should contact my provider if I have any unexpected bleeding, chest pain, or dyspnea."	✗	
"I will be sure to go to the lab for frequent blood tests needed while I'm on this drug."		✗
"I will take this capsule as prescribed and follow up with my provider."	✗	

Rationale

All of these statements are correct and show the client's understanding about taking dabigatran, except there is no need for ongoing blood tests. Dabigatran is a direct thrombin inhibitor used to treat DVT and PE. By blocking thrombin in the blood, this drug prevents clot development. Therefore there is no need for frequent lab tests such as platelet count, prothrombin time, and INR.

CJ Cognitive Skill: Evaluate Outcomes
Reference: McCuistion et al., 2023, pp. 534–535

Unfolding Case Study 13.2

Thinking Exercise 13.2.1

Answer

      ○ SpO$_2$
      ○ Increased rigidity
      ○ Slowed gait
      ✗ Blood pressure
      ✗ Visual hallucinations
      ○ Bilateral foot and ankle edema
      ✗ Dizziness and light-headedness

Rationale

The client has low blood pressure, which could result in inadequate perfusion (blood flow) to vital organs and subsequent organ failure. Therefore the nurse would immediately follow up on the client's blood pressure. The client also recently experienced dizziness and light-headedness that almost resulted in a fall. This finding is a major safety concern and therefore needs immediate follow-up. Hallucinations indicate possible psychosis, which is concerning and could result in client harm. This finding is associated with Parkinson disease (PD); it is also an adverse effect seen in clients who have been taking carbidopa/levodopa combinations for 1 to 2 years. Slower gait and increase rigidity are common in clients who have PD and are not potentially life threatening. Therefore these findings do not require immediate follow-up but would be assessed at a later time. The SpO$_2$ is slightly below normal limits for a young adult, but most older adults function well at levels between 90% to 95%.
CJ Cognitive Skill: Recognize Cues
Reference: Linton & Matteson, 2023, pp. 395–398; McCuistion et al., 2023, pp. 231–232

Thinking Exercise 13.2.2

Answer

The nurse would recognize that the client is ***most likely*** experiencing **psychotic episodes** and **orthostatic hypotension**.

Rationale

The client experienced hallucinations, which are psychotic behaviors; delusions are also psychotic behaviors. In psychosis, the client is not "in touch with reality." The changes in the client's blood pressures based on body position meet the definition of orthostatic hypotension: the blood pressure decreases between 10 and 15 mm Hg or more when the client changes from a lying to standing position. There is no indication that the client has dehydration except for low blood pressure. However, dehydration usually causes tachycardia to compensate for the low blood pressure. This client's heart rate is below 100 beats/min. Other than dependent foot and ankle edema, there are no other indications that the client has heart failure.
CJ Cognitive Skill: Analyze Cues
Reference: Linton & Matteson, 2023, pp. 395–398

Thinking Exercise 13.2.3

Answer

The nurse determines that the ***priority*** for care at this time is to manage the client's **orthostatic hypotension** because the client is at high risk for **falls**.

Rationale

The nurse prioritizes care by ensuring client safety. There is no indication that the client has any issues with airway, breathing, or circulation (ABCs). However, the client is at risk for falls because of light-headedness and dizziness, which are most likely caused by orthostatic hypotension. Falls in older adults often result in potentially life-threatening fractures or other trauma. However, foot and ankle edema, hallucinations, and immobility are not necessarily potentially life threatening.

CJ Cognitive Skill: Prioritize Hypotheses
Reference: Linton & Matteson, 2023, pp. 395–398

Thinking Exercise 13.2.4

Answer

- ○ Send the client to the nearby lab to draw blood for multiple tests.
- ○ Send the client to the nearby imaging center for a head CT.
- ✗ Plan for direct client admission to the acute care hospital.
- ○ Prescribe an antipsychotic medication to manage hallucinations.
- ○ Instruct the family member to purchase an automated blood pressure machine for home.
- ✗ Encourage the client to drink plenty of fluids.

Rationale

The client is hypotensive with a risk for falls. This finding may be associated with PD or with taking the maximum dosage of carbidopa/levodopa for a prolonged period. Sending the client home on an antipsychotic drug and a blood pressure machine or sending the client to the lab or imaging center is not safe because of the risk for falls from light-headedness and dizziness. Therefore the best action is to send the client directly to the acute care hospital for admission and evaluation. The nurse would encourage the client to drink plenty of fluids to increase blood volume. There is no indication that the client has kidney or cardiac impairment, so there is no known contraindication for increasing fluid intake.

CJ Cognitive Skill: Generate Solutions
Reference: Linton & Matteson, 2023, pp. 395–398

Thinking Exercise 13.2.5

Answer

POTENTIAL NURSING ACTIONS	INDICATED	NOT INDICATED
Document frequent orthostatic blood pressure checks	✗	
Place the client on nothing by mouth (NPO) status		✗
Begin supplemental oxygen via NC		✗
Hold the client's carbidopa/levodopa	✗	
Remind the client to use the call light for assistance to get out of bed	✗	

Rationale

In the hospital setting, the client's safety is essential. Therefore the nurse would frequently remind the client about the need to use the call light when needing to be out of bed. To determine if the hypotension and hallucinations are adverse effects of the medication used to control the client's PD (carbidopa/levodopa), the drug would be discontinued. If these findings continue, they are likely associated with the disease process rather than the medication. The client's blood pressure, especially when changing position, would be monitored and documented to determine if it was improving. There is no reason

why the client would need to be NPO. Instead, the client would receive additional fluids to increase blood volume and increase the client's blood pressure. Given the client's SpO$_2$ and lack of respiratory distress, there is also no need for supplemental oxygen.
CJ Cognitive Skill: Take Actions
Reference: Linton & Matteson, 2023, pp. 395–398

Thinking Exercise 13.2.6
Answer

CLIENT FINDINGS	IMPROVED	NOT IMPROVED
Standing BP 110/69 mm Hg	X	
No light-headedness when changing positions	X	
No bowel movement during hospital stay		X
Occasional resting tremors and increased stiffness		X
No hallucinations or delusions during hospital stay	X	

Rationale

The client's orthostatic blood pressures have markedly increased, which is a major improvement. This increase has prevented further episodes of light-headedness when changing body positions. The client has not experienced any further hallucinations during the hospital stay, which also shows improvement in the client's condition. However, the client has more resting tremors and stiffness, which shows worsening of signs and symptoms. The client has not been able to have a bowel movement while in the hospital for 3 days, which is a new symptom and indicates a worsened condition.
CJ Cognitive Skill: Evaluate Outcomes
Reference: Linton & Matteson, 2023, pp. 395–398

Stand-Alone Thinking Exercise 13.1
Answer

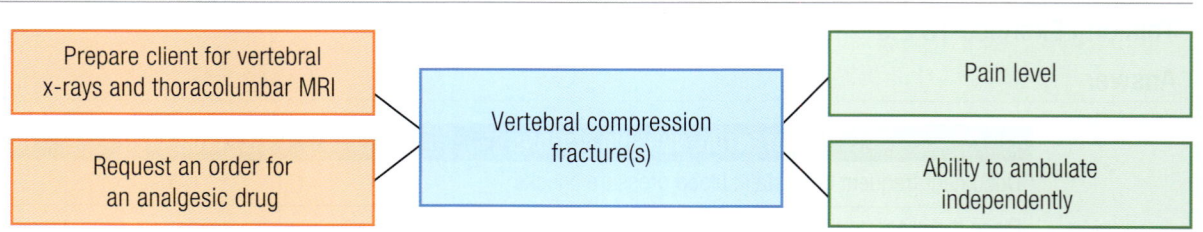

Rationale

Clients who have severe osteoporosis often experience fragility fractures, especially wrist, hip, and vertebral fractures. Compression fractures of the vertebrae occur most often after an event that stresses the area such as lifting, bending, or other exertion. This client experienced severe back pain after using a vacuum cleaner. The pain caused by vertebral microcompression fractures often worsens when the client moves or changes position. Often referred to as *renal colic*, the pain caused by one or more kidney stones is also sudden and typically excruciating, especially when the stone moves. Metastatic bone cancer commonly occurs when a client has a history of breast cancer. However, the pain is usually slower in onset and initially less painful than the sensation the client is experiencing. The client likely does not have a herniated lumbar disk because there is no report of radiating pain down into the buttock or leg. To address the severe pain associated with vertebral fracture(s), the nurse would request an analgesic. The client would need to have imaging procedures to determine if one or more fractures exist and where the fracture(s) is/are. Many clients have more than one fracture at the same time. Once the treatment plan is decided, physical therapy may or not be contacted to help the client after any procedure to treat the fracture. Nurses do not obtain consent for surgery—this is the responsibility of the surgeon. Surgery would be the last resort to treat this client's condition. There is no indication that the client would need a cystoscopy. After treatment, the nurse and interprofessional health care team would ensure that the client has minimal pain and continues to ambulate and perform ADLs independently. The client's condition does not involve muscle strength or infection. Additionally, the client likely has chronic hypocalcemia, which is usually managed with calcium supplements. Monitoring this level is not useful in clients who have severe osteoporosis.

CJ Cognitive Skill: Recognize Cues, Analyze Cues, Prioritize Hypotheses, Generate Solutions, Take Actions, Evaluate Outcomes

Reference: Linton & Matteson, 2023, pp. 903–905, 912–931

Stand-Alone Thinking Exercise 13.2

Answer

Monitor urine quantity and quality			Pain level
Prepare client for pelvic x-rays and abdominal CT scan	Pelvic fracture(s)		Mobility status

Rationale

Although older adults usually fracture their pelvis as a result of falling, this client had a motor vehicle accident that resulted in this condition. The client has abdominal pain, which is the most common finding when experiencing a fractured pelvis. If the client had peritonitis, the client would have a fever and a rigid abdomen. If the client had a small bowel obstruction, the client would have abdominal pain and frequent vomiting, especially after any oral intake. This client does not have these findings. Hemothorax is an emergency that occurs from chest trauma, not abdominal trauma. Therefore hemothorax is not a cause of the client's pain. Pelvic fractures can cause organ perforation, especially perforation of the bladder. Therefore the nurse would monitor the client's voiding pattern and quality of the urine. Anuria, oliguria, and/or hematuria are common findings in clients who have pelvic fractures. Pelvic fractures are confirmed through imaging studies including x-rays and abdominal CT. Management of pelvic fractures depends on whether the fracture is displaced and if the site of the fracture is weight bearing. After treatment for the client's fracture, the nurse would monitor the client's mobility and pain levels. Monitoring blood pressure, bowel sounds, or SpO_2 does not indicate the effectiveness of the client's care related to the fracture.

CJ Cognitive Skill: Recognize Cues, Analyze Cues, Prioritize Hypotheses, Generate Solutions, Take Actions, Evaluate Outcomes

Reference: Linton & Matteson, 2023, pp. 929, 1291

Answers With Rationales for Thinking Exercises

Unfolding Case Study 14.1

Thinking Exercise 14.1.1

Answer

- ○ 3+ Pitting edema
- ○ Bile-colored emesis
- ✗ Bilateral coarse crackles auscultated
- ○ Decreased appetite due to nausea
- ○ FSBG 128 mg/dL (7.1 mmol/L)
- ✗ Oriented to self and family only
- ○ Paresthesia in bilateral lower extremities

Rationale

The nurse must differentiate normal findings associated with the client's chronic health conditions and findings that indicate a potential acute illness or a complication of chronic disease. The nurse would identify shallow and labored respirations with bilateral coarse crackles as an acute and potentially life-threatening respiratory finding, especially because the client is also disoriented. Inadequate ventilation and/or oxygen perfusion leads to tissue and organ death. Although the client's SpO$_2$ is within normal limits, confusion is often an initial first sign of inadequate oxygenation in older adults. The nurse would immediately follow up on respiratory and neurologic findings. Lower extremity pitting edema is a complication of chronic kidney disease (CKD), and paresthesia is a complication of chronic diabetes mellitus. Neither finding is life threatening. Decreased appetite, nausea, and vomiting are important findings, but they do not indicate a life-threatening condition requiring emergent intervention and therefore would be managed after following up on respiratory and cardiac findings. The finger stick blood glucose (FSBG) level is within normal limits for a client with type 2 diabetes mellitus.
CJ Cognitive Skill: Recognize Cues
Reference: Linton & Matteson, 2023, pp. 90–94, 861–863

Thinking Exercise 14.1.2

Answer

The client is **most likely** experiencing **pulmonary edema** as evidenced by **shallow, labored respirations** and **coarse crackles**.

Rationale

The client findings are classic signs of pulmonary edema including shallow, labored respirations, auscultated coarse crackles, and disorientation (especially in older adults). Pulmonary edema is a life-threatening complication of CKD caused by decreased cardiac function and fluid overload. Oliguria contributes to fluid retention but is not evidence of pulmonary edema. Deep vein thrombosis manifests as pain, swelling, and redness in one leg. This client's pitting edema is bilateral, not unilateral, and there is no indication of redness or pain in the client's lower extremities. Classic signs of small bowel obstruction are nausea and vomiting (possibly projectile vomiting) along with abdominal distention, tenderness, and guarding. The client is experiencing some of these findings, but not to the extent that the nurse would suspect small bowel obstruction.

CJ Cognitive Skill: Analyze Cues
Reference: Linton & Matteson, 2023, pp. 861–863

Thinking Exercise 14.1.3

Answer

The nurse determines the *priority* for care at this time is emergent hemodialysis due to **pulmonary edema with respiratory distress** and **hyperkalemia with ECG changes**.

Rationale

The client's chronic kidney condition apparently has been previously managed with diuretics. Current findings indicate that this treatment plan is no longer working, and the client is experiencing life-threatening complications. Emergent hemodialysis is required when experiencing pulmonary edema with respiratory distress and/or symptomatic hyperkalemia with ECG changes. Pulmonary edema inhibits oxygen perfusion leading to respiratory failure and organ death. Hyperkalemia, especially extremely high serum potassium levels (>6.5 mEq/L [>6.5 mmol/L]), can cause ECG changes leading to ineffective contractions and cardiac arrest. Hemodialysis will remove both fluid and potassium from the body, minimizing these life-threatening conditions. Pitting edema and oliguria are signs that the current treatment plan is not working and the client is retaining fluid. But these findings are not life threatening and therefore are not the primary reason for emergent hemodialysis. Other abnormal laboratory findings are caused by CKD and diabetes mellitus and are not reasons for emergent hemodialysis.

CJ Cognitive Skill: Prioritize Hypotheses
Reference: Linton & Matteson, 2023, pp. 861–866; Pagana et al., 2023, pp. 50, 179, 296, 451, 675, 707, 749, 803

Thinking Exercise 14.1.4

Answer

CLIENT CONDITIONS	POTENTIAL NURSING ACTIONS
Fluid volume excess related to fluid retention because of kidney dysfunction	✗ Accurately calculate daily fluid intake from all sources. ✗ Obtain daily weights at the same time using the same scale. ✗ Assess vital signs, respiratory effort, and lung sounds every 4 hours.
Inadequate nutrition related to anorexia, nausea, vomiting, and dietary restrictions	✗ Collaborate with a registered dietary nutritionist to educate the client and family on nutritional needs and restrictions. O Provide the client with protein shakes between each meal. O Teach the client to use salt substitutes.
Potential for injury related to acute confusion, bone demineralization, and peripheral neuropathy	✗ Assess skin and bony areas for pressure wounds and unusual surface bumps or depressions. ✗ Facilitate frequent client rounding to reorient and provide basic care needs. ✗ Teach assistive nursing personnel the correct use of lift sheets to reposition the client in bed.

Rationale

The nurse would assess the client's fluid status by obtaining daily weights and reviewing intake and output. All sources of fluid must be included in daily fluid intake calculations. The nurse would also frequently monitor the client for symptoms of fluid overload including shallow respirations, auscultated crackles, decreased SpO_2, and increased heart rate, respiratory rate, and blood pressure. Diets for clients with CKD are complicated and unique to the individual. The nurse would collaborate with a registered dietary nutritionist to develop a dietary plan and educate the client and family on nutritional needs and restrictions. Protein is generally restricted based on the degree of kidney impairment, the severity of the symptoms, and medical treatments such as hemodialysis. Therefore the nurse would not provide supplemental protein shakes between meals. Salt substitutes frequently contain potassium and would be contraindicated for a client with CKD. Clients with CKD are at risk of acute confusion related to the effects of uremia on the nervous system, pressure wounds due to peripheral neuropathy, infection related to impaired malnutrition and immune response, and fractures/fragile bones due to bone resorption from excessive phosphorous levels. To prevent injury, the nurse would collaborate with the registered nurse and assistive nursing personnel for frequent client rounding to reorient and provide basic care needs. The nurse would use a lift sheet to reposition the client and would teach assistive nursing personnel the correct use to minimize bone fractures and dislocations. Additionally, the nurse would assess for early signs of pressure wounds and any unusual surface bumps or depressions over bony areas.

CJ Cognitive Skill: Generate Solutions

Reference: Linton & Matteson, 2023, pp. 861–869; Pagana et al., 2023, pp. 50, 179, 296, 451, 675, 707, 749, 803

Thinking Exercise 14.1.5

Answer

- O Alert the Rapid Response Team.
- ✗ Assist the client when ambulating to the bathroom.
- O Hold the next dose of losartan-hydrochlorothiazide.
- O Obtain a bedside FSBG reading.
- O Prepare to administer an IV bolus of 0.9% normal saline.
- ✗ Remind the client to use the call bell prior to rising from the bed.
- ✗ Request assistance to obtain orthostatic vital signs.

Rationale

The nurse would recognize that the client's light-headedness is most likely a postdialysis complication caused by excessive intravascular fluid being removed and a slow response by the body to resume fluid hemostasis and adapt with position changes. Light-headedness may also be a sign of hypoglycemia, but the client is not experiencing nausea, diaphoresis, or pallor, which are classic signs of hypoglycemia. The client's light-headedness subsides and the blood pressure is within normal limits when lying in bed; therefore this is not an urgent situation, and there is no need to contact the Rapid Response Team. The nurse would assess orthostatic vital signs to evaluate heart rate and blood pressure changes during standing, sitting, and lying positions. The nurse would not delegate assessment of orthostatic vital signs to assistive nursing personnel but must request assistance to safely position the client during each part of the procedure. The nurse may offer oral fluids within the prescribed restriction limit but would not plan to administer an IV fluid bolus because the blood pressure is within normal limits. The client is at risk of falling; therefore the nurse would remind the client to use the call light prior to rising from the bed and would assist the client when ambulating. Losartan-hydrochlorothiazide is generally administered once a day in the morning. There are no data to suggest the next dose of this blood pressure medication needs to be held.

CJ Cognitive Skill: Take Actions

Reference: Linton & Matteson, 2023, pp. 861–869; Clayton et al., 2022, pp. 355–379

Thinking Exercise 14.1.6

Answer

DATA COLLECTION FINDING	IMPROVED	NOT IMPROVED
Alert and oriented × 4	✗	
BP 135/60 mm Hg	✗	
Denies nausea	✗	
FSBG 188 mg/dL (10.4 mmol/L)		✗
No adventitious lung sounds	✗	

Rationale

The client is currently alert and oriented × 4, which is an improvement from the emergency department assessment 2 days ago, when the client was drowsy and oriented to self and family only. Other improvements include normal blood pressure, equal and unlabored respirations, and no adventitious lung sounds. Additionally, the client is no longer nauseated and expresses interest in eating. The client's blood glucose level has increased since admission, which may be due to the body's response to recent stressors. The nurse may need to request sliding-scale insulin to manage glucose levels during hospitalization.

CJ Cognitive Skill: Evaluate Outcomes

Reference: Linton & Matteson, 2023, pp. 861–869

Unfolding Case Study 14.2

Thinking Exercise 14.2.1

Answer

History and Physical	Nurses' Notes	Orders	Progress Notes

1000: Client made appointment due to new-onset urinary frequency and urgency. Client is alert and oriented × 4. Expresses embarrassment regarding urinary symptoms stating, "I have had trouble initiating urination for a while, but recently I have been voiding without warning, especially during the night." Client confirms postvoid dribbling and denies pain or burning with urination. Health history includes type 2 diabetes mellitus, hypertension, hyperlipidemia, and COPD. Current medications are metformin, losartan, amlodipine, and simvastatin. VS: T 98.5°F (36.9°C), HR 61 beats/min, RR 14 breaths/min, BP 138/66 mm Hg, SpO$_2$ 94% on RA. Denies pain. FSBG 132 mg/dL (7.3 mmol/L).

Rationale

The nurse must acknowledge the client's concern with new-onset urinary symptoms and prioritize following up on urinary frequency, urinary urgency, nocturia, and postvoid dribbling. Trouble initiating urination is not a new symptom for the client. Health history and medication are not of immediate concern because they do not directly relate to the current urinary symptoms. The client's vital signs and FSBG are within normal range for the client's age and health history.

CJ Cognitive Skill: Recognize Cues

Reference: Linton & Matteson, 2023, p. 1094

Thinking Exercise 14.2.2

Answer

The nurse recognizes that the client is *most likely* experiencing **benign prostatic hyperplasia**.

Rationale

Benign prostatic hyperplasia (BPH) and renal calculi can both manifest with urinary frequency, urgency, and incontinence due to urethral obstruction. The client's age and gender increase the risk of BPH, an enlargement of the prostate gland and a common age-related physiologic change. Additional symptoms of BPH, which the client is experiencing, include a weak urinary stream, nocturia, and post-micturition dribble. The client does not have specific risk factors for renal calculi (kidney stones) and is not experiencing flank or abdominal pain, which usually accompanies calculi. The client's history of hypertension and diabetes mellitus increases the risk of intrarenal failure, but current findings do not correlate with acute kidney disease. Pyelonephritis (inflammation of the kidneys) manifests with high fever, chills, nausea, vomiting, dysuria, and flank pain. The client is not experiencing these symptoms. Therefore the client is most likely experiencing BPH.
CJ Cognitive Skill: Analyze Cues
Reference: Linton & Matteson, 2023, pp. 844–845, 848–849, 856–858, 1094

Thinking Exercise 14.2.3

Answer

The nurse determines the *priority* for care at this time is improving **urinary elimination** to prevent complications such as **urinary retention** and **urinary tract infection**.

Rationale

The pathophysiology of BPH involves the abnormal overgrowth of prostate tissue that leads to an enlarged prostate gland, which causes bladder outlet obstruction and lower urinary tract symptoms. Badder outlet obstruction results in urinary retention and residual urine or stasis urine, which increases the risk of urinary tract infection (UTI). Treatment of BPH focuses on improving urinary elimination to decrease urinary retention, residual urine, and UTIs. Increasing detrusor (bladder) muscle strength can initially help urine push past the enlarged prostate gland, but thickened detrusor muscles are unable to overcome chronic hyperplasia and ultimately contribute to greater urinary retention and chronic UTIs. Increasing fluid intake also increases the client's risk for BPH complications including bladder distention and hydronephrosis.
CJ Cognitive Skill: Prioritize Hypotheses
Reference: Linton & Matteson, 2023, pp. 1094–1096

Thinking Exercise 14.2.4

Answer

POTENTIAL ORDERS	INDICATED	NOT INDICATED
Behavior modification to promote bladder emptying and minimize urge incontinence	✗	
Daily urinary self-catheterization to prevent bladder distention		✗
Drug therapy with an alpha$_1$-adrenergic antagonist and/or a 5-alpha-reductase inhibitor	✗	
Fluid restriction of less than 1200 mL per day		✗
Preoperative teaching for transurethral resection of the prostate (TURP)		✗

Rationale

Treatment for BPH ranges from careful monitoring to surgery. This client is symptomatic but not experiencing complications; therefore surgical intervention would not be included in the initial plan of care. The nurse would anticipate behavior modification and drug therapy to be ordered. Behavioral modifications include avoiding bladder irritants and diuretics, avoiding drinking large amounts of fluids at one time, and utilizing a variety of voiding strategies. Fluids are not restricted due to the risk for a UTI. Instead, the client would be instructed to drink a total of 1500 mL to 2000 mL of fluids daily, spacing the liquids throughout the day rather than consuming large amounts at one time. Voiding strategies may include scheduled voiding and double voiding in which the client voids, waits several minutes, and voids again to help empty the bladder. Pharmacologic treatment usually involves an alpha$_1$-adrenergic antagonist, which relaxes smooth muscle in the bladder neck, or a 5-alpha-reductase inhibitor, which reduces prostate size. These medications may also be prescribed in combination. The client may require catheterization if acute urinary retention causes bladder distention, but catheterization is not used to prevent distention, and the client would not be performing self-catheterization. The nurse would instruct the client to contact the physician if unable to void and the bladder becomes distended.

CJ Cognitive Skill: Generate Solutions
Reference: Linton & Matteson, 2023, pp. 1094–1096

Thinking Exercise 14.2.5

Answer

○ Assist the client to develop a schedule for voiding every 3 to 4 hours while awake.
✗ Ask the client to keep a journal with fluid intake and urinary symptoms.
✗ Have the client rise slowly from the bed and lie down if feeling dizzy.
○ Instruct the client to stop taking medications if impotence or sexual dysfunction occurs.
✗ Obtain a baseline serum prostate-specific antigen (PSA) level.
✗ Instruct the client to restrict fluids 2 hours before bedtime.
✗ Teach the client to urinate as soon as the urge to void is felt.

Rationale

BPH symptoms may be triggered by bladder irritants such as alcohol, caffeine, and artificial sweeteners. To help identify specific triggers for the client, the nurse would ask the client to keep a journal of fluid intake (types, amounts, and times of ingestion) and urinary symptoms (frequency, volume, and other symptoms). The nurse would also instruct the client to void promptly when the urge is felt and avoid drinking fluids for 2 hours before bedtime to reduce nighttime voiding. To prevent urge incontinence, the nurse would assist the client to develop a schedule for voiding every 90 to 120 minutes while awake. Doxazosin, an alpha$_1$-adrenergic antagonist, may cause dizziness and orthostatic hypotension, especially with initial doses. The nurse would warn the client about this possible adverse effect and teach the client to rise slowly and to lie down if symptoms occur. Finasteride, a 5-alpha-reductase inhibitor, can cause a decrease in serum PSA levels, even in the presence of prostate cancer. Therefore a baseline PSA level would be obtained prior to the first dose, and PSA levels would be monitored closely throughout drug therapy. Any sustained increase in PSA levels while receiving finasteride must be investigated, including consideration of prostate cancer and noncompliance with therapy. Impotence, decreased libido, and decreased volume of ejaculate are adverse effects that appear in a small number of male clients receiving finasteride. The nurse would explain that these adverse effects may occur but tend to be self-limiting. The nurse would instruct the client to not discontinue the medication and consult the health care provider if the problem becomes unacceptable.

CJ Cognitive Skill: Take Actions
Reference: Linton & Matteson, 2023, pp. 1094–1096; Clayton et al., 2022, pp. 661–664

Thinking Exercise 14.2.6

Answer

History and Physical	Nurses' Notes	Orders	Progress Notes

1000: Client made appointment due to new-onset urinary frequency and urgency. Client is alert and oriented × 4. Expresses embarrassment regarding urinary symptoms stating, "I have had trouble initiating urination for a while, but recently I have been voiding without warning, especially during the night." Client confirms postvoid dribbling and denies pain or burning with urination. Health history includes type 2 diabetes mellitus, hypertension, hyperlipidemia, and COPD. Current medications are metformin, losartan, amlodipine, and simvastatin. VS: T 98.5°F (36.9°C), HR 61 beats/min, RR 14 breaths/min, BP 138/66 mm Hg, SpO$_2$ 94% on RA. Denies pain. FSBG 132 mg/dL (7.3 mmol/L).

1020: Physician at bedside, updated on client findings. Physical and diagnostic examination completed. Client diagnosed with BPH.

1100: Prescription for combination drug therapy with finasteride and doxazosin received. Client teaching provided.

2 Weeks Later
0910: Telemedicine follow-up call. Client alert and oriented. Reports drowsiness and light-headedness for a few days after starting drug therapy, but symptoms have subsided with no episodes of dizziness or orthostatic hypotension in the past few days. Client reports attempting to void every 90 minutes while awake and using the double-voiding technique with each attempt. Postmicturition dribble continues, but episodes of urge incontinence have stopped. Client also reports that limiting evening fluid intake has decreased nocturia, allowing for several hours of uninterrupted sleep every night. VS: T 98.6°F (37°C), HR 63 beats/min, RR 12 breaths/min, BP 132/65 mm Hg, SpO$_2$ 95% on RA. Denies bladder distention and burning or pain with urination. FSBG 144 mg/dL (8 mmol/L).

Rationale

Drug therapy may require more than 6 to 12 months to achieve a therapeutic response, but behavioral changes can create more immediate favorable client outcomes. The client has implemented a urination schedule, utilized the double-voiding technique, and decreased evening fluids. These modifications have resulted in decreased nocturia and incontinence, both signs of improvement. The client experienced adverse effects with initial doses of medication, but these effects were self-limiting and have stopped. A lack of dizziness and orthostatic hypotension is not a therapeutic effect but demonstrates medication tolerance with no adverse effects, which is an improvement.
CJ Cognitive Skill: Evaluate Outcomes
Reference: Linton & Matteson, 2023, pp. 1094–1096

Stand-Alone Thinking Exercise 14.1

Answer

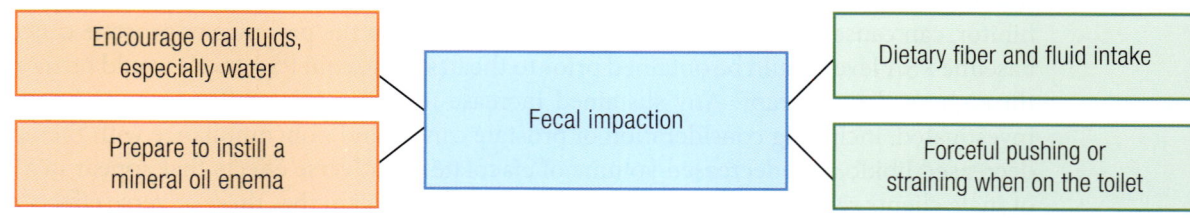

Rationale

The client is an older adult who reported not having a bowel movement for the past 3 days and has attempted, unsuccessfully, to evacuate stool multiple times this evening. The nurse would recognize inability to defecate as the client's priority concern and determine that the client is most likely experiencing fecal impaction, the retention of a mass of stool in the rectum that the client is unable to evacuate by regular peristaltic activity. Manifestations of fecal impaction are strong urge to defecate, pressure on the rectum, abdominal bloating, and liquid stool that may trickle around the impaction and be mistaken for diarrhea. If agency protocol permits, the nurse may assess for impaction by inserting a gloved, lubricated finger into the rectum. The fecal mass is usually easily felt and may be very hard or soft. Removing the fecal mass is the goal of treatment. The nurse would prepare to instill a mineral oil enema to soften the hard stool followed by a soap suds enema to clean out the rectum. The nurse would also encourage the client to drink ample water and may administer docusate or sorbitol to soften the stool for evacuation. To prevent future impaction, the nurse would teach the client to eat high-fiber foods, including plenty of raw fruits and vegetables and whole-grain products; drink adequate amounts of fluids, especially water; and exercise regularly. Walking is a great way for older adults to remain active and promote bowel motility. The nurse would monitor daily intake of dietary fiber and water. The client's light-headedness occurred while sitting on the toilet and is most likely a vagal nerve response to straining or "bearing down" to evacuate stool. This is not the result of orthostatic hypotension, which would have occurred when the client originally rose from the bed or chair to walk to the bathroom. To promote safety, the nurse would teach the client to avoid straining during defecation and would monitor for forceful pushing or straining when the client is on the toilet. The nurse would also remind the client to use the call bell and wait for assistance prior to ambulating to the bathroom. The toilet or a bedside commode creates a more natural position and increases the potential for a successful bowel movement. A bedpan would not be used for this client.

CJ Cognitive Skills: Recognize Cues, Analyze Cues, Prioritize Hypotheses, Generate Solutions, Take Actions, Evaluate Outcomes

Reference: Linton & Matteson, 2023, pp. 205, 231–238, 789–792

Stand-Alone Thinking Exercise 14.2

Answer

- ✗ Anticipate the need for straight catheterization to obtain a sterile urine sample.
- ✗ Cleanse the perineum and apply barrier cream after each incontinence episode.
- ✗ Collaborate with the interdisciplinary team to provide constant client supervision.
- ○ Contact the stroke alert or Rapid Response Team.
- ✗ Keep the bed in the lowest position with the call bell within reach.
- ○ Recommend a 1000-mL IV fluid bolus.
- ✗ Schedule client toileting every 60 to 90 minutes.

Rationale

The nurse must recognize acute changes in client findings. Although the client has a history of dementia, the client's level of consciousness and orientation have diminished significantly from the established baseline. Acute confusion or delirium, especially in older adults, may be caused by a variety of health issues but is most commonly associated with an acute infection. An analysis of client findings should lead the nurse to suspect a UTI. Classic symptoms of UTI include urgency, frequency, dysuria, hematuria, nocturia, bladder spasms, low-grade fever, and dark, tea-colored, or cloudy urine. Atypical UTI manifestations in the older adult include hypotension, tachycardia, urinary incontinence, poor appetite, drowsiness, frequent falls, and delirium. The nurse must take actions to protect the client from injury including falls and skin breakdown. Cleansing and applying barrier cream to the client's perineum will help prevent excoriation and ulcers. The client is most likely not experiencing a stroke due to clear speech and equal movement of extremities; therefore contacting the stroke alert or Rapid Response Team is not required. The nurse would report client findings to the physician and anticipate orders for diagnostic testing (blood and urine cultures) and antibiotics. The nurse would also closely monitor intake and output and may encourage oral fluids within established restrictions. Due to the client's history of heart failure, intravenous fluids may be contraindicated. If dehydration occurs and IV fluids are prescribed, the nurse must carefully monitor the client for signs of congestion and respiratory distress.

CJ Cognitive Skills: Recognize Cues, Analyze Cues, Priority Hypotheses, Generate Solutions, Take Actions

Reference: Linton & Matteson, 2023, pp. 222–236, 842–843

Answers With Rationales for Thinking Exercises

Unfolding Case Study 15.1

Thinking Exercise 15.1.1

Answer

- ○ 2+ nonpitting edema of feet
- ○ Pain rated 7/10
- ○ Blistered skin on both hands
- ○ Oriented × 2 (person and situation)
- ✗ Soot around nares and mouth
- ○ BP 135/82 mm Hg
- ✗ SpO_2 90% on RA

Rationale

Client findings that require immediate follow-up are life threatening or potentially life threatening. Soot is a black, powdery substance containing carbon particles that results from incomplete combustion of organic materials during a fire. The presence of soot around the nares and mouth suggests the client likely inhaled fumes and soot when trying to put out the fire. This foreign substance may have entered the lungs, which could become life threatening. An SpO_2 of 90% is low and, combined with possible inhalation of soot and other toxic substances, could also become a life-threatening condition. Pain, foot edema, and blistered skin are not life threatening and can wait to be managed. Even though the client's blood pressure is elevated, it is not at a life-threatening level. Blood pressure and heart rate often increase due to the body's sympathetic response (increased adrenalin) to trauma or a major life event. The client's cognitive state is also not life threatening.

CJ Cognitive Skill: Recognize Cues
Reference: Linton & Matteson, 2023, pp. 1161–1162, 1291

Thinking Exercise 15.1.2

Answer

The client is most at risk for having **a smoke inhalation injury** because the client has **soot around the nares and mouth**.

Rationale

In view of the presence of soot around the client's nares and mouth, the client is most at risk for lung injury caused by smoke inhalation. There is no evidence that the client has third-degree burns. Blistering is associated with second-degree burns; skin redness indicates first-degree burns. Both first- and second-degree burns are partial-thickness burns. A blood pressure of 135/82 mm Hg is elevated but is not high enough to indicate hypertensive crisis. If the client were experiencing hypovolemic shock, the blood pressure would be very low, and the heart rate would likely be above 100 beats/min.

CJ Cognitive Skill: Analyze Cues
Reference: Linton & Matteson, 2023, pp. 1161–1162, 1291

Thinking Exercise 15.1.3

Answer

Based on the client's risk for complications, the *priority* for client care is to anticipate the need for potential **respiratory** support.

Rationale

The client is at risk for lung injury related to smoke inhalation. Therefore the client's potential priority is the need for respiratory support to maintain lung function. The client's nausea may be the result of the sympathetic nervous system response. The client has decreased pedal pulses, increased capillary refill time, and foot edema, but these findings are commonly seen in older adults due to the normal physiologic changes of aging. Therefore cardiac, vascular, or gastrointestinal support would likely not be a priority for client care.
CJ Cognitive Skill: Prioritize Hypotheses
Reference: Linton & Matteson, 2023, pp. 1161–1162, 1291

Thinking Exercise 15.1.4

Answer

✗ Administer supplemental oxygen therapy.
✗ Place the client in an upright sitting position.
○ Administer acetaminophen for elevated temperature.
✗ Monitor respiratory rate and SpO_2 at least every hour.
○ Administer an oral loop diuretic such as furosemide.
○ Observe burned areas for signs of infection.

Rationale

Given the client's probable smoke inhalation injury and the most current client findings, the nurse would plan interventions that would provide respiratory support. Nursing actions that are appropriate for improving lung function include administering supplemental oxygen and placing the client in an upright sitting position to promote lung expansion. To determine the client's respiratory status, the nurse would need to frequently monitor the client's respiratory rate and SpO_2 level. The client does not have a fever and therefore would not need acetaminophen. The client likely has dependent edema, which improves when sleeping. There is no evidence of heart or kidney disease; therefore the client would not require diuretic therapy. Clients with partial-thickness burns are prone to infection. However, infection tends to occur several days after the initial burn injury and is not an appropriate nursing action at this time in the emergency department.
CJ Cognitive Skill: Generate Solutions
Reference: Linton & Matteson, 2023, pp. 1161–1169

Thinking Exercise 15.1.5

Answer

BODY SYSTEM	NURSING ACTIONS
Respiratory	✗ Request a bedside chest x-ray. ✗ Consult respiratory therapy. ○ Suction the client using a sterile catheter.
Neurologic	✗ Request a carbon monoxide blood test. ✗ Transfer client care to the registered nurse. ✗ Monitor neurologic status every hour.
Integumentary	✗ Apply an antimicrobial dressing to second-degree burn areas. ○ Elevate both arms above the heart. ○ Plan to admit the client to the acute burn unit.

Rationale

The client's condition is worsening, including the client's vital signs and respiratory and neurologic function. Therefore the primary responsibility for client care would transfer to the registered nurse with assistance of the licensed practical nurse (LPN) or licensed vocational nurse (LVN). When smoke inhalation injury is suspected, the provider orders a chest x-ray, which may be repeated as the client's condition changes. The nurse would notify respiratory therapy for a client consult to support lung function. Respiratory therapy often includes treatments with bronchodilators and/or corticosteroids to open airways, decrease inflammation, and promote breathing. There is no need to suction the client at this time because the client's cough is nonproductive (dry). Given that the client has a smoke inhalation injury, the client is at high risk for inhalation of carbon monoxide (CO), a potentially life-threatening odorless gas produced by the fire. Therefore taking a blood level of CO would be an appropriate nursing action. CO poisoning can cause headache, decreased level of consciousness, and cognitive decline. The client is already disoriented and restless, indicating neurologic change. Therefore the nurse would monitor the client's neurologic status frequently. An antimicrobial dressing would be appropriate for the second-degree burn areas to help prevent infection. Elevating the arms would inhibit adequate blood flow and would not be appropriate. The client's burns are not severe enough to require admission to a burn specialty unit, but the client would be hospitalized.

CJ Cognitive Skill: Take Actions

Reference: Linton & Matteson, 2023, pp. 1161–1169, 1294

Thinking Exercise 15.1.6

Answer

History and Physical	Nurses' Notes	Orders	Laboratory Results

2230: Client brought to ED by friend after trying to extinguish a fire caused by a propane heater in a tent encampment for unhoused individuals. Friend unable to provide health history or information about whether the client takes medications but states client is a veteran who served in Vietnam. Client appears unkempt with poor hygiene; alert and oriented × 2 (person and situation). Ragged torn coat sleeves carefully removed to inspect skin. Palms of both hands blistered and swollen. Lower arms from hands to elbows reddened and slightly swollen. Reports pain rated 7/10 and "waves of nausea." Smudges on face and soot around nares and mouth. No adventitious or abnormal lung sounds. Denies dyspnea or shortness of breath. Peripheral pulses 2+, except for pedal pulses, which are barely palpable. Cap refill >3 sec; 2+ nonpitting edema in both feet. Able to move all extremities. Abdomen soft and round with active bowel sounds present in all quadrants. VS: T 99°F (37.2°C), HR 92 beats/min and regular, RR 20 breaths/min, BP 135/82 mm Hg, SpO$_2$ 90% on RA.

2310: Blood drawn for CMP and CBC. Peripheral IV access established in left forearm in nonburned area. NS infusing at 100 mL/h. Continues to be alert and oriented × 2. Pain medication administered. Reports feeling a "little short of breath" but has less nausea. Slight inspiratory wheezing auscultated throughout lung fields. Wound care provided. VS: T 99°F (37.2°C), HR 100 beats/min and regular, RR 22 breaths/min, BP 138/84 mm Hg, SpO$_2$ 88% on RA.

2355: Alert but disoriented and restless. Cannot follow conversation. Continues to have wheezing, which is worsening. VS: T 99°F (37.2°C), HR 108 beats/min and irregular, RR 30 breaths/min and shallow, BP 150/92 mm Hg, SpO$_2$ 89% on 4 L/min O$_2$ via NC.

0010: Bedside chest x-ray performed. Bronchodilator via nebulizer administered by RT. Blood drawn for stat carbon monoxide level.

0045: Alert and oriented × 2. Able to follow conversation and respond appropriately. Occasional wheezing. No smoke inhalation injury noted on chest x-ray. Antimicrobial dressings applied to both hands. VS: T 98.6°F (37°C), HR 88 beats/min and regular, RR 20 breaths/min, BP 148/88 mm Hg, SpO$_2$ 95% on 4 L/min O$_2$ via NC.

Rationale

The client's condition has improved as a result of collaborative actions by the health care team. The client's neurologic status has returned to baseline, wheezing has improved, and the SpO_2 is now within usual range while on oxygen therapy. The client is no longer tachycardic or tachypneic as evidenced by a heart rate below 100 beats/min and a respiratory rate of 20 breaths/min. The client's body temperature remains in the usual range, but the blood pressure remains elevated.

CJ Cognitive Skill: Evaluate Outcomes
Reference: Linton & Matteson, 2023, pp. 1161–1169, 1294

Unfolding Case Study 15.2

Thinking Exercise 15.2.1

Answer

- O 6/10 sacral area pain
- O Decreased appetite
- O Hypoactive bowel sounds
- ✗ Elevated temperature
- O Tachycardia
- O Tachypnea
- ✗ Low blood pressure
- ✗ Elevated FSBG
- ✗ Warm and reddened skin around wound

Rationale

Client findings that require immediate follow-up are those which are or could be potentially life threatening. In this older adult's case, an elevated temperature of 100.8°F (38.2°C) could indicate dehydration and lead to hypovolemia or hypovolemic shock. The client's low blood pressure also supports possible dehydration. When older adults become dehydrated, they often become acutely confused due to lack of oxygen supply to the brain (hypoxia). Tachycardia and tachypnea are findings that help compensate for hypotension and do not require follow-up at this time. The client's blood glucose is elevated and could lead to a potentially life-threatening diabetic complication known as *hyperglycemic hyperosmolar syndrome*. Therefore the FSBG requires immediate follow-up. The warm and reddened skin around the client's pressure injury indicates spread of the local infection to a systemic infection. This change needs immediate attention and follow-up to prevent potentially life-threatening complications. Pain and anorexia are not life threatening and can be followed up later. Poor food and fluid intake could be associated with the client's hypoactive bowel sounds.

CJ Cognitive Skill: Recognize Cues
Reference: Linton & Matteson, 2023, pp. 94–95, 1158–1161

Thinking Exercise 15.2.2

Answer

- ✗ Sepsis
- O Heart failure
- O Bowel obstruction
- ✗ Dehydration
- ✗ Malnutrition
- O Hypoglycemia

Rationale

Because the client likely has a systemic infection as evidenced by cellulitis around the sacral pressure injury and a fever, the client is at risk for sepsis and potentially septic shock, which are life-threatening conditions. The client is also at risk for dehydration and malnutrition due to poor appetite. Tachycardia and low blood pressure indicate that the client likely has dehydration. There is no evidence that the client has or is at risk for heart failure or bowel obstruction. The client's FSBG shows hyperglycemia rather than hypoglycemia.

CJ Cognitive Skill: Analyze Cues
Reference: Linton & Matteson, 2023, pp. 94–95, 1158–1161

Thinking Exercise 15.2.3

Answer

The *priority* for the client's care is to prevent or monitor for **sepsis**.

Rationale

The client likely has a systemic infection as evidenced by fever, cellulitis, and dehydration. The priority for the nurse is to plan and implement care that helps prevent sepsis. If the client has signs and symptoms associated with sepsis, the nurse would carefully monitor the client for this complication. Sepsis is the body's unexpected response to a systemic infection and can cause organ failure and eventually death. High lactic acid levels help confirm a diagnosis of sepsis. Clients who are older than 65 years of age and have chronic diseases such as diabetes mellitus are at especially high risk for sepsis. This client could develop protein deficiency or electrolyte imbalance due to poor food intake and loss of wound drainage, but these complications are not as life threatening as sepsis. At this time, bone is not exposed in the pressure injury; however, the client could develop osteomyelitis if the infection spreads to the bone. This complication can become chronic and require treatment for many months. However, it is less life threatening than other complications.

CJ Cognitive Skill: Prioritize Hypotheses
Reference: Linton & Matteson, 2023, pp. 94–95, 160, 1158–1161

Thinking Exercise 15.2.4

Answer

POTENTIAL NURSING ACTION	INDICATED	NOT INDICATED
Administer antibiotic therapy per agency protocol.	X	
Start IV fluids via peripheral IV access.	X	
Administer supplemental oxygen therapy via nasal cannula.		X
Take and record vital signs every 4 hours.	X	
Request consults with a registered dietitian nutritionist and a certified wound specialist.	X	

Rationale

The client's infection and likely dehydration require IV fluids and antibiotics as soon as possible. At a skilled nursing facility, the nurse would monitor vital signs frequently, at least every 4 hours. A wound specialist is essential to prescribe the appropriate wound care to help heal the pressure injury, which will be a long-term process. A registered dietitian nutritionist is needed to help plan a diet high in protein and vitamin C for tissue healing. Supplemental enteral nutrition may also be needed between meals for additional protein and calories. At this time, there is no indication for supplemental oxygen therapy.

CJ Cognitive Skill: Generate Solutions
Reference: Linton & Matteson, 2023, pp. 94–95, 1158–1161

Thinking Exercise 15.2.5

Answer

- ✗ "A foam dressing that is covered with a clear adhesive layer will be used with the wound VAC device."
- ✗ "The wound VAC device will be connected to a pump that removes drainage and air pressure from the wound and promotes healing."
- ○ "The foam dressing is changed once a month for most clients who have pressure injuries."
- ✗ "An alarm will sound if the wound VAC system is not working properly."
- ✗ "The nurse will monitor the amount and quality of the drainage from the wound frequently."

Rationale

All of these statements would be included when reinforcing health teaching, except for the frequency of changing the foam dressing. For most clients, the dressing needs to be changed every few days, not once a month.

CJ Cognitive Skill: Take Actions
Reference: Linton & Matteson, 2023, pp. 298–299, 1158–1161

Thinking Exercise 15.2.6

Answer

The client's condition has **improved** as evidenced by **decreased body temperature** and **decreased wound size**.

Rationale

The client's condition has improved as a result of a positive response to the collaborative plan of care. The client's systemic infection is resolving as evidenced by slow wound healing and a return to the usual range for body temperature. The client's blood glucose has also decreased. Blood glucose tends to increase in the presence of infection but decreases when infection is resolving. Except for body temperature, the other vital signs have remained in the same range. The client continues to have a stage 4 pressure injury with drainage, although the characteristics of the drainage are changing.

CJ Cognitive Skill: Evaluate Outcomes
Reference: Linton & Matteson, 2023, pp. 298–299, 1158–1161

Stand-Alone Thinking Exercise 15.1

Answer

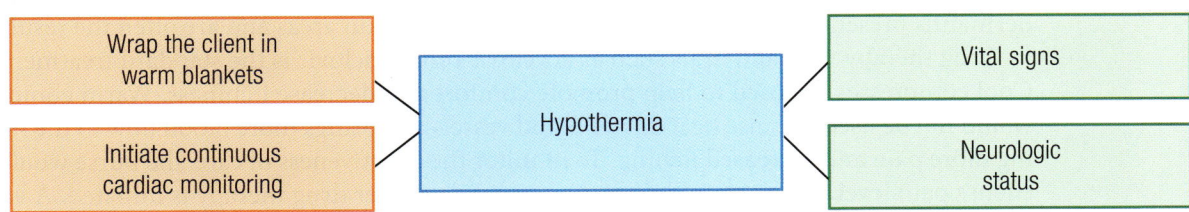

Rationale

Hypothermia is a decrease in core body temperature to below 95°F (35°C) that is usually caused by prolonged exposure to cold temperatures or immersion in very cold water. Hypothermia can cause major organ failure, including cardiac dysrhythmias, and eventually death if not treated. This client was shoveling snow for more than 30 minutes before experiencing signs and symptoms associated with hypothermia. Clients with hypothermia often appear dazed, are acutely disoriented and confused, and shiver to generate body heat. Vital signs are usually decreased. This client presented with all of these findings. In addition, the client's speech is slurred, pupils are dilated, and muscles are rigid. Frostbite usually affects the nose, cheeks, fingers, and toes, and it causes lack of blood supply leading to tissue necrosis. There is no evidence that the client has frostbite. Although the client's bowel sounds are hypoactive, there are no other findings associated with bowel obstruction. Pulmonary embolus is usually characterized by chest pain and dyspnea. This client does not appear to have these findings. Clients who have hypothermia need to be rewarmed slowly by wrapping them in blankets (torso before extremities). Continuous cardiac monitoring is needed to identify cardiac dysrhythmias. Tissue debridement is not necessary because the client does not have frostbite. Antibiotic therapy is not necessary because the client does not have an infection at this time. To assess the effectiveness of the plan of care, the nurse would continue monitoring vital signs for an increase in body temperature and collect data about neurologic status. The client does not report pain; the SpO_2 is below 95% but is commonly between 90% and 94% in older adults without respiratory distress. It would not be helpful to monitor the client's prothrombin time or INR level.

CJ Cognitive Skills: Recognize Cues, Analyze Cues, Prioritize Hypotheses, Generate Solutions, Take Actions, Evaluate Outcomes

Reference: Linton & Matteson, 2023, pp. 1292–1294

Stand-Alone Thinking Exercise 15.2

Answer

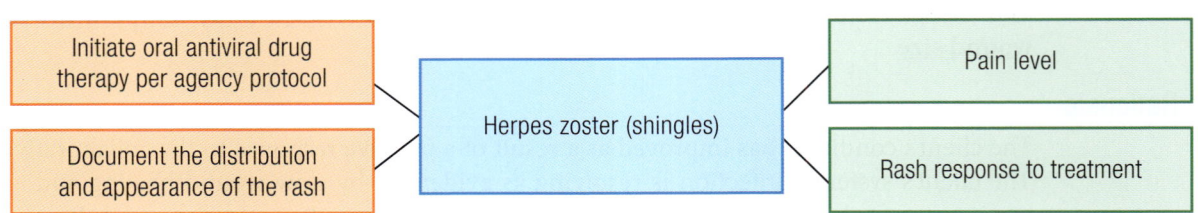

Rationale

Herpes zoster, also known as *shingles,* is caused by the same virus (varicella-zoster) that causes chickenpox. In many individuals, the virus remains dormant in nerve tissue until it is triggered later in life. Older adults and those who are immunocompromised are the most at risk for this condition. The infection begins as a painful and itchy rash most often seen on the chest, abdomen, or back. The nurse would document the distribution and appearance of the rash before treatment begins. Crusts form on the blisterlike lesions, which are contagious to individuals who have not been exposed to the virus for about 7 to 10 days. These crusts would not be removed. Melanoma is a serious cancerous skin condition that appears as one lesion without pain or itchiness. Both eczema (atopic dermatitis) and contact dermatitis present as rashes that occur on one or more skin areas and are often the result of allergies.

Drug therapy with antivirals such as acyclovir or famciclovir is the standard treatment for shingles. Cool compresses are used to help promote comfort and decrease itchiness. Warm compresses or heat would not be used because heat dilates blood vessels and brings more blood flow to the rash area, causing more pain and increased itching. To monitor the effectiveness of care, the nurse would monitor the client's pain level, which should decrease several days after drug therapy is initiated. A variety of analgesics, antidepressants, and antiepileptic drugs are used to manage the pain associated with shingles. These medications may also be used to manage postherpetic neuralgia, a common complication of shingles in older adults. Blood pressure, white blood cell count, and body temperature are usually not affected by herpes zoster infection.

CJ Cognitive Skills: Recognize Cues, Analyze Cues, Prioritize Hypotheses, Generate Solutions, Take Actions, Evaluate Outcomes

Reference: Linton & Matteson, 2023, pp. 1143–1144, 1153–1154, 1157

Answers With Rationales for Thinking Exercises

Unfolding Case Study 16.1

Thinking Exercise 16.1.1

Answer

- ⊙ Approximated incision
- ⊙ Bradycardia
- ✗ Extremity numbness
- ⊙ Heberden nodes
- ✗ Increased fatigue
- ⊙ Portable electric heater
- ✗ Report of feeling cold
- ⊙ Standard 4-point walker

Rationale

The nurse would recognize manifestations of the client's chronic health conditions and treatments such as Heberden nodes, which are associated with osteoarthritis, and bradycardia, which is most likely caused by cardiac medications including atenolol, a beta-adrenergic blocker, and nifedipine, a calcium channel blocker. These findings are expected and would not require immediate follow-up by the nurse. Additionally, the client's wound assessment is within normal limits, and use of a standard 4-point walker after hip surgery is common for an older adult. The nurse would recognize unexpected findings such as increased fatigue, extremity numbness, and reports of feeling cold besides having multiple blankets and a portable electric heater. These findings are vague and may be caused by several different conditions or complications. Therefore the nurse would follow up on them immediately. The client is using a portable electric heater to stay warm, but there is no concern with the actual heater. The heater cord is tucked under the couch, and the room is free from clutter, both reducing fall hazards.

CJ Cognitive Skill: Recognize Cues
Reference: Linton & Matteson, 2023, pp. 567–570, 687–691, 988–990

Thinking Exercise 16.1.2

Answer

CLIENT FINDINGS	ANEMIA	HEART FAILURE	HYPOTHYROIDISM
Fatigue	✗	✗	✗
Nonpitting edema		✗	✗
Frequent headaches	✗		
Weight gain		✗	✗
Extremity numbness	✗		✗

Rationale

The client's symptoms are related to several conditions including anemia, hypothyroidism, and heart failure. All three conditions result in fatigue and activity intolerance: anemia due to a lack of oxygen transportation to organs, hypothyroidism due to decreased metabolic rate, and heart failure due to decreased cardiac output and oxygen perfusion. Clients who have anemia or hypothyroidism experience frequent headaches and numbness in the extremities. Headaches caused by inadequate thyroid hormones are most reported as migraines, and headaches associated with anemia are caused by inadequate oxygen perfusion to the brain. Numbness in the extremities is also related to inadequate oxygen perfusion in clients with anemia and is related to peripheral neuropathy in clients with hypothyroidism. Nonpitting edema and weight gain are both manifestations of hypothyroidism and heart failure. Edema and weight gain in a client with heart failure are related to fluid retention. In a client with hypothyroidism, weight gain is related to a decreased metabolic rate, and edema is related to myxedema and generally present on the face, hands, and feet.

CJ Cognitive Skill: Analyze Cues
Reference: Linton & Matteson, 2023, pp. 567–570, 687–691, 988–990

Thinking Exercise 16.1.3

Answer

The nurse recognizes that the client is *most likely* experiencing **hypothyroidism**. The nurse would recommend **hormone replacement therapy**.

Rationale

Thyroid hormone levels in the body are regulated by a feedback loop. When hormone levels are low, the anterior pituitary gland releases thyroid-stimulating hormone (TSH), which stimulates the thyroid gland to increase the production of triiodothyronine (T_3) and thyroxine (T_4) and increase hormone levels back to normal. When the thyroid gland fails to respond and does not produce thyroid hormones, T_3 and T_4 levels decrease or remain low, and the anterior pituitary gland continues to produce TSH at elevated levels. The client's low T_4 level and elevated TSH level along with clinical manifestations such as fatigue, cold intolerance, weight gain, frequent headaches, paresthesia, and nonpitting edema of the hands and feet support that the client is most likely experiencing hypothyroidism. The client is also experiencing manifestations of anemia, but laboratory tests demonstrate normal hemoglobin and hematocrit levels. The client has risk factors for heart failure including advanced age and hypertension. Common manifestations of heart failure including cool extremities, weak peripheral pulses, dyspnea, and pulmonary congestion are not present. The client's B-type natriuretic peptide (BNP) is also within normal limits. BNP correlates well with left ventricular pressures and is a good marker for congestive heart failure. Pharmacologic treatment for hypothyroidism is administration of oral thyroid replacement hormones. The other treatments would not be appropriate for the client at this time.

CJ Cognitive Skill: Prioritize Hypotheses
Reference: Linton & Matteson, 2023, pp. 567–570, 687–691, 988–990; Pagana et al., 2023, pp. 475, 479, 624, 851, 857

Thinking Exercise 16.1.4

Answer

POTENTIAL NURSING ACTION	INDICATED	NOT INDICATED
Teach the client about hormone replacement therapy.	✗	
Encourage the client to integrate periods of rest during activities of daily living.	✗	
Assist the client in bathing twice a day to decrease skin drying.		✗
Consult a registered dietitian nutritionist for diet and food option recommendations.	✗	
Wear a surgical mask during home health visits to minimize the risk of infection transmission.		✗

Rationale

The nurse would teach the client when to take the hormones, when to expect a therapeutic response, and when to report side effects or adverse reactions to the health care provider. The client is experiencing increased fatigue and is at risk for activity intolerance. Rest periods during activities of daily living will enable the client to conserve energy and complete more activities. Impaired skin integrity frequently occurs in clients with hypothyroidism due to dry skin and inactivity. The nurse would teach the client to assess the skin daily, use soap-free and nondrying products to bathe, avoid daily tub baths and showers, and change position at least every 2 hours. The client's decreased metabolic rate may cause increased weight and nutritional deficits. Consulting a registered dietitian nutritionist would assist the client to make food choices to prevent unwanted weight gain while meeting nutritional needs. Hypothyroidism is not an infectious condition and does not cause immunosuppression. Therefore wearing a mask would not be not indicated for the client at this time.

CJ Cognitive Skill: Generate Solutions
Reference: Linton & Matteson, 2023, pp. 988–992

Thinking Exercise 16.1.5—Pharmacology

Answer

- ✗ "Constipation may result from hypothyroidism. Increasing your fluid and fiber intake may help with this condition."
- ✗ "Fatigue and mental slowness are symptoms of hypothyroidism and should improve with treatment."
- ○ "If hormone replacement therapy is not successful, the health care provider may recommend surgical intervention."
- ○ "Laboratory tests will be rechecked in 6 weeks, and you can stop taking levothyroxine if levels are normal."
- ✗ "The best time to take your levothyroxine is 30 to 60 minutes before breakfast."
- ○ "You may take a sedative or tranquilizer if you are having difficulty sleeping through the night."

Rationale

Constipation is a common manifestation of hypothyroidism. Eating a high-fiber diet with fresh fruits and raw vegetables along with increasing fluid intake and activity will help the client manage bowel issues. Levothyroxine would be administered at the same time each day and on an empty stomach. Taking it 30 to 60 minutes before breakfast each morning is the best time to take the drug. Most symptoms associated with hypothyroidism will resolve once hormone levels, including fatigue and mental slowness, have been corrected. The client will most likely need lifelong thyroid hormone replacement therapy and should not expect to stop taking levothyroxine when laboratory results indicate normal hormone levels. There are no surgical interventions to treat hypothyroidism. Thyroidectomy is a treatment for hyperthyroidism, not hypothyroidism. Sedatives, opioids, and tranquilizers can precipitate a potentially fatal myxedema coma in clients with hypothyroidism and would not be appropriate for the client at this time. The nurse would teach the client to contact the health care provider if insomnia, agitation, tachycardia, or any other symptoms of hyperthyroidism develop.

CJ Cognitive Skill: Take Actions
Reference: Linton & Matteson, 2023, pp. 988–992; Clayton et al., 2022, pp. 597–600

Thinking Exercise 16.1.6

Answer

History and Physical	Nurses' Notes	Orders	Laboratory Results

Postoperative Day 4

1245: Initial home health visit after left hip arthroplasty. Client's health history includes osteoarthritis, hypertension, and a recent fall. Medications include acetaminophen, atenolol, and nifedipine. Client is lying on a couch covered in multiple blankets. Room is free from clutter, standard 4-point walker within client's reach, and cord for portable electric heater tucked under the couch. Client alert and oriented × 4. Reports feeling more fatigued than normal. Sits upright when asked and moves all extremities equally. Denies surgical pain but reports frequent headaches, joint stiffness, and extremity numbness. Heart tones regular. Pulses 2+ throughout. Nonpitting edema present in bilateral hands and feet. Respirations equal and unlabored with no adventitious breath sounds. Client denies chest pain or dyspnea. Skin warm and dry. Heberden nodes present on bilateral hands. Client reports feeling cold and asks spouse to turn up the heater. Left hip incision well approximated. No redness or swelling present. Client confirms active participation in home PT activities. VS: T 97.6°F (36.4°C), HR 58 beats/min and regular, BP 129/66 mm Hg, RR 14 breaths/min, SpO$_2$ 96% on RA. Noted weight gain of 10 lb (4.5 kg) since annual physical 6 months ago.

1315: Provider notified. Laboratory tests ordered. Phlebotomy procedures completed, and samples prepared for transport to laboratory.

Postoperative Day 5

0900: Client prescribed levothyroxine 50 mcg orally every morning. Follow-up home visit scheduled.

Postoperative Day 6

0920: Follow-up home health visit. Client alert and oriented × 4. Sitting at dining table finishing breakfast. Client states, "I had two cups of coffee and a glass of prune juice. I feel optimistic about a bowel movement today." VS: T 97.4°F (36.3°C), HR 57 beats/min and regular, BP 133/70 mm Hg, RR 15 breaths/min, SpO$_2$ 97% on RA. Denies pain. Incision well approximated, no redness or swelling noted. Client reports ambulating with walker to mailbox at front of house yesterday afternoon. Spouse present. Health teaching provided related to hypothyroidism and levothyroxine administration.

3 Weeks After Surgery

1115: Follow-up clinic visit. Client alert and oriented × 4. Participates in PT three times weekly and reports needing to nap after each PT session. Respirations equal and unlabored. Lung fields clear throughout. Heart tones regular, pulses 2+ throughout, and no edema noted. Client denies paresthesia. Skin warm and dry. Reports eating well and having a bowel movement this morning. VS: T 98.6°F (37°C), HR 59 beats/min and regular, BP 134/62 mm Hg, RR 12 breaths/min, SpO$_2$ 96% on RA. Denies pain including headaches and surgical pain. No change in weight since surgery.

Rationale

Treatment with oral thyroid replacement therapy usually takes 6 weeks to correct hormone levels, but clients usually begin to see improvement within 2 to 3 weeks. Increased body temperature and normal bowel elimination are positive signs that the client's metabolic rate is increasing. The client's denial of pain indicates that the client is no longer experiencing headaches. A lack of edema and paresthesia also indicates that the client is improving.

CJ Cognitive Skill: Evaluate Outcomes

Reference: Linton & Matteson, 2023, pp. 988–992; Clayton et al., 2022, pp. 597–600

Unfolding Case Study 16.2

Thinking Exercise 16.2.1

Answer

History and Physical	Nurses' Notes	Orders	Laboratory Results

1215: The nurse is requested by a visitor to the client's room. Upon arrival, the client is alert and observed wandering around the room without a shirt on. Oriented to self only. Skin warm and dry. Jaundice present. 2+ pitting edema present in bilateral lower extremities. Respirations labored. Abdomen distended with spider angiomas present. Client reorients to place and some situations, follows simple commands, and moves extremities equally. Facial features are symmetrical. Asterixis noted in bilateral hands. Client sits in a chair for a few minutes before rising and wandering again. Speaks loudly, "Get out of my house. I do not need your help." Equal movement in all extremities, but gait is unstable. VS: T 98.7°F (37°C), HR 92 beats/min, RR 18 breaths/min, BP 115/60 mm Hg, SpO$_2$ 94% on RA. Health history includes spinal disk herniation with diskectomy, chronic back pain, and hepatic cirrhosis.

Rationale

The nurse must recognize signs and symptoms that are abnormal and then differentiate expected and unexpected findings based on the client's past medical history. The client's acute confusion, unstable gait, and asterixis (a coarse tremor characterized by rapid, nonrhythmic extensions and flexions in the wrists and fingers) are priority concerns because acute changes in cognition and neuromuscular function are frequently life threatening. The client's labored respirations are also concerning as this finding may indicate a cardiac or respiratory condition. Other abnormal findings including jaundice, pitting edema, and distended abdomen with spider angiomas are important, but they are not life threatening and may be associated with the client's history of hepatic cirrhosis.

CJ Cognitive Skill: Recognize Cues
Reference: Linton & Matteson, 2023, pp. 799–804

Thinking Exercise 16.2.2

Answer

The nurse recognizes that the client is *most likely* experiencing **hepatic encephalopathy** as manifested by **mental confusion** and **asterixis**.

Rationale

The client has a history of hepatic cirrhosis. Client findings related to liver cirrhosis are mental confusion, jaundice, pitting edema, abdominal distention (ascites), and spider angiomas. The client's clinical manifestations indicate that the client is most likely experiencing hepatic encephalopathy, a complication of liver cirrhosis that is often associated with elevated ammonia levels and characterized by progressive changes in level of consciousness, thinking processes, and the neuromuscular system. Client findings that correlate with hepatic encephalopathy are mental confusion and asterixis, difficulty concentrating or short attention span, coordination or balance problems, and anxiety or irritability. Mental confusion also correlates with ischemic stroke, but other common symptoms of stroke are not present. Similarly, alcohol-induced psychosis manifests with mental confusion and behavior changes, but the client is not experiencing hallucinations or a loss of touch with reality, which are common symptoms of psychosis. The client was able to reorient for a short period.

CJ Cognitive Skill: Analyze Cues
Reference: Linton & Matteson, 2023, pp. 418–421, 799–804, 1266

Thinking Exercise 16.2.3

Answer

- ✗ Vital sign changes/abnormalities
- ○ Impaired skin integrity
- ○ Inadequate nutrition
- ✗ Ineffective ventilation
- ○ Infection
- ✗ Potential for injury

Rationale

Clinical manifestations and laboratory results indicate that the client has several complications of chronic liver cirrhosis. To prevent life-threatening complications, the nurse would focus interventions on providing effective ventilation, achieving fluid balance, monitoring vital signs for changes/abnormalities that indicate hemodynamic stability, and ensuring client safety. Manifestations of hepatic encephalopathy increase the client's risk for falls and other injuries. Therefore the nurse would prioritize safety and implement care to prevent injury. Client findings indicate respiratory distress including low SpO_2 level, labored respirations, and diminished breath sounds. The client's ascites (fluid collected within the peritoneal cavity) may also affect ventilation by pressing the abdominal wall up against the diaphragm, especially when lying flat. These findings would lead the nurse to prioritize ineffective ventilation and risk for respiratory failure. In addition to client safety and ventilation concerns, the nurse would prioritize vital sign changes/abnormalities. The client's vital signs, including heart rate and blood pressure, indicate an acute change from the client's status a couple of hours earlier. Tachycardia and a borderline low blood pressure are most likely caused by decreased intravascular fluid. This may be due to a shift of fluid from intravascular to extravascular spaces, which is caused by increased hydrostatic pressure from portal hypertension and the damaged liver's inability to produce albumin (decreased protein levels). Pitting edema and ascites are signs of this fluid shift. Vital sign changes may also be caused by a loss of blood due to gastrointestinal bleeding. Gastroesophageal varices occur when esophageal veins become distended from increased portal vein pressure. Varices have weak vascular walls and rupture easily, causing massive bleeding into the gastrointestinal tract. The nurse would take actions to address the client's vital sign changes to prevent cardiovascular collapse. The client is at risk for impaired skin integrity, nutritional deficiencies, and infection, but these are not life threatening and not a priority at this time.

CJ Cognitive Skill: Prioritize Hypotheses
Reference: Linton & Matteson, 2023, pp. 799–804

Thinking Exercise 16.2.4

Answer

PRIORITY CONDITIONS	POTENTIAL NURSING ACTIONS
Potential for injury	✗ Collaborate with assistive nursing personnel to check on the client frequently. ✗ Monitor changes in level of consciousness and orientation. ○ Obtain an order for soft wrist restraints to prevent client falls.
Hemodynamic instability	✗ Accurately measure and record intake and output. ✗ Frequently assess vital signs. ✗ Monitor hemoglobin and hematocrit levels.
Respiratory distress	✗ Initiate supplemental oxygen to keep SpO_2 >92% ✗ Measure abdominal girth daily. ○ Position the client in the supine position with the head of the bed elevated no more than 30 degrees.

Rationale

Nursing actions for acute confusion from hepatic encephalopathy and elevated ammonia levels focus on maintaining client safety and slowing or stopping the accumulation of ammonia. The nurse would collaborate with assistive nursing personnel to ensure frequent rounding and would closely monitor and assess the client's neurologic status for progression of cognitive decline and therapeutic responses once pharmacologic therapy is initiated. As an alternative to restraints, the nurse would implement continuous direct or indirect supervision based on the client's level of confusion. Fluid imbalances in clients with hepatic cirrhosis are complicated to manage. The client is intravascularly dehydrated but has excess fluid in the extravascular spaces. Pharmacologic treatment may include a combination of IV fluids, diuretics, and albumin. To manage these therapies, the nurse would frequently assess vital signs, ensure that intake and output is measured and recorded properly, and effectively communicate client findings to the registered nurse and health care provider. The nurse would also monitor hemoglobin and hematocrit levels to assess for potential gastrointestinal bleeding as a cause of hemodynamic instability. Respiratory support for this client includes providing supplemental oxygen to maintain a normal SpO_2 level, measuring abdominal girth daily, and positioning the client with the head of the bed elevated at least 30 degrees or as high as the client desires to improve breathing.

CJ Cognitive Skill: Generate Solutions
Reference: Linton & Matteson, 2023, pp. 799–804

Thinking Exercise 16.2.5—Pharmacology

Answer

✗ Assist the physician to contact the client's medical power of attorney.
✗ Collaborate with assistive nursing personnel to ensure safe access for toileting.
○ Hold oral medications until after the procedure.
✗ Increase the flow of supplemental oxygen.
✗ Monitor serum electrolyte levels.
○ Obtain the client's signature on a consent form for abdominal paracentesis.
✗ Weigh the client prior to administering medications.

Rationale

The client's SpO_2 is lower than desired. Therefore the nurse would need to increase the flow of supplemental oxygen using a high-flow nasal cannula and would continue to monitor and titrate oxygen as needed. Lactulose is frequently prescribed to reduce ammonia levels in the body. Lactulose is a viscous, sticky, sweet-tasting liquid that is given either orally or by nasogastric tube. It has a laxative effect and rids the intestinal tract of toxins that contribute to encephalopathy. The nurse would collaborate with assistive nursing personnel to ensure safe access for toileting. Diuretic therapy is administered to reduce fluid accumulation and prevent cardiopulmonary problems. The nurse would plan to monitor daily weights, measure intake and output, and assess electrolyte levels to evaluate outcomes and prevent complications from diuretic therapy. Paracentesis is an invasive procedure performed to remove abdominal fluid. The procedure requires consent, but the client is only oriented to self and therefore cannot sign a consent form. The nurse would assist the physician to contact the client's medical power of attorney. The physician must explain the situation and procedure and answer any questions prior to obtaining a phone consent. The client would not need to be NPO prior to the procedure. Some medications are held prior to an invasive procedure, but this client's medications would not need to be held and could cause further cardiac and respiratory complications if held.

CJ Cognitive Skill: Take Actions
Reference: Linton & Matteson, 2023, pp. 799–804

Thinking Exercise 16.2.6

Answer

CLIENT STATEMENTS	UNDERSTANDING	NO UNDERSTANDING
"I will ask the assistive care staff to help manage my medications."	✗	
"I will bathe in tepid water, vigorously scrubbing with mild soap to manage dry skin."		✗
"I will consult the physician before taking any over-the-counter medications."	✗	
"I will eat small but frequent, low-protein meals throughout each day."		✗
"I will sleep in my recliner because I am most comfortable there."	✗	

Rationale

Clients with chronic illnesses frequently have difficulty managing their medications due to polypharmacy or side effects. The client with hepatic cirrhosis may be discharged on lactulose and diuretic therapy, which result in frequent bowel and urine elimination and may be unpleasant. It is essential that the client continues to take all medications, even if feeling better, to prevent complications of liver failure. Asking the assistive care staff to help manage medications demonstrates that the client is dedicated to proper administration of prescribed therapies. Many medications including over-the-counter medications and herbal treatments are metabolized by the liver, and some are toxic to the liver. The nurse would teach the client to take only medications that are approved by the physician. Good nutrition is essential for clients with liver disease. The nurse would teach the client to eat a balanced diet and follow nutritional guidance provided by the registered dietitian nutritionist. Protein restriction, previously prescribed to prevent accumulation of ammonia, is no longer recommended. The registered dietitian nutritionist will most likely recommend normal or increased protein to prevent malnutrition. Additionally, the nurse would encourage the client to eat small, frequent meals in a pleasant dining environment to manage anorexia, a common symptom of liver failure. Pruritus (itching) is also common in clients with chronic liver disease, and the natural response is to scratch, which may cause breaks in the skin. The nurse would teach the client to bathe in tepid water with a mild soap and then pad dry. Scrubbing the skin may cause injury and is contraindicated. Lubricating and topical antipruritic lotions may be applied after bathing. The client may sleep wherever is comfortable. There are no restrictions on where or how the client sleeps.

CJ Cognitive Skill: Evaluate Outcomes
Reference: Linton & Matteson, 2023, pp. 799–804

Stand-Alone Thinking Exercise 16.1

Answer

The nurse recognizes that the client is *most likely* experiencing **metabolic syndrome**. The nurse would *prioritize* health teaching focused on **dietary intake** and **physical activity**.

Rationale

Metabolic syndrome is the term used to describe a condition that involves impaired glucose tolerance, hypertension, and dyslipidemia (elevated triglycerides, low HDL cholesterol, and high LDL cholesterol). Obesity, as determined by body mass index (BMI) and waist-to-hip ratio, increases the client's risk for metabolic syndrome. Long-term effects of metabolic syndrome are atherosclerosis, ischemic heart disease, left ventricular hypertrophy, and type 2 diabetes mellitus. Pharmacologic management of metabolic syndrome focuses on controlling blood glucose levels, lowering lipids, and treating hypertension. In addition to teaching clients about medications, the nurse would provide health education focused on lifestyle changes to promote weight loss. In obese clients, weight loss improves cardiovascular condition and insulin sensitivity and promotes a sense of well-being. In collaboration with a registered dietitian nutritionist, the nurse would remind the client to eat more vegetables, whole grains, and omega-3 fatty acids and to avoid processed foods and foods that are high in sugar, simple carbohydrates, and saturated fats. The nurse would also teach the client to integrate exercise into a regular routine and to participate in at least 150 minutes of moderate to strenuous physical activity each week. The nurse would assist the client to set reasonable goals for exercise, starting slowly and building in intensity and duration over time. Emotional support and monitoring of blood pressure and glucose are important in the management of metabolic syndrome but are not as essential as interventions focused on diet and physical activity.
CJ Cognitive Skill: Recognize Cues, Analyze Cues, Priority Hypotheses, Generate Solutions, Take Actions
Reference: Linton & Matteson, 2023, pp. 679, 999–1022; Pagana et al., 2023, pp. 451, 461, 556, 870

Stand-Alone Thinking Exercise 16.2

Answer

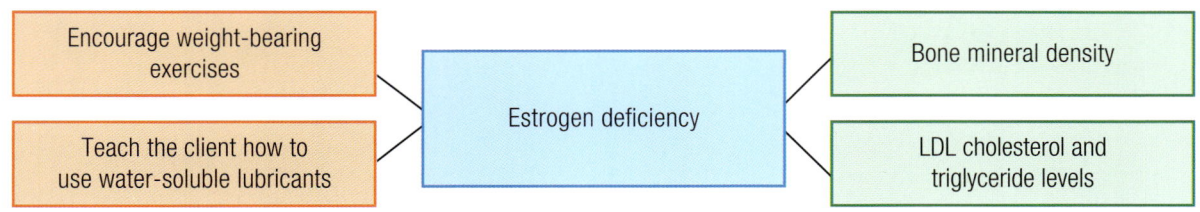

Rationale

Common symptoms of adrenal insufficiency are fatigue, muscle weakness, loss of appetite, and weight loss. The client is not experiencing any of these symptoms. Diabetes insipidus, a deficiency of antidiuretic hormone from the posterior pituitary gland, is characterized by excessive output of dilute urine that results in symptoms of dehydration including thirst, hypotension, tachycardia, and dizziness. The client reported urinary stress incontinence, not excessive urination. Additionally, the client's vital signs do not indicate dehydration or diabetes insipidus. Deficiencies in estrogen and parathyroid hormones can increase the risk of fractures, but the client is not experiencing any neuromuscular symptoms associated with hypoparathyroidism. The client is experiencing additional symptoms of estrogen deficiency or menopause. Natural menopause occurs gradually with aging; ovulation ceases, and estrogen production declines. This change of life, known as the *perimenopausal period*, commonly occurs between 45 and 55 years of age and is frequently associated with hot flashes, night sweats, irregular menses, fatigue, and emotional instability. The menopausal period begins when the client has not menstruated for a full 12 months. Complications of menopause are related to decreased estrogen.

Without estrogen, the uterus becomes smaller, the vagina shortens, and vaginal tissues become drier. Supporting pelvic structures relax, causing some females to have stress incontinence. Significant loss of bone mass may occur, leading to fragile bones. The nurse would provide health education to prevent complications of menopause and promote self-care and personal well-being. Teaching would include the value of weight-bearing exercises in slowing bone loss, the use of water-soluble lubricants before intercourse to relieve vaginal dryness and pain, Kegel exercises to increase pelvic wall tone, and drinking at least eight glasses of water daily to prevent urinary tract infections. The nurse would assess for osteoporosis including bone mineral density based on the client's age, state of menopause, and recent fracture. The nurse would also monitor the client's LDL cholesterol and triglyceride levels. Estrogen helps regulate lipid metabolism in the liver; therefore the menopausal decrease in estrogen levels leads to higher LDL cholesterol and triglyceride levels. Elevated cholesterol increases the client's risk for cardiovascular disease. Monitoring the client's heart rate and rhythm, urine specific gravity, and cognition is not a priority at this time.

CJ Cognitive Skills: Recognize Cues, Analyze Cues, Prioritize Hypotheses, Generate Solutions, Take Actions, Evaluate Outcomes

Reference: Linton & Matteson, 2023, pp. 969–970, 972–976, 993–996, 1074–1075; Leifer & Little, 2023, pp. 282–287

Answers With Rationales for Thinking Exercises

Unfolding Case Study 17.1

Thinking Exercise 17.1.1

Answer

History and Physical	Nurses' Notes	Orders	Laboratory Results

1400: Client presents for a routine appointment to follow up on multiple medical conditions including hypertension, hyperlipidemia, and congestive heart failure. Current medications are carvedilol, digoxin, simvastatin, and furosemide. The client is a widower and lives independently. Alert and oriented × 4. Respirations equal and unlabored. Fine crackles auscultated in bilateral lower lobes of lungs. Productive cough present with scant pale secretions expectorated. Denies shortness of breath. Skin warm and dry with generalized nonpitting edema and 1+ pitting edema in bilateral feet and ankles. A scabbed wound is present on right knee and surrounded by yellowish-green bruising. Client reports a recent fall, stating, "I tripped over a chair in my kitchen several days ago. I must need a stronger prescription for my glasses because I didn't even see that the chair was pulled out." Reports vision has recently become blurry, "as if there are smudges on my eyeglasses" and is also experiencing double vision. Client confirms driving during the day, but has not driven at night for several years due to difficulties seeing after dark. Denies eye redness, pain, and drainage. Abdomen soft and round with bowel sounds present in all quadrants. Last bowel movement yesterday morning. Client reports occasional urinary incontinence, stating, "I have to stay close to a bathroom in the morning to prevent an accident." VS: T 98.4°F (36.8°C), HR 58 beats/min and regular, RR 13 breaths/min, BP 133/45 mm Hg, SpO2 95% on RA. Client denies pain.

Rationale

The nurse must differentiate expected findings related to the client's health history and medication regimen from unexpected findings that indicate a complication or change in status. Fine crackles and pitting edema are common findings for a client who has congestive heart failure. These findings could indicate a potential complication, but the client denies shortness of breath, has unlabored respirations, and SpO2 levels are within normal limits. Therefore, these findings would not be an immediate concern at this time. The client is taking several medications for hypertension and heart failure that slow cardiac conduction and account for the bradycardia. The client is alert and oriented, has warm skin with normal capillary refill, and blood pressure within normal limits. These findings indicate that the client is perfusing adequately with a slower than normal heart rate. Client statements regarding occasional incontinence do not require immediate follow-up. Urinary incontinence is more common in older adults than younger adults due to age-related weakening of pelvic muscles, and the client has adapted activities of daily living (ADLs) to accommodate for diuretic therapy in the morning. The nurse would also recognize difficulty seeing after dark as a chronic issue that started several years ago and would not prioritize this finding for immediate follow-up. The nurse would recognize acute changes in the client's vision, including blurry and double vision, as abnormal findings that must be addressed. The nurse would also prioritize client safety and follow up on the recent fall as well as visual acuity for driving a motor vehicle.

CJ Cognitive Skill: Recognize Cues
Reference: Linton & Matteson, 2023, pp. 1174–1188

Thinking Exercise 17.1.2

Answer

The nurse recognizes that the client's vision changes are ***most likely*** caused by a **condition of the eye**.

Rationale

Visual acuity declines with age-related changes to the structure and function of the eye. Older adults commonly experience drier eyes and difficulty seeing near objects, maintaining gaze focused on a single object, and adjusting to dark environments. Blurry and double vision do not result from normal age-related changes. Neurologic vision impairment results from a brain injury and may manifest with vision and eye movement problems. Common causes of brain injury are stroke, anoxic events, brain tumors, neurologic infection, and traumatic brain injury. The client does not have any symptoms or history associated with these brain injuries. Several conditions of the eye affect visual sensory perception including glaucoma, cataracts, and retinopathy. Clients with a health history of hypertension, diabetes mellitus, thyroid problems, and cardiac disease are at higher risk for conditions affecting the eye and vision. The client's symptoms and health history lead the nurse to conclude that the client is most likely experiencing a condition of the eye.
CJ Cognitive Skill: Analyze Cues
Reference: Linton & Matteson, 2023, pp. 1174–1188

Thinking Exercise 17.1.3

Answer

The ***priority*** for the client's care at this time is to **assess safety risks** because the client is experiencing **impaired visual perception**.

Rationale

The client is experiencing blurry and double vision, which indicates impaired visual sensory perception and increases the client's risk of injury. Many clients live with reduced vision for years and only seek assistance when their vision causes a safety concern or interferes with ADLs. The client is alert and oriented and should be able to identify when ADLs can no longer be performed safely and independently due to impaired visual sensory perception. Therefore the nurse would engage the client in a personal assessment of vision issues and safety risks. Urinary incontinence and pitting edema increase the client's risk for skin breakdown and infections, but there are no findings to indicate that these are current issues for the client.
CJ Cognitive Skill: Prioritize Hypotheses
Reference: Linton & Matteson, 2023, pp. 1174–1188

Thinking Exercise 17.1.4

Answer

POTENTIAL NURSING ACTIONS	INDICATED	NOT INDICATED
Assist with programming the client's phone with automatic dialing of emergency numbers.	X	
Collaborate with the case management nurse for admission to a skilled nursing facility.		X
Encourage installation of handgrips in the bathroom and a nonskid surface on the shower floor.	X	
Identify a friend or family member who will assist to organize daily drugs in different shape containers.	X	
Provide information about food delivery services including groceries and prepared meals.	X	

Rationale

There are many changes the client can make to ensure safety and independence with impaired visual sensory perception including interventions for personal care, medication administration, food preparation, and communication. The nurse would encourage the client to install handgrips in the bathroom and a nonskid surface on the shower floor and to eliminate throw rugs and other fall risks such as long appliance cords and footstools. The client is on several prescribed medications. To ensure that medications are administered safely, the nurse would assist the client to identify a friend or family member who can visit weekly and organize drugs for each day and time into differently shaped containers that are labeled properly with black, raised lettering. Driving, even during the day, is a safety concern. Therefore the nurse would advise the client to ask a family member or friend to provide rides to the grocery store or to utilize delivery services for groceries and prepared meals. Finally, the nurse would assist the client to program the phone with vocal commands and automatic dialing for emergency numbers such as the fire department, police, relatives, and friends. Currently, the nurse is focused on safe, independent living. There are no client findings that indicate the client needs inpatient skilled nursing services.

CJ Cognitive Skill: Generate Solutions
Reference: Linton & Matteson, 2023, pp. 1211–1213

Thinking Exercise 17.1.5

Answer

○ Administer supplemental oxygen.
○ Assess the client's pupil response and visual acuity.
○ Assist the client to clear the airway by blowing the nose.
✗ Ensure that the client can properly instill eyedrops.
○ Position the head of the bed lower than 30 degrees.
✗ Reinforce activity restrictions.
✗ Review prescribed eyedrops and administration schedule.

Rationale

Because the client is stable and will most likely be discharged within an hour after surgery, nursing interventions must focus on reinforcing prescription eyedrops and the planned schedule for administration. The client must closely adhere to the prescribed regime and use proper technique to instill eyedrops. If the client is unable to instill eyedrops, the nurse would confirm that the daughter understands and can perform the administration procedures. The nurse would also reinforce activity restrictions. The client must refrain from driving until vision is clear. Cooking and light housekeeping are permitted, but vacuuming should be avoided for several weeks because of the forward flexion involved and the rapid, jerky movements required. Finally, the nurse would take actions to prevent an increase in intraocular pressure (IOP) including teaching the client to keep the head of the bed elevated; avoid sneezing, coughing, and blowing the nose; and avoid bending at the waist or straining to have a bowel movement. The client's SpO_2 is within the normal range for an older adult, therefore supplemental oxygen is not required. After cataract surgery, pupillary light response may be impaired for several months. Therefore the nurse would not shine a light into the client's eye to check pupil response but would advise the client to wear dark glasses outdoors and in brightly lit environments until the pupil responds appropriately to light.

CJ Cognitive Skill: Take Actions
Reference: Linton & Matteson, 2023, pp. 1211–1213

Thinking Exercise 17.1.6

Answer

- ✗ Headache and nausea
- ○ Bloodshot sclera
- ○ Scratchy, sandlike feeling in eye
- ✗ Swollen eyelid
- ○ Took acetaminophen for pain
- ○ Vision remains blurry

Rationale

Mild eye discomfort and itchiness, a bloodshot appearance, and *slightly* swollen eyelids are normal findings after cataract surgery. However, significant swelling that prevents the client from opening the eyelid and a headache with nausea are not normal and may be signs of postoperative complications including increased IOP and infection. Signs of increased IOP are severe eye pain, headache, nausea, and vomiting. Signs of infection include increased eye redness and swelling, decreased vision, and increased tears and photophobia. Yellow or green drainage also indicates an infection. Mild eye discomfort may be controlled with acetaminophen or acetaminophen with oxycodone as prescribed. The nurse would intervene if the client took aspirin for pain as this could cause bleeding due to its effects on blood clotting. Clients usually experience a dramatic improvement in vision within 1 day of surgery, but the final best vision would not occur until 4 to 6 weeks after surgery. Slightly blurry vision the day after surgery is normal.
CJ Cognitive Skill: Evaluate Outcomes
Reference: Linton & Matteson, 2023, pp. 1211–1213

Unfolding Case Study 17.2

Thinking Exercise 17.2.1

Answer

- ○ Blood glucose level
- ○ Blood pressure
- ✗ Diabetic foot ulcer
- ○ Lower extremity edema
- ✗ Visual disturbances
- ○ Weight loss

Rationale

The nurse must follow up on the client's diabetic foot ulcer and visual disturbances. Diabetic foot ulcers are among the most common complications for clients with diabetes mellitus and can lead to serious outcomes including osteomyelitis and amputation. Ulcers are usually the result of poor glycemic control, neuropathy, peripheral vascular disease, and/or improper foot care. The nurse must complete further assessments to evaluate these underlying causes to develop an effective plan of care for the client. Additionally, the client's visual disturbances are not normal age-related changes and therefore require follow-up. Impaired visual sensory perception occurs with a variety of conditions and is most likely contributing to the client's complication of diabetes mellitus. The client's blood pressure, FSBG level, and generalized lower extremity edema are not concerning based on the client's age and health history. The client is overweight (normal BMI is 18.5–24.9), therefore the weight loss is a positive finding.
CJ Cognitive Skill: Recognize Cues
Reference: Linton & Matteson, 2023, pp. 1174–1188

Thinking Exercise 17.2.2

Answer

CLIENT FINDINGS	CATARACT	GLAUCOMA	RETINOPATHY
Blurry vision	✗	✗	✗
Spots in visual field		✗	✗
Vision-impairing ADLs	✗	✗	✗
Halos around lights		✗	

Rationale

A cataract is the clouding of a normally clear lens of the eye. Early signs of cataract development are blurred vision and decreased color perception. As lens cloudiness continues, double vision occurs, and the client may have difficulty with ADLs. Glaucoma is an eye condition that causes damage to the optic nerve. Glaucoma manifests gradually with patchy blind spots in vision, blurry vision, mild eye aching, and occasional headaches. Later signs include seeing halos around lights and having decreased visual sensory perception that interferes with ADLs. Retinopathy is caused by damage to the blood vessels in retinal tissues. Early signs include blurred vision, dark spots or floaters in the visual field, and difficulty perceiving colors. Retinopathy affects central vision; Decreased visual perception can interfere with ADLs and ultimately lead to blindness.

CJ Cognitive Skill: Analyze Cues
Reference: Linton & Matteson, 2023, pp. 1002–1004, 1174–1188, 1211–1218

Thinking Exercise 17.2.3

Answer

The nurse recognizes that the client is ***most likely*** experiencing **glaucoma** and will ***prioritize*** health teaching regarding **medication therapy** to **prevent further loss** of visual sensory perception.

Rationale

The client is most likely experiencing glaucoma based on symptoms and diagnostic results. Although some client findings are associated with the conditions of cataract and retinopathy, current symptoms are more closely aligned with glaucoma. Primary open-angle glaucoma, the most common form of primary glaucoma, usually affects both eyes and develops slowly with gradual loss of visual fields. Glaucoma is most commonly caused by increased IOP. Diagnostic findings indicate increased IOP in both eyes. Diagnostic tests demonstrate the client's lens and retina are normal. Positive diagnostic findings for cataracts would reveal a cloudy lens with opacity making it difficult to see the retina. Red reflux may also be absent and the pupil bluish white. Change in the retina including edema and possibly bleeding would be signs of retinopathy.

The nurse would anticipate a variety of ophthalmic drugs to be prescribed to reduce IOP and delay or prevent further damage to the optic nerve. Medication therapy does not reverse damage to the optic nerve and will not restore visual sensory perception back to normal. Surgery may be done if drug therapy is not effective in managing eye pressure. Maintaining normal blood glucose levels and blood pressure may help prevent further sensory loss but lifestyle changes are not a priority at this time. Instead, the nurse must focus on educating the client about each prescribed drug and proper techniques for safe administration. Close adherence to the prescribed dosage schedule is essential to receiving the maximum therapeutic effect.

CJ Cognitive Skill: Prioritize Hypotheses
Reference: Linton & Matteson, 2023, pp. 1002–1004, 1174–1188, 1211–1218

Thinking Exercise 17.2.4—Pharmacology

Answer

✗ "Avoid touching the drug container tip to any part of the eye."
○ "Contact the provider if you experience tearing and mild burning immediately after instillation."
○ "Hold medications if you experience severe eye pain and/or headache."
✗ "Perform good handwashing before administering eyedrops."
✗ "Place pressure on the corner of the eye near the nose immediately after instillation."
✗ "These drugs decrease intraocular pressure by limiting the production and increasing the drainage of fluid within the eye."
✗ "Wait 5 to 10 minutes between administration of each medication."

Rationale

The health teaching would focus on each eyedrop medication and the prescribed schedule. The medications are prescribed to reduce IOP. Bimatoprost, a prostaglandin agonist, reduces IOP by dilating blood vessels in the trabecular mesh, which then collects and drains aqueous humor. Timolol maleate is an adrenergic agonist and reduces IOP by limiting the production of aqueous humor and dilating the pupil to improve the flow of fluid to its absorption site. The benefit of drug therapy only occurs when eyedrops are instilled on time and not skipped for any reason. The nurse would teach the client to contact the provider if experiencing severe eye pain and/or headache as these are signs of increased IOP. Eyedrops may cause tearing, mild burning, blurred vision, and a reddened sclera for a few minutes after instilling the drug. These symptoms are not concerning and would not need to be reported to the provider. Proper administration of eyedrops includes administering only one drug at a time and waiting 5 to 10 minutes between instillation of different drugs to prevent one drug from diluting another drug. To prevent infection, the nurse would stress performing good handwashing, keeping the eyedrop container tip clean, and avoiding touching the tip to any part of the eye. Additionally, the nurse would teach the technique of punctual occlusion (placing pressure on the corner of the eye near the nose) immediately after instillation to prevent systemic absorption of the drug.
CJ Cognitive Skill: Generate Solutions
Reference: Linton & Matteson, 2023, pp. 1214–1217; Clayton et al., 2022, pp. 690–692

Thinking Exercise 17.2.5

Answer

✗ Check finger stick blood glucose level.
✗ Complete medication reconciliation.
✗ Encourage rising and changing positions slowly.
○ Recommend discontinuation of bimatoprost eyedrops.
○ Recommend discontinuation of timolol eyedrops.
✗ Reinforce teaching related to punctual occlusion.
○ Suggest that the client wear dark glasses.

Rationale

Medications prescribed for glaucoma therapy can be absorbed systemically and cause systemic problems. Client findings indicate that this adverse effect has occurred. Timolol maleate is a beta-adrenergic blocker and can cause a decrease in heart rate and blood pressure if absorbed systemically. The client is experiencing bradycardia, lower-than-normal blood pressure, and orthostatic hypotension (light-headedness when rising from the bed or sitting positions). The nurse would promote safety by encouraging the client to rise and change positions slowly. The nurse would also reinforce teaching related to punctual occlusion to prevent further systemic problems. The client has a history of diabetes and is at higher risk for hypoglycemia due to prescribed medications masking hypoglycemia symptoms. The nurse would request a blood glucose check and teach the client to check blood glucose levels more frequently. The nurse would not recommend discontinuing eyedrops but would complete a medication reconciliation to ensure that there are no contradictions or synergistic effects from other medications that could cause complications.

CJ Cognitive Skill: Take Actions
Reference: Linton & Matteson, 2023, pp. 1214–1217; Clayton et al., 2022, pp. 690

Thinking Exercise 17.2.6

Answer

The client's condition has ***worsened*** as evidenced by **decreased appetite** and **insomnia**.

Rationale

The reality of the loss of vision can be distressing for a client and cause conditions of anxiety and/or depression. Client findings of decreased appetite and insomnia may be signs of depression and may indicate that the client is not effectively adapting to vision changes. Impaired visual sensory perception does not need to create a loss of independence. The nurse would assist the client and spouse to adapt activities so the client can be more independent. The nurse would also recommend a mental health professional consultation to provide counseling and support to the client during this time of transition. Bimatoprost eyedrops can cause eye color darkening and lengthening of eyelashes. This is not an adverse effect. Other findings indicate that the client's condition is improving or is unchanged.

CJ Cognitive Skill: Evaluate Outcomes
Reference: Linton & Matteson, 2023, pp. 1214–1217; Clayton et al., 2022, pp. 690–692

Stand-Alone Thinking Exercise 17.1

Answer

The ***priority*** interventions for the client's care at this time would focus on improving the client's ability to **communicate effectively** and **adapt to changes in social interactions** due to **impaired hearing**.

Rationale

The client's behavior would lead the nurse to suspect hearing impairment. The client leans in and turns one ear toward the speaker, asks the speaker to repeat statements, speaks while others are speaking, turns the television up very loudly, and mishears statements (old versus cold). Additionally, the client does not like social situations with background noise such as family engagements and eating at a restaurant. The client is consistently alert and oriented, follows directions when provided in a quiet, one-on-one environment, and performs ADLs independently. Therefore the client is most likely aware of the hearing impairment but refuses to admit this loss. There is no evidence that the client has dementia; the client is oriented × 4. Clients with hearing impairment frequently suffer from severe social isolation due to embarrassment or an inability to adapt to the environment to effectively interact in social situations. Hearing impairment has already alienated the client from family and friends who could support the client during postoperative and cancer therapies. The nurse would prioritize interventions that improve the client's ability to communicate effectively and adapt to changes in social interactions.

CJ Cognitive Skills: Recognize Cues, Analyze Cues, Prioritize Hypotheses
Reference: Linton & Matteson, 2023, pp. 1189–1201

Stand-Alone Thinking Exercise 17.2

Answer

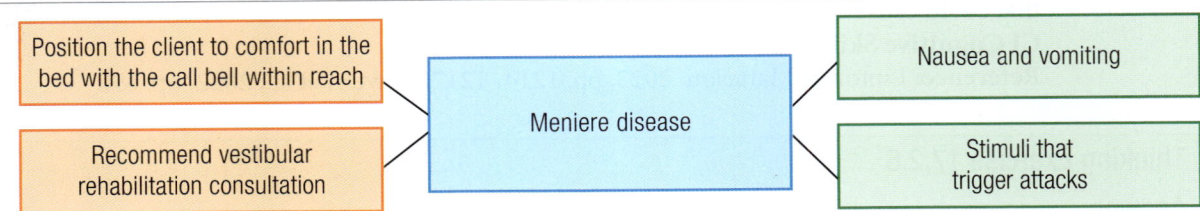

Rationale

Hearing loss can occur with all potential conditions, but vertigo attacks, as described by the client, only occur with Meniere disease, a disorder of the labyrinth. Client findings associated with Meniere disease are caused by an accumulation of fluid in the inner ear and include frequent, acute vertigo attacks accompanied by pallor, diaphoresis, nausea, and vomiting; hearing loss, especially low-frequency sounds; and a feeling of fullness in the ear. External otitis is an infection or inflammation of the lining of the external ear canal and manifests with red, swollen, and tender ear, dizziness, fever, drainage, and hearing loss. Mastoiditis, a complication of chronic otitis media, occurs when a middle ear infection extends into the mastoid bone. Symptoms of mastoiditis are redness, swelling, tenderness and pain behind the ear, thick purulent drainage from the ear, headache, malaise, fever, and hearing loss. Presbycusis is a natural, age-related hearing loss and does not present with any other symptoms.

Client safety is a priority concern in the emergency department and upon discharge because attacks are unpredictable. The nurse would position the client to comfort, raise the bed rails, put the bed in the lowest position, provide the call bell, and encourage the client to ask for assistance when getting out of bed. The nurse would also monitor for signs of vertigo, nausea, and vomiting. The nurse would collaborate with the client to identify and monitor substances and stimuli that trigger vertigo attacks. Medical management of Meniere disease involves complex medication therapy including benzodiazepines, antihistamines, antiemetics, anticholinergics, vasodilators, and/or diuretics. A low-sodium diet may also be prescribed to increase the length of time between attacks by reducing edema in the inner ear. A high-calorie, low-fat diet is not required. The nurse would encourage the client to drink plenty of water, take small sips if feeling sick or nauseated, and refrain from beverages containing caffeine and alcohol. The nurse would also recommend a consultation for vestibular rehabilitation, a variety of cognitive and physical therapies used to help the client develop tolerance and live successfully with vertigo. Positive pressure therapy, biofeedback, self-hypnosis, and relaxation techniques are all integrated into vestibular rehabilitation. Surgical treatment is only advised when all other measures have failed. Currently, there is no need to admit the client for surgery.

CJ Cognitive Skills: Recognize Cues, Analyze Cues, Prioritize Hypotheses, Generate Solutions, Take Actions, Evaluate Outcomes

Reference: Linton & Matteson, 2023, pp. 1223–1231

Answers With Rationales for Thinking Exercises

Thinking Exercise 18.1.1

Answer

- ○ Both feet cool
- ○ Pedal pulses 1+ and equal
- ✗ Trying to get out of bed
- ○ Diminished bowel sounds
- ✗ Screaming and crying

Rationale

The client is an older adult who was admitted from the PACU after a major surgery. The client likely had general anesthesia as part of a multimodal sedation approach, which would slow bowel sounds. Therefore this finding is expected and would not require immediate follow-up. The coolness of both feet and decreased pedal pulses are also not of immediate concern because these findings are expected in an older adult due to arteriosclerosis and atherosclerosis. However, the client's behaviors of trying to climb out of bed, screaming, and crying are *not* normal changes associated with aging but are seen in older adults after surgery, especially fractured hip repair surgery. These findings need immediate follow-up to keep the client safe and less anxious.

CJ Cognitive Skill: Recognize Cues
Reference: Halter & Fratena, 2023, pp. 208–212

Thinking Exercise 18.1.2

Answer

Based on the collected data, the client ***most likely*** has **delirium**.

Rationale

Based on the client findings, the client most likely has a neurocognitive condition known as *delirium*, also called *acute delirium*. Delirium is an acute condition or syndrome that is usually reversible if the causative factors can be removed or resolved. Examples of common factors that can contribute to or cause delirium include pain, sedating medications, hypoxia, an unfamiliar environment, infection, dehydration, and immobilization. This client is likely experiencing operative pain, is immobilized in an unfamiliar environment, and received sedation during surgery. The client is not hypoxic because the SpO_2 on oxygen is 95%, which is within the normal range. The family reported that the client was alert and oriented prior to surgery, which validates that the client does not have dementia. *Dementia* is a broad term used to describe chronic cognitive deterioration and impairment. This client's cognitive status changed rather quickly as a result of surgery and other associated factors. There is no evidence that the client is experiencing clinical depression, which is typically manifested by sad mood, sleep disturbances, changes in appetite, and apathy.

CJ Cognitive Skill: Analyze Cues
Reference: Halter & Fratena, 2023, pp. 104–108, 208–212

Thinking Exercise 18.1.3

Answer

The *priority* for the client's care at this time is to ensure <u>safety</u> because the client is <u>at risk for falls</u>.

Rationale

The client who has delirium is disoriented and often manifests behaviors that could jeopardize the client's safety. Having recent orthopedic surgery, an IV, and an indwelling urinary catheter require the client to stay in bed until the client is assisted in getting out of bed for the first time. Additionally, the client is drowsy and should not be out of bed without assistance and supervision to prevent a fall with possible injury. The client is not hypoxic as evidenced by the SpO_2 of 95%. The client's slowed peristalsis and resulting diminished bowel sounds are expected and not an issue at this time.

CJ Cognitive Skill: Prioritize Hypotheses

Reference: Halter & Fratena, 2023, pp. 208–212

Thinking Exercise 18.1.4

Answer

POTENTIAL NURSING ACTIONS	INDICATED	NOT INDICATED
Darken the client's room to prevent overstimulation.		✗
Ask the family to stay with the client as long as possible.	✗	
Use soft restraints to prevent IV catheter dislodgement.		✗
Frequently reorient the client to reality.	✗	
Administer medication for pain per agency protocol.	✗	

Rationale

Clients with delirium are disoriented, and they often display behaviors that threaten their safety. Therefore the client needs constant supervision, which may be provided by family members. Staff members on an orthopedic unit do not have the time for one-on-one observation. Restraints would only be used as a last resort because they can cause complications and injury. Additionally, restraints can increase client anxiety and restlessness. Darkening the room is not recommended because the client's vision could be impaired, thus increasing anxiety and other behavioral findings. Pain can increase anxiety and delirium and would be managed promptly and effectively. The nurse would also frequently reorient the client to reality to help with reversal of cognitive changes.

CJ Cognitive Skill: Generate Solutions

Reference: Halter & Fratena, 2023, pp. 208–212

Thinking Exercise 18.1.5

Answer

✗ Use simple and short sentences when communicating with the client.
✗ Ensure that the client wears glasses and hearing aids, if appropriate.
✗ Monitor the client for hallucinations or delusions.
✗ Ensure that staff members introduce themselves at each encounter with the client.
○ Request an order for medication for agitation and confusion.

Rationale

The client experiencing delirium has limited short-term memory and needs assistance with being reoriented to reality. Therefore staff members would reintroduce themselves at each encounter with the client and monitor for psychotic behaviors such as hallucinations and delusions. If the client cannot see or hear what is happening in the environment, the client may become more anxious and disoriented. Therefore the nurse would check to determine if the client usually wears glasses or uses one or more hearing aids to improve communication and prevent worsening of confusion that could occur due to lack of sensory input. Ensuring effective and accurate communication is essential when talking with a client who has delirium. Therefore using simple and short sentences is recommended. Drug therapy would not be given to calm the client because it could increase drowsiness, disorientation, and confusion.

CJ Cognitive Skill: Take Actions
Reference: Halter & Fratena, 2023, pp. 208–212

Thinking Exercise 18.1.6

Answer

History and Physical	Nurses' Notes	Orders	Laboratory Results

Admission to Orthopedic Unit

1520: Client returned from PACU following a left hip open reduction and internal fixation (ORIF) for a fracture caused by falling down the stairs at home. According to family, prior to surgery client lived alone, was independent in ADLs, and was alert and oriented × 4. Currently drowsy and disoriented. Unable to follow conversation. When performing the admission assessment, client began screaming and crying; tried to get out of bed. Family holding client's hand and offering reassurance to help calm client. IV lactated Ringer's solution infusing at 100 mL/h in right forearm. Lungs clear throughout; abdomen soft and round with diminished bowel sounds in all quadrants. Left hip surgical dressing dry and intact. Indwelling urinary catheter draining clear yellow urine. Pedal pulses 1+ and equal. Both feet cool and move equally. SCDs in place. VS: T 98°F (36.7°C), HR 80 beats/min and regular, RR 16 breaths/min, BP 115/62 mm Hg, SpO$_2$ 95% on 3 L/min O$_2$ via NC.

1640: Client very restless and moaning; picking at covers and IV dressing. Family states client grimaces when staff repositions the client.

1705: Acetaminophen and gabapentin administered for pain with assistance of family. Family states they plan to stay overnight to prevent client from getting out of bed unsupervised. Client tolerating sips of water and juice. Refused dinner tray; swiped hand and knocked tray off of overbed table.

4 Days Later

0915: Client alert and oriented × 4. Able to follow conversation. Scheduled to be discharged today to rehabilitation unit. No adventitious or abnormal breath sounds throughout, but breath sounds in left lower lung diminished when compared with right lung. Abdomen soft and round with active bowel sounds in all quadrants. Ambulates with walker and supervision to bathroom, but states feeling "a little short of breath" after that activity; voiding clear yellow urine without difficulty. Pedal pulses 1+ and equal. Both feet cool and move equally. VS: T 100.6°F (38.1°C), HR 102 beats/min and regular, RR 24 breaths/min, BP 122/70 mm Hg, SpO$_2$ 89% on RA.

Rationale

The client's cognitive status has markedly improved, but the client's respiratory status has declined or worsened. After walking to the bathroom, the client has shortness of breath; breath sounds in the left lung are diminished, and the client has an elevated temperature. Additionally, the client has tachycardia, tachypnea, and a low SpO_2. The expected SpO_2 for an older adult is above 90%, depending on agency protocol, provider preference, and individual client health condition. All of these findings suggest a possible lung infection such as pneumonia.

CJ Cognitive Skill: Evaluate Outcomes
Reference: Linton & Matteson, 2023, pp. 509–511

Unfolding Case Study 18.2

Thinking Exercise 18.2.1

Answer

- O Obesity
- O Blood pressure
- ✗ Memory lapses
- O Weight loss
- ✗ Forgetting words
- O Peripheral pulses

Rationale

The client has experienced recent cognitive changes that are affecting the client's life and work. Memory lapses and forgetfulness are *not* normal changes associated with aging. Therefore these findings require immediate follow-up. The client is obese and has lost weight following a diet. However, weight loss is a positive outcome, and neither obesity nor weight loss requires immediate follow-up. Peripheral pulses are normal at 2+, but the client's blood pressure is elevated. While blood pressure would require follow-up at a later time, the level of hypertension is not life threatening. The client has a history of hypertension, and an elevated blood pressure is not unusual.

CJ Cognitive Skill: Recognize Cues
Reference: Halter & Fratena, 2023, pp. 212–217

Thinking Exercise 18.2.2

Answer

Based on the assessment findings, the client ***most likely*** has <u>**early-stage dementia**</u>.

Rationale

Dementia is a broad term for chronic, global cognitive impairment and deterioration. The most common cause of dementia is Alzheimer disease, which has three stages as the client deteriorates. In the early stage of the condition, the client recognizes the cognitive changes, including difficulty remembering words and names, difficulty with planning and organization, losing or misplacing items, and challenges in performing tasks. This client presents with many of these findings but is still able to function. There is no evidence that the client currently has clinical depression, which is manifested by sad mood, sleep disturbances, appetite changes, and apathy. Clients who have acute delirium are not able to communicate or function.

CJ Cognitive Skill: Analyze Cues
Reference: Halter & Fratena, 2023, pp. 212–217

Thinking Exercise 18.2.3

Answer

The *priority* for the client's care at this time is **improving cognition** to **help the client maintain employment**.

Rationale

The priority for client care is to improve the client's memory, forgetfulness, and organizational skills. These findings are likely negatively affecting the client's personal and work life. As a hairstylist, the client would need to plan and organize appointments, supplies, and other aspects of the business. There is no evidence that the client is at risk for falls or that the client is not getting adequate nutrition.
CJ Cognitive Skill: Prioritize Hypotheses
Reference: Halter & Fratena, 2023, pp. 212–226

Thinking Exercise 18.2.4

Answer

POTENTIAL NURSING ACTIONS	INDICATED	NOT INDICATED
Use a reliable mental status tool to assess cognition.	✗	
Reinforce teaching about cholinesterase inhibitors.	✗	
Prepare the client for admission to an inpatient mental health unit or facility.		✗
Refer the client to a neuropsychologist or other qualified mental health care professional.	✗	

Rationale

The client has a cognitive impairment that would be assessed to serve as a baseline. A number of reliable tools, such as the Montreal Cognitive Assessment (MoCA), are evidence-based tools that provide an accurate assessment of a client's condition. The client likely has Alzheimer disease for which cholinesterase inhibitors are frequently prescribed, especially in the early and middle stages of the condition. The client would benefit from a complete evaluation by a neuropsychologist or other qualified health care professional who specializes in neurocognitive disorders. The client would not require admission to an inpatient mental health unit or facility.
CJ Cognitive Skill: Generate Solutions
Reference: Halter & Fratena, 2023, pp. 212–226

Thinking Exercise 18.2.5—Pharmacology

Answer

○ "Take this drug on an empty stomach first thing each morning."
✗ "Do not take nonsteroidal anti-inflammatory drugs (NSAIDs) while taking donepezil."
✗ "Report a pulse below 60 beats/min to the provider as soon as possible."
✗ "This drug should help improve your memory, but it may not return to your usual level."
○ "Donepezil can only be taken during the early stage of Alzheimer dementia."

Rationale

Donepezil is a cholinesterase inhibitor prescribed for clients who have any stage of Alzheimer disease (AD), not just for those in the early stage. This drug, like others in its class, slows the breakdown of cholinesterase, an enzyme that prevents the effectiveness of acetylcholine in the brain. Clients with AD are thought to have a deficiency of acetylcholine. Donepezil can improve memory and other cognitive changes but may not return the client to the usual baseline level. All of the drugs in this classification can cause gastrointestinal distress, especially nausea, vomiting, and diarrhea. Therefore the nurse would teach the client to take the drug with food and not on an empty stomach. NSAIDs can also cause gastrointestinal distress and should be avoided when taking donepezil. Although not common, clients taking cholinesterase inhibitors can develop bradycardia and/or incontinence. Therefore the nurse would report these side effects to the provider as soon as possible.

CJ Cognitive Skill: Take Actions
Reference: Halter & Fratena, 2023, pp. 413–414, 417

Thinking Exercise 18.2.6

Answer

History and Physical	Progress Notes	Nurses' Notes	Laboratory Results

1120: Client scheduled for annual physical examination today. Has long-term history of low back pain, osteoarthritis, clinical depression, and hypertension. Is widowed, and works full-time as a hairstylist. Reports having memory lapses, which have increased in the past few months. Client concerned about sometimes having difficulty remembering words or names. Feels more disorganized lately. Remains independent in ADLs. Denies feeling sad, having sleep disturbances, or having a change in appetite. Denies suicidal ideation. Has been on a low-carbohydrate diet for several months and lost 15 lb (6.8 kg). Currently weighs 184 lb (83.5 kg); height 64 inches (162.6 cm); BMI 31.6. Lungs clear throughout; abdomen soft and round with active bowel sounds in all quadrants. Peripheral pulses 2+ and equal. All extremities move freely. Strong hand grip. No tremors or weakness. VS: T 98.2°F (36.8°C), HR 72 beats/min and regular, RR 18 breaths/min, BP 145/82 mm Hg, SpO$_2$ 96% on RA.

1215: Referral to neuropsychologist. Prescription for donepezil to begin immediately.

2-Month Follow-Up Visit
0830: Follow-up visit after client diagnosed with early-stage dementia, probably Alzheimer disease, and starting donepezil 2 months ago. Client states feeling that memory is better with fewer lapses and beginning to feel more organized at work and home. Fewer problems with remembering words and names since starting drug therapy. Continuing diet, but has lost only 3 lb (1.4 kg) during the past 2 months. Is frustrated that weight loss has slowed, and considering joining an established weight-loss program.

Rationale

The client's cognitive status seems to be improving as evidenced by a report of fewer memory lapses, fewer problems remembering words and names, and beginning to feel more organized at work and home. These positive changes demonstrate that the treatment plan has been effective.

CJ Cognitive Skill: Evaluate Outcomes
Reference: Halter & Fratena, 2023, pp. 212–226

Stand-Alone Thinking Exercise 18.1

Answer

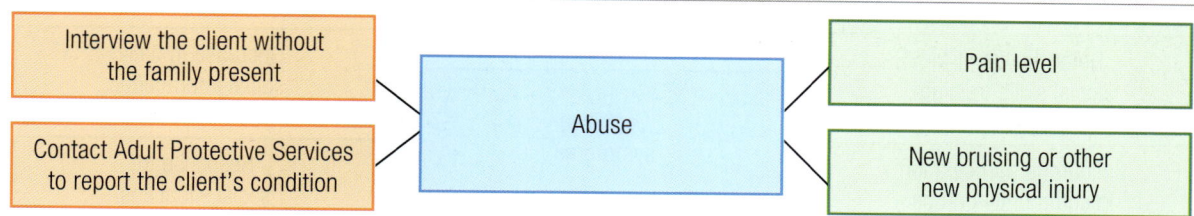

Rationale

The client presents with findings that indicate likely elder abuse, including a recent right wrist injury and old bruising on the torso. Elder abuse could be life threatening and requires immediate follow-up by the nurse. There is no evidence of neglect because the client gained weight and has a well-groomed appearance. There is also no evidence that the client is experiencing anxiety or depression, but the nurse would screen for these conditions later. To address the client's likely abuse, the nurse would collect more data in a private interview with the client to determine if the abuse was caused by family caregivers. Then the nurse would contact the appropriate agency, such as Adult Protective Services (APS), to report the suspected abuse. To determine if the plan was effective, the nurse would monitor the client for additional physical injury or emotional abuse. The nurse would also monitor pain level because elder abuse can cause pain and discomfort.

CJ Cognitive Skills: Recognize Cues, Analyze Cues, Prioritize Hypotheses, Generate Solutions, Take Actions, Evaluate Outcomes

Reference: Halter & Fratena, 2023, pp. 303–306

Stand-Alone Thinking Exercise 18.2

Answer

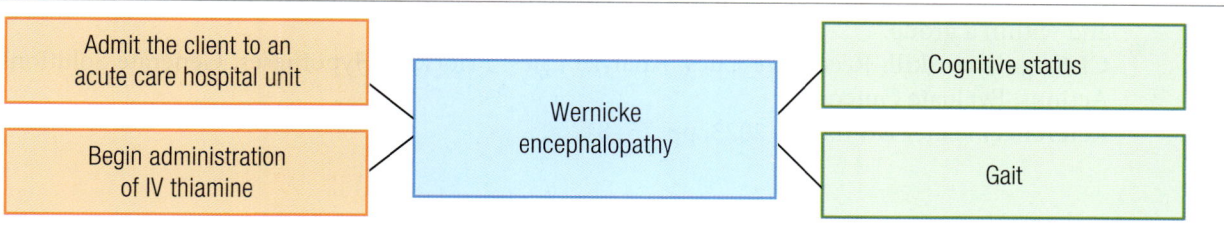

Rationale

Clients who have been heavy drinkers for many years can have a thiamine deficiency, which causes temporary or permanent memory impairment, altered gait, confusion, and a variety of eye changes, including unequal pupils with sluggish response to light. Although Wernicke encephalopathy is a reversible condition, it is a medical emergency requiring admission to acute care for daily IV administration of thiamine for 1 to 2 weeks. Once the client's thiamine level has returned to normal range, the client's clinical findings usually improve. Untreated Wernicke encephalopathy can progress to Korsakoff syndrome, which is a much more severe and chronic condition requiring many months of thiamine therapy. This client's signs and symptoms began a few days ago, and the client does not have the more severe condition associated with long-term heavy alcohol consumption. There is no evidence that the client has dementia because the client findings began 2 days ago. Delirium can occur in clients who are alcoholics, but it tends to occur most commonly when alcohol is withdrawn. The nurse and health care team would monitor the client's cognitive status and gait, which were impaired prior to treatment.

CJ Cognitive Skills: Recognize Cues, Analyze Cues, Prioritize Hypotheses, Generate Solutions, Take Actions, Evaluate Outcomes

Reference: Halter & Fratena, 2023, pp. 192–195

Stand-Alone Thinking Exercise 18.3

Answer

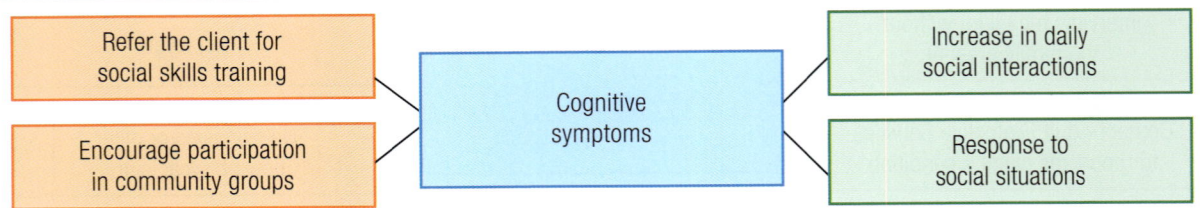

Rationale

Clients who are diagnosed with schizophrenia usually have many different types of symptoms that progress in a rather predictable manner over time. Positive symptoms refer to behaviors that should not be present and tend to occur in the acute phase of the condition. Common positive symptoms include hallucinations, delusions, and disorganized thinking. Negative symptoms refer to human behaviors and qualities that should be present but are not. Examples include apathy, lack of verbalization, and an inability to feel joy or pleasure. Affective symptoms manifest as unstable emotions and mood. Many clients who have schizophrenia also experience primary clinical depression and/or substance use disorder. Cognitive symptoms tend to occur in clients who have had schizophrenia for a large portion of their lives. These symptoms prevent clients from functioning in various aspects of their lives and include alterations in working memory, attention, social skills, and reasoning/problem solving. There is no evidence that the client has any of these symptom types except for cognitive symptoms. Appropriate actions for the client with cognitive symptoms include increasing opportunities for individual social interactions, referring the client for social skills training, and encouraging participation in community groups. The client does not require admission to an acute mental health facility or a change in drug therapy. There is also no evidence that the client is at risk for suicide or suicidal ideation. The nurse and family would follow up to determine the client's response to social situations following social skills training and ensure that the client has increased opportunities for social interactions, both individual and within a group.

CJ Cognitive Skill: Recognize Cues, Analyze Cues, Prioritize Hypotheses, Generate Solutions, Take Actions, Evaluate Outcomes

Reference: Halter & Fratena, 2023, pp. 75–81

Answers With Rationales for Thinking Exercises

Unfolding Case Study 19.1

Thinking Exercise 19.1.1

Answer

- ○ Left-sided weakness
- ○ Slurred speech
- ✗ Occasional dizziness
- ✗ Feeling sad and "moody"
- ○ Insomnia
- ✗ Weight loss

Rationale

The client is experiencing occasional dizziness when ambulating, which could lead to injury from a fall. Therefore this finding requires immediate follow-up to determine the cause of the client's dizziness. Feeling sad and "moody" is of immediate concern because the client's emotional state could affect progress during rehabilitation and after discharge to home. The client's unintended weight loss is likely from a lack of appetite. This finding requires immediate follow-up because the client needs adequate nutrition for healing and strength to ensure continued rehabilitation and progress at home. Left-sided weakness and slurred speech were the result of the client's stroke 4 weeks ago and are expected client findings following a right cerebral ischemic stroke. Therefore these findings would not require immediate follow-up. Insomnia can be life threatening if it continues for a long period. Many clients have difficulty sleeping at inpatient facilities but are able to rest and sleep better at home. Therefore insomnia would not require immediate follow-up at this time.

CJ Cognitive Skill: Recognize Cues
Reference: Halter & Fratena, pp. 106–107

Thinking Exercise 19.1.2

Answer

The client is likely experiencing secondary **depression** as a result of the client's **stroke**.

Rationale

The client's findings are consistent with depression, especially feeling sad and "moody," sleep disturbance, anger/agitation, and loss of appetite. Some clients experience depression as a result of having a catastrophic or traumatic health event, such as a stroke. In this case, the depression would not be considered the primary disorder but rather a secondary condition. Clients who are anxious tend to excessively worry, but there is no indication that the client is experiencing this behavior. There is also no indication that the client has bipolar disorder, although depression is commonly seen in clients who have that condition.

CJ Cognitive Skill: Analyze Cues
Reference: Halter & Fratena, pp. 106–107

Thinking Exercise 19.1.3

Answer

The *priority* for the client's care at this time is to assess for **suicide risk**.

Rationale

The client is an older adult with weakness and dizziness who is at risk for falling. However, the client also likely has depression as a result of neurologic changes from a catastrophic health event, which places the client at risk for suicide. Suicide attempts are life threatening, therefore suicide risk is the priority for the client's care at this time. The client may also be at risk for inadequate nutrition, but the client has only lost 5 lb (2.3 kg) in the past 2 weeks.

CJ Cognitive Skill: Prioritize Hypotheses
Reference: Halter & Fratena, p. 110

Thinking Exercise 19.1.4

Answer

POTENTIAL NURSING ACTIONS	INDICATED	NOT INDICATED
Consult with the social worker for evaluation.	X	
Assess the client for suicide risk.	X	
Frequently reorient the client to reality.		X
Request drug therapy for the client's condition.	X	
Remind the client and spouse that the client is independent in ambulation.		X

Rationale

The client's mental/emotional state should be evaluated by a health care professional. Social workers, depending on their credentialing, have the ability to evaluate this client and assess the client's risk for suicide or suicidal ideation. Drug therapy likely would be indicated to help with mood stabilization. Reminding the client and spouse of the client's progress would not help decrease sadness, agitation/ anger, or moodiness. There is no indication that the client is out of touch with reality or experiencing psychosis. Therefore orienting the client to reality would not be indicated.

CJ Cognitive Skill: Generate Solutions
Reference: Halter & Fratena, pp. 110–117

Thinking Exercise 19.1.5—Pharmacology

Answer

X "This drug will be started at a low dose to determine the best dosage for you."
O "When you feel better, you can discontinue this drug whenever you want."
X "This drug is taken orally several times a day with food to help prevent nausea."
O "While taking this drug, you won't need to see your counselor or therapist."
X "Monitor your blood pressure and pulse, and contact your provider if they significantly increase."

Rationale

Venlafaxine is a serotonin-norepinephrine reuptake inhibitor (SNRI) that can result in dose-dependent increases in blood pressure and heart rate because of its blockage of norepinephrine reuptake. This problem is more likely to occur at higher doses. Therefore the drug is started at a low dose that can be increased slowly as needed to manage depression. The nurse would teach the client and family how to monitor the client's blood pressure and pulse and to inform the provider if these values significantly increase. Venlafaxine can also cause gastrointestinal distress including nausea; taking the drug with

food can help minimize this side effect. The drug would not be discontinued unless this process is supervised by a qualified health care professional. Antidepressants take 1 to 2 weeks to produce an effect but can take up to 6 weeks for clients to experience their full benefit. Therefore counseling or therapy would begin immediately while the client is waiting for the drug to work.
CJ Cognitive Skill: Take Actions
Reference: Halter & Fratena, pp. 371–372

Thinking Exercise 19.1.6

Answer

History and Physical	Nurses' Notes	Orders	Laboratory Results

Acute Rehabilitation Unit

0845: Client very concerned about planned discharge to home with spouse later this week after being at acute rehabilitation facility for 4 weeks following a right cerebral ischemic stroke. Reports having trouble sleeping most nights and a declining appetite in the past 2 weeks resulting in an unintended 5-lb (2.3-kg) weight loss. Is worried about the future and retirement. Client is owner of a construction company, but currently has left-sided weakness and slurred speech. Walks independently with a walker, but has occasional dizziness. Feels sad most mornings, but is "moody" during the day. Spouse visiting later today.

1310: Spouse expresses concern about client's mental and emotional state. Client reports sadness and anger because of inability to provide for the family. Client has had several anger outbursts when spouse visits.

1625: Social worker in to visit spouse and family. Suicide risk assessment conducted; currently not at risk.

1800: Antidepressant drug therapy initiated. Health teaching about drug provided to both client and spouse.

Follow-up Provider Visit—4 Weeks After Discharge

0945: Client and spouse at provider's office for follow-up visit after discharge from acute rehabilitation facility. Client reports feeling less sad and less moody since being on venlafaxine. Had several episodes of nausea when first starting medication, but has had no nausea for the past 2 weeks. Spouse reports that client has worked in office 2 to 3 days a week, and construction business is "doing well." Client not able to drive yet, but has been using a cane independently for ambulation for the past week. Attends psychotherapy at least once a week.

Rationale

Several changes in client findings have occurred over the past 4 weeks. First, the client's emotional state has improved as indicated by reporting feeling less sad and less moody since being on the antidepressant. The client's physical condition also has improved as evidenced by walking with a cane compared with relying on a walker 4 weeks ago.
CJ Cognitive Skill: Evaluate Outcomes
Reference: Halter & Fratena, pp. 106–117

Unfolding Case Study 19.2

Thinking Exercise 19.2.1

Answer

History and Physical	Nurses' Notes	Orders	Laboratory Results

2145: Client admitted to ED via ambulance after family found client on floor. Was unresponsive at home when paramedics arrived. Family reported client may have taken a large number of oxycodone tablets because prescription bottle is empty. Increased level of consciousness noted after naloxone administration. On ED admission, client drowsy but oriented × 4. When asked about what happened, client started crying and repeated several times, "I don't want to be a burden to anyone. Please just let me die." Family explained that client has recently experienced worsening chronic pain from metastatic bone cancer. Client frequently expresses hopelessness and wonders if cancer treatment should continue because current "last resort" cancer drug causes extreme nausea and fatigue.

Rationale

The client's mental and emotional state is very concerning, especially the feelings of hopelessness and wanting to die. These findings could be life threatening and therefore require immediate follow-up. The client's drowsiness would be expected because the client apparently took a large number of oxycodone tablets.

CJ Cognitive Skill: Recognize Cues
Reference: Halter & Fratena, pp. 253–262

Thinking Exercise 19.2.2

Answer

The client is at highest risk for __suicide__ because the client __had a suicide attempt__.

Rationale

Clients who attempt suicide have the highest risk for another suicide attempt, a potentially life-threatening condition. Older adults are also at risk for falling, but this risk would not be the potential highest-risk condition. There is no evidence that the client is at risk for cognitive decline except that the client is of advanced age. Older adults have the highest incidence of delirium and dementia.

CJ Cognitive Skill: Analyze Cues
Reference: Halter & Fratena, pp. 253–262

Thinking Exercise 19.2.3

Answer

The *priority* need for the client at this time is to __maintain safety__.

Rationale

Because the client is at high risk for another suicide attempt, the priority need for this client is to maintain the client's safety and the safety of others. Managing pain is also an important client need, but unless the client is safe, this need would not be relevant. There is no evidence that the client is at risk for cognitive impairment.

CJ Cognitive Skill: Prioritize Hypotheses
Reference: Halter & Fratena, pp. 253–262

Thinking Exercise 19.2.4

Answer

✗ Identify the client's risk for another suicide attempt.
✗ Determine the level of suicide precautions that are needed for the client at this time.
✗ Identify the client's support system and protective factors.
✗ Collaborate with the family to plan for possible client discharge to home with them.
✗ Prepare the family for possible admission to an inpatient acute psychiatric unit.
○ Request psychoactive drug therapy to sedate the client to prevent another suicide attempt.

Rationale

Clients who attempt suicide may be managed in the community or in an acute inpatient setting. The decision about the plan of care is determined by assessing the client's support system, risk factors, protective factors, and level of suicide precautions that are needed based on that assessment. The client's support system may include a religious or spiritual leader or beliefs and family/friends. In addition to a suicide attempt, other risk factors include a history of suicide in the family, substance use, mood disorder, and chronic illness causing chronic pain. Examples of protective factors include having close family relationships and good problem-solving skills. The level of suicide precautions is determined

by analyzing risk factors and protective factors. It would not be appropriate to provide drug therapy to sedate older adults to prevent another suicide attempt. In this case, the drug would be considered a chemical restraint, which can lead to adverse effects for older adults.
CJ Cognitive Skill: Generate Solutions
Reference: Halter & Fratena, pp. 253–262

Thinking Exercise 19.2.5

Answer

- ✗ Teach the client and family about prescribed antidepressant drug therapy.
- ✗ Teach the family about behaviors associated with worsening depression or suicide risk.
- ◯ Schedule a follow-up visit for the client in 6 to 8 weeks.
- ✗ Provide the client and family with crisis or emergency hotline information.
- ✗ Identify social supports for client and the need to contact them.
- ✗ Teach the client and family the importance of professional counseling as soon as possible.

Rationale

The client is an older adult who would likely be more comfortable with staying with family rather than being admitted to an unknown unit or agency. Clients and family in the home environment need education on the treatment plan and support services or resources they can use in case of a crisis or emergency. Social supports would also be identified. The treatment plan would likely include antidepressant drug therapy. The client should start professional counseling or psychotherapy as soon as possible and attend these sessions on a regular basis. Drug therapy begins to work in 1 to 2 weeks, but the client would not feel its full benefit for 4 to 6 weeks or longer. Because the client attempted suicide, waiting 6 to 8 weeks for a follow-up visit is too long. Instead, the first follow-up visit would be in about 1 week with frequent visits thereafter until the drug therapy is fully effective.
CJ Cognitive Skill: Take Actions
Reference: Halter & Fratena, pp. 253–262

Thinking Exercise 19.2.6

Answer

CLIENT FINDINGS	IMPROVED	NOT IMPROVED
Mood and affect	✗	
Appetite		✗
Pain control	✗	
Suicidal ideation	✗	

Rationale

The client's emotional state has improved as evidenced by stating a feeling of less hopelessness when compared with 1 week earlier. The client states having no thoughts of suicide, which is another improvement. The client is now using fentanyl patches as treatment for chronic cancer pain from metastatic bone cancer. These patches are effective in reducing pain according to the client. This statement indicates that the client's pain control has improved. The client's appetite remains poor, which shows no improvement.
CJ Cognitive Skill: Evaluate Outcomes
Reference: Halter & Fratena, pp. 253–262

Stand-Alone Thinking Exercise 19.1

Answer

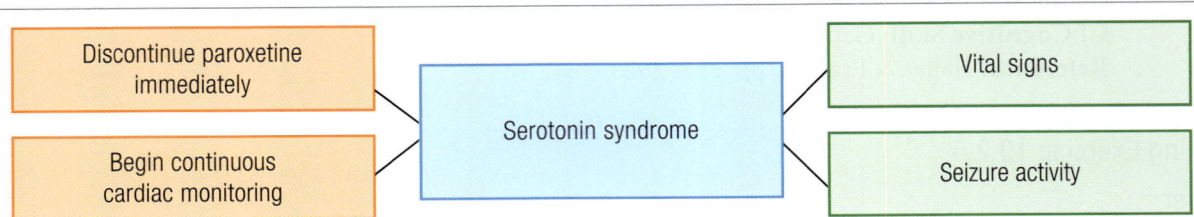

Rationale

The client is taking paroxetine, which is a selective serotonin reuptake inhibitor (SSRI). A relatively rare and potentially life-threatening toxic effect of SSRIs is serotonin syndrome, which is caused by overactivation of central serotonin receptors resulting from either a high dose or interaction with other drugs, such as cough and cold medications and opioids. Signs and symptoms of serotonin syndrome include tachycardia, fever, elevated blood pressure, delirium, seizures, abdominal pain and diarrhea, and mood swings. If this syndrome is not successfully treated, the client could experience shock, apnea, and eventually death. This client has most of the common signs and symptoms of serotonin syndrome. Gastroenteritis presents as gastrointestinal distress and possible fever, but the other client findings are not consistent with this condition. Dementia presents with chronic confusion, which the client does not have. Dementia usually does not affect vital signs or cause gastrointestinal distress. Thyroid storm occurs when the thyroid gland secretes an excessive amount of thyroid hormones. This client has an underactive thyroid gland for which medication is used to replace natural hormones. Because serotonin syndrome is caused by SSRIs, the nurse would immediately discontinue the paroxetine. Additionally, the nurse would begin continuous cardiac monitoring because the condition is potentially life threatening. The client's temperature is not high enough to require a cooling blanket at this time, but it could be needed if the temperature increases. There is no need to perform a mental status assessment at this time because the client's mental status should improve after the serotonin syndrome is effectively managed. There is no need to draw a TSH level because the client's condition is not related to thyroid function. The nurse would continue to monitor vital signs for any changes that could indicate severe hyperthermia or shock. The nurse would also monitor for any seizure activity, which could lead to status epilepticus, a life-threatening complication. The client's abdominal pain level or stool count or quality would not be the most important parameters to measure when compared with vital signs that could indicate shock or another life-threatening complication. The client's SpO_2 is in the normal range for older adults (above 90%), and the client does not have respiratory distress. Therefore monitoring the peripheral arterial oxygen level would not be indicated at this time.

CJ Cognitive Skills: Recognize Cues, Analyze Cues, Prioritize Hypotheses, Generate Solutions, Take Actions, Evaluate Outcomes

Reference: Halter & Fratena, pp. 365–371

Stand-Alone Thinking Exercise 19.2

Answer

Based on the collected data, the client is most likely experiencing **drug toxicity**.

Rationale

Valproic acid is a mood-stabilizing drug used to treat mania associated with bipolar disorder. This drug has a black box warning about hepatotoxicity, including fatalities, that can occur in the first 6 months after starting it. Hepatotoxicity can be detected by monitoring liver function tests (LFTs), including bilirubin and liver enzymes. This client's LFTs are all well above the normal reference range. Valproic acid can also affect platelets and coagulation studies, as seen by the decline in this client's platelet count. There are no physical findings indicating the client is experiencing hepatitis or bleeding. There are no client behaviors consistent with depression.

CJ Cognitive Skill: Analyze Cues
Reference: Halter & Fratena, pp. 358–359

Answers With Rationales for Thinking Exercises

Unfolding Case Study 20.1

Thinking Exercise 20.1.1

Answer

History and Physical	Nurses' Notes	Orders	Laboratory Results

1010: Client presents at 19 weeks' gestation for initial prenatal visit. Obstetric history: G4P3. Medical history: asthma, depression, and atopic dermatitis. Alert and oriented × 4. Reports feeling stressed, stating, "I didn't plan on getting pregnant again. I can't afford another child." Respirations equal and unlabored with mild expiratory wheezing noted on auscultation. Skin warm with dry, inflamed areas noted on bilateral hands and right lower arm. Bowel sounds present in all quadrants. Denies nausea, vomiting, excessive thirst, and dysuria. Reports urinary frequency. Fetal heart tones auscultated in lower abdomen with client in semi-Fowler's position; Fetal HR 116 beats/min. Fundal height 19 cm. Client reports signs of positive quickening. Client works 32 hours weekly as a retail clerk, lives with spouse and three children, and denies extended family or support systems outside of the home. VS: T 98.6°F (37°C), HR 84 beats/min and regular, RR 16 breaths/min, BP 124/74 mm Hg, SpO$_2$ 96% on RA.

Rationale

The nurse would recognize late prenatal care, feelings of stress, financial concerns, and lack of support systems outside of the home as risk factors for immediate follow-up. Early prenatal care is associated with improved outcomes for both the client and infant. The first trimester is considered 0 to 13 weeks' gestation, and it is recommended to start prenatal care in the first trimester. Late prenatal care is often associated with social factors such as lack of insurance or inadequate support systems that prohibit seeking medical care. The nurse would assess social factors, following up on the client's verbalized concerns, to promote positive outcomes for the client and fetus. Additionally, the nurse will follow up on the client's history of depression. Clients who have a history of depression before pregnancy are at high risk for depression during pregnancy. The nurse must follow up to determine if the client is currently experiencing any signs or symptoms of depression during this pregnancy. Other client findings are within normal limits or not priority concerns at this time.

CJ Cognitive Skill: Recognize Cues
Reference: Leifer & Little, 2023, pp. 47–84

Thinking Exercise 20.1.2

Answer

The nurse recognizes that the client is *most likely* experiencing **self-care deficit** as manifested by **delayed prenatal care** and **not bathing or eating**.

Rationale

The client reports giving all energy to the care of children and not taking time for self-care. Delaying prenatal care, not taking prenatal vitamins, and failing to bathe or eat daily are signs indicating that the client is not taking time for self-care. Self-care deficit during pregnancy occurs more frequently in low-income families and those without social support and resources, and it can lead to significant maternal and fetal complications including perinatal and maternal death. The nurse must identify self-care deficit as the client's greatest risk and focus care on improving self-care activities including hygiene, nutrition, and prenatal care. The client's lack of self-care may be exacerbated by depression, but there is no evidence of suicidal ideation or domestic violence.

CJ Cognitive Skill: Analyze Cues
Reference: Leifer & Little, 2023, pp. 47–84

Thinking Exercise 20.1.3

Answer

The *priority* for the client's care at this time is **anticipatory guidance** and **community resources** to address the physical, emotional, and psychological changes that occur with pregnancy.

Rationale

The nurse's primary goal is to help the client anticipate how the body will be changing and how to respond to changes in such a way that promotes well-being of both the client and fetus. Health teaching and anticipatory guidance will help the client prepare for the expected physical, emotional, and psychosocial changes that occur during pregnancy and take steps to prevent highly probably complications. Community resources may also assist the client to accept and adapt to pregnancy and receive necessary support during all intrapartum stages.

CJ Cognitive Skill: Prioritize Hypotheses
Reference: Leifer & Little, 2023, pp. 47–84

Thinking Exercise 20.1.4

Answer

- O "Ask your doctor to discontinue sertraline during your pregnancy."
- ✗ "Drink plenty of water between meals, but limit your fluid intake with meals."
- ✗ "Keep a 24-hour intake diary to assess your current eating patterns."
- ✗ "Participate in 30 minutes of mild to moderate exercise 5 days per week."
- O "Schedule an appointment to receive the varicella vaccination."
- ✗ "Take a prenatal vitamin every day."
- O "Treat yourself to a spa day, and soak in a hot tub or sit in a sauna to relax."
- O "Use a food guide to plan two to three large daily meals that include iron and protein-rich foods."

Rationale

There is a high correlation between maternal diet and fetal health, therefore the nurse would assist the client in understanding the value of eating a healthy, balanced, nutrient-dense diet. The nurse must reinforce the client's nutritional needs and the use of a food guide, such as MyPlate, to ensure that the client is eating essential nutrients every day. The nurse may also advise the client to keep a 24-hour intake diary to assess current eating patterns and identify opportunities for improvement. Nausea is common during pregnancy, so the nurse would reinforce strategies to reduce or improve the client's tolerance of nausea/vomiting such as reducing fluids when eating and avoiding eating large amounts at one time. Additionally, the nurse would reinforce the importance of taking daily prenatal vitamins, avoiding alcohol, and limiting caffeine intake. Mild to moderate exercise is beneficial during a normal pregnancy, but vigorous exercise should be avoided. The nurse would reinforce 30 minutes of mild to moderate exercise 5 days per week to improve the client's ability to cope with the emotional, physical, and psychological changes and prevent excess weight gain during pregnancy. Although the client may benefit from a spa day, the use of a hot tub or sauna during pregnancy is contraindicated; maternal body temperature should not exceed 100.4°F (38°C). Live attenuated vaccines, such as measles, mumps, rubella, or varicella, are contraindicated during pregnancy as they have teratogenic effects on the fetus. Inactivated vaccines, such as influenza, Tdap, hepatitis B, and COVID-19 vaccines, have protective qualities for the client during pregnancy and reduce the passage of illness to the newborn.

CJ Cognitive Skill: Generate Solutions
Reference: Leifer & Little, 2023, pp. 47–84

Thinking Exercise 20.1.5

Answer

- ○ Administer supplemental oxygen.
- ○ Elevate the client's legs above the heart.
- ○ Massage the client's lower back.
- ✗ Monitor vital signs until symptoms subside.
- ○ Obtain a finger stick blood glucose (FSBG) level.
- ○ Provide an emesis bag to collect any vomitus.
- ✗ Reposition client to the lateral side-lying position.

Rationale

Supine positioning of a pregnant client may cause the uterus to expand and exert pressure on the vena cava, which can create a hypotensive reaction for both the client and fetus. Pallor, dizziness, faintness, breathlessness, tachycardia, sudden nausea, and diaphoresis are all signs of supine hypotension. The nurse must immediately reposition the client to the side-lying or lateral position to remove pressure on the vena cava. Elevating the client's legs above the heart does not alleviate vena cava pressure. Prolonged or repetitive compression of the vena cava can reduce placental circulation, which may result in intrauterine growth restriction. The nurse will remain with the client and continue to monitor the client until symptoms subside and vital signs stabilize to within normal limits. The client is not experiencing hypoxia, and therefore supplemental oxygen is not needed. Massaging the lower back and providing an emesis bag may provide the client with comfort, but these items do not address the hypotensive condition being experienced by the client and fetus.

CJ Cognitive Skill: Take Actions
Reference: Leifer & Little, 2023, pp. 56–58

Thinking Exercise 20.1.6

Answer

CLIENT FINDINGS	IMPROVED	NOT IMPROVED
Arranged time for self-care	✗	
Collaborated with a registered dietitian nutritionist	✗	
Expresses financial concerns		✗
Eats small, nutrient-dense meals and snacks	✗	
Fundal height 21 cm		✗

Rationale

The client has taken many steps to improve self-care and engage community resources for support. Arranging for children to attend an after-school program and collaborating with a registered dietitian nutritionist demonstrate that the client has engaged community resources for support. Using newly arranged time for self-care and eating small, nutrient-dense meals and snacks throughout the day are also significant improvements for this client. The client continues to express concerns about being able to afford the newborn. The client's financial situation has not worsened, but the concern has not been addressed and therefore is not improved. Fundal height should reflect the client's weeks in gestation within one-half week. The client's fundal height is currently less than expected (23 cm), which suggests that the fetus is potentially not growing appropriately. The nurse would recognize this as a worsening condition and collaborate with the health care team to perform additional testing and monitoring for intrauterine growth restriction.

CJ Cognitive Skill: Evaluate Outcomes
Reference: Leifer & Little, 2023, pp. 47–120

Unfolding Case Study 20.2

Thinking Exercise 20.2.1

Answer

- O Apgar scores
- ✗ Blood pressure
- O Erythematous and swollen incision
- ✗ Heart rate
- ✗ Soft fundus at umbilicus
- O Temperature

Rationale

The nurse must recognize that the client's fundus is not firm. After a full-term birth, the uterus should be easily palpated through the abdominal wall as a firm mass about the size of a grapefruit. If the uterus does not contract appropriately, the fundus may feel soft or boggy. This finding is caused by one of several potentially life-threatening complications and requires immediate follow-up. The nurse would also recognize the client's abnormal heart rate and blood pressure. Tachycardia and low blood pressure are signs of decreased circulating volume or hypovolemia and require immediate follow-up to prevent shock and other life-threatening complications. The client's temperature and incisional assessment are not within normal limits and could be signs of infection. The nurse would prioritize these findings after stabilizing the client's vital signs and addressing the soft fundus. The newborn's Apgar scores are within normal limits.

CJ Cognitive Skill: Recognize Cues
Reference: Leifer & Little, 2023, pp. 250–257

Thinking Exercise 20.2.2

Answer

CLIENT FINDINGS	POSTPARTUM INFECTION	POSTPARTUM HEMORRHAGE
Red and swollen incision	✗	
Fever	✗	
Narrowing pulse pressure		✗
Soft fundus		✗
Tachycardia	✗	✗

Rationale

Infection is a common complication after childbirth. Tissue trauma during labor, surgical incisions, cracks in the nipples of the breasts, and an increased vaginal pH after birth are all risk factors for infection. Postpartum infections may be localized or spread causing peritonitis and sepsis. Client findings that suggest a possible postpartum infection are fever; tachycardia; abdominal tenderness; and redness, swelling, and drainage from surgical wounds. Postpartum hemorrhage is a loss of more than 500 mL after vaginal birth or 1000 mL after cesarean birth that results in signs or symptoms of hypovolemia. The client's estimated cesarean blood loss was 1200 mL. Client findings that suggest postpartum hemorrhage are light-headedness, tachycardia, decreased blood pressure, and narrowing pulse pressure (systolic pressure decreases while diastolic pressure increases).

CJ Cognitive Skill: Analyze Cues
Reference: Leifer & Little, 2023, pp. 250–257

Thinking Exercise 20.2.3

Answer

The nurse recognizes that the client is *most likely* experiencing postpartum **hemorrhage** resulting from **uterine atony**.

Rationale

There are no signs indicating that the client is experiencing any type of mood disorder including postpartum depression. Although some of the client findings are consistent with a postpartum infection, initial signs of a postsurgical infection usually do not manifest for several days after the procedure. It would be very unlikely for the client to be experiencing a wound infection from a cesarean section that occurred 8 hours ago. It is much more likely that the client findings are the result of postpartum hemorrhage. Early postpartum hemorrhage occurs within the first 24 hours after birth and most commonly results from vaginal injury, hematoma, or uterine atony. The client had a cesarean section, therefore vaginal injury and hematoma are unlikely causes of the postpartum bleeding. Uterine atony, or inadequate uterine muscle tone, manifests as a soft or boggy uterus and may result from bladder distention, an overdistended uterus due to a large baby or a multiple-baby pregnancy, multiparity, cesarean birth, and medications used during labor. The client has several risk factors for postpartum hemorrhage resulting from uterine atony.

CJ Cognitive Skill: Prioritize Hypotheses
Reference: Leifer & Little, 2023, pp. 250–257

Thinking Exercise 20.2.4

Answer

Based on the client's condition, the most appropriate potential nursing actions are **massaging the uterus** and **promoting breast-feeding**.

Rationale

The client is experiencing postpartum hemorrhage resulting from uterine atony. Bladder distention is an easily corrected cause of uterine atony, but the client recently voided and therefore a full bladder is not the likely cause. The nurse would instead prioritize massaging the uterus until it is firm and promoting breast-feeding, which simulates the secretion of oxytocin and causes uterine contractions. Additional interventions may include a dilute oxytocin (Pitocin) IV infusion, uterine tamponade or packing, and surgical intervention if bleeding cannot be stopped. The client does not need to remain on bed rest but would be advised to ask for assistance when rising from a chair or getting out of bed until vital signs return to normal. An ice pack can be used to treat perineal swelling, which may occur in both vaginal and cesarean deliveries; it is not used to treat uterine atony.

CJ Cognitive Skill: Generate Solutions
Reference: Leifer & Little, 2023, pp. 250–257

Thinking Exercise 20.2.5

Answer

○ "Breast-feeding will delay the return of ovulation, which will provide reliable contraception for several months."

✗ "Contact your provider if you notice a foul smell from your vaginal discharge or experience increasing pain."

○ "It is common to feel a huge range of emotions for several months after delivery including feelings of not enjoying your life."

✗ "Postpartum bleeding will continue for several weeks and become increasingly lighter in color and flow."

✗ "Shower daily, and continue perineal care until the flow of bleeding stops."

✗ "Take it easy for the next few weeks. Start with low-impact activities, and progress slowly."

Rationale

Postpartum bleeding (lochia) is commonly heavy and bright red for the first few days before transitioning to a lighter flow, more like a period. This period-like flow can last up to 2 weeks before becoming a light-beige discharge, which can last an additional 2 to 3 weeks. The nurse would teach the client to contact the provider if bleeding saturates a pad every hour for multiple hours, a clot larger than a baseball is passed, vaginal discharge has a foul smell, or the client experiences increasing pain or fever of 100.4°F (38°C) or higher. A well-balanced diet and moderate exercise promote healing and recovery. The nurse would teach the client to start slowly with low-impact activities and progress to moderate activities over several weeks. A daily shower and perineal care provide essential hygiene and promote refreshing and positive physical and emotional feelings. Ovulation may resume within weeks of delivery, and breast-feeding is not a reliable contraceptive. The nurse must emphasize the risk of getting pregnant and encourage the client to use contraception when resuming sexual intercourse. It is common to feel a huge range of emotions for a couple of weeks following delivery, but not for several months. The nurse would encourage the client to contact the provider if after a couple of weeks the client still feels anxious or overwhelmed, feels that they cannot handle the baby, does not feel love for the baby, or cannot sleep. These are symptoms of postpartum mood disorder, and the client would need additional support.

CJ Cognitive Skill: Take Actions

Reference: Leifer & Little, 2023, pp. 243–245

Thinking Exercise 20.2.6

Answer

History and Physical	Nurses' Notes	Orders	Laboratory Results

1010: G3P2 client delivered a viable male at 38 weeks' gestation via repeat cesarean section for breech presentation. Apgar scores 6, 8, and 9 at 1, 5, and 10 minutes, respectively. Weight 6 lb, 4 ounces (2.8 kg). Cord blood sent for typing. Estimated blood loss 1200 mL.

1130: Transferred to mother-newborn care unit. Client alert and oriented × 4. VS: T 99.3°F (37.3°C), HR 89 beats/min and regular, RR 14 breaths/min, BP 112/62 mm Hg, SpO$_2$ 96% on RA. Partner at bedside and exhibiting appropriate bonding with newborn.

1600: Client alert and oriented × 4. Cradling newborn with skin-to-skin contact. Respirations equal and unlabored with no adventitious breath sounds. Skin warm and dry with 1+ pitting edema in bilateral lower extremities. Abdomen round with bowel sounds present in all quadrants. Positive flatus and tenderness noted with light palpation. Abdominal incision well-approximated with staples intact. Erythema, swelling, and moderate amount of serosanguineous drainage present. Fundus soft at umbilicus. Moderate amount of lochia rubra noted, no clots. Client uses toilet with standby assist due to reports of light-headedness. Voids 775 mL dark-yellow urine; no burning or difficulty urinating. VS: T 100.6°F (38.1°C), HR 112 beats/min and regular, RR 16 breaths/min, BP 94/69 mm Hg, SpO$_2$ 95% on RA.

1620: Fundal massage performed until midline and firm. Client tolerated well. Client and newborn positioned for breast-feeding. Lactation consultant at bedside.

2030: Client alert and oriented × 4. Newborn sleeping in bassinet at bedside. Abdomen soft and nontender. Incision erythematous but well-approximated with staples intact. No drainage or swelling noted. Fundus midline and firm. Denies light-headedness. Ambulates to the toilet and voids clear, yellow urine without difficulty. Light amount of lochia rubra with several small clots noted on perineal pad. Reviewed plan for discharge home in the morning.

Ambulatory Clinic: 3 Days After Hospital Discharge

1210: Client arrives for postpartum follow-up appointment and staple removal of lower abdominal incision. Alert and oriented × 4. Reports breast-feeding every 2–3 hours including during the night and taking naps during the day when the newborn sleeps. Eats small snacks throughout the day, but has not felt hungry enough to eat a full meal. Abdomen soft, round, and nontender. Denies having a bowel movement since discharge. Lower abdominal incision well approximated. No redness or drainage noted. VS: T 98.6°F (37°C), HR 75 beats/min and regular, RR 14 breaths/min, BP 124/66 mm Hg, SpO$_2$ 97% on RA. Denies pain. Reports a scheduled appointment with the lactation clinic this afternoon and with the obstetrician in 10 days.

Rationale

The nurse would evaluate the client's physiologic and psychological transition to becoming a new parent by assessing the client's ability to develop a positive bond with the newborn, take appropriate care of self, and provide care to the newborn. The client's report of breast-feeding and taking naps when the newborn sleeps are signs the client is effectively transitioning. Breast-feeding every 1 to 3 hours including during the night is important for the growth of the newborn and for the breast-feeding parent to build an adequate supply of milk and ensure breast-feeding success. Breast-feeding, especially throughout the night, can be exhausting. Napping when the newborn sleeps promotes rest for the client and ensures that the client is available to provide care when the newborn is awake. Statements regarding scheduling appropriate follow-up appointments at the lactation clinic and with the obstetrician also indicate an effective transition. The client's dietary intake is concerning and would be further assessed by the nurse to ensure that the nutritional needs of the client and newborn are being met.

CJ Cognitive Skill: Evaluate Outcomes

Reference: Leifer & Little, 2023, pp. 243–247

Stand-Alone Thinking Exercise 20.1

Answer

✗ Consult with a registered dietitian nutritionist.
✗ Provide a balanced diet divided into three meals and three to four snacks daily.
○ Administer glargine insulin 5 units subcutaneously twice a day.
✗ Administer glucose tablets or another oral fast-acting sugar as needed.
✗ Instruct the client on proper methods for obtaining and monitoring FSBG levels.
✗ Administer regular insulin subcutaneously per sliding scale before meals.
✗ Teach the client about signs and symptoms of hyperglycemia and hypoglycemia.

Rationale

Laboratory findings from the 3-hour glucose tolerance tests indicate that the client is not producing enough insulin to maintain normal carbohydrate metabolism. During pregnancy, hormones produced by the placenta (estrogen and progesterone) and increased prolactin levels increase the resistance of cells to insulin and increase the breakdown of insulin. Both processes can lead to accumulation of glucose in the blood and risk for fetal organ damage from resulting hyperglycemia. The nurse would anticipate a diagnosis of gestational diabetes mellitus and physician orders focused on managing blood glucose levels. The nurse would expect to assist the client to properly obtain and monitor FSBG levels and administer insulin subcutaneously. Although oral antihyperglycemic medication may be used to manage glucose levels in clients with gestational diabetes mellitus, current research suggests that use of regular and fast-acting insulins is highly effective and leads to better maternal and fetal outcomes. Glargine insulin is not recommended for use during pregnancy because of variations in basal insulin needs during pregnancy. The nurse must recognize that the client is experiencing episodes of hypoglycemia as manifested by dizziness, chills, and clamminess. The nurse would expect to reinforce teaching on signs and symptoms of both hyperglycemia and hypoglycemia and ways to divide daily food intake over multiple meals and snacks, including a snack before bedtime to minimize the risk of hypoglycemia. Additionally, the nurse would also expect orders for a registered dietitian nutritionist consultation and for the client to always carry glucose tablets or another fast-acting sugar source for use when hypoglycemia symptoms are present.
CJ Cognitive Skills: Recognize Cues, Analyze Cues, Prioritize Hypotheses, Generate Solutions
Reference: Leifer & Little, 2023, pp. 104–107

Stand-Alone Thinking Exercise 20.2—Pharmacology

Answer

The nurse recognizes that the client is *most likely* experiencing **preeclampsia** and would anticipate administration of **magnesium sulfate** and **hydralazine**.

Rationale

Hyperemesis gravidarum is excessive nausea and vomiting that significantly interfere with food intake and fluid balance. Hyperemesis gravidarum manifests as weight loss, dehydration, electrolyte imbalances, and acid-base imbalances. Placenta previa occurs when the placenta develops in the lower part of the uterus rather than the upper part. Painless vaginal bleeding is the main characteristic of placenta previa. The client findings do not correlate with hyperemesis gravidarum or placenta previa. Preeclampsia is an increase in blood pressure and proteinuria that occurs after 20 weeks' gestation in a client who had normal blood pressure before pregnancy. The client does not have a history of hypertension and exhibited normal blood pressure early in pregnancy, but is now experiencing sustained hypertension; the client's blood pressure was greater than 160/110 mm Hg on more than one occasion. The client's urine is also positive for protein. Other manifestations associated with preeclampsia are headache, dizziness, visual disturbances, peripheral edema, and excess weight gain of more than 4 lb (1.8 kg) in 1 week during the second or third trimester. Several drugs are used to treat preeclampsia.

Antihypertensive drugs, such as hydralazine, are used to reduce blood pressure when it reaches a level that might cause intracranial bleeding, usually greater than 160/110 mm Hg. Magnesium sulfate is also prescribed to trigger cerebral vasodilation, reduce potential ischemia generated by cerebral vasospasm, and prevent seizures caused by severe hypertension. The nurse would anticipate administration of these medications. Primary care of the client would be transferred to the registered nurse, but the nurse can assist by closely monitoring the client's blood pressure and communicating to the registered nurse and physician if blood pressure readings remain elevated.

CJ Cognitive Skills: Recognize Cues, Analyze Cues, Prioritize Hypotheses, Generate Solutions
Reference: Leifer & Little, 2023, pp. 90–102; Willihnganz et al., 2022, pp. 378, 438, 626–643

Stand-Alone Thinking Exercise 20.3

Answer

| Assist the client to the knee-chest position | → | | → | Fetal heart rate |
| Apply supplemental oxygen | | Prolapsed umbilical cord | | Fetal movement |

Rationale

Premature labor occurs when regular contractions result in opening of the cervix after 20 weeks' gestation and before 37 weeks' gestation. The client is full term at 39 weeks' gestation. Hypotonic labor is caused by decreased uterine muscle tone and results in contractions that are too weak to be effective during active labor. Clients who experience this dysfunction usually begin labor normally, but contractions diminish after 4 cm of cervical dilation, when the pace of labor is expected to accelerate. The client's cervix is dilated 5 cm, and uterine contractions remain normal. Contractions are reported every 4 to 5 minutes, with each lasting 40 to 60 seconds and increasing in intensity. Uterine rupture, a tear in the uterine wall, occurs when the muscle cannot withstand the pressure inside and manifests with abdominal and chest pain, cessation of contractions, and abdominal or absent fetal heart tones. The client has no signs or symptoms of uterine rupture. Prolapse occurs when the umbilical cord slips downward in the pelvis after the membranes rupture and becomes compressed, decreasing oxygen to the fetus. When the cord is visible at the vaginal opening, the cord is considered completely prolapsed. The client is most likely experiencing an occult prolapse, which is not visible but is suspected due to abnormal fetal heart rates and previous membrane rupture. Nursing care for a prolapsed cord focuses on displacing the fetus upward to stop compression against the pelvis. The knee-chest position can accomplish this displacement. The nurse may also provide supplemental oxygen to increase oxygen availability to the fetus. The nurse would never attempt to replace the cord; this is contraindicated and could cause significant harm to the client and fetus. The nurse would prioritize monitoring the client for signs of fetal hypoxia, which include decreased fetal heart rate and decreased fetal movement. Continuous fetal heart monitoring and engaging the client to identify fetal movement is essential to evaluate if interventions have resolved the umbilical cord prolapse.

CJ Cognitive Skills: Recognize Cues, Analyze Cues, Prioritize Hypotheses, Generate Solutions, Take Actions, Evaluate Outcomes
Reference: Leifer & Little, 2023, pp. 196–206

Answers With Rationales for Thinking Exercises

Unfolding Case Study 21.1

Thinking Exercise 21.1.1

Answer

The nurse recognizes that the client's **SpO₂ level** requires *immediate* follow-up by the health care team.

Rationale

The nurse would recognize that the client's vital signs are not within normal limits. Vital signs of a healthy newborn are T 97.1°F to 99.8°F (36.2°C–37.7°C), HR 110 to 160 beats/min, RR 40 to 60 breaths/min, and $SpO_2 > 94\%$ on RA. Although all of these vital signs are concerning, the nurse would prioritize the SpO_2 level, immediately addressing the client's hypoxia. Other vital signs may naturally correct once the SpO_2 level is within normal limits or would be subsequently addressed by the health care team. Ballard scores are used to determine gestational age. There are no interventions for the scores. The Apgar score is a standardized method of evaluating the newborn's condition immediately after delivery. The nurse would not follow up on the actual Apgar score but instead would use it as additional data to support the client's respiratory and oxygenation findings as priorities.
CJ Cognitive Skill: Recognize Cues
Reference: Leifer & Little, 2023, pp. 296–298, 320–333

Thinking Exercise 21.1.2

Answer

- ○ Asphyxia
- ✗ Cold stress
- ✗ Fluid and electrolyte imbalances
- ○ Phenylketonuria
- ○ Polycythemia
- ✗ Respiratory distress syndrome
- ○ Spina bifida

Rationale

The client's gestational age, Ballard score, and clinical findings indicate a preterm birth, which increases the newborn's risk for many complications. The preterm client is at risk for cold stress resulting from lack of brown fat and other natural temperature-control mechanisms and from fluid and electrolyte imbalances due to immature kidneys. Additionally, the preterm client is at risk for respiratory distress syndrome, a condition caused by lung immaturity and resulting in reduced gas exchange. Asphyxia and polycythemia are common complications of the postterm client due to chronic hypoxia caused by a deteriorated placenta. Spina bifida is a congenital defect, and phenylketonuria is a genetic disorder. Neither are complications of preterm birth.
CJ Cognitive Skill: Analyze Cues
Reference: Leifer & Little, 2023, pp. 320–334, 349

Thinking Exercise 21.1.3

Answer

The nurse determines the *priority* for care at this time is **humidified oxygen** administered via **warm incubator**.

Rationale

The client is experiencing inadequate respiratory function and hypoxia as manifested by low SpO_2 level, tachypnea (RR >60 breaths/min), nasal flaring, grunting, and intercostal and sternal retractions. Supplemental oxygen is required to increase the client's SpO_2 level. The oxygen must be warmed and humidified to prevent drying of the mucous membranes. A warmed incubator is a good way to administer this oxygen, especially because the client is also experiencing cold stress. Signs and symptoms of cold stress are bradycardia (HR <110 beats/min), tachypnea, and mottling of the skin. The nurse would initiate intravenous fluids and gastric feedings if the client is unable to orally ingest adequate fluids and nutrition. Although kangaroo care via skin-to-skin contact is important for client-parent bonding, the client's unstable vital signs must be addressed first.

CJ Cognitive Skill: Prioritize Hypotheses
Reference: Leifer & Little, 2023, pp. 320–333

Thinking Exercise 21.1.4

Answer

CLIENT CONDITIONS		POTENTIAL NURSING ACTIONS
Fluid and electrolyte imbalance	✗ ✗ ✗	Assess the status of fontanelles and tissue turgor. Document urine output by weighing the client's wet diapers. Monitor serum calcium and glucose levels.
Poor control of body temperature	✗ ✗ O	Adjust the incubator to maintain optimal body temperature. Monitor respirations for periods of apnea. Place a skin probe on the client's abdomen below the diaper.
Respiratory distress	✗ ✗ O	Assess arterial blood gas results. Initiate continuous pulse oximetry. Maintain emergency respiratory equipment at the bedside.

Rationale

Immature kidneys in a preterm client lead to improper elimination of body wastes, electrolyte imbalances, and dehydration. The nurse would carefully monitor the client for signs of dehydration as well as overhydration because intravenous fluids are being administered. The nurse would assess the status of fontanelles, tissue turgor, daily weight, and urine output. Subtracting the weight of a dry diaper from the weight of the client's wet diaper is used to determine urine output. Additionally, the nurse would monitor serum calcium and glucose levels. Hypocalcemia is common among preterm and sick newborns due to an immature parathyroid gland. Clients stressed by hypoxia or birth trauma are at high risk for hypocalcemia. The preterm client may also have insufficient stores of glycogen and fat, which increases the risk of hypoglycemia. A skin probe is used to monitor the temperature of preterm clients. The nurse would place the probe on the right upper quadrant of the client's abdomen, ensuring that it is not directly over a bony prominence or under the diaper. The nurse would adjust the temperature of the incubator to keep the client's body temperature within normal limits (97.1°F–98.6°F [36.2°C–37°C]). The nurse would also monitor the client for signs and symptoms of cold stress including increased respiratory rate with periods of apnea. Newborns receiving oxygen therapy must be monitored closely for oxygen toxicity. The nurse would initiate continuous pulse oximetry to monitor SpO_2 levels and assess the arterial blood gas to determine if ventilation and perfusion are adequate. Emergency equipment should be readily available in case suctioning or mechanical bag-valve-mask ventilation is required.

CJ Cognitive Skill: Generate Solutions
Reference: Leifer & Little, 2023, pp. 320–333

Thinking Exercise 21.1.5

Answer

✗ Assess bowel sounds and monitor for the passage of meconium.
✗ Consult a certified lactation consultant for suck-training exercises.
✗ Encourage manual expression of breast milk after feeding attempts.
✗ Evaluate the strength of the client's suck reflex.
○ Initiate gavage feedings via nasogastric tube.
✗ Use a small, soft nipple with a large hole when bottle-feeding.
✗ Wake the client and promote breast-feeding every 2 to 3 hours.

Rationale

The ability to coordinate breathing, sucking, and swallowing develops at 32 to 36 weeks' gestation. Therefore the preterm client born at 34 weeks' gestation may have trouble sucking. Signs of ineffective sucking are latching on and then letting go of the breast repeatedly, pushing away or resisting latch-on, and falling asleep or sucking for only a few minutes. The nurse would initially assess bowel sounds and monitor for the passage of meconium, which are signs of intestinal readiness for feeding. The nurse would also assess the strength of the client's suck reflex by placing a clean finger in the client's mouth and touching the roof of the mouth. There are several exercises that can be used to strengthen the client's ability to suck. The nurse would consult a certified lactation consultant to teach the parents suck-training exercises, positions that may assist the client to latch, and other strategies to promote effective breast-feeding. Most newborns will learn to breast-feed effectively if given time. Therefore the nurse would encourage the parent to wake the client and attempt to breast-feed every 2 to 3 hours. Some clients may require supplemental bottle-feeding while strengthening the suck reflex. Bottle-feedings should occur after each attempt to breast-feed, and a small, soft nipple with a large hole should be used to minimize the energy and effort required for sucking. Breast milk is ideal, therefore the nurse would encourage the parent to manually express breast milk for the preterm client's bottle. Gavage feedings via a nasogastric tube may be required if the client is unable to manage fluid and calorie needs with breast or bottle feedings, but all other options would be implemented first for the preterm client born at 34 weeks' gestation. Finally, the nurse would monitor the client's intake, output, and daily weights to evaluate fluid and nutritional outcomes.

CJ Cognitive Skill: Take Actions
Reference: Leifer & Little, 2023, pp. 320–333

Thinking Exercise 21.1.6

Answer

DATA COLLECTION FINDINGS	IMPROVING	NOT IMPROVING
Breast-feeding		✗
Fluid balance	✗	
Oxygenation	✗	
Temperature		✗

Rationale

The client's fluid balance and oxygenation status are improving. Skin and neurologic findings as well as heart rate, respiratory rate, and SpO_2 levels on room air indicate that oxygenation issues are improving. Additionally, respiration and ventilation efforts have improved; the client is no longer presenting with nasal flaring, grunting, or intercostal and sternal retractions. Urine intake and output are within normal limits and demonstrate adequate fluid balance. It is normal for a newborn to lose 7% to 10% of birth weight during the first few days after birth. This weight loss does not indicate a fluid imbalance.

The nurse would expect the client to regain lost weight within the next 2 weeks. Breast-feeding and temperature control have not improved. The client remains unable to effectively breast-feed and continues to need supplemental bottle feedings. The client also requires a bedside warmer to maintain a normal body temperature. The client's temperature decreased from 98.2°F (36.7°C) to 97.1°F (36.1°C) during the 30-minute feeding.

CJ Cognitive Skill: Evaluate Outcomes
Reference: Leifer & Little, 2023, pp. 320–333

Unfolding Case Study 21.2

Thinking Exercise 21.2.1

Answer

- ✗ Auscultated breath sounds
- ✗ Last diaper change
- ○ Length of feeding
- ✗ Level of consciousness
- ○ Parent's expressed frustration
- ✗ Quality of respirations
- ○ Vital signs

Rationale

The nurse would recognize all options as requiring follow-up by the nurse but would prioritize the client's physiologic complications before addressing parental teaching and psychosocial needs. Lethargy, anuria (no urine for more than 6 hours), audibly wet respirations, frequent coughing, and rhonchi auscultated throughout the lung fields are signs of potential life-threatening conditions for the newborn and require immediate follow-up to prevent respiratory, circulatory, and neurologic complications. The client's vital signs are currently within normal limits and do not require immediate follow-up but would be monitored closely.

CJ Cognitive Skill: Recognize Cues
Reference: Leifer & Little, 2023, pp. 289–318

Thinking Exercise 21.2.2

Answer

The nurse recognizes that client findings are ***most likely*** caused by __aspiration__ and __dehydration__.

Rationale

The client findings are consistent with aspiration and dehydration. The client has several risk factors for aspiration including cleft lip and palate and lying supine after feeding. Inadequate oral pressure and compensatory muscle movements due to the client's cleft lip and palate affect all phases of swallowing and increase the client's risk of aspiration and respiratory distress. Signs of aspiration during feeding include weak sucking, choking, coughing, tachypnea, and milk leaking from the nasal passages. Client findings consistent with respiratory distress are wet or gurgle-sounding respirations, cough, and auscultated rhonchi or rales. Additional signs of respiratory distress include tachypnea, nasal flaring, retractions, cyanosis, and grunting. Clients with cleft lip and palate are also at risk for dehydration due to difficulty with adequate oral fluid intake. Signs of dehydration in a newborn are decreased urine output, lethargy, and depressed fontanelles. Urine output for a newborn should be 1 to 2 mL/kg/h. Maple syrup urine disease is a defect in the metabolism of amino acids. An infant with maple syrup urine disease appears healthy at birth but soon develops feeding difficulties, loss of Moro reflex, hypotonia, irregular respirations, convulsions, and a sweet aroma from urine, sweat, and cerumen. Although the client is experiencing respiratory distress, the client's Moro reflex is intact, muscle tone is normal, and no maple syrup odor is noted. Cephalohematoma is a collection of blood between the surface of the cranial bone and the periosteal membrane, usually caused by trauma during birth. No client findings suggest this condition. Trisomy 21 syndrome, the most common type of Down syndrome, is a chromosomal abnormality consisting of three number 21 chromosomes rather than two. Typical manifestations of Down syndrome in an infant are an upward slant of the canthal folds of the eyes, a protruding tongue, and a short, thick neck. Although clients may experience more than one birth defect, client findings are not caused by the additional chromosome 21.

CJ Cognitive Skill: Analyze Cues
Reference: Leifer & Little, 2023, pp. 291, 328, 343–344, 350–353

Thinking Exercise 21.2.3

Answer

The nurse determines the *priority* for care at this time is to manage the client's **airway**. The nurse's *priority* action would be to **place the client in the high-Fowler position**.

Rationale

The nurse would prioritize airway management and place the client in an upward or high-Fowler position to ensure that the airway is patent and decrease additional aspiration of breast milk. The client may be held in this position or placed in an upright car seat so other interventions may be implemented. Care for the client may include nasal and oral suctioning to remove trapped milk as well as supplemental oxygen if SpO_2 levels drop further. Intubation, mechanical ventilation, endotracheal suctioning, and transfer to the neonatal intensive care unit may also be necessary. The nurse would prioritize fluid resuscitation after stabilizing the client's airway and breathing. Care plans for client nutrition and surgical repair of orofacial clefts are important but would not take precedence over the client's airway, breathing, and circulatory needs.

CJ Cognitive Skill: Prioritize Hypotheses
Reference: Leifer & Little, 2023, pp. 321–326, 341–344

Thinking Exercise 21.2.4

Answer

○ "Breast-feeding is the best way to meet your baby's nutritional needs."
✗ "Feedings should be about 30 minutes or less to prevent exhaustion and calorie loss."
○ "Milk leaking from the client's nose and mouth during feedings is a sign of choking."
✗ "Place your baby in an upright, sitting position to prevent the backflow of milk."
✗ "Tilt the bottle so the nipple is always filled and pointed down away from the cleft."
✗ "Use the specialized cleft palate bottle provided to you by the lactation consultant."
✗ "You should burp your baby two to three times during feedings."

Rationale

Clients with a cleft lip are usually able to breast-feed with some modifications. In most cases, clients with both cleft lip and cleft palate are unable to breast-feed. The parent may choose to attempt breast-feeding but must be aware that it may be necessary to bottle-feed to meet developmental weight and nutritional outcomes. Specially designed feeding bottles and teats are used to help the client draw milk from the bottle when naturally generated negative intraoral pressure is insufficient. The parent would be taught to position the client in an upright position to prevent backflow, to keep the bottle tilted so the nipple is always filled with milk and pointed down away from the cleft, and to feed for no longer than 30 minutes to prevent exhaustion and loss of calories that the baby needs. The nurse would also reinforce that babies with oral cleft need to be burped more often because they take in more air while feeding. Burping 2 to 3 times during each feeding is recommended. Additionally, some milk escaping

through the nose is common and expected. This is not a sign of choking, and holding the baby in a more upright position will lessen the amount of milk coming through the nose.
CJ Cognitive Skill: Generate Solutions
Reference: Leifer & Little, 2023, pp. 341–344

Thinking Exercise 21.2.5

Answer

○ Assess pain using the Wong-Baker FACES® scale.
○ Carefully position the client on the abdomen to rest.
○ Encourage the client to use a pacifier.
✗ Ensure that the client is adequately swaddled.
✗ Gently cleanse the suture line with sterile water.
○ Provide tube feedings until the incision heals.

Rationale

Cheiloplasty repairs the client's cleft lip and is usually scheduled when the infant is about 3 months of age. Priorities after cheiloplasty are similar to most surgical procedures and focus on pain management, wound care, and infection prevention. Gently cleansing the suture line with sterile water promotes wound healing by preventing crust formation and infection. The nurse would prioritize assessing pain and discomfort and administering medications for pain and sedation as needed. Using the Wong-Baker FACES® scale would not be appropriate for the newborn client. The nurse would use the FLACC (faces, legs, activity, cry, consolability) scale to assess the client's pain. Care should be taken to protect the client's fragile lip and surgical incision for several weeks after surgery. The nurse would ensure that the client is properly swaddled to provide comfort, restore warmth, and prevent the infant from scratching the incision. The infant would not be positioned on the abdomen due to the risk of rubbing the incision on the hard surface. Similarly, a pacifier would not be used due to the increased pressure exerted on the back of the surgical wound during sucking. Oral nutrition would be resumed after surgery with specialized nipples for bottle feedings.
CJ Cognitive Skill: Take Actions
Reference: Leifer, 2023, pp. 341–344

Thinking Exercise 21.2.6

Answer

CLIENT STATEMENTS	UNDERSTANDING	NO UNDERSTANDING
"Cuddling with my baby will provide emotional support for us both."	✗	
"I will administer children's aspirin to manage my baby's pain."		✗
"It is important to prevent bumping or scratching of the lip and nose areas."	✗	
"Now that the cleft lip is fixed, I can breast-feed instead of using the bottle."		✗
"I will use a cotton-tipped applicator to gently cleanse the sutures and apply topical ointment."	✗	

Rationale

Embracing and cuddling with the infant provides emotional support and bonding for both the parent and client. This may also help comfort and console the client, who is unable to obtain the usual satisfaction from sucking. The nurse would reinforce cradling and swaddling strategies that prevent accidental bumping of the clients facial incisions. Soft arm or elbow restraints, such as a Logan bow, may also help prevent the client from rubbing or scratching the incision. The surgical procedure repaired only the client's cleft lip. Palatoplasty, repair of the cleft palate, is usually scheduled when the baby is 10 to 12 months of age. Because the palate is still open, the infant would most likely not be able to establish the suction required to breast-feed. The nurse would reinforce teaching regarding the use of specialized cleft palate nipples for client feedings. The client's parents would be taught to keep the surgical area and suture line clean. A cotton-tipped applicator should be used to cleanse the sutures and apply a coating of topical antibiotic ointment after each feeding. Aspirin is not recommended for children as it can cause Reye syndrome. The client will most likely be prescribed acetaminophen or an opioid medication for short-term management of surgical pain.

CJ Cognitive Skill: Evaluate Outcomes
Reference: Leifer & Little, 2023, pp. 341–344

Stand-Alone Thinking Exercise 21.1

Answer

DATA COLLECTION FINDINGS	IMPROVING	NOT IMPROVING
Breast-feeding		✗
Jaundice	✗	
Level of consciousness	✗	
Temperature		✗
Weight		✗

Rationale

The client is experiencing hyperbilirubinemia as manifested by elevated total bilirubin level, changes in level of consciousness (early signs of encephalopathy and kernicterus), and jaundice of the skin, sclera, and urine. Hyperbilirubinemia occurring in a breast-feeding newborn over 24 hours after birth is most likely caused by a lack of caloric and fluid intake. The client is having trouble latching, has not eaten in several hours, and is exhibiting symptoms of inadequate intake including decreased urination and stooling. The client has also lost weight since birth, but the amount of neonatal weight lost is within normal limits: 5% to 10% of birth weight within the first 48 hours. The nurse recognizes the client's primary problems and collaborates with the health care team to implement appropriate care: a lactation consultant to assist the parent and client with breast-feeding and phototherapy to promote bilirubin excretion through the skin. Client findings that indicate the treatment plan is effective and the client is improving are (1) improved level of consciousness from lethargic to easily aroused and (2) jaundice now localized to the face and sclera. Although the client is latching and feeding for 5 to 10 minutes on each breast, the client's dietary intake has not improved to a normal feeding schedule (every 2–3 hours). Additionally, the recommended frequency for breast-feeding in the management of early-onset jaundice is every 1.5 to 2 hours. The nurse must engage the parent in feeding the client more frequently. The client's temperature has also decreased significantly and is no longer within normal limits (97.7°F–100°F [36.5°C–37.5°C]). Further interventions are needed to help the newborn maintain an adequate temperature.

CJ Cognitive Skills: Recognize Cues, Analyze Cues, Prioritize Hypotheses, Generate Solutions, Take Actions, Evaluate Outcomes
Reference: Leifer & Little, 2023, pp. 305, 328, 355–356

Stand-Alone Thinking Exercise 21.2

Answer

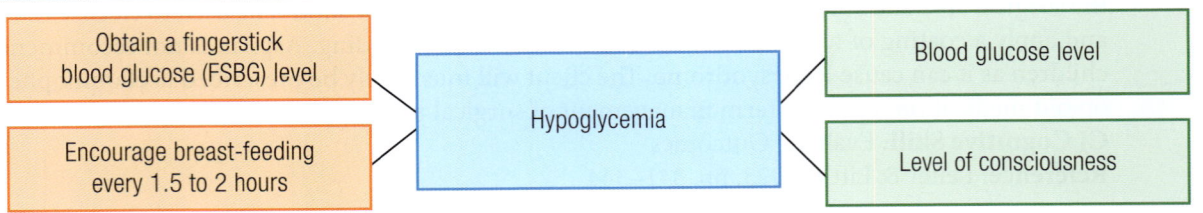

Rationale

The nurse would recognize the client's birth weight as above normal. Infants whose weight is greater than the 90th percentile for gestational age are classified as large for gestational age. The client's weight is within the 95th percentile and is most likely caused by maternal diabetes and poor glycemic control during pregnancy. This condition is termed *macrosomia* and increases the client's risk for numerous complications including birth trauma, hypoglycemia, hypocalcemia, hyperbilirubinemia, and neonatal sepsis. The client is most likely experiencing hypoglycemia as manifested by irritability; weak, high-pitched cry; diaphoresis; tremors; and tachypnea. The nurse would obtain the client's finger stick blood glucose (FSBG) level and collaborate with the registered nurse to provide care. A glucose level less than 40 mg/dL (term) and 30 mg/dL (preterm) is considered hypoglycemic in a newborn and would be treated with dextrose 10% administered intravenously via a slow, continuous drip or on an intermittent schedule every 2 to 3 hours. The nurse would plan to monitor glucose levels frequently and may implement continuous glucose monitoring. The nurse would also encourage breast-feeding every 1.5 to 2 hours because the client is tolerating feeding. Frequent breast-feeding helps the newborn maintain blood glucose levels within normal limits. The client is experiencing mild respiratory distress (tachypnea and nasal flaring), but SpO_2 levels remain within normal limits. Therefore supplemental oxygen would not be needed at this time. Hypoglycemia-induced convulsions are a life-threatening complication of newborn hypoglycemia. The nurse would monitor for decreased level of consciousness (lethargy and stupor), tremors, and other signs of seizure activity. Phenylketonuria (PKU) is a genetic disorder that causes severe cognitive delay that presents between 4 and 6 months of age. A blood test is used to detect PKU, but symptoms would not be present within the first few hours of life. Isoimmunization occurs with Rh and ABO incompatibilities, which are not present. Swaddling the client in a blanket, monitoring urinary output, and preventing heat loss are interventions for all newborns and not specific to macrosomia or hypoglycemia.

CJ Cognitive Skills: Recognize Cues, Analyze Cues, Prioritize Hypotheses, Generate Solutions, Take Actions, Evaluate Outcomes

Reference: Leifer & Little, 2023, pp. 326–327

Answers With Rationales for Thinking Exercises

Unfolding Case Study 22.1

Thinking Exercise 22.1.1

Answer

History and Physical	Nurses' Notes	Orders	Laboratory Results

1540: Child transferred to PACU following tonsillectomy and adenoidectomy for recurrent upper respiratory infections; parent at bedside. Child placed in side-lying position; ice collar in place. Child whimpering and stating throat hurts "a lot." No nausea or vomiting. Small amount of pinkish drainage from mouth on tissue. Eating a few ice chips. IV infusing in left forearm. VS: 99°F (37.2°C), HR 100 beats/min, RR 24 breaths/min, BP 98/50 mm Hg, SpO$_2$ 94% on RA. Acetaminophen administered per agency protocol.

1645: Child dozing intermittently; restless at times. Swallowing frequently while sleeping. VS: 98.6°F (37°C), HR 104 beats/min, RR 24 breaths/min, BP 94/50 mm Hg, SpO$_2$ 93% on RA.

Rationale

Any child is at risk for complications after a tonsillectomy. Frequent swallowing while sleeping and restlessness are findings that require immediate follow-up because the child could be experiencing a potentially life-threatening postoperative complication. Pinkish drainage is not unusual immediately after surgery. The vital signs are within normal range for the child's age at this time, but the nurse would monitor these values on an ongoing basis because they could change. The child's pain is not life threatening, but the nurse administered acetaminophen.
CJ Cognitive Skill: Recognize Cues
Reference: Leifer & Little, 2023, p. 606

Thinking Exercise 22.1.2

Answer

The client is ***most likely*** experiencing **hemorrhage** as evidenced by **restlessness** and **frequent swallowing**.

Rationale

Bleeding (hemorrhage) is the most common postoperative complication associated with tonsillectomy. Frequent swallowing while sleeping is an early indication of bleeding after this type of surgery. Restlessness could be related to pain or bleeding, possibly caused by lack of perfusion to the brain. The child's temperature is within normal range, and there is no other indication of infection. Sleep apnea is often associated with enlarged tonsils in a child, but the child had a tonsillectomy.
CJ Cognitive Skill: Analyze Cues
Reference: Leifer & Little, 2023, p. 606

Thinking Exercise 22.1.3

Answer

The *priority* for client care at this time is to prevent **hypovolemic shock**.

Rationale

Any client who is experiencing hemorrhage is at risk for fluid deficit and potential hypovolemic shock. Lack of circulating blood within the body decreases perfusion to major body organs and results in subsequent shock. Infection, including pneumonia, is not a commonly occurring complication, but it can occur as early as 24 to 48 hours after surgery and as late as 2 weeks postoperatively. Therefore infection at the surgical site or in the respiratory tract would not be the priority for client care at this time.
CJ Cognitive Skill: Prioritize Hypotheses
Reference: Leifer & Little, 2023, p. 606

Thinking Exercise 22.1.4

Answer

POTENTIAL NURSING ACTIONS	INDICATED	NOT INDICATED
Transfer care of the client to the registered nurse.	✗	
Decrease the IV infusion rate.		✗
Observe the client carefully for bleeding.	✗	
Monitor vital signs every 30 minutes.	✗	
Report relevant client findings to the surgeon.	✗	

Rationale

This client likely has a potentially life-threatening hemorrhage, which would be managed by the registered nurse. The registered nurse would manage the care of any client with an unstable condition, but the licensed vocational nurse/licensed practical nurse (LVN/LPN) can assist with care. The nurse would carefully observe the client for any signs of oral bleeding and frequently monitor vital signs to assess for indications of fluid deficit. Because the client may experience or is experiencing fluid deficit, the nurse would increase the IV infusion rate per agency protocol, not decrease. All client findings related to postoperative hemorrhage should be reported to the surgeon as soon as possible.
CJ Cognitive Skill: Generate Solutions
Reference: Leifer & Little, 2023, p. 606

Thinking Exercise 22.1.5

Answer

✗ Monitor the client for indications of fluid overload after increasing the IV infusion rate.
○ Encourage the client to drink fluids to prevent dehydration.
✗ Keep the client in the sitting position with the head elevated.
✗ Administer the ordered opioid medication for pain management.
✗ Prepare the parent and client for a possible treatment procedure in the operating suite.

Rationale

Although it is appropriate to increase the IV infusion rate to prevent fluid deficit, too many fluids can quickly cause circulatory overload in a young child. Therefore the nurse would monitor the client for this complication. The client may need an invasive intervention to stop bleeding, such as electrocautery. This procedure and similar treatments are performed in the operating suite under sedation. Therefore the nurse would not encourage the client to drink fluids prior to another visit to the operating suite.

To prevent aspiration of blood, the client would be kept in the sitting position so the head is elevated. The acetaminophen did not effectively manage the client's pain. Therefore the nurse would administer an opioid to achieve better pain control. Crying and whimpering irritate the throat and can increase or cause bleeding.
CJ Cognitive Skill: Take Actions
Reference: Leifer & Little, 2023, p. 606

Thinking Exercise 22.1.6

Answer

The client's condition has **improved** as evidenced by **no additional bleeding**.

Rationale

The client experienced bleeding as a result of having a tonsillectomy. The nurse increased the client's IV infusion rate and frequently monitored the client's vital signs for indications of fluid deficit and possible hypovolemic shock. As a result, there was no additional bleeding noted, and vital signs remained stable. Therefore the client's condition improved because there was no additional bleeding. The client's pain was better managed by administering an opioid drug because the client rated the pain as 1/10 rather than 5/10 on the FACES scale. A pain rating of 1/10 indicates that the pain "hurts a little bit," and a rating of 5/10 indicates that the pain "hurts the worst." The parent, not the client, experienced the anxiety.
CJ Cognitive Skill: Evaluate Outcomes
Reference: Leifer & Little, 2023, pp. 486–487, 606

Unfolding Case Study 22.2

Thinking Exercise 22.2.1

Answer

- ✗ Temperature
- ✗ Heart rate
- ✗ Respiratory rate
- ✗ Blood pressure
- ○ SpO$_2$
- ○ Weight
- ○ Skin turgor/mucous membranes
- ✗ Decreased urine output

Rationale

This newborn infant has been vomiting and therefore losing body fluids. The client has fewer wet diapers as a result of less fluid being retained, which indicates a decrease in urine output. This finding requires immediate follow-up because the client may have kidney impairment, dehydration, urinary obstruction, or another potentially life-threatening condition. The client's axillary temperature is above 99°F (37.2°C), which indicates a fever. A fever in a newborn infant can be life threatening and requires immediate follow-up. The client's heart rate and respiratory rate are elevated above normal range for age and require immediate follow-up because these changes could indicate a life-threatening condition. The infant's blood pressure is lower than expected, which may decrease perfusion (blood flow) to major organs—also a potentially life-threatening condition. The client's weight loss, poor skin turgor, and dry mucous membranes are not immediately life threatening but indicate a fluid deficit from frequent vomiting. The SpO$_2$ is above 90%, which is within the expected range.
CJ Cognitive Skill: Recognize Cues
Reference: Leifer & Little, 2023, pp. 664–666, 676–677

Thinking Exercise 22.2.2

Answer

- ✗ Urinary tract infection
- ✗ Electrolyte imbalance
- ○ Intussusception
- ✗ Aspiration pneumonia
- ✗ Urinary calculi

Rationale

Any client with decreased urinary output usually has a more concentrated urine. Concentrated urine can lead to urinary tract infection and/or urinary calculi (stones). Decreased body fluid also changes the concentration of electrolytes in the blood, causing electrolyte imbalances, especially low serum sodium. Vomiting also causes sodium loss because sodium is a large component of gastric juices. Vomitus can be aspirated by the infant and cause the development of pneumonia. Intussusception is a telescoping or slipping of one part of the small intestine into another part just below it. It usually occurs in children between 3 months and 2 years of age. This condition is not a complication of fluid deficit.

CJ Cognitive Skill: Analyze Cues
Reference: Leifer & Little, 2023, pp. 664–666, 676–677, 668, 693–695

Thinking Exercise 22.2.3

Answer

The *priority* for the client's care at this time is to prevent **major organ dysfunction**.

Rationale

The infant is experiencing fluid deficit (dehydration) from loss of fluids via frequent vomiting. As a result of hypovolemia, major organs may not be adequately perfused. Without adequate blood flow, major body organs, such as the kidneys, heart, and brain, cannot properly function due to lack of oxygen. Organ failure is a life-threatening condition. If the vomiting continues over time, the infant could become malnourished, which can result in delayed physical and mental development. Excessive or prolonged vomiting can result in metabolic alkalosis because the stomach contains hydrochloric acid, which is lost. The infant is not at risk for metabolic acidosis. Although a urinary tract infection can occur when a client is dehydrated, preventing this condition is not the priority for care.

CJ Cognitive Skill: Prioritize Hypotheses
Reference: Leifer & Little, 2023, pp. 664–666

Thinking Exercise 22.2.4

Answer

POTENTIAL NURSING ACTIONS	INDICATED	NOT INDICATED
Establish peripheral IV access for fluids.	✗	
Continue to feed the infant as usual.		✗
Draw labs per orders.	✗	
Prepare for emergency surgery.	✗	
Document the diaper count per agency protocol.	✗	

Rationale

Pyloric stenosis is an obstruction of the lower end of the stomach (pylorus) caused by either frequent spasms of the pyloric sphincter or hypertrophy of the circular muscles of the pylorus. Symptoms usually begin when the infant is 2 or 3 weeks of age. Vomiting is the most common finding in this condition. To relieve the obstruction, emergency surgery (pyloromyotomy) is performed. Labs should be drawn to correct any electrolyte imbalances, and IV access would be established. The nurse would not feed the infant because this would cause more vomiting due to the obstruction, and the infant should be NPO if surgery is planned in the next few hours.
CJ Cognitive Skill: Generate Solutions
Reference: Leifer & Little, 2023, pp. 664–666

Thinking Exercise 22.2.5

Answer

✗ Monitor vital signs every 1 to 2 hours.
○ Connect the nasogastric tube to low continuous suction.
○ Place the infant in the prone position.
✗ Assess the infant for pain, and manage accordingly.
✗ Advise the parents that the infant can be fed as usual later today.
○ Insert an indwelling urinary catheter to assess output.
✗ Take daily weights each morning before feeding.

Rationale

As for any client having surgery, the nurse would monitor vital signs frequently immediately after the procedure and manage the client's pain. For this client, the nurse would use the Neonatal Infant Pain Scale (NIPS) to assess pain level and guide appropriate and effective pain control. For the pyloromyotomy procedure, the muscle is cut, but the small bowel is not affected. Therefore a nasogastric tube for decompression would not be needed. The infant is placed in the sitting (Fowler) position rather than the prone position to facilitate drainage. The infant is fed as soon as possible with precautions, including frequent burping and lying the infant on the right side after feeding to facilitate digestion and movement of the feeding into the small intestine. Overfeeding is avoided. A diaper count is maintained rather than inserting a urinary catheter that can cause a urinary tract infection. Daily weights are carefully recorded to indicate fluid balance and nutritional status.
CJ Cognitive Skill: Take Actions
Reference: Leifer & Little, 2023, pp. 487, 664–666

Thinking Exercise 22.2.6

Answer

CLIENT FINDINGS	IMPROVED	NOT IMPROVED
Feeding	✗	
Heart rate		✗
Weight	✗	
Temperature		✗

Rationale

The infant's condition of pyloric stenosis has improved as evidenced by taking and retaining bottle feedings along with gaining weight. However, the infant's temperature has worsened, and the infant now has a fever. The infant's heart rate has increased, most likely due to the fever causing increased metabolism. The infant may have an infection, which should be identified and managed as soon as possible.

CJ Cognitive Skill: Evaluate Outcomes
Reference: Leifer & Little, 2023, pp. 664–666

Unfolding Case Study 22.3

Thinking Exercise 22.3.1

Answer

BODY SYSTEMS	CLIENT FINDINGS
Respiratory	✗ Occasional dyspnea ○ Decreased SpO$_2$
Skin/musculoskeletal	✗ Thoracic and abdominal rash ✗ Joint pain and swelling
Metabolic	✗ Fever ○ Fatigue

Rationale

The child has several findings that require immediate follow-up because they could indicate potentially life-threatening conditions. Although the child is not currently experiencing respiratory distress, the report of occasional dyspnea on exertion requires immediate follow-up because it could worsen. The SpO$_2$ is within normal range at this time. Joint pain and swelling are not expected for a child and are concerning because these findings could affect mobility and quality of life. Although rashes are typically not life threatening, a rash extending over the chest and abdomen could suggest a possible communicable condition and pose an issue related to body image and self-concept for the preadolescent. Therefore the rash requires immediate follow-up. A fever also requires immediate follow-up because if it continues or worsens, the child could experience fluid and electrolyte imbalances.

CJ Cognitive Skill: Recognize Cues
Reference: Leifer & Little, 2023, pp. 633–635

Thinking Exercise 22.3.2

Answer

CLIENT FINDINGS	RUBELLA (GERMAN MEASLES)	SYSTEMIC JUVENILE IDIOPATHIC ARTHRITIS	RHEUMATIC FEVER
Fever	✗	✗	✗
Rash	✗	✗	✗
Fatigue		✗	✗
Pain that moves from joint to joint			✗

Rationale

All of the client findings are consistent with rheumatic fever. Rheumatic fever is an inflammatory, autoimmune systemic condition that occurs as a complication of untreated group A beta-hemolytic streptococcus throat infection. This disorder ranges from mild to severe and occurs 1 to 6 weeks after the strep throat infection. Classic findings include migratory polyarthritis, skin rash, chorea, fever, abdominal pain, fever, fatigue, and carditis (inflammation of the heart). Rubella, also known as German measles, is a communicable disease that commonly presents with fever and rash. Joints are usually not affected. Children with juvenile idiopathic arthritis, especially when systemic, have low-grade fever, fatigue, rash, and joint involvement. However, the joint pain and swelling do not move from joint to joint, and at least five joints are involved at one time.

CJ Cognitive Skill: Analyze Cues
Reference: Leifer & Little, 2023, pp. 585–586, 633–635, 744–748

Thinking Exercise 22.3.3

Answer

The **priority** for the client's care is to monitor for findings associated with **heart failure** because the client's condition can cause **carditis**.

Rationale

Based on the analysis of relevant findings, the child likely has rheumatic fever. Rheumatic fever can cause inflammation of the heart, a condition called *carditis*. This condition can be fatal because it can lead to heart enlargement and failure. The myocardium, pericardium, epicardium, and heart valves are affected most often. Therefore the priority for the nurse would be to monitor for findings associated with heart failure, including cyanosis, tachycardia, and tachypnea. Rheumatic fever does not cause pyelonephritis (kidney infection) resulting in acute kidney injury. Respiratory failure can occur as a result of carditis, depending on the heart tissues that are affected. Pneumonia is not a common finding associated with rheumatic fever.

CJ Cognitive Skill: Prioritize Hypotheses
Reference: Leifer & Little, 2023, pp. 633–635

Thinking Exercise 22.3.4

Answer

✗ Draw blood for anti-streptolysin O (ASO) titer.
✗ Perform an electrocardiogram.
✗ Draw blood for erythrocyte sedimentation rate.
○ Prepare to transfer the client to an acute care pediatric unit.
✗ Anticipate an order for one of the penicillin drugs.

Rationale

Several lab tests can help confirm a diagnosis of rheumatic fever, including ASO, ESR, and C-reactive protein. These tests are markers for inflammation and support the presence of systemic inflammation. An ECG helps confirm if the heart is affected by the condition. Cardiac involvement can be fatal. One of the penicillins is typically prescribed to manage the client's underlying strep infection. This client seems to have a milder case of rheumatic fever and therefore would likely not be admitted to the acute care unit.

CJ Cognitive Skill: Generate Solutions
Reference: Leifer & Little, 2023, pp. 633–635

Thinking Exercise 22.3.5—Pharmacology

Answer

✗ "Take medications with food because they can cause gastrointestinal distress, especially diarrhea."

○ "Make arrangements to have the penicillin injection given every 28 days."

✗ "Even if the client is feeling better, be sure to give all of the prescribed doses."

○ "Penicillin V potassium will help relieve the client's joint pain and fever."

✗ "Inform the health care provider if the client has any allergies to penicillin or other antibiotics."

✗ "Call the clinic if the client experiences any episodes of bleeding or excessive bruising."

✗ "The client will need to take a prophylactic antibiotic prior to any medical or dental procedure."

Rationale

Penicillins, such as penicillin V potassium and amoxicillin, are commonly used to treat strep infections. These drugs do not work to treat pain, but body temperature and joint pain should decrease as the infection resolves. Before penicillin is prescribed, the nurse would ensure that the prescriber is aware of any allergies to penicillin or other antibiotics. Penicillin V potassium is an oral drug and would not be administered via injection; the entire prescription should be taken no matter how the child feels. In addition to treatment with penicillin, the child should take a prophylactic antibiotic prior to any invasive medical or dental procedure. Naproxen is a nonsteroidal anti-inflammatory drug that can help relieve joint pain by decreasing inflammation. Bleeding is an adverse effect that should be immediately reported to the prescriber.

CJ Cognitive Skill: Take Actions

Reference: Leifer & Little, 2023, pp. 633–635; Willihnganz, et al., 2022, pp. 740–742

Thinking Exercise 22.3.6

Answer

History and Physical	Nurses' Notes	Orders	Laboratory Results

Pediatric Clinic Initial Visit

1740: Child brought to clinic by grandparent, who is the child's legal guardian. Grandparent reports that child has had joint pain that moves from one joint to another and a rash on the chest and abdomen for several days. Child reports lack of appetite, fatigue, and occasional dyspnea on exertion. Grandparent reports that the child had a very sore throat with a "little fever" about 3 weeks ago but does not have a sore throat now. Did not take child for medical attention 3 weeks ago due to lack of health insurance. Borrowed money from a family member to pay for today's clinical visit. Child currently presents with swollen knee joints bilaterally and left wrist redness and swelling, but can move all extremities. Reddened circular rash on anterior thorax and abdomen noted. No adventitious breath sounds throughout lung fields. No respiratory distress; denies chest pain. VS: T 102.6°F (39.2°C), HR 90 beats/min and regular, RR 20 breaths/min, BP 100/62 mm Hg, SpO_2 95% on RA.

1815: Blood drawn for BMP, ASO titer, and ESR. ECG performed: Normal sinus rhythm. No abnormalities noted.

1850: Health teaching for child discharge to home with grandparent. Advised grandparent to allow child to rest and play quietly. Prescription for penicillin V potassium and naproxen; given discount coupons for drugs.

Pediatric Clinic Follow-Up Visit—2 Weeks Later

0830: Follow-up visit for rheumatic fever diagnosed 2 weeks ago and treated at home with drug therapy and rest. Grandparent reports that child wanted to visit with friends and go to school, so did not rest as much during drug therapy as intended. Took all of the antibiotic doses as prescribed. Joint pain and swelling decreased; rash barely visible. Yesterday, child had several episodes of shortness of breath and chest discomfort. Appetite remains poor. Has intermittent fevers, mostly in the evenings. VS: 99.4°F (37.4°C), HR 88 beats/min and irregular, RR 26 breaths/min, BP 104/56 mm Hg, SpO_2 91% on RA.

Rationale

Some of the client findings have improved, including decreased joint pain and swelling as well as a less-visible rash. Other findings have stayed the same, such as fever (although now intermittent) and poor appetite. The findings that indicate worsening of the client's condition are chest discomfort, tachypnea, and dyspnea. Additionally, the peripheral oxygen saturation rate (SpO_2) has decreased from 95% to 91%. This decline indicates early hypoxemia and should be managed to prevent the SpO_2 from decreasing below 90%.

CJ Cognitive Skill: Evaluate Outcomes
Reference: Leifer & Little, 2023, pp. 633–635

Stand-Alone Thinking Exercise 22.1

Answer

Stop the blood transfusion	→		→	SpO_2
Increase the oxygen rate	→	Fluid overload	→	Vital signs

Rationale

Fluid (circulatory) overload is always a possibility when children receive infusions. Client findings associated with fluid overload include dyspnea, chest pain or discomfort, cyanosis, crackles, and cough. In more severe cases, neck veins may become distended. The child demonstrated some of these findings after the blood transfusion began. There are no findings that indicate an allergic reaction such as chills, itching, fever, or headache. Most blood transfusion reactions occur within 10 to 15 minutes after the transfusion begins. The child's vital signs do not indicate hypovolemia or hypovolemic shock. In these conditions, the child would have hypotension and tachycardia. There are also no findings that indicate an acute exacerbation of leukemia, which typically includes fever, pallor, bruising, leg and joint pain, fatigue, and lymph node enlargement. The most important nursing action for a client with fluid overload is to stop the source of the extra fluid (not decrease the flow rate); in this case, the blood transfusion would be stopped. The child's SpO_2 decreased as a result of fluid overload. The nurse would increase the flow of oxygen to help perfuse major organs. The nurse would not administer diphenhydramine because this drug is given for allergic reactions. The nurse would place the child in the sitting position rather than the supine position to facilitate ease in breathing. The nurse would frequently monitor the child's vital signs and SpO_2 to determine the effectiveness of the plan of care. Urine output is not a reliable indicator of effectiveness because the kidneys compensate by attempting to remove the extra body fluid, which results in increased output. The presence of bleeding and hemoglobin/hematocrit values would be important if the child had an exacerbation of acute lymphoblastic leukemia.

CJ Cognitive Skills: Recognize Cues, Analyze Cues, Prioritize Hypotheses, Generate Solutions, Take Actions, Evaluate Outcomes
Reference: Leifer & Little, 2023, pp. 95, 650, 652–653

Stand-Alone Thinking Exercise 22.2

Answer

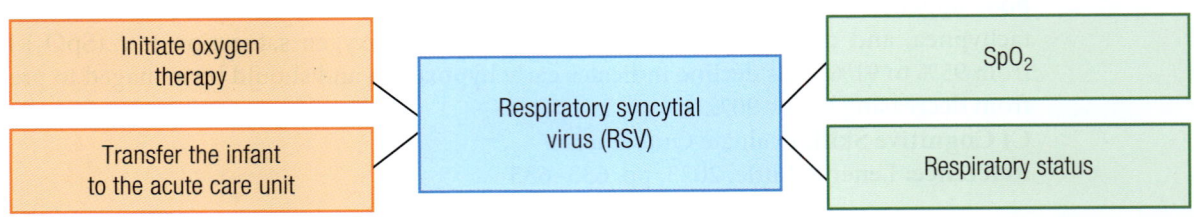

Rationale

Respiratory syncytial virus (RSV) is the most common cause of viral pneumonia in infants and toddlers. Infants between 2 and 7 months of age can become very ill because they have small airways that can easily become obstructed with mucus. In severe cases, nasal flaring and chest retractions to help with breathing are present. In addition to difficulty breathing, young children typically have fever, cough, and rhinorrhea (clear nasal drainage). Croup is a syndrome of several conditions in which a "barking" cough with stridor is present. Epiglottitis is a medical emergency in which the client has swelling above the larynx that can cause complete airway obstruction. The client does not have a cough or fever; instead, the client is anxious, apprehensive, and often sits up with the mouth open. This infant does not have these classic findings. Asthma is also not an infection; it is a condition that causes intermittent constriction of the airways of the lungs. The client has a cough and difficulty breathing but does not have a fever. The immediate nursing action for this infant would be to begin oxygen therapy to increase the SpO_2 so it is between 90% and 95%. Due to the severity of respiratory distress, the infant would also be admitted to the acute care hospital and evaluated for increased respiratory support. The clinic is not equipped to place the infant on mechanical ventilation if needed. Amoxicillin is used to manage bacterial infections; RSV is a virus. Infants are not able to use an inhaler due to their developmental stage. The nurse would monitor SpO_2 levels and respiratory status to determine which support measures are required. Wheezing and nasal drainage are expected with RSV. Arterial blood gas studies are painful and not needed.

CJ Cognitive Skills: Recognize Cues, Analyze Cues, Prioritize Hypotheses, Generate Solutions, Take Actions, Evaluate Outcomes

Reference: Leifer & Little, 2023, pp. 599–600, 602–603, 607–609

Answers With Rationales for Thinking Exercises

Unfolding Case Study 23.1

Thinking Exercise 23.1.1

Answer

○ Body temperature
○ Heart rate
✗ Distended abdomen
○ Blood pressure
○ Lack of appetite
✗ Right lower quadrant abdominal pain

Rationale

The client has a distended abdomen with acute right lower quadrant pain, which could indicate a potentially life-threatening condition such as bowel obstruction or inflammation/infection. Therefore these findings require immediate follow-up. The client's lack of appetite and low-grade fever are not potentially life threatening and would not require immediate follow-up. The client's heart rate and blood pressure are within normal limits.
CJ Cognitive Skill: Recognize Cues
Reference: Leifer & Little, 2023, pp. 680–681

Thinking Exercise 23.1.2

Answer

The complication for which the client is **most** at risk is **perforated appendix**.

Rationale

The appendix is a small appendage attached to the ascending colon (cecum) that can collect fecal matter. As a result, it can become inflamed and infected with swelling and growth of pathogenic organisms causing pain and distention. Abdominal pain is often increased when the client moves the right leg. Rupture or perforation of the appendix can occur within 36 hours of the onset of acute right lower quadrant abdominal pain. Release of fecal matter and other debris into the abdominal cavity can then lead to peritonitis and septicemia, which are potentially life-threatening conditions. The client could become dehydrated, but intravenous fluids are being administered to prevent this potential complication. Loss of sodium (hyponatremia) is most likely to occur when a client experiences profuse or prolonged vomiting. This client has not reported any vomiting at this time. If the client had a small bowel obstruction, profuse vomiting would usually occur.
CJ Cognitive Skill: Analyze Cues
Reference: Leifer & Little, 2023, pp. 680–681

Thinking Exercise 23.1.3

Answer

The *priority* for client care at this time is to **observe for signs of peritonitis**.

Rationale

When an inflamed appendix ruptures, the client often experiences decreased pain initially. However, the contents of the appendix irritate the peritoneum and cause peritoneal inflammation (peritonitis) and eventually infection. The client's temperature and serum white blood cell count would then increase, and the client would be at risk for sepsis. If the client is treated early, life-threatening complications such as sepsis may be avoided. Managing the client's pain and nutritional status is not as important as monitoring for peritonitis. Changes in the client's SpO_2 would not be expected as a result of appendicitis for an adolescent.
CJ Cognitive Skill: Prioritize Hypotheses
Reference: Leifer & Little, 2023, pp. 680–681

Thinking Exercise 23.1.4

Answer

The nurse anticipates that the client will have **emergency surgery** because the client could develop **peritonitis**.

Rationale

Appendicitis is the most common reason for emergency surgery in childhood and adolescence. The client's body temperature has increased, and the client has chills. These changes in findings indicate that the client's condition is worsening, and emergency surgery to remove the appendix and irrigate the abdominal cavity is required to prevent peritonitis and sepsis. Enemas are never indicated when a client has appendicitis. A nasogastric tube is not usually inserted because appendectomies are typically performed laparoscopically. The client is not at risk for constipation from appendicitis. If peritonitis occurs and becomes severe, the client could experience paralytic ileus, which would result in diminished or absent bowel sounds, not hyperactive bowel sounds.
CJ Cognitive Skill: Generate Solutions
Reference: Leifer & Little, 2023, pp. 680–681

Thinking Exercise 23.1.5

Answer

- ✗ Keep the client NPO with an intravenous fluid infusion.
- ○ Obtain informed consent for abdominal surgery.
- ✗ Place the client in the sitting or semireclining position.
- ○ Administer an opioid analgesic for abdominal pain.
- ✗ Observe the abdomen for rigidity and increased distention.
- ✗ Monitor vital signs every 30 to 60 minutes.
- ✗ Check for body jewelry, and cover or remove it.

Rationale

The client is scheduled for emergency surgery and would require preoperative preparation, including remaining NPO. Because the appendix likely perforated, the nurse would place the client in the sitting position to keep the contents released by the appendix in the lower abdomen and prevent spread throughout the entire abdominal cavity. The nurse would observe the abdomen for boardlike rigidity and increased distention, which are classic findings associated with peritonitis. Vital signs should be monitored frequently to be able to detect potential sepsis very early to prevent negative outcomes.

The nurse would also follow agency protocol regarding body jewelry to remove it or, if it does not interfere with surgery, possibly cover it with tape or another material. The individual responsible for obtaining informed consent for surgery is the surgeon, not the nurse. Strong analgesics would not be given because they can mask potential worsening abdominal pain. Acute pain is a warning sign that the client is experiencing a complication or potentially life-threatening condition.

CJ Cognitive Skill: Take Actions
Reference: Leifer & Little, 2023, pp. 534–535, 680–681

Thinking Exercise 23.1.6

Answer

Based on current client findings, the nurse determines that the client's condition has **improved**.

Rationale

The client currently has minimal abdominal pain, and the client's abdomen is soft rather than distended. All vital signs, including body temperature, are now within normal limits. Because these findings are all normal, the client's condition is considered to be improved. It has not remained the same or worsened when compared with findings on admission to the emergency department.

CJ Cognitive Skill: Evaluate Outcomes
Reference: Leifer & Little, 2023, pp. 536, 680–681

Unfolding Case Study 23.2

Thinking Exercise 23.2.1

Answer

BODY SYSTEMS	CLIENT FINDINGS
Respiratory	✗ Occasional expiratory wheezing ○ Deep, rapid respirations ✗ Cough and chest congestion
Integumentary/metabolic	✗ Temperature ✗ Finger stick blood glucose (FSBG) ○ Fruity breath
Cardiovascular	○ Fatigue ✗ Heart rate ✗ Blood pressure

Rationale

The child has type 1 diabetes mellitus and is at risk for complications that should be identified and managed promptly to prevent potential life-threatening conditions. The nurse would be very concerned about the client's blood glucose level, which is well above 200 mg/dL (11.1 mmol/L), indicating the presence of acute hyperglycemia. This could lead to dehydration and metabolic acidosis if left untreated, therefore the client's finger stick blood glucose level requires immediate follow-up. The client's vital signs are abnormal, including fever, tachycardia, tachypnea, and hypotension. These changes require immediate follow-up because the client has acute hyperglycemia. The client's fruity breath; deep, rapid respirations; and fatigue are consistent with acute hyperglycemia in clients who have type 1 diabetes mellitus. However, these findings are not life threatening or potentially life threatening. The client has respiratory changes including chest congestion and wheezing at times. The nurse would recognize that these findings require immediate follow-up to prevent worsening of these findings, which could continue to increase the client's blood glucose level.

CJ Cognitive Skill: Recognize Cues
Reference: Leifer & Little, 2023, pp. 730–731

Thinking Exercise 23.2.2

Answer

    ✗ Hyperglycemia
    ✗ Ketoacidosis
    ○ Hyponatremia
    ✗ Dehydration
    ✗ Hyperkalemia

Rationale

Based on the laboratory results, the client has an increase in serum potassium (hyperkalemia) and glucose (hyperglycemia) but does not have a decreased sodium (hyponatremia). The serum sodium level is within normal limits. The client also has ketoacidosis, a type of metabolic acidosis, as evidenced by the presence of ketones in the urine, low serum pH, and a low bicarbonate level. A decreased pH shows that the client has acidosis. Bicarbonate is a base that helps maintain acid-base balance in the body and is often low when the client has metabolic acidosis. The client who has diabetic ketoacidosis is often dehydrated. The client's increased BUN, tachycardia, and hypotension are consistent with dehydration.
CJ Cognitive Skill: Analyze Cues
References: Leifer & Little, 2023, pp. 730–731; Pagana et al., 2023, pp. 101, 150, 296, 451, 707, 803, 910

Thinking Exercise 23.2.3

Answer

The *priority* for the client's care at this time is to manage the client's **diabetic ketoacidosis**.

Rationale

The client is experiencing diabetic ketoacidosis, a potentially life-threatening acute complication, which is the priority for care at this time. When this condition is managed, the client's potassium level and fluid balance should be restored. The client does not have chronic kidney disease because the serum creatinine is within normal range. As a waste product of protein metabolism, creatinine is a major indicator of kidney function. The kidneys normally eliminate most creatinine in urine, leaving only a small amount. However, when kidney function declines, the amount of creatinine excreted decreases, leaving an increased amount in the blood. The client's sodium is also normal, so the client does not have hyponatremia. The client's respiratory condition would be managed but is likely not life threatening at this time.
CJ Cognitive Skill: Prioritize Hypotheses
References: Leifer & Little, 2023, pp. 730–731; Pagana et al., 2023, pp. 101, 150, 296, 451, 707, 803, 910

Thinking Exercise 23.2.4

Answer

POTENTIAL NURSING ACTIONS	INDICATED	NOT INDICATED
Monitor a continuous regular insulin infusion.	✗	
Administer antibiotic therapy per agency protocol.		✗
Encourage oral fluids including water.	✗	
Administer a 5%D/0.45% NS intravenous infusion.		✗
Perform rapid testing for respiratory infections.	✗	

Rationale

The client needs intravenous regular insulin to decrease blood glucose and treat diabetic ketoacidosis. Intravenous and oral fluids are also essential for managing dehydration. However, the intravenous fluid being administered would not contain dextrose because it increases blood glucose. Antibiotic therapy would not be administered until a respiratory infection is confirmed. Antibiotics are used for bacterial infections; the client could have a viral infection. Rapid testing for influenza, COVID-19, and respiratory syncytial virus (RSV) would be indicated to determine if the client has a respiratory virus.

CJ Cognitive Skill: Generate Solutions

References: Leifer & Little, 2023, pp. 730–731; Pagana et al., 2023, pp. 101, 150, 296, 451, 707, 803, 910

Thinking Exercise 23.2.5

Answer

○ Begin antiviral therapy per PED protocol.
✗ Redraw labs to monitor for changes.
✗ Monitor finger stick blood glucose (FSBG) levels every 30 to 60 minutes.
✗ Begin continuous cardiac monitoring.
○ Initiate supplemental oxygen therapy.

Rationale

Potassium is needed in the body to maintain adequate skeletal and cardiac muscle function. An increased level of this electrolyte can cause muscle weakness and life-threatening cardiac dysrhythmias. Therefore the nurse would provide continuous cardiac monitoring to detect any problems and manage these conditions early. Labs would be redrawn to monitor blood glucose and electrolyte levels. The nurse would also frequently monitor FSBG levels. Antiviral therapy would not be administered until the results of the rapid testing for common respiratory infections are available. Supplemental oxygen therapy is not needed because the client has a peripheral oxygen saturation (SpO_2) of 95% and no report of dyspnea. The normal SpO_2 value should be 95% or higher.

CJ Cognitive Skill: Take Actions

References: Leifer & Little, 2023, pp. 730–731; Pagana et al., 2023, pp. 101, 150, 296, 451, 707, 803, 910

Thinking Exercise 23.2.6

Answer

History and Physical	Nurses' Notes	Orders	Laboratory Results

1400: Child brought to PED by family after school nurse notified them of child's new-onset drowsiness, abdominal pain, cough, nasal congestion, and increased thirst. Child has had type 1 diabetes mellitus for 8 years, which has been controlled by glargine and lispro insulin for the past year. Planning to obtain a continuous glucose monitoring system to use with an insulin pump next year. No other medical history or medications. Family reports that child attended a large birthday party this past weekend where "several kids had colds or some sort of respiratory illness." Child reports feeling very tired and wanting to sleep. Drowsy but oriented × 4. Face flushed; lips reddened and dry. Breath smells fruity. Occasional expiratory wheezing; deep rapid respirations. Abdomen soft and round with bowel sounds present × 4. All pulses 2+; cap refill <3 sec. Skin turgor poor; skin and mucous membranes dry. VS: 102.6°F (39.2°C), HR 112 beats/min, RR 30 breaths/min, BP 90/48 mm Hg, SpO_2 95% on RA. Denies dyspnea. FSBG 285 mg/dL (15.8 mmol/L).

1420: Labs drawn, and peripheral IV access established in right forearm.

1515: PED physician notified of lab results.

1520: Orders received. Rapid bedside testing negative for COVID, RSV, and influenza.

1645: Continuous regular insulin infusing per protocol. Child less drowsy; oriented × 4. Face remains flushed; lips dry. Breath continues to smell fruity. No report of abdominal pain. Continues with occasional coughing and nasal congestion. VS: 100.6°F (38.1°C), HR 102 beats/min, RR 26 breaths/min, BP 100/52 mm Hg, SpO_2 97% on RA, FSBG 188 mg/dL (10.4 mmol/L). Repeat labs drawn.

Rationale

After the nurse initiated the plan of care, the client's level of consciousness improved because the client became less drowsy. All vital signs improved, although the client continues to have a low-grade fever, tachycardia, and tachypnea. The client's FSBG decreased to below 200 mg/dL (11.1 mmol/L]), which also shows an improvement in the client's condition. Repeat labs would be drawn to assess fluid and electrolyte balance.
CJ Cognitive Skill: Evaluate Outcomes
References: Leifer & Little, 2023, pp. 730–731; Pagana et al., 2023, pp. 101, 150, 296, 451, 707, 803, 910

Unfolding Case Study 23.3

Thinking Exercise 23.3.1

Answer

✗ Fever
○ Tachycardia
○ Tachypnea
○ SpO$_2$
✗ Headache
✗ Nausea and vomiting
✗ Neck stiffness
○ Enlarged calf muscles
○ Duchenne muscular dystrophy

Rationale

The client has a high fever with nausea and vomiting, which can lead to dehydration due to fluid loss, a potentially life-threatening condition. Therefore these findings would require immediate follow-up. Headache combined with neck stiffness implies a possible central nervous system (brain) condition, which could also be life threatening. The client has had Duchenne muscular dystrophy for many years and has learned to live with the disorder. As expected in clients with muscular dystrophy, the calf muscles are enlarged. The client has tachycardia, but it is not at a life-threatening level. The client's respiratory rate is only slightly increased, and the SpO$_2$ is only slightly below 95%. Therefore these findings do not require immediate follow-up.
CJ Cognitive Skill: Recognize Cues
Reference: Leifer & Little, 2023, pp. 551–552

Thinking Exercise 23.3.2

Answer

The client *most likely* has **meningitis** as evidenced by **neck stiffness** and **fever**.

Rationale

Meningitis is inflammation of the covering of the brain and spinal cord (meninges) caused by pathogens that can enter the body via the bloodstream, ear, sinuses, teeth, and lungs. The classic findings for clients who have this condition result from intracranial irritation and include headache, drowsiness, vomiting, irritability, restlessness, and neck stiffness (nuchal rigidity). This client has most of these findings, which are consistent with meningitis. Tachycardia is likely the result of increased metabolism due to a fever. The client is not hypotensive because the systolic blood pressure is over 90 mm Hg. The SpO$_2$ is only slightly below 95%, which is the expected value for an adolescent. A brain tumor does not typically manifest as acute findings but rather has a slower onset. There is no evidence that the client experienced an injury to the head, which is the cause of traumatic brain injury.
CJ Cognitive Skill: Analyze Cues
Reference: Leifer & Little, 2023, pp. 551–552

Thinking Exercise 23.3.3

Answer

The *priority* for client care at this time would be to **manage the central nervous system infection**.

Rationale

If the client's infection (meningitis) is not managed or does not respond to management, the client may develop increased intracranial pressure or seizures. These complications can be life threatening. If the infection is treated as soon as possible, the client's headache and nausea/vomiting should improve. The nurse cannot prevent a decreasing level of consciousness but can detect changes early to report to the registered nurse.

CJ Cognitive Skill: Prioritize Hypotheses
Reference: Leifer & Little, 2023, pp. 551–552

Thinking Exercise 23.3.4

Answer

POTENTIAL NURSING ACTIONS	INDICATED	NOT INDICATED
Prepare for probable lumbar puncture.	✗	
Obtain peripheral venous access.	✗	
Start high-flow oxygen via facemask.		✗
Monitor for seizure activity.	✗	
Place the client on Droplet Precautions.	✗	

Rationale

A lumbar puncture allows the laboratory examination of cerebrospinal fluid (CSF) to determine the pathogen causing the client's likely meningitis. Peripheral venous access is needed for hydration and possible medication administration, depending on the type of meningitis the client has. Because the client is at risk for seizures from cranial irritation, the nurse would observe for seizures. If a seizure occurs, the nurse would turn the client on the side if possible and prevent injury. The nurse would document the client's activity during the seizure and the length of the seizure and would report this to the provider. Droplet Precautions requiring a well-fitted facemask or respirator are needed in addition to Standard Precautions when providing care for the client who has meningitis. High-flow oxygen is not indicated for this client because there is no evidence that the client is experiencing respiratory distress.

CJ Cognitive Skill: Generate Solutions
Reference: Leifer & Little, 2023, pp. 551–552

Thinking Exercise 23.3.5

Answer

✗ Administer antibiotic therapy per protocol.
○ Place the client on protective (reverse) isolation.
✗ Administer antiseizure drug therapy.
○ Monitor vital signs every 8 to 12 hours.
✗ Monitor neurologic status frequently.
○ Keep the room as brightly lit as possible.

Rationale

The CSF analysis confirmed the client's condition of meningococcal meningitis, and the client was placed in a private room. This type of meningitis is bacterial and requires intravenous antibiotic therapy and Droplet Precautions, not protective (reverse) precautions. The nurse would take vital signs at least every 4 hours (not every 8–12 hours) to monitor for response to treatment and for the presence of early sepsis. The nurse would also monitor the client's neurologic status every 4 hours to note any changes, especially in level of consciousness. Protective (reverse) precautions are used to protect the client from infection; this client already has an infection. Antiseizure medication is often ordered to prevent seizures that can occur in clients who have meningitis. The client's private room allows a quiet environment in which the client can rest. Many clients who have meningitis have photophobia, and bright lights cause discomfort. Therefore the room would also be kept dimly lit or as dark as possible depending on what the client prefers.

CJ Cognitive Skill: Take Actions
Reference: Leifer & Little, 2023, pp. 551–552

Thinking Exercise 23.3.6

Answer

CURRENT CLIENT FINDINGS	IMPROVED	NOT IMPROVED
Headache pain rated 2/10	✗	
Alert and oriented × 4	✗	
Temperature 99.4°F (37.4°C)	✗	
Heart rate 88 beats/min	✗	
Blood pressure 146/92 mm Hg		✗

Rationale

All of the client's current findings show improvement in the client's condition, including less headache pain, decreased body temperature, and return to normal range for heart rate. In addition, the client's level of consciousness has improved because the client is now completely alert. However, the client's blood pressure is now higher than the usual range for the client's age.

CJ Cognitive Skill: Evaluate Outcomes
Reference: Leifer & Little, 2023, pp. 551–552

Stand-Alone Thinking Exercise 23.1

Answer

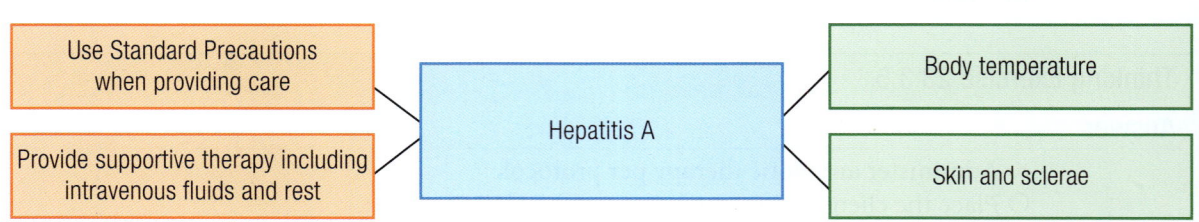

Rationale

Hepatitis A is the most common type of viral hepatitis and is caused by water, food, or medical equipment that has been contaminated by fecal material. Common findings of hepatitis A include severe headache, anorexia, right upper quadrant abdominal pain, nausea, vomiting, and anorexia. Many clients also have jaundice, light- or clay-colored stools, and dark urine caused by increased circulating bilirubin from the inflamed liver. This disorder usually resolves, but clients may need supportive care such as intravenous or oral fluids to prevent or manage dehydration and rest for healing to occur. Preventing transmission of hepatitis A includes good handwashing, especially after toileting. If caring for the client in a health care setting, Standard Precautions would be used to prevent transmission of the infection. There is no indication that the client needs supplemental oxygen or hemodialysis. A hepatitis A vaccine is available but is not needed because the infection provides antibodies to the condition in the future. To determine the effectiveness of care and the body's ability to heal itself, the nurse would monitor the skin and sclerae for decreased yellowish coloration as well as the client's body temperature, which should return to normal limits. The client's SpO_2 is within normal range, and there is no indication that the client's kidney function, as indicated by serum creatinine, was affected by the virus. Appetite is a very subjective client finding that could be affected by many factors. An increased appetite does not imply that the client's condition has improved.

CJ Cognitive Skill: Recognize Cues, Analyze Cues, Prioritize Hypotheses, Generate Solutions, Take Actions, Evaluate Outcomes

References: Leifer & Little, 2023, p. 746; Linton & Matteson, 2023, pp. 794–797

Stand-Alone Thinking Exercise 23.2

Answer

The *priority* need for client care at this time is to **ensure adequate tissue perfusion** because the client most likely has **sickle cell anemia**.

Rationale

Sickle cell disease is an inherited condition in which there is a defect in an individual's hemoglobin. The severe form of sickle cell disease is sickle cell anemia. Typical clinical findings of this condition include finger swelling, chronic anemia, fatigue, anorexia, joint and abdominal pain, and muscle spasms. The client's chronic anemia has worsened as evidenced by decreased red blood cells, hemoglobin, and hematocrit. Clients who have leukemia typically have a low red blood cell count, but they also have a low platelet count and an abnormally high white blood cell count. Hemophilia is a bleeding disorder; this client does not have findings associated with unusual bleeding. Clients who have thalassemia have chronic anemia but also have jaundice, dark urine, and slow developmental growth. This client is at risk for sickle cell crisis, which can be fatal due to organ failure caused by lack of adequate blood flow and oxygen to body cells. Therefore the priority at this time would be to ensure adequate perfusion (blood flow) to major organs of the body to prevent life-threatening complications. Pain, fever, and inadequate nutrition are not immediately life threatening.

CJ Cognitive Skill: Recognize Cues, Analyze Cues, Prioritize Hypotheses

References: Leifer & Little, 2023, pp. 643–644, 646–653; Pagana et al., 2023, 476, 479, 688, 749, 946

References

Cooper, K. & Gosnell, K. (2023). *Foundations and adult health nursing* (9th ed.). St. Louis: Elsevier.

Halter, M. J. & Fratena, C. A. (2023). *Varcarolis' manual of psychiatric nursing care: An interprofessional approach* (7th ed.) St. Louis: Elsevier.

Leifer, G. & Little, K. (2023). *Introduction to maternity and pediatric nursing* (9th ed.). St. Louis: Elsevier.

Linton, A. D. & Matteson, M. A. (2023). *Medical-surgical nursing* (8th ed.). St. Louis: Elsevier.

McCuistion, L. E., Vuljoin-DiMaggio, K., Winton, M. B., & Yeager, J. J. (2023). *Pharmacology: A patient-centered nursing process approach* (11th ed.). St. Louis: Elsevier.

Morrison-Valfre, M. (2023). *Foundations of mental health care* (8th ed.). St. Louis: Elsevier.

Pagana, K. D., Pagana, T. J., & Pagana, T. N. (2023). *Mosby's diagnostic and laboratory test reference* (16th ed.). St. Louis: Elsevier.

Willihnganz, M. J., Gurevitz, S. L., & Clayton, B. D. (2022). *Basic pharmacology for nurses* (19th ed.). St. Louis: Elsevier.